# OTOLARYNGOLOGY
## HEAD & NECK
### SURGERY

## CLINICAL REFERENCE GUIDE

### Fourth Edition

D0888314

# OTOLARYNGOLOGY
## HEAD **&** NECK
### S U R G E R Y

## CLINICAL REFERENCE GUIDE

### Fourth Edition

Raza Pasha, MD
Justin S. Golub, MD

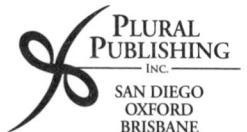

PLURAL
PUBLISHING
— INC. —
SAN DIEGO
OXFORD
BRISBANE

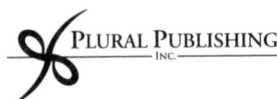

PLURAL PUBLISHING
INC.

5521 Ruffin Road
San Diego, CA 92123

e-mail: info@pluralpublishing.com
Web site: http://www.pluralpublishing.com

Copyright © by Plural Publishing, Inc. 2014

Typeset in 9/11 Adobe Garamond by Achorn International, Inc.
Printed in the United States of America by McNaughton & Gunn, Inc.

17 16 15    2 3 4 5

## NOTICE TO THE READER

Care has been taken to confirm the accuracy of the indications, procedures, drug dosages, and diagnosis and remediation protocols presented in this book and to ensure that they conform to the practices of the general medical and health services communities. However, the authors, editors, and publisher are not responsible for errors or omissions or for any consequences from application of the information in this book and make no warranty, expressed or implied, with respect to the currency, completeness, or accuracy of the contents of the publication. The diagnostic and remediation protocols and the medications described do not necessarily have specific approval by the Food and Drug administration for use in the disorders and/or diseases and dosages for which they are recommended. Application of this information in a particular situation remains the professional responsibility of the practitioner. Because standards of practice and usage change, it is the responsibility of the practitioner to keep abreast of revised recommendations, dosages, and procedures.

**Library of Congress Cataloging-in-Publication Data**

Pasha, R., author.
  Otolaryngology : head & neck surgery : clinical reference guide / Raza Pasha,
Justin S. Golub. — Fourth edition.
       p. ; cm.
  Includes bibliographical references and index.
  ISBN-13: 978-1-59756-532-5 (alk. paper)
  ISBN-10: 1-59756-532-6 (alk. paper)
  I. Golub, Justin S., author. II. Title.
  [DNLM: 1. Otorhinolaryngologic Diseases—surgery. 2. Face—surgery. 3. Head—surgery. 4. Neck—surgery. 5. Otorhinolaryngologic Surgical Procedures.  WV 168]
  RF46
  617.5'1059—dc22
                                                                    2013028078

# CONTENTS

*Cody A. Koch, Timothy D. Doerr, Robert H. Mathog, and Raza Pasha*

# FOREWORD TO THE FIRST EDITION

This text promises to be a vital addition to the armamentarium of knowledge available to every individual aspiring to understand the pathophysiology and management of disorders in Otolaryngology—Head and Neck Surgery. Dr. Pasha and his co-authors have done a brilliant job of organizing their thoughts so that readers will have no problems seeking out the disorder they hope to understand. This work will succeed where others have not simply because it does what every book hopes to do, that is, it addresses the needs of the reader. I plan to have a copy available for all my residents and medical students, as well as the primary care residents who rotate through our service.

It is a stroke of intelligence that should survive for many years in our armamentarium.

Harold C. Pillsbury, MD
Professor and Chief
Otolaryngology—Head and Neck Surgery
The University of North Carolina at Chapel Hill

# PREFACE TO THE FIRST EDITION

Most students and practitioners of medicine may be overwhelmed in their initial endeavors to understand the field of Otolaryngology—Head and Neck Surgery. The sheer quantity of information from the anatomy of the temporal bone to head and neck reconstruction strategies may be difficult to comprehend and organize.

This reference book provides a state-of-the-art, comprehensive overview that captures the essential facts relative to various Otolaryngology topics. All chapters are co-authored by nationally recognized subspecialty experts. Each chapter follows a uniform outline to facilitate systematic development of in-depth knowledge of head and neck pathologies and to afford quick reviews at a glance. Its comprehensive content provides the depth required for written and oral standardized tests.

In addition, the material presented provides practitioners with current step-by-step management protocols for patients with common clinical problems such as dysphonia, dysphagia, head and neck trauma, upper airway obstruction, and head and neck cancer. Each work-up includes differential diagnoses, symptomatology, pathophysiology, complications, and alternative treatment plans that are consistent with accepted standards of care.

Chapter 1 offers a complete review of rhinology, paranasal sinuses, and immunology, including clinical protocols regarding nasal obstruction. Chapter 2 addresses salivary gland pathology and management strategies. Chapter 3 discusses the anatomy, physiology, and pathological conditions associated with Laryngology, including complete clinical work-ups of dysphonia and upper airway obstruction. Chapter 4 provides a comprehensive review of general otolaryngological disorders such as pharyngitis, thyroid disease, and sleep apnea. Chapter 5 discusses management of the head and neck cancer patient by anatomical site. Chapter 6 reviews diseases of the ear and temporal bone, including management protocols for hearing loss, dizziness, and facial nerve injuries. Chapter 7 offers the fundamental principles for aesthetic and reconstruction surgery of the head and neck. Finally, Chapter 8 introduces the essential concepts of managing the head and neck trauma patient.

# ACKNOWLEDGMENTS TO THE FIRST EDITION

This reference guide required the guidance and contributions of many individuals to whom I must express my appreciation. Some are formal contributors, others have provided support in more subtle ways unknown to them.

To my mentors, Dr. James Paul Dworkin and Dr. Robert J. Meleca, who encouraged the conception of this project and who have graciously provided editorial comments: Without your expert advice this project could not have been possible.

To Dr. Robert H. Mathog and the faculty of Wayne State University Department of Otolaryngology—Head and Neck Surgery who provided the foundation of my education: I am forever grateful for their scholarly guidance and their contribution to this material.

To Candice Janco, Kristin Banach, Sandy Doyle, indexer Pam Rider, and the staff of Singular who had the faith and patience with this first-time author and who helped in many decisions along the path to publication.

To Loralee McAuliffe, who created splendid illustrations from sketchy line drawings and illegible handwriting.

To Dr. Harry Kim for his expertise in editing our review of radiation oncology and to Dr. Margie Crawford for her expertise in reviewing audiology and vestibular testing.

To my graduating colleagues of 2001: Syed, Sam, and Greg, who encouraged my endeavor from the onset and on whom I have relied for so many things over the past years.

To my closest friends of Detroit: Doug and Kristin, Faye, Olmina (Maria), Joe and Rielly, Jimmy, Dave, Ramin, Steve, Teresa and Norm, Joe and Paula, all of whom have provided a family away from home.

Finally, to my loving family to whom I dedicate this book: Everything I have ever accomplished and ever will accomplish goes to their credit.

Thank you all.

—*Raza Pasha*

# PREFACE TO THE SECOND EDITION

This time in office, the messages were different . . . a physician from Turkey? A residency director in California? My "Contact Us" hyperlink registered a number of hits from systems outside of the Greater Houston circle requesting additional copies of the "Pocket Pasha." After being dropped by my original publishing company, having 2 years' worth of updates stolen from my car, starting my private practice, and officially resigning from checking the status box, "Single," to the one of "Married," I pretty much had sequestered any remnants of the first edition to a shadow box in my office waiting room. Graciously, I did not have to wait as long to realize the full potential of the first edition, nor its postresidency boom in interest; albeit, this occurred the day after it was out of press and no longer available.

As a result of the positive response to the first edition, and gratefully by request, I present the second edition. The augmented pages contain updated information specifically in regards to General Otolaryngology, Rhinology, and Endocrinology. In addition, the Head and Neck Cancer, Neurotology/Otology, Trauma, and Facial Plastic/Reconstructive chapters have undergone academic facelifts. I have retained the same format of its predecessor, excising only the pharmacology section, which was not user friendly. A more functional index further augments the second edition for another generation of residents, medical students, and clinicians.

Please send your comments, errors, or suggestions for upcoming editions to rpasha@PashaMD.com

# ACKNOWLEDGMENTS TO THE SECOND EDITION

I am indebted to many people—the list has as much depth and is as vivid as the circumstances, mentors, friends, and family in my life have been thus far.

I graciously thank my wonderful staff. Angie Cano, Angel Rodriquez, Tracey Kaderka, Claudia Ramirez, and Monica Lerma who provide a smooth running ship, encouraging and enabling me to complete this latest project.

The patient people of Plural Publishing, especially Sandy Doyle who has been present since the inception of the first edition.

The Boys of Houston, Zahid, Taseer, Poorang, Soroush, Umair, Kraig, Rodney, Ed, and Zephyr. You have all been unwavering in your friendship, confidence, and support of all projects I heap on to my plate.

Finally, to my wonderful wife, Mamta, and family who provide the baseline of my happiness and who are the best "springboard from which to launch beyond myself." It is your intrepid courage, your omnipresent love, your sage thoughts, your reckless abandon, and your belief in who I am, that sustains me. I look to you all for inspiration, the true mentors of my life. Thank you.

Thank you all once again.

—*Raza Pasha*

# PREFACE TO THE THIRD EDITION

You would have thought that I'm the chump responsible for an off-shore oil spill by the number of hate E-mails I have received. Almost daily, my inbox was torpedoed with charming one-liners in the form of multilingual expletives and lots of exclamation marks. You guys did a commendable job on slamming the index of the last edition. Hopefully we have recalibrated all the elements in this edition, so please no more cyber grumbles.

## Hear Ye, Hear Ye

Loyal subjects of the great ENT fiefdom, heed my word: we need to be more integrated into sleep medicine. Sleep is as controversial as it comes and as surgeons, we are getting clobbered. Our data are stale and not convincing to the many critics who wave the wand of the almighty CPAP wizard for every snorer, mouth breather, and overworked truck driver. As with allergy in sinus surgery or audiology in otology, we need to speak the language and be part of the great debate. As vanguard surgeons, we cannot consider the sleep apneic without recognizing the narcoleptic. At the same time, a sleep study is more than an AHI and a CPAP level.

I'm offering Chapter 5, Sleep Medicine and Sleep Apnea Surgery, as a crusade to my readers. Admittedly, some parts may be over the top. Read the chapter. Absorb the concepts. Then highlight the OSAS and sleep test section for your exam. I purposely want to be cutting edge and cover the basics of sleep medicine and not just OSAS surgery. You may thank me later.

## Moving Ahead

It has been an incredible experience creating this pocket book. I especially have enjoyed working with Dr. Golub, the resident on the ground per se. As I become more and more removed from residency, I invite all of you to be part of the fourth edition. If you have corrections, additions, illustrations, charts, appendix notes, or any other essentials, collect them, verify them, and then provide your source and visit my Web site, PashaMD.com. You may upload your information for consideration for the next edition under the tab, "Residents and Practitioners."

We want to continue to produce a book that is less self-indulgent and more about you, the student, the practitioner, the resident who is pounding the dirt and is too overwhelmed to read through 50 pages of historical references on odontogenic cysts before getting to the one-sentence summary point. Our aim is to deliver just the facts, so that you get through preoperative interrogations, morning round grilling, and exams based in minutia. We have done our job well if we are able to get you home in time to enjoy the more important things in life; family, friends, and cable programming.

# ACKNOWLEDGMENTS TO THE THIRD EDITION

As always I have to thank God, family, and friends for guiding me through this venture with both encouragement and forgiveness. But I would be remiss if I did not acknowledge a few essential ingredients that lent their flavor and dimension to making this text more robust.

By far, I would like to recognize our fresh infusion of scholarly blood in the form of our newest contributor and cyber collegue, Justin Golub. Pending a face-to-face encounter with Dr. Golub, I have formulated my own version of him: A young academician ensconced in a makeshift laboratory-cave buried high within the formidable Washington mountains. Cloaked in all the mystery of Charlie to his Angels, Dr. Golub is recognized by his voice alone and a series of communiques via Outlook. Although we have yet to meet in person, our minds have already taken the liberty to do so. Justin and I share the same intuition, drive, and impetuous flow of thought in creating this book. My "hands on" experience garnered by my years in the trenches coupled with Justin's full-time immersion in academia, we have succeeded in stocking this book with the most current and relevant information. I look forward to both working with and meeting Justin for the fourth edition.

I also need to shoutout to a handful of new coauthors who helped overhaul a few chapters, Neil Tanna, Joseph Goodman, and Douglas Sidell. In keeping with the same dose of incognito as Justin, these writers and revisers were diligent in their efforts to take an already phenomenal text and make it better.

Another key reviewer was Vishad Nabili, a microvascular and reconstructive fellow from UCLA, who uploaded the latest and greatest in H&N Cancer.

I'd also like to recognize those individuals comprising the Accuracy Police, who were kind (read: obsessed) enough to point out blunders, bloopers, fiction, and outright lies that occasionally appeared in the second edition. The sheriff of this fact-finding force, Talal Al-Khatib from McGill University, not only ferreted out significant errors but also caught wind of the less notable grammatical goofs, extra letters, gratuitous spaces, widgets, and dingbats.

I'll even give John Ramsay a plug. He educated me on the grammatical analysis and root form of "stridorous," which gets flagged on every medical spell-checker I've used. FYI . . . "stridulous" is the Latin adjective, "stridor" is the noun.

Thank you also to Plural Publishing for supporting this project and letting me have my way with the cover and agreeing on the color change. Black is so bad.

So, with that, I hope you enjoy, maybe even rally around this piece of literary canon for a Pulitzer. In any case, we worked hard and we worked smart to bring you the ins and outs of all the latest, greatest, and often exam-tested ENT facts.

Peace.

*—Raza Pasha*

# PREFACE TO THE FOURTH EDITION

This fourth edition evens out my staggered, shadow-boxed display in my office waiting room. It also satisfies an essential update and provides an introduction to our more than welcomed Little People chapter for those of you entrenched in transmittable conjunctivitis and the everlasting cold/influenza rotation.

As for me, I've spent the last few years as a target for academics and skeptics alike lecturing cross-country on "hot button" topics such as indications of in-office balloon sinuplasty and the surgical management of sleep apnea. Should you ever find yourself with a desire to nettle to the brink of combat, walk into a rhinology conference and brag about how balloon sinuplasty is the greatest thing since electrocautery. Better yet, whisper to your pulmonologist colleague that you operated on his 23-year-old bachelor referral last week by jerking his 4+ tonsils without offering him a CPAP machine. "What?!!! You didn't even have the decency to offer him a dental appliance so he can experience referred otalgia and teeth shifting first?!?"

No worries though. You'd be pressed to find any controversial points in this handbook. No need for naked disclosures. We're once again, no nonsense. We've kept to the highlights so you can pass your boards and possibly prevent an occasional cauliflower ear now and then.

No specific acknowledgments section this year since a well-deserved Justin Golub is now blazed in the front of the book and authors are credited within.

Deeply entrenched in midlife, with three sprouting legacies, my time is apportioned between soccer matches, Super Mario marathons, and piano recitals. I dream about Mary's Little Lamb as an adjuvant remedy for psycho-physiological insomnia. The fourth edition is a product of my free time and I was tempted to include illustrations of the cochlear labyrinth crafted by my 5-year-old. Wanting to minimize distractions and leaving something for inclusion in the fifth edition, I opted to leave those out.

Thanks for your support.

—*Raza Pasha*

**Help us make this book even better!**

We welcome any tips, suggestions, or corrections. Please email PashaGolubGuide@gmail.com.

We regret if we cannot respond to all emails, but we will consider every comment.

# CONTRIBUTORS

*Italic lines indicate areas of author's contributions*

**Syed F. Ahsan, MD, FACS**
Neurotologist
Henry Ford Medical Center
Clinical Assistant Professor
Interim Residency Program
    Director
Wayne State University
Department of Otolaryngology
Detroit, MI
*Chapter 8*

**Richard L. Arden**
William Beaumont Hospital
Troy, Michigan
*Chapter 9*

**Dennis I. Bojrab, MD**
CEO and Director of Research
Michigan Ear Institute
Professor of Otolaryngology
Oakland University William
    Beaumont School of Medicine
Rochester Hills, MI
Clinical Professor of
    Otolaryngology and
    Neurosurgery
Wayne State University
Detroit, MI
Founding President
American CISEPO (Canada
    International Scientific
    Exchange Program)
Toronto, Canada
*Chapter 8*

**Don L. Burgio, MD, FACS**
Chief
Otology/Neurotology
Valley ENT
Scottsdale, AZ
*Chapter 8*

**Anthongy J. Cornetta, MD, FACS**
Attending
Otolaryngology-Head and Neck
    Surgery
Huntington Hospital
North Shore–Long Island Jewish
    Health System
Huntington, NY
*Chapter 2*

**Valerie Cote, MD, FRCS (C)**
Pediatric Otolaryngologist
Division of Otolaryngology-
    Head and Neck Surgery
Connecticut Children's Medical
    Center
Hartford, CT
Assistant Professor
University of Connecticut
Farmington, CT
*Chapter 10*

**Timothy D. Doerr, MD, FACS**
Associate Professor
Residency Program Director
Head of Facial Plastic Surgery
Department of Otolaryngology-
    Head and Neck Surgery
University of Rochester Medical
    Center
Rochester, NY
*Chapter 11*

**James P. Dworkin**
Professor
Department of Otolaryngology
Detroit Medical Center
Detroit, MI
College of Osteopathic Medicine
Michigan State University
East Lansing, MI
*Chapter 3*

**Justin S. Golub, MD**
Otology/Neurotology/Skull Base
   Surgery Fellow
Clinical Instructor
Department of Otolaryngology-
   Head and Neck Surgery
University of Cincinnati
Cincinnati Children's Hospital
   Medical Center
Cincinnati, OH
*Chapters 1, 3, 5, 6, 7, 8, 9, and 10*

**Joseph F. Goodman, MD**
Division of Otolaryngology-
   Head and Neck Surgery
George Washington University
Washington, DC
*Chapter 9*

**Amanda Hu, MD, FRCSC**
Assistant Professor
Laryngologist
Department of Otolaryngology-
   Head and Neck Surgery
Drexel University College of
   Medicine
Philadelphia Ear, Nose and
   Throat Associates
Philadelphia, PA
*Chapter 3*

**Peggy E. Kelley, MD, FACS,
FAAP**
Associate Professor
Director
Voice, Vascular Malformation,
   and Microtia Clinics

Division of Pediatric
   Otolaryngology
Children's Hospital Colorado
Department of Otolaryngology
University of Colorado, Denver
Aurora, CO
*Chapter 10*

**Cody A. Koch, MD, PhD**
Clinical Instructor
Department of Otolaryngology-
   Head and Neck Surgery
University of Washington
Seattle, WA
Koch Facial Plastic Surgery
Des Moines, IA
*Chapter 11*

**Steven C. Marks, MD**
Private Practice
Havre de Grace, Maryland
*Chapter 1*

**Robert H. Mathog, PhD, MD**
Professor and Chairman
Department of
   Otolaryngology-Head and
   Neck Surgery
Wayne State University
Karmanos Hospital
Harper Hospital
Detroit, MI
Oakwood Hospital
Dearborn, MI
Crittenton Hospital
Rochester Hills, MI
*Chapter 11*

**Robert J. Meleca, MD, FACS**
Grand Rapids ENT, PC
Grand Rapids, MI
*Chapter 3*

**Vishad Nabili, MD, FACS**
Diplomate, ABFPRS
Associate Professor

Clinical Head and Neck Surgery
Residency Program Director
Department of Head and Neck
   Surgery
University of California, Los
   Angeles
Los Angeles, CA
*Chapter 7*

**Henry C. Ou, MD**
Associate Professor
Pediatric Otolaryngology-Head
   and Neck Surgery
Seattle Children's Hospital
University of Washington
Virginia Merrill Bloedel Hearing
   Research Center
Seattle, WA
*Chapter 10*

**Richard Chan Woo Park, MD**
Assistant Professor
Department of Otolaryngology-
   Head and Neck Surgery
Rutgers New Jersey Medical
   School
Newark, New Jersey
*Chapter 7*

**Raza Pasha, MD**
Medical Director
Pasha Snoring and Sinus Center
Altus Healthcare Management
   Services
Houston, TX
Oprex Surgery Center
Beaumont, TX
*Chapters 1, 2, 3, 4, 5, 6, 7, 8, 9,
   10, and 11*

**Jeremy Prager, MD**
Assistant Professor Pediatric
   Otolaryngology
University of Colorado
Denver, CO
Staff Otolaryngologist

Co-Director, Aerodigestive
   Program
Children's Hospital Colorado
Aurora, Colorado
*Chapter 10*

**Robert T. Sataloff, MD, DMA,
FACS**
Professor and Chairman
Department of Otolaryngology-
   Head and Neck Surgery
Senior Associate Dean for
   Clinical Academic Specialties
Drexel University College of
   Medicine
Chairman
The Voice Foundation
Chairman
American Institute for Voice and
   Ear Research
Philadelphia, PA
*Chapter 2*

**Terry Y. Shibuya, MD, FACS**
Co-Director SCPMG Head and
   Neck Tumor Board
Co-Director SCPMG Skull Base
   Surgery Center of Excellence
Full-Time Partner
Department of Head and Neck
   Surgery
Southern California Permanente
   Medical Group
Orange County, CA
Assistant Clinical Professor
Department of Otolaryngology-
   Head and Neck Surgery
University of California Irvine
   School of Medicine
Irvine, CA
*Chapter 6*

**Douglas R. Sidell, MD**
Cincinnati Children's Hospital
Cincinnati, Ohio
*Chapter 8*

**Robert J. Stachler**
Senior Staff
Otolaryngology-Head and Neck
    Surgery
Henry Ford Medical Group
Division Chief
Lakeside Medical Center
Clinical Associate Professor
Wayne State University
Department of Otolaryngology-
    Head and Neck Surgery
Detroit, MI
*Chapters 3 and 6*

**Mas Takashima, MD, FACS**
Director
Otolaryngology Section
Sleep Medicine Fellowship
Baylor College of Medicine
Houston, TX
*Chapter 5*

**Neil Tanna, MD, MBA**
Associate Professor
Plastic Surgery and
    Otolaryngology
Hofstra North Shore–LIJ School
    of Medicine
Huntington, NY

Division of Plastic and
    Reconstructive Surgery
New York Head and Neck
    Institute
New York, NY
*Chapters 8 and 9*

**George H. Yoo, MD, FACS**
Chief Medical Officer
Karmanos Cancer Center
Professor
Departments of Otolaryngology-
    Head and Neck Surgery and
    Oncology
Wayne State University School
    of Medicine
Detroit, MI
*Chapter 7*

**Richard Zoumalan, MD**
Private Practice
Beverly Hills, CA
Cedars-Sinai Medical Center
West Hollywood, CA
Clinical Instructor
UCLA and USC Schools of
    Medicine
Los Angeles, CA
*Chapter 9*

# COMMON ABBREVIATIONS IN OTOLARYNGOLOGY–HEAD AND NECK SURGERY

| | |
|---|---|
| 3D | 3 dimensional |
| 5-FU | 5-fluorouracil |
| A-E | aryepiglottic |
| AA | arytenoid abduction |
| ABG | arterial blood gas, air bone gap |
| ABR | auditory brainstem response |
| AC | air conduction |
| ACE | angiotensin converting enzyme |
| AHI | apnea-hypopnea index |
| AI | apnea index |
| AIDS | acquired immunodeficiency syndrome |
| AJCC | American Joint Commission on Cancer |
| ALD | assisted listening device |
| ALS | amyotrophic lateral sclerosis |
| ANA | antinuclear antibody |
| AOM | acute otitis media |
| APAP | autotitrating positive airway pressure |
| ASA | aspirin |
| ASSR | auditory steady-state response |
| AVM | arteriovenous malformation |
| BAEP | brainstem auditory evoked potential |
| BAER | brainstem auditory evoked response |
| BAHA | bone-anchored hearing aid |
| BC | bone conduction |
| BCC | basal cell carcinoma |
| BID | twice a day |
| BiPAP | bilevel positive airway pressure |
| BMT | bilateral myringotomy and tubes |
| BOA | behavioral observation audiometry |
| BPPV | benign paroxysmal positional vertigo |
| BTE | behind the ear |
| BUN | blood urea nitrogen |
| CAPE-V | Consensus Auditory-Perceptual Evaluation of Voice |
| CBC | complete blood count |
| cGy | centigray |
| CHL | conductive hearing loss |
| CIC | completely in canal |
| CMV | cytomegalovirus |
| CN | cranial nerve |
| CNS | central nervous system |
| COM | chronic otitis media |
| COMMANDO | combined mandibulectomy and neck dissection operation |

| | | | |
|---|---|---|---|
| CPA | cerebellopontine angle, conditioned play audiometry | ECMO | extracorporeal membrane oxygenation |
| CPAP | continuous positive airway pressure | ECoG | electrocochleography |
| CROS | contralateral routing of sound | ECS | extracapsular spread |
| CRP | C-reactive protein | EEG | electroencephalography |
| CSA | central sleep apnea | EGFR | epidermal growth factor receptor |
| CSF | cerebrospinal fluid | | |
| CT | computed tomography | EJV | external jugular vein |
| CTA | computed tomographic angiography | EMG | electromyogram |
| | | END | elective neck dissection |
| CVA | cerebrovascular accident | ENG | electronystagmography |
| cVEMP | cervical vestibular evoked myogenic potential | ENoG | electroneuronography |
| | | EOG | electrooculography |
| | | ESR | erythrocyte sedimentation rate |
| CXR | chest x-ray | | |
| dB | decibel | ESS | endoscopic sinus surgery |
| dB HL | decibel hearing level | | |
| dB SL | decibel sensation level | ET | eustachian tube, endotracheal |
| dB SPL | decibel sound pressure level | | |
| | | ETT | endotracheal tube |
| DCR | dacryocystorhinostomy | FB | foreign body |
| | | FEES | functional endoscopic evaluation of swallowing |
| DDx | differential diagnosis | | |
| DL | direct laryngoscopy | | |
| DLB | direct laryngoscopy and bronchoscopy | | |
| | | FEESST | functional endoscopic evaluation of swallowing with sensory testing |
| DLBE | direct laryngoscopy, bronchoscopy, and esophagoscopy (panendoscopy) | | |
| | | | |
| DPOAE | distortion product otoacoustic emissions | FESS | functional endoscopic sinus surgery |
| Dx | diagnosis | | |
| EAC | external auditory canal | FEV | forced expiratory volume |
| EBV | Epstein-Barr virus | | |
| ECA | external carotid artery | FNA | fine-needle aspiration |
| ECG | electrocardiogram | | |

| | | | |
|---|---|---|---|
| FOM | floor of mouth | IAC | internal auditory canal |
| FTA-ABS | fluorescent treponemal antibody-absorption test | ICA | internal carotid artery |
| FTSG | full-thickness skin graft | ICP | intracranial pressure |
| | | IFN | interferon |
| GABHS | group A ß-hemolytic streptococci | Ig | immunoglobulin |
| | | IHC | inner hair cell, immunohisto-chemistry |
| GCS | Glasgow Coma Scale | | |
| GERD | gastroesophageal reflux disease | IJV | internal jugular vein |
| | | IL | interleukin |
| GI | gastrointestinal | IM | intramuscularly |
| GRBAS | grade, roughness, breathiness, asthenia, strain | IMF | intermaxillary fixation (see MMF) |
| | | IMRT | intensity-modulated radiation therapy |
| GSPN | greater superficial petrosal nerve | IS | incudostapedial (joint) |
| Gy | gray | | |
| H&N | head and neck | ISSNHL | idiopathic sudden sensorineural hearing loss |
| HA | hearing aid, headache | | |
| HBO | hyperbaric oxygen | ITC | in the canal |
| HFSNHL | high frequency sensorineural hearing loss | ITE | in the ear |
| | | ITM | in the mouth |
| | | IVIG | intravenous immunoglobulin |
| HHT | hereditary hemorrhagic telangiectasia | JNA | juvenile nasopharyngeal angiofibroma |
| HINT | hearing-in-noise test | | |
| HIV | human immunodeficiency virus | KTP | potassium titanyl phosphate |
| | | LAD | lymphadenopathy |
| HL | hearing level, hearing loss | LARP | left anterior, right posterior semicircular canal pair |
| HNSCC | head and neck squamous cell carcinoma | | |
| | | LCA | lateral cricoarytenoid muscle |
| HPV | human papilloma virus | | |
| HSV | herpes simplex virus | LDH | lactate dehydrogenase |
| I&D | incision and drainage | | |

| | | | |
|---|---|---|---|
| LDL | loudness discomfort level | MRND | modified radical neck dissection |
| LEMG | laryngeal electromyography | MRSA | methicillin resistant *Staphyloccocus aureus* |
| LES | lower esophageal sphincter | MSLT | multiple sleep latency test |
| LFT | liver function test | MWT | maintenance of wakefulness test |
| LMA | laryngeal mask airway | Mφ | macrophage |
| LP | lumbar puncture | NCCN | National Comprehensive Cancer Network |
| LPR | laryngopharyngeal reflux | | |
| LSPN | lesser superficial petrosal nerve | ND | neck dissection |
| | | NET | nerve excitability test |
| LTB | laryngotracheo-bronchitis | NF | neurofibromatosis |
| | | NHL | non-Hodgkin's lymphoma |
| MBS | modified barium swallow | NIHL | noise-induced hearing loss |
| MBSS | modified barium swallow study | NOE | naso-orbitoethmoid |
| MCL | medial canthal ligament | NP | nasopharynx |
| | | NPC | nasopharyngeal carcinoma |
| MDL | microdirect laryngoscopy | NPO | nothing by mouth |
| MDLB | microdirect laryngoscopy and bronchoscopy | NREM | nonrapid eye movement |
| | | NSAID | nonsteroidal anti-inflammatory drug |
| ME | middle ear | | |
| MEE | middle ear effusion | NSTI | necrotizing soft tissue infection |
| MEN | multiple endocrine neoplasia | OAE | otoacoustic emissions |
| MHL | mixed hearing loss | OC | oral cavity |
| MMA | maxillomandibular advancement | OCR | ossicular chain reconstruction |
| MMF | maxillomandibular fixation | OE | otitis externa |
| | | OHC | outer hair cell |
| MND | modified neck dissection | OM | otitis media |
| MRA | magnetic resonance angiography | OMC | ostiomeatal complex |
| | | OME | otitis media with effusion |
| MRI | magnetic resonance imaging | OP | oropharynx |

| | | | |
|---|---|---|---|
| ORIF | open reduction internal fixation | PPI | proton-pump inhibitor |
| ORL | otorhinolaryngology | PSG | polysomnography |
| OSA | obstructive sleep apnea | PT | prothrombin time |
| | | PTA | pure-tone average, peritonsillar abscess |
| OSAS | obstructive sleep apnea syndrome | PTH | parathyroid hormone |
| OTC | over-the-counter | PTT | partial thromboplastin time |
| OTE | over-the-ear | | |
| oVEMP | ocular vestibular evoked myogenic potential | PVFD | paradoxical vocal fold motion disorder |
| OW | oval window | PVFM | paradoxical vocal fold motion |
| PB max | phonetically balanced maximum | QOL | quality of life |
| PCA | posterior cricoarytenoid muscle | RALP | right anterior, left posterior semicircular canal pair |
| PCR | polymerase chain reaction | RAST | radioallergosorbent test |
| PDT | percutaneous dilational tracheotomy | RDI | respiratory disturbance index |
| PE | physical examination, pressure equalization, pulmonary embolus | REM | rapid eye movement |
| | | RERA | respiratory effort-related arousal |
| PEEP | positive end-expiratory pressure | RF | rheumatoid factor, radiofrequency |
| PEG | percutaneous endoscopic gastrostomy | RFFF | radial forearm free flap |
| PET | pressure equalization tube, positron emission tomography | RLN | recurrent laryngeal nerve |
| | | RPA | retropharyngeal abscess |
| PLM | periodic leg movement | RSTL | relaxed skin tension line |
| PLMD | periodic limb movement disorder | RTOG | Radiation Therapy Oncology Group |
| | | RW | round window |
| PORP | partial ossicular replacement prosthesis | Rx | treatment |
| | | SC | subcutaneous |
| | | SCC | squamous cell carcinoma, semicircular canal |

| | |
|---|---|
| SCM | sternocleidomastoid |
| SDB | sleep-disordered breathing |
| SIADH | syndrome of inappropriate antidiuretic hormone |
| SL | sensation level |
| SLE | systemic lupus erythematosus |
| SLN | superior laryngeal nerve |
| SLP | superficial lamina propria, speech-language pathologist |
| SMAS | superficial musculoaponeurotic system |
| SMG | submandibular gland |
| SNHL | sensorineural hearing loss |
| SPL | sound pressure level |
| SQ | subcutaneous |
| SML | suspension microlaryngoscopy |
| SRT | speech (spondee) reception threshold |
| SSD | single sided deafness |
| SSNHL | sudden sensorineural hearing loss |
| SSx | signs and symptoms |
| STSG | split-thickness skin graft |
| T&A | tonsillectomy and adenoidectomy |
| TA | thyroarytenoid muscle |
| TB | tuberculosis |
| TCA | tricyclic antidepressant, trichloroacetic acid |
| TEOAE | transiently evoked otoacoustic emissions |
| TEP | tracheoesophageal puncture |
| TFT | thyroid function test |
| TGDC | thyroglossal duct cyst |
| TID | three times a day |
| TL | total laryngectomy |
| TLM | transoral laser microsurgery |
| TM | tympanic membrane |
| TMJ | temporomandibular joint |
| TNF | tumor necrosis factor |
| TNM | tumor, node, metastasis |
| TORCH | toxoplasmosis, other, rubella, cytomegalovirus, herpes simplex virus |
| TORP | total ossicular replacement prosthesis |
| Trach | tracheostomy, tracheotomy, tracheostomy tube, tracheotomy tube |
| TSH | thyroid-stimulating hormone |
| TVC | true vocal cord |
| TVF | true vocal fold |
| U/S | ultrasound |
| UARS | upper airway resistance syndrome |
| UES | upper esophageal sphincter |
| UP3 | uvulopalato-pharyngoplasty |

| | | | |
|---|---|---|---|
| UPPP | uvulopalato-pharyngoplasty | VNG | videonystagmography |
| URI | upper respiratory infection | VOR | vestibulo-ocular reflex |
| VBI | vertebrobasilar insufficiency | VPI | velopharyngeal insufficiency |
| VC | vocal cord | VRA | visual response audiometry |
| VCD | vocal cord dysfunction (see PVFD) | VZV | varicella zoster virus |
| VDRL | venereal disease research laboratory | W/U | workup |
| VEMP | vestibular evoked myogenic potential | XRT | radiation therapy |
| VF | vocal fold | YAG | yttrium aluminium garnet |
| VFSS | videofluoroscopic swallow study | ZMC | zygomaticomaxillary complex |

*In the Name of God, the Merciful Redeemer, the Merciful Benefactor*

Dedicated to my Ever Expanding Family:

Dad, Mom, Mamta, Aramay Ocean, Zaedyn Bear, Ayla Sofia, Little Brother (Nasir), Anita, Jamie, Tasnim, Imran, Jazair, Rahul Uncle, Swati Auntie, Dave, Rumi, and Zephyr

*—Raza*

To my wife, Katrina, for her infinite support and patience; to Lily for keeping me always recharged; and to my mother, Carol, father, Larry, and sister, Danielle, for their continued kindness and encouragement even from afar.

*—Justin*

# CHAPTER

# Rhinology and Paranasal Sinuses

Justin S. Golub, Steven C. Marks, and Raza Pasha

# ANATOMY OF THE NOSE AND PARANASAL SINUSES

## Paranasal Sinus Anatomy

### Lateral Nasal Wall (Figure 1–1)

- **Turbinates (Conchae)**: three to four shelves (inferior, middle, superior, and supreme [normal variant]) covered by erectile mucosa, serve to increase the interior surface area
- **Meatuses**: three spaces located beneath each turbinate; superior meatus provides drainage for the sphenoid and posterior ethmoid sinuses; middle meatus provides drainage for the frontal, anterior ethmoid, and maxillary sinuses; inferior meatus contains the orifice of the nasolacrimal duct
- **Uncinate Process**: sickle-shaped thin bony part of the ethmoid bone, covered by mucoperiosteum, medial to the ethmoid infundibulum and lateral to the middle turbinate
- **Ethmoid Infundibulum**: pyramidal space that houses the drainage of the maxillary, anterior ethmoid, and frontal sinuses; superior attachment of uncinate determines spatial relationship of frontal sinus drainage (80% attach to the lamina papyracea resulting in frontal sinus drainage medial to the uncinate, 20% attach to the skull base or middle turbinate resulting in frontal sinus drainage lateral to the uncinate and into the infundibulum)
- **Semilunar Hiatus**: gap that empties the ethmoid infundibulum, located between the uncinate process and the ethmoid bulla
- **Sphenopalatine Foramen**: posterior to inferior attachment of the middle turbinate, contains sphenopalatine artery, sensory nerve fibers, and secretomotor fibers (parasympathetic fibers from vidian nerve to pterygopalatine ganglion)
- **Concha Bullosa**: an aerated middle turbinate, may result in nasal obstruction
- **Paradoxical Middle Turbinate**: a middle turbinate that is "turned" medially instead of laterally
- **Ostiomeatal Complex**: region referring to the anterior ethmoids containing the ostia of the maxillary, frontal, and ethmoid sinuses; lateral to the middle turbinate
- **Nasal Fontanelles**: areas of the lateral nasal wall where no bone exists, located above the insertion of the inferior turbinate, may be the site of accessory maxillary ostia
- **Nasolacrimal Duct and Sac**: duct is located lateral to the anterior uncinate process, sac is lateral to the agger nasi cell and opens into the inferior meatus via **Hasner's valve**

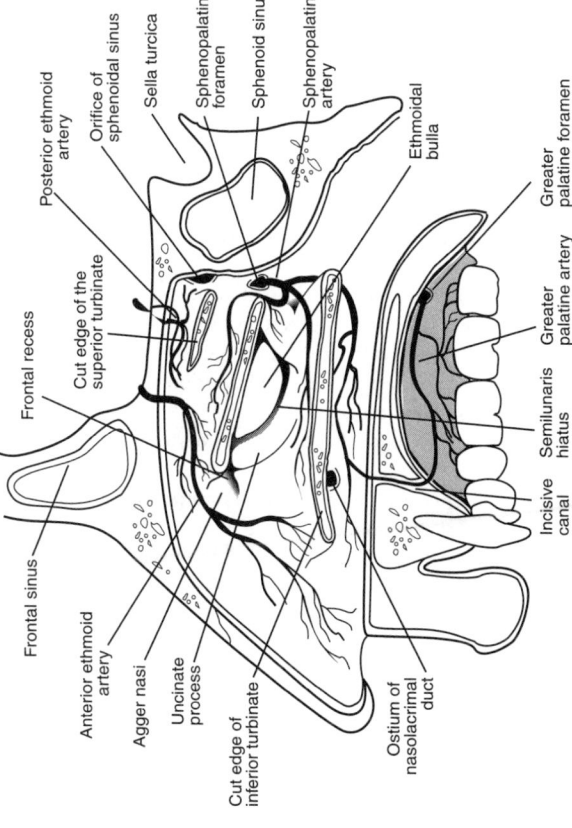

**FIGURE 1–1.** Anatomy of the lateral nasal wall including vascular supply.

Posterior ethmoid artery

Orifice of sphenoidal sinus

Sella turcica

Sphenopalatine foramen

Sphenoid sinus

Sphenopalatine artery

Ethmoidal bulla

Greater palatine foramen

Greater palatine artery

Semilunaris hiatus

Incisive canal

Cut edge of the superior turbinate

Frontal recess

Frontal sinus

Anterior ethmoid artery

Agger nasi

Uncinate process

Cut edge of inferior turbinate

Ostium of nasolacrimal duct

## Frontal Sinus

- <u>Embryology</u>: does not appear until 5–6 years old
- <u>Volume at Adult</u>: 4–7 mL by 12–20 years old (5–10% underdeveloped)
- <u>Drainage</u>: frontal recess via the anterior middle meatus either medial or lateral to the uncinate
- <u>Vasculature</u>: supraorbital and supratrochlear arteries, ophthalmic (cavernous sinus) and supraorbital (anterior facial) veins
- <u>Innervation</u>: supraorbital and supratrochlear nerves (CN $V_1$)
- <u>X-ray</u>: lateral and Caldwell view
- **Frontal Recess**: drainage space between the frontal sinus and semilunar hiatus; bounded by the posterior wall of the agger nasi cell, lamina papyracea, and middle turbinate
- **Frontal Sinus Infundibulum**: space that drains into frontal recess, superior to the agger nasi cells
- **Foramina of Breschet**: small venules that drain the sinus mucosa into the dural veins
- **Frontal Cells**: anterior ethmoid cells that pneumatize the frontal recess, may cause obstruction or persistent disease, posterior to the agger nasi cell, 4 types as defined by Bent and Kuhn
  <u>Type I</u>: single cell above agger nasi cell but below the floor of the frontal sinus (infundibulum)
  <u>Type II</u>: multiple cells above agger nasi cell may invade into the frontal sinus
  <u>Type III</u>: single large cell that extend supraorbitally through the floor of the frontal sinus, attaches to the anterior table
  <u>Type IV</u>: single isolated cell that is within the frontal sinus

## Maxillary Sinus

- <u>Embryology</u>: first to develop in utero, biphasic growth at 3 and 7–18 years old
- <u>Volume at Adult</u>: typically 15 mL (largest paranasal sinus)
- <u>Drainage</u>: ethmoid infundibulum (middle meatus, 10–30% have accessory ostium)
- <u>Vasculature</u>: maxillary and facial artery, maxillary vein
- <u>Innervation</u>: infraorbital nerve (CN $V_2$)
- <u>X-ray</u>: Water's view
- <u>Adjacent Structures</u>: lateral nasal wall, alveolar process of maxilla (contains second bicuspid and first and second molars), orbital floor, posterior maxillary wall (contains pterygopalatine fossa housing the maxillary artery, pterygopalatine ganglion, and branches of CN V)

# Ethmoid Sinus

- <u>Embryology</u>: three to four cells at birth (most developed paranasal sinus at birth), formed from 5 ethmoturbinals (1 = agger nasi, uncinate; 2 = middle turbinate; 3 = superior turbinate; 4–5 = supreme turbinate; may vary by source)
- <u>Volume at Adult</u>: 10–15 aerated cells, total volume of 2–3 mL (adult size at 12–15 years old)
- <u>Drainage</u>: anterior cells drain into the ethmoid infundibulum (middle meatus), posterior cells drain into the sphenoethmoidal recess (superior meatus)
- <u>Vasculature</u>: anterior and posterior ethmoid arteries (from ophthalmic artery), maxillary and ethmoid veins (cavernous sinus)
- <u>Innervation</u>: anterior and posterior ethmoidal nerves (from nasociliary nerve, CN $V_1$)
- <u>X-ray</u>: lateral and Caldwell view
- <u>Adjacent Structures</u>: skull base, anterior ethmoid artery (roof of anterior ethmoid cells), nasal cavity, orbit
- **Agger Nasi Cells**: most anterior of anterior ethmoid cells found anterior and superior to the middle turbinate attachment to the lateral wall, the posterior wall of the agger nasi cells forms the anterior wall of the frontal recess
- **Ethmoid Bulla**: the largest of the anterior ethmoid cells that lies above the infundibulum, the anterior ethmoid artery courses the roof of this cell
- **Basal (Ground) Lamella of the Middle Turbinate**: posterior bony attachment of the middle turbinate that **separates anterior and posterior ethmoid cells**; **anterior** part inserts vertically into the crista ethmoidalis, **middle** part inserts obliquely into the lamina papyracea, and the **posterior** third attaches to the lamina horizontally
- **Onodi Cells**: ethmoid cells that pneumatize lateral or posterior to anterior wall of the sphenoid, commonly mistaken as sphenoid cells, optic nerve or carotid artery may indent into the lateral wall
- **Haller Cells**: ethmoid cells that extend into maxillary sinus above the ostium, pneumatize the medial and inferior orbital walls
- **Lamina Papyracea**: lateral thin bony wall of the ethmoid sinus, separates orbit from ethmoid cells as a part of the medial orbital wall
- **Fovea Ethmoidalis**: roof of ethmoid sinus

# Sphenoid Sinus

- <u>Embryology</u>: evagination of nasal mucosa into sphenoid bone
- <u>Volume at Adult</u>: 0.5–8 mL (adult size at 12–18 years old)

- <u>Drainage</u>: sphenoethmoidal recess in the superior meatus
- <u>Vasculature</u>: sphenopalatine artery (from maxillary artery), maxillary vein (pterygoid plexus)
- <u>Innervation</u>: sphenopalatine nerve (parasympathetic fibers and CN $V_2$)
- <u>X-ray</u>: lateral and submentovertex (basal)
- <u>Adjacent Structures</u>: pons, pituitary (sella turcica), carotid artery (lateral wall, **25% dehiscent**), optic nerve (lateral wall, **5% dehiscent**), cavernous sinus (laterally), CN $V_2$ and VI, clivus, septal branch of the sphenopalatine artery (inferior aspect of the sphenoid os)

# Nasal Anatomy

## Nasal Cartilage

- **Upper Lateral Cartilage**: inferior to nasal bone
- **Lower Lateral (Greater) Alar Cartilage**: paired cartilage inferior to the upper lateral cartilage, composed of lateral and medial crura
- **Lesser Alar Cartilage**: small cartilagenous plates that are lateral to the lower lateral alar cartilage

## Nasal Septum (Figure 1–2)

- **Quadrangular Cartilage**: septal cartilage
- **Perpendicular Plate of the Ethmoid**: projects from cribriform plate to septal cartilage
- **Vomer**: posterior and inferior to perpendicular plate
- **Nasal Crest (Maxillary and Palatine Bone)**: trough of bone that supports the septal cartilage
- **Anterior Nasal Spine**: bony projection anterior to piriform aperture

## Sensory Innervation

### External Innervation

- supratrochlear and infratrochlear nerves (CN $V_1$): nasal dorsum
- external nasal branch of anterior ethmoid (CN $V_1$): nasal tip
- infraorbital nerve (CN $V_2$): malar, lateral nose, and subnasal regions

### Internal Innervation

- internal nasal branch of anterior ethmoid (CN $V_1$): anterosuperior nasal cavity
- posterior ethmoid nerve (CN $V_1$): posterior nasal cavity
- sphenopalatine nerve (CN $V_2$): posterior and inferior nasal cavity
- superior alveolar nerves (CN $V_2$)

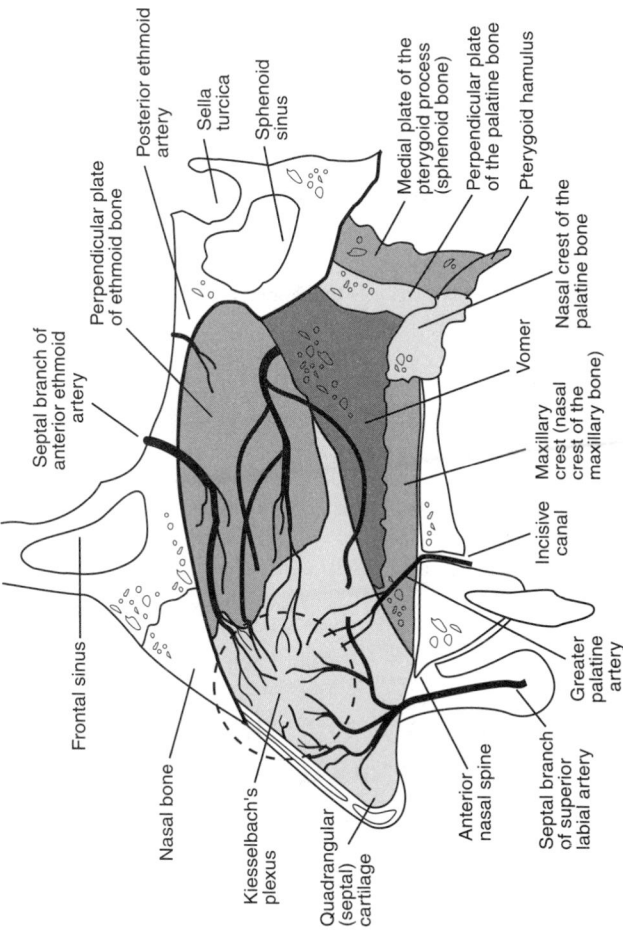

**FIGURE 1–2.** Anatomy of the septum including vascular supply.

Frontal sinus

Nasal bone

Kiesselbach's plexus

Quadrangular (septal) cartilage

Anterior nasal spine

Septal branch of superior labial artery

Septal branch of anterior ethmoid artery

Perpendicular plate of ethmoid bone

Posterior ethmoid artery

Sella turcica

Sphenoid sinus

Medial plate of the pterygoid process (sphenoid bone)

Perpendicular plate of the palatine bone

Pterygoid hamulus

Nasal crest of the palatine bone

Vomer

Maxillary crest (nasal crest of the maxillary bone)

Incisive canal

Greater palatine artery

## Vascular Anatomy (*see* Figures 1–1 and 1–2)

### *External Carotid Artery Branches*

#### Maxillary Artery (Internal Maxillary Artery)
- descending palatine artery → greater palatine and lesser palatine arteries
- sphenopalatine artery → sphenopalatine foramen (posterior to the middle turbinate) → medial (nasoseptal) and lateral nasal artery (middle and inferior turbinates)

#### Facial Artery
- superior labial artery → nasal septum and alar branches
- lateral nasal artery
- angular artery

### *Internal Carotid Artery → Ophthalmic Artery*

- anterior ethmoid artery (larger than the posterior ethmoid artery) → lateral nasal wall and septum
- posterior ethmoidal artery → superior concha and septum
- dorsal nasal artery → external nose

### *Venous System*

- greater palatine vein → posterior facial vein (external jugular vein) and cavernous sinus
- septal vein drains → anterior facial vein (internal jugular vein)
- sphenopalatine vein → cavernous sinus and maxillary vein (internal jugular vein)
- anterior and posterior ethmoidal veins → ophthalmic veins (cavernous sinus)
- angular vein → anterior facial vein (internal jugular vein)

# PHYSIOLOGY OF THE NOSE AND PARANASAL SINUSES

## Physiology of the Nasal Airway

### Nasal Cycle and Respiratory Airflow

- nasal airflow is regulated through the volume of the venous sinusoids (capacitance vessels) in the nasal erectile tissue (located primarily in the inferior turbinate and to a lesser extent in the anterior septum)

- the hypothalamus continuously stimulates a sympathetic tone (via the superior cervical sympathetic ganglia) to maintain a level of nasal vasoconstriction
- inspired air is warmed to body temperature and is humidified to almost 100% humidity
- Nasal Flow = Pressure / Resistance; flow may be laminar (normal) or turbulent (may cause eddied currents that may be perceived as nasal obstruction)
- **Sneeze Reflex**: induced by allergens, ammonia, viral infections, exercise, and other irritants, which stimulate trigeminal afferents; complex efferent input results in a slow inspiratory phase, glottic and velopharyngeal closure (increases subglottic pressure), followed by a sudden glottic opening (sneeze)
- Regulation Response Types
    1. **Asymmetric Congestive Response (The Nasal Cycle)**: normal physiologic congestion/decongestion cycle alternating between nasal sides every 2–7 hours
    2. **Symmetric Congestive Response**: temporary bilateral congestion induced by exercise, changes in body position, hyperventilation, cold air, sulfur, histamine, and other irritants; lasts 15–30 minutes

## Microvasculature

- regulates nasal volume, humidity, and heat exchange
- **Resistance Vessels**: arterioles and precapillary sphincters, regulate blood flow to the nasal mucosa
- **Subepithelial Capillaries**: fenestrated vessels allow for transport of solutes and fluids
- **Venous Sinusoids**: capacitance vessels, determine blood volume and nasal congestion
- **Arteriovenous Anastomoses**: regulate nasal blood flow by allowing blood to flow directly from the resistance vessels to the venous sinusoids

## Regulation of Nasal Microvasculature

- Sympathetic Innervation: provides vasoconstrictor tone to arteries and capacitance veins, mediated through **norepinephrine** (primary neurotransmitter), **neuropeptide Y** (a weak vasoconstrictor, enhances effects of norepinephrine), and avian pancreatic polypeptide (APP)
- Parasympathetic Innervation: controls secretions and dilates resistance vessels, mediated through **acetylcholine** (primary

neurotransmitter), **vasoactive intestinal peptide** (VIP), and **peptide histamine isoleucine** (PHI)

## Mucociliary System

- Function: humidification, cleaning of inspired air, eliminating debris and excess secretion from paranasal sinuses and nasal airway
- Mucociliary Flow: mass motion of the mucous blanket in the paranasal sinuses at 1 cm/minute (eg, migration in the maxillary sinus begins at the floor of maxillary sinus → natural ostium → nasal cavity → nasopharynx)
- **Components**
  1. **Ciliated, Pseudostratified Columnar Epithelium**: anterior border begins at limen nasi
  2. **Double-Layered Mucous Blanket**: deep, less viscous, serous periciliary fluid (sol phase) and superficial, more viscous, mucous fluid (gel phase)
  3. **Mucus-Producing Glands**: goblet cells (columnar cells, basal nucleus, secretory granules at lumen end), deep and superficial seromucinous glands (serous or mucous acini with cuboidal-lined duct complexes), and intraepithelial glands (20–50 mucous cells around a single duct)
- Major Composition of Nasal Mucus: 95% water, 3% glycoproteins (mucin), 2% salts, immunoglobulins (IgA), lysozymes (bacteriolytic), and lactoferrin (bacteriostatic)

## Olfactory Physiology

- olfaction requires turbulent airflow from the anterior nares or the choanae
- pungent odors (vinegar, ammonia) may be perceived through **trigeminal nerve fibers** (via substance P pain fibers)
- Olfactory Epithelial Cell Types
  1. **Ciliated Olfactory Receptor Cells**: club-shaped bipolar neurons with axons that synapse to the olfactory bulb
  2. **Microvillar Cells**: neuronal cells of unknown function
  3. **Supporting Cells**: sustenacular cells
  4. **Basal Cells**: allow capability of olfactory fiber regeneration (unlike most other sensory cells)
- Olfactory Mechanism: odorant enters olfactory cleft → odorant dissolves in mucus → odorant binding proteins (OBP) concentrate the solubilized odorant → binds to olfactory receptor at the sensory cilia → stimulates a specific G-protein (cAMP-dependent) cascade for depolarization → synaptic connections form a complex network

of secondary neurons (suggesting peripheral processing) before entering the brain (dentate and semilunate gyri)
- each odorant receptor cell detects a single type of odorant; there are hundreds of types of receptor cells

# EVALUATION FOR NASAL OBSTRUCTION
## History and Physical Exam
### History

- <u>Character of Nasal Obstruction</u>: onset and duration, constant versus intermittent, unilateral (tumors, normal nasal cycle) versus bilateral obstruction, associated mouth breathing, snoring, anosmia/hyposmia/taste disturbances, tearing (nasolacrimal duct obstruction or allergy)
- <u>Contributing Factors</u>: potential toxin and allergen exposure, known drug allergies, medications (*see* Table 1–1), history of immunodeficiency, asthma, rhinosinusitis, otitis media, allergy, sleep disturbances, facial trauma or surgery
- <u>Associated SSx</u>: allergic component (sneezing, itchy and watery eyes, clear rhinorrhea), sinus involvement (facial pain, headaches), acute infection (fevers, malaise, purulent or odorous nasal discharge, pain)
- <u>H&N</u>: sore throat, postnasal drip, cough, ear complaints, halitosis, ocular pain, hoarseness
- think "KITTENS" for differential diagnosis (*see* Table 1–2)

---

**TABLE 1–1.** Common Classifications of Drugs That Cause Rhinorrhea and Nasal Congestion

- **Antihypertensives**
- **Psychotropic Medications**
- **Oral Contraceptives**
- **Chronic Nasal Decongestants:** rhinitis medicamentosa
- **Cocaine:** local vasoconstriction
- **Tobacco:** irritates mucosa and impairs ciliary clearance
- **Antithyroid Medication**
- **Aspirin:** activates peripheral chemoreceptors
- **Marijuana**

---

**TABLE 1–2.** Differential Diagnosis of Nasal Obstruction: KITTENS Method

| (K) Congenital | Infectious & Idiopathic | Toxins & Trauma | Tumor (Neoplasia) | Endocrine | Neurologic | Systemic |
|---|---|---|---|---|---|---|
| Neurogenic tumors | Infectious rhinitis | Nasal and septal fractures | Papillomas | Diabetes | Vasomotor rhinitis | Granulomatous diseases |
| Congenital nasopharyngeal cysts | Rhinoscleroma | Medication side effects (rhinitis medicamentosa) | Nasal polyps | Hypothyroidism | | Vasculitis |
| | Chronic sinusitis | | Hemangiomas | Pregnancy | | Allergy |
| Teratoma | Adenoid hyperplasia | Synechia | Pyogenic granulomas | | | Cystic fibrosis |
| Choanal atresia | | Environmental irritants | Juvenile nasopharyngeal angiofibromas | | | |
| Nasoseptal deformities | | Septal hematomas | Malignancy | | | |
| | | Foreign bodies | | | | |

## Physical Exam

- <u>External Nasal Exam</u>: external deformities (firmness, tenderness on palpation), nasal flaring, nasal airflow
- <u>Anterior Rhinoscopy/Nasal Endoscopy</u>: examine twice (with and without topical decongestion), quality of turbinates (hypertrophic, pale, blue), quality of nasal mucosa, nasal septum, ostiomeatal complex obstruction, foreign bodies, nasal masses, choanal opening
- <u>Quality of Nasal Secretions</u>: purulent or thick (infectious), watery and clear (vasomotor rhinitis, allergy), salty and clear (CSF leak)
- <u>H&N Exam</u>: facial tenderness, tonsil and adenoid hypertrophy, cobblestoned posterior pharynx, cervical adenopathy, otologic exam

## Ancillary Tests

- **Allergy Evaluation**: (*see* pp. 35–37)
- **Paranasal X-ray**: may be considered for screening, high rate of false negatives, largely replaced by CT/MRI
- **CT/MRI of Paranasal Sinus**: indicated if obstruction may be secondary to nasal masses, polyps, or for workup of chronic rhinosinusitis; MRI preferred if suspect tumors, intracranial involvement, or complicated rhinosinusitis
- **Biopsy**: indicated for any mass suspicious for malignancy, avoid biopsy of vascular neoplasms (juvenile nasopharyngeal angiofibroma, sarcomas) or encephaloceles
- **Rhinomanometry**: provides an objective measurement of airway resistance, largely not utilized in clinical practice since highly time-consuming, not cost-effective, and inaccurate
- **Ciliary Biopsy and Mucociliary Clearance Tests**: electron microscopy and ciliary motility studies for ciliary defects
- **Nasal Secretion Protein, Glucose, or $\beta_2$-transferrin**: evaluate for CSF leak
- **Culture and Sensitivity**: directed nasal swab, surgically obtained cultures may be indicated for complicated acute rhinosinusitis and resistant chronic rhinosinusitis
- **Pulmonary Function Tests**: consider if suspect coexisting reactive airway disease
- **Olfactometry**: qualitative and quantitative testing of olfactory substances, largely not utilized in clinical practice

# NASAL DISEASES

## Congenital Nasal Disorders (see pp. 541–542)

## Inflammatory Nasal Masses

### Nasal Folliculitis and Furuncles

- <u>Pathogenesis</u>: a pyoderma (purulent skin disease) secondary to *Staphylococcus* or *Streptococcus*, typically arises from a hair follicle (**folliculitis**), may organize to form pus with a central core (**furuncle** or boil); a carbuncle is a group of furuncles
- <u>SSx</u>: intranasal tenderness, reddening and edema of nasal vestibule, sensation of tension at tip of nose, fever
- <u>Dx</u>: clinical exam, culture
- <u>Complications</u>: septal abscess, septal chondritis, saddle nose deformity, cavernous sinus thrombosis
- <u>Rx</u>: oral antibiotic and triple-antibiotic ointment may be used initially, avoid manipulation, incision and drainage for abscess formation, intravenous antibiotics for recalcitrant disease

### Septal Abscess

- <u>Pathophysiology</u>: usually secondary to trauma (causing septal hematoma, which is a nidus for infection) or a furuncle
- <u>SSx</u>: widened septum, nasal obstruction, severe pain, fever, erythema in nasal vestibule
- <u>Complications</u>: intracranial extension (cavernous sinus thrombosis, meningitis), septal chondritis, saddle nose deformity due to cartilage necrosis
- <u>Rx</u>: aggressive management with incision and drainage and consideration of intravenous antibiotics

### Rhinophyma

- <u>Pathophysiology</u>: massive hypertrophy and hyperplasia of sebaceous glands (form of acne rosacea), associated with *Demodex folliculorum* (face mite)
- typically afflicts white 40–60-year-old males, **not** associated with alcohol, associated with facial flushing
- <u>SSx</u>: begins with **acne rosacea** with a flush reaction in adolescence, skin becomes oily, cystic, and thick; later stages form large pits, fissures, lobulations, and pedunculation deforming the nose into a large lobular swelling of the nasal tip, may cause nasal obstruction

- <u>Dx</u>: clinical exam
- may house occult basal cell carcinoma
- <u>Rx</u>: preventive therapy includes cleansing the skin with defatting detergents, anti-inflammatory agents, antibiotics, benzoyl peroxide lotions, and isotretinoin; nasal deformity may only be treated surgically (partial or full-thickness excision [decortication] using laser, Bovie, dermabrasion, or scalpel followed by skin grafts)

## Rhinoliths/Nasal Foreign Bodies

- <u>Pathophysiology</u>: concretions secondary to encrustation of foreign body or longstanding nasal crusting may form **rhinoliths**
- <u>SSx</u>: unilateral, purulent rhinorrhea, pain, epistaxis
- most common cause of pediatric unilateral rhinorrhea
- <u>Dx</u>: anterior rhinoscopy, imaging, or nasal endoscopy
- <u>Complications</u>: secondary infection
- <u>Rx</u>: removal (may require general anesthetic, may trigger epistaxis)

## Nasal (Sinonasal) Polyposis

- <u>Pathophysiology</u>: unclear, may be secondary to abnormal cellular homeostasis from chronic inflammation resulting in polypoidal degeneration, typically arises from lateral nasal wall
- <u>Samter's Triad</u> (**8–10%** of nasal polyposis patients)
  1. **asthma**
  2. **aspirin sensitivity**
  3. **nasal polyposis**
- associated with chronic rhinosinusitis (~50%), allergic rhinitis, cystic fibrosis (up to 40%), trauma, and metabolic diseases
- must also consider the potential of an encephalocele, glioma, or inverted papilloma
- <u>SSx</u>: smooth, pale, intranasal clustered grapelike masses (usually bilateral), nasal obstruction, anosmia/hyposomia, postnasal drip, rhinorrhea
- <u>Dx</u>: anterior rhinoscopy, nasal endoscopy, CT of paranasal sinuses (nonenhancing nasal mass, partial or complete sinus opacification, may reveal expansion of superior nasal fossa), allergy testing
- <u>Histopathology</u>: **pseudostratified respiratory epithelium** with three types of stroma: **edematous** (few inflammatory cells with edematous stroma), **inflammatory** (predominantly inflammatory cells), **fibrous** (collagen stroma); eosinophilia predominates
- <u>Complications</u>: exacerbation of rhinosinusitis, proptosis, diplopia, bone erosion, osteitis, meningitis

## *Management*

- **Medical Management**: aggressive allergy management, long-term nasal corticosteroid sprays, oral corticosteroids (may be considered 3–4 times per year and preoperatively, although surgery is preferred over chronic use), avoidance of aspirin (if intolerant), cromolyn spray, consider lipoxygenase pathway inhibitors for aspirin-sensitive patients (*controversial*)
- **Polypectomy**: effective in short term (high rate of recurrence), provides a biopsy specimen
- **Functional Endoscopic Sinus Surgery (FESS)**: treatment of choice for persistent and severe symptoms; includes polypectomy, complete sphenoethmoidectomy, antrostomy for ventilation and drainage; polypoid specimen should be sent as specimen to evaluate for potential underlying tumor; recurrence common
- **Recurrent or Severe Sinonasal Polyposis**: requires frequent monitoring, consider comprehensive (revision) endoscopic approaches, consider daily oral corticosteroids (low-dose) or high-dose corticosteroid nasal saline irrigations (**budesonide**), corticosteroid eluding stents (*new*)

## Antrochoanal Polyp

- <u>Pathophysiology</u>: retention cyst from maxillary sinus that protrudes through the antrum and may enter the choana and nasopharynx
- <u>SSx</u>: unilateral obstructing polyp
- <u>Histopathology</u>: not associated with eosinophilia or typical inflammatory markers of nasal polyposis
- <u>Rx</u>: endoscopic removal including the pedicled site within the maxillary sinus

# Benign Tumors

## Keratotic Papilloma (Benign Squamous Papilloma, Schneiderian Papilloma, Vestibular Wart)

- <u>Pathophysiology</u>: benign lesion arises from squamous or Schneiderian (nasal) epithelium, associated most commonly with **HPV 6, 11**
- low malignant potential
- subtypes include fungiform (most common, originates from nasal septum), inverted (*see below*) and cylindrical (originates from nasal wall)
- <u>SSx</u>: verrucous lesion, commonly on nasal vestibule, often multiple, painless

- <u>Dx</u>: anterior rhinoscopy, nasal endoscopy, biopsy confirms diagnosis
- <u>Rx</u>: simple excision or laser ablation; for septal keratotic papillomas a cuff of normal mucoperichondrium should be taken with lesion to avoid recurrence

## Inverted Papilloma

- <u>Pathophysiology</u>: arises from proliferation of reserve cells in **Schneiderian mucosa** associated with HPV 6, 11, and EBV; benign pathology but locally aggressive behavior
- more common in males
- often misdiagnosed as a nasal polyp (polyps are more translucent, bilateral, and less vascular)
- <u>SSx</u>: **unilateral polyp** (obstruction or rhinosinusitis), epistaxis, rhinorrhea, diplopia, typically presents on the lateral nasal wall (rarely on the nasal septum), may be associated with a hyperinflammatory nasal polyp
- <u>Dx</u>: CT of paranasal sinuses reveals erosion into lateral nasal wall or extension into maxillary or ethmoid sinuses, may reveal calcifications; MRI may be considered for extensive involvement or for recurrence; biopsy confirms diagnosis (must check imaging study prior to biopsy to avoid possible vascular or brain injury)
- <u>Histopathology</u>: **endophytic growth of epithelium**, cristae-laden senescent mitochondria, inflammatory cells throughout epithelium
- <u>Complications</u>: 10% malignant degeneration from lateral wall lesions (rare from nasal septum), extension into sinuses, orbit (blindness, diplopia, proptosis), or intracranial cavity and skull base
- <u>Rx</u>: adequate en bloc excision typically requires a **medial maxillectomy** or **midface degloving** (less common), **endoscopic excision** more common with modern techniques, radiation not recommended (unless associated with malignant degeneration); recurrence varies widely and depends on adequacy of resection, rare recurrence after 2 years

## Juvenile Nasopharyngeal Angiofibroma (JNA)

- most common vascular mass in nose, most common nasopharyngeal benign neoplasm
- exclusive to **adolescent males**
- <u>Pathophysiology</u>: benign yet aggressive vascular tumor, etiology unknown (may have hormonal element since exclusive to adolescent males)
- slow growing, locally invasive, may spread intracranially, does not metastasize

- <u>SSx</u>: smooth purplish lobulated mass in nasopharynx or lateral nasal wall (posterior aspect of the middle turbinate near the **sphenopalatine foramen**), recurrent unilateral **epistaxis** (may be bilateral), rhinorrhea, nasal obstruction, anosmia, headache, facial swelling, proptosis
- <u>Dx</u>: CT/CTA/MRI/MRA of paranasal sinuses (mass with extension into pterygomaxillary fissure), carotid angiography, **avoid biopsy**
- <u>Histopathology</u>: benign, encapsulated, composed of **vascular** tissue and fibrous stroma, abundant mast cells
- <u>Complications</u>: extension into sinuses, orbit (blindness, diplopia, proptosis), or intracranial and skull base
- <u>Fisch's Classification</u>: **I**—limited to nasal cavity; **II**—extends into pterygomaxillary (pterygopalatine) fossa or sinuses with bony destruction; **III**—invades infratemporal fossa, orbit, or parasellar area; **IV**—extends into cavernous sinus, optic chiasmal region, or pituitary fossa
- <u>Managament</u>
  1. **Endoscopic Surgery**: avoids facial incision and dividing bone for access; may be considered with tumors limited to the ethmoids, maxillary sinus, sphenoid sinus, sphenopalatine foramen, pterygomaxillary fossa, nasopharynx, or limited infratemporal fossa involvement, consider preoperative embolization
  2. **Open Surgical Approaches**: type I or II tumors may be approached through a transpalatal, transmaxillary, sphenoethmoidal, or lateral rhinotomy route; infratemporal, midface degloving, facial translocation, and subcranial approaches may be considered for advanced disease; consider preoperative embolization
  3. **Radiation and Chemotherapy**: limited use due to potential complications (eg, malignant transformation, growth retardation, hypopituitarism, cataracts); considered for residual tumors, intracranial extension, or nonoperative candidates; chemotherapy considered for failed surgical and radiation therapies
  4. **Hormonal Therapy**: eg, estrogen, flutamide, may decrease tumor size and vascularity, not routine

## Other Benign Tumors

- **Benign Salivary Gland Tumors**: rare, pleomorphic adenoma most common; <u>Rx</u>: local excision
- **Hemangioma**: most often presents at Little's area (Kiesselbach's plexus, caudal septum) or inferior turbinate; <u>Rx</u>: excision with cuff of normal mucoperichondrium, may consider preoperative embolization
- **Pyogenic Granuloma**: friable polypoid lesion (usually on septum, may be secondary to trauma), difficult to distinguish from

hemangioma, presents with epistaxis and unilateral obstruction, may present during pregnancy ("pregnancy tumor"); <u>Rx</u>: excision although most resolve
- **Hemangiopericytoma**: arises from pericytes, 10% malignant degeneration; <u>Rx</u>: excision, 50% recur
- **Osteoma**: common benign tumor, slow growing, usually asymptomatic, multiple lesions associated with **Gardner syndrome** (malignant degeneration of intestinal polyps); <u>Rx</u>: excision for symptomatic lesions otherwise may observe with serial imaging
- **Chordoma**: arises from notochord of nasopharynx, may produce obstructive symptoms or involve cranial nerves; <u>Rx</u>: excision

## Malignancy (*see* pp. 309–315)

# Systemic Diseases Affecting the Nose

## Granulomatous Diseases (*see also* pp. 242–244)

- **Sarcoidosis**: cobblestoning of sinonasal mucosa from granulomatous inflammation, dryness, crusting, epistaxis, or septal perforation
- **Granulomatosis with Polyangiitis (GPA)**: *see following*
- **Langerhans Cell Histiocytosis**: nasal mass, epistaxis, or septal perforation
- **Nasal Extranodal NK/T-Cell Lymphoma**: clear to purulent rhinorrhea, septal perforation, epistaxis, "midline" facial destructive lesions

## Vasculitic Diseases (*see also* pp. 249–251)

- **Granulomatosis with Polyangiitis (GPA; Wegener's Granulomatosis)**: inflamed friable mucosa, ulcerative septal perforation, saddle nose deformity, epistaxis
- **Polyarteritis Nodosa**: nasal mucosal lesions
- **Lupus Erythematosus**: ulcerated nasal septum (nasal perforation)

# Nasal Anatomic Abnormalities

## Nasal Valvular Obstruction

- **Valvular Collapse**: a dynamic obstruction due to weak structural support of the nasal valve, results in obstruction during inhalation
- **Bernoulli's Principle**: the narrowest segment (nasal valves) accelerates nasal airflow resulting in a decrease in intraluminal pressure causing collapse

- <u>Causes</u>: congenital, trauma, iatrogenic (excessive cartilage removal at intercartilaginous junction and lateral crus), aging, caudal septal deflection, facial nerve paralysis (loss of nasal dilators), topical nasal decongestants
- <u>SSx</u>: nasal airway obstruction on inspiration (valvular collapse), crusting, epistaxis, recurrent rhinosinusitis, hyposmia
- <u>Dx</u>: anterior rhinoscopy, nasal endoscopy, **Cottle maneuver** (pulling superiorly on medial maxilla skin to open valve, if improves airway suggests external valve collapse)

### External Nasal Valve Boundaries

- forms **nasal vestibule**
- <u>Boundaries</u>
  1. **nasal alar cartilage** (superior and lateral walls)
  2. **caudal septum and medial crura (columella)** (medial wall)
  3. **nasal sill** (inferior wall)

### Internal Nasal Valve Boundaries

- forms **limen nasi**
- narrowest part of nasal airway (**50% of total nasal resistance**)
- <u>Boundaries</u>
  1. caudal edge of **upper lateral cartilage** (superior wall)
  2. **dorsal septum** (medial wall)
  3. anterior edge of the **inferior turbinate** (lateral wall)

### External Nasal Valve Obstruction Management

- **Nasal Breathing Strips**: can be used at night
- **Septoplasty**: addresses significant caudal deviation
- **Suspension Sutures**: suture that is suspended from lateral crus to the orbital rim
- **Cartilaginous Spreader Grafts**: address defects of the lateral nasal wall, cartilage placed between upper lateral cartilage and septum
- **Onlay Batten Grafts**: augments lateral wall support of the alar cartilage during inspiration, placed under the edges of the lower lateral cartilage
- **Columellar Strut**: cartilage placed in between medial crura, improves tip ptosis
- **Caudal Extension Graft**: cartilage placed at the caudal portion of the septum, repositions the tip, lengthens the nose to support the external nasal valve
- **Rim Graft**: cartilage placed in caudal alar region
- **Functional Septorhinoplasty**: a septoplasty combined with the above mentioned techniques to address nasal obstruction

## Internal Nasal Valve Obstruction Management

- medically treat underlying cause (eg, infectious, allergy), surgery for mechanical obstruction
- **Septoplasty**: addresses a dorsal septal deflection (the most common cause of internal nasal valve obstruction)
- **Inferior Turbinate Reduction**: *see following*
- **Butterfly Graft**: curved cartilage placed under the upper lateral cartilage

## Surgical Management of the Septum

- **Submucous Resection**: obstructing cartilaginous and bony portion of the nasal septum is removed
- **Septoplasty**: removal of deviated cartilaginous and bony septum with reinsertion after remodeling and repositioning (preserves support system, less risk of perforation)
- Indications: nasal obstruction (deviated nasal septum), epistaxis, chronic rhinosinusitis (when septum is obstructing), access for transseptal sphenoidotomy, associated pain from an impacted spur (contact point headaches, *controversial*), septal neoplasm (rare), improve CPAP compliance
- Complications: perforation, saddle nose deformity (over resecting cartilage anteriorly), cribriform plate fracture, septal hematoma, anosmia, septal abscess, bleeding

## Surgical Management of the Inferior Turbinate

- **Inferior Turbinate Outfracturing**: easy technique, poor long-term results
- **Intramural Cautery/Coblation/Radiofrequency Ablation**: easy technique, may be done in the office, poor long-term benefit
- **Partial Turbinate Reduction (Submucosal Resection)**: various techniques to remove turbinate bone while preserving the medial mucosa, excellent long-term benefit
- **Total Turbinectomy**: rarely recommended due to high risk of atrophic rhinitis
- Indications: nasal obstruction, chronic rhinosinusitis (middle turbinectomy may be considered if obstructing or with severe polypoidal degeneration), surgical access (middle turbinectomy may be required for CSF leak repair or to access the sphenoid sinus)
- Complications: bleeding, **atrophic rhinitis (empty nose syndrome**; *see* p. 43)

## Septal Perforation

- <u>Causes</u>: septoplasty (most common cause, >50%, particularly if bilateral opposing tears in septal flaps), trauma (nose picking), cocaine use, infection (tertiary syphilis), malignancy, granulomatous disease, vasculitis, corticosteroid nasal spray
- <u>Dx</u>: anterior rhinoscopy; consider biopsy of granulation tissue or abnormal mucosa to evaluate for malignancy, sarcoidosis, tuberculosis, and other granulomatous diseases
- <u>SSx</u>: crusting, epistaxis, whistling (small perforations), obstructive sensation from turbulent flow, may be asymptomatic
- <u>Rx</u>: manage if symptomatic
  1. **Nasal Hygiene**: moisture to reduce crusting and bleeding (saline irrigation, petroleum ointment, emollients, humidity), avoid digital manipulation
  2. **Silastic Button**: easily inserted in office, various sizes available, tolerance varies, crusting may occur around button
  3. **Surgical Repair**: often challenging; includes sliding or rotating mucoperichondrial flaps with or without a fascial graft; contraindicated for large perforations (approximately >2 cm of vertical height)

## Septal Hematoma

- <u>Pathophysiology</u>: hemorrhage (from trauma or recent septal surgery) collects beneath mucoperichondrium and mucoperiosteum resulting in elevation of the mucosa off the cartilaginous septum (loss of cartilaginous vascular supply)
- <u>SSx</u>: unilateral obstruction (may be bilateral), compressible cherry-like or bluish septal swelling, nasal pain, nasal tip tenderness
- <u>Complications</u>: septal abscess, cavernous sinus thrombosis, saddle nose deformity due to cartilage necrosis
- <u>Rx</u>: immediate evacuation of hematoma followed by nasal packing to prevent reaccumulation, antibiotic prophylaxis

# Olfactory Dysfunction

## Introduction

- impairs quality of life (loss of both smell and taste), safety risks (ingestion of spoiled food, inability to smell environmental dangers such as smoke or gas leak), may interfere with profession (chefs, firefighters)
- 80% of taste disorders are primary smell disorders

### *Classification of Olfactory Dysfunction*

- **Anosmia**: no sense of smell (eg, traumatic shearing of olfactory neurons, congenital)
- **Hyposmia (Microsmia)**: reduced sense of smell (eg, smokers, postmenopausal, elderly)
- **Hyperosmia**: heightened sense of smell (eg, hunger, cystic fibrosis, Addison's disease)
- **Phantosmia**: perception of odors that are not present (olfactory hallucinations)
- **Dysosmia**: distorted perception of smell (may occur during degeneration and recovery)
- **Parosmia**: change in the quality of an olfactory cue (eg, flowers smell rancid)

### *Anatomy and Physiology*

- *see also* pp. 10–11
- the olfactory nerve (**CN I**) is the major carrier of olfactory information, other contributions are from the trigeminal nerve (**CN V**, noxious stimuli, role in reflexes such as halting of inhalation) and the nervus terminalis (possible role in pheromone detection, exact function unknown)
- <u>Main Olfactory Pathway</u>: odorant molecule (odorant binding protein) → odorant receptor cell (within olfactory cleft) → CN I → cribriform plate → olfactory bulb → second order neurons
- olfactory receptor cells have varying ability to regenerate (usually incomplete, less with age)

## Evaluation

### *History and Physical Exam*

- <u>Quality of Olfactory Dysfunction</u>: classification (anosmia, hyposmia, phantosmia, dysosmia, parosmia, hyperosmia), single-sided (obstructing, traumatic, infectious) versus bilateral olfactory loss
- <u>Timing of Onset</u>: gradual (sinonasal disease, tumor) versus sudden (trauma)
- <u>Contributing Factors</u>: history of URI, rhinosinusitis, allergy, trauma, toxins, medications, smoking
- <u>Associated SSx</u>: changes in sense of taste, other cranial nerve involvement (diplopia, hearing loss, hoarseness, etc)
- <u>Social History</u>: smoking, cocaine, huffing (inhalant abuse), work and environmental exposure
- <u>Physical Exam</u>: rhinologic and sinus evaluation including nasal endoscopy to evaluate for obstruction, otologic examination to

evaluate for injury to the chorda tympani, full neurologic workup to determine other possible coexisting defects

### Diagnostic Tests

- <u>CT of Paranasal Sinuses</u>: mainstay for complicated olfaction disorders or unclear etiology
- <u>MRI</u>: examine olfactory bulb and tracts for masses
- <u>Olfactory Tests</u>: includes scratch and sniff identification tests such as the **UPSIT (University of Pennsylvania Smell Identification Test**; fast and reliable; scored 0–40; <6 malingering, 6–18 total anosmia, >33–34 normal), odor vials (including ammonia); can monitor progression, recovery/response to treatment, or help detect malingering; often required for medicolegal purposes; electrophysiologic tests (eg, odor event-related potentials and electroolfactogram) largely confined to research
- <u>Labs</u>: thyroid function, tests for mineral/vitamin deficiencies
- <u>Biopsy</u>: sampling of olfactory epithelium, risk of further damage, largely confined to research
- <u>Taste Testing</u>: not routinely utilized

## Causes and Treatment

### Obstructive Nasal and Paranasal Disease

- **most common** etiology of anosmia
- <u>Pathophysiology</u>: obstruction may compromise airflow to olfactory bulb
- <u>Common Causes</u>: mucosal edema, allergies, tumors (eg, nasopharyngeal carcinoma), nasoseptal deformities, polyps
- <u>Rx</u>: address underlying cause, relieve obstruction

### Upper Respiratory Infection

- second most common etiology of anosmia
- may cause parosmia
- <u>Pathophysiology</u>: may be secondary to viral-induced neuronal injury, epithelial damage, or obstruction
- <u>Rx</u>: no effective treatment, may trial steroids to reduce inflammation, observation

### Head Trauma

- third most common etiology of anosmia
- <u>Pathophysiology</u>: shearing forces injure the axons of olfactory neurons at the cribriform plate (more common in occipital injuries),

damage to brain regions that mediate olfaction may also occur (eg, olfactory bulbs and tracts)
- Rx: no effective treatment, observation

### Other Causes

- Congenital: familial dysautonomia, Kallmann syndrome (autosomal dominant; hypogonadotrophic; anosmia secondary to incomplete olfactory bulb and stalk, hypothalamus, or olfactory epithelium)
- Neurologic Tumors: temporal or frontal lobe lesions, esthesioneuroblastoma, meningioma, pituitary adenoma
- Neurologic Disease: Parkinson's, Alzheimer's (typically causes parosmia), multiple sclerosis, epilepsy
- Aging Effects (Presbyosmia): common (75% prevalence of olfactory dysfunction in >80 years old), includes age-related sensorineural degeneration and cumulative damage from diverse repeated insults (viral, toxic, etc)
- Medications and Toxins: smoke, cigarettes (cessation often results in improved function over years, may be exacerbating agent), sulfur dioxide, putrid gases, cocaine, cadmium, heavy metals (eg, intranasal zinc), radiation, chemotherapy
- Medical: hypothyroidism, mineral/vitamin deficiencies
- Surgical Iatrogenic: trauma to olfactory epithelium, sinonasal surgery, transphenoidal pituitary resection

### General Treatment Principles

- treatment often limited, address underlying cause whenever possible
- critical to emphasize **safety precautions** (working **smoke and gas detectors**, always **check expiration dates** before drinking/eating)
- may consider short trial of intranasal or systemic steroids to address any inflammation-induced causes
- encourage smoking cessation as may exacerbate other causes of olfactory dysfunction

# Epistaxis

## Nasal Arterial Plexus

### Kiesselbach's Plexus (Little's Area)

- **most common** site of epistaxis (90%)
- confluence of vessels at the **anterior** nasal septum
- susceptible to bleeding due to the fragile mucosa and tight adherence to underlying mucosa affording little resistance to mechanical stress

- Contributing Arteries
  1. internal carotid → ophthalmic → **anterior ethmoid**
  2. external carotid → facial → **superior labial**
  3. external carotid → maxillary → descending palatine → **greater palatine**
  4. external carotid → maxillary → **sphenopalatine** (terminal branches)

### Woodruff's Plexus

- common source of **posterior** bleeds
- confluence of vessels on the lateral wall, posterior to the inferior/middle turbinates
- Contributing Arteries
  1. external carotid → maxillary → **sphenopalatine**
  2. external carotid → **ascending pharyngeal**

## Evaluation

### History

- after evaluating the ABCs (airway, breathing, intravenous access), ideally should perform a systematic evaluation of the patient prior to controlling the bleeding (may not be possible for heavy bleeding; consider phenylephrine or oxymetazoline-soaked cotton pledgets as a temporizing procedure)
- Characterize Epistaxis: estimate amount of blood loss, duration of bleeding, intermittent versus continuous bleeding, and side of bleeding
- Epistaxis History: previous episodes (frequency, magnitude, duration), inciting factors, hospitalizations, self-resolution versus need for packing or other management
- Medical History and Blood Dyscrasias: hypertension, atherosclerosis, leukemia, idiopathic thrombocytopenic purpura, von Willebrand disease, renal and hepatic failure, anemia, hemophilia (higher risk of arterial, pulsatile bleeding), Osler-Weber-Rendu
- Medications: antiplatelet medications (ASA, NSAIDs), anticoagulants (warfarin, heparin), herbal medicine (garlic, ginkgo, ginseng)
- Social History: cocaine, other intranasal drugs, alcoholism, smoking
- Toxin Exposure: ammonia, sulfuric acid, gasoline, phosphorus (associated with nasal dryness and crusting)
- Other Contributing Factors: previous septal or nasal surgery, recent trauma to nasal bone or septum, facial skeleton, dry environment,

home CPAP/ventilators or oxygen, high altitude living, symptoms of allergy, rhinosinusitis, rhinitis, URI (typically short-lived bleeding)

## *Physical Exam and Initial Ancillary Tests*

- check vital signs, especially blood pressure
- patient should sit up with body tilted forward to allow blood to be spit out and not swallowed
- initial attempt to stop/slow bleeding by applying continuous pressure to nasal alae for several minutes
- apply vasoconstrictive (phenylephrine, oxymetazoline, 4% cocaine) and, if necessary, topical anesthetic agents (lidocaine)
- acquire adequate lighting (head lamp), nasal speculum, bayonet forceps, Frazier and Yankhauer suctions to suction clot from nose and nasopharynx and aid visualization
- attempt to localize active bleeding; examine for excoriations, foreign bodies, masses, nasoseptal deformities, etc
- examine oropharynx for clot (risk of airway compromise and aspiration)
- endoscopic exam for chronic or recurrent epistaxis without an obvious bleeding source
- <u>Labs</u>: PT/PTT, bleeding time, liver function tests, creatinine, CBC, type and cross

## Causes

- trauma (eg, nose picking and vigorous nose blowing) and mucosal dehydration (eg, winter, dry climate) are the most common causes of **anterior epistaxis**
- hypertension, aspirin (and other platelet-inhibiting medications), and alcohol abuse account for the most common causes of **refractory epistaxis**
- hypertension is a common cause of **posterior epistaxis**
- nasoseptal deformities may result in epistaxis secondary to the drying effects of turbulent airflow
- think "KITTENS" for differential diagnosis (*see* Table 1–3)

## *Osler-Weber-Rendu Syndrome (Hereditary Hemorrhagic Telangiectasia)*

- <u>Pathophysiology</u>: autosomal dominant defect in contractile elements (elastic and muscular layers) of vessels, results in telangiectasias and arteriovenous malformations in multiple organs
- <u>SSx</u>: friable mucosa, numerous visceral and mucosal telangiectasias (tongue, oral mucosa, colon, lung), intermittent epistaxis (typically

**TABLE 1–3.** Differential Diagnosis of Epistaxis: KITTENS Method*

| (K) Congenital | Infectious & Idiopathic | Toxins & Trauma | Tumor (Neoplasia) | Endocrine | Systemic |
|---|---|---|---|---|---|
| Nasoseptal deformities | Infectious rhinitis/ sinusitis | Nasal picking | Juvenile nasopharyngeal angiofibroma | Pheochromocytoma (hypertensive crisis) | Allergy (allergic rhinitis) |
| Osler-Weber-Rendu | Mucosal dehydration | Nasal and septal fractures | Other benign or malignant sinonasal tumors | | Anticoagulants (aspirin/NSAID abuse, warfarin, heparin) |
| Congenital coagulopathy (hemophilia, von Willebrand disease) | | Septal perforation | | | Coagulopathy (renal/ hepatic failure, alcoholism, leukemia, platelet disorders, *see* Congenital) |
| | | Foreign body | | | |
| | | Nasal prongs (O$_2$ cannula), CPAP | | | Hypertension |
| | | Iatrogenic (recent nasal surgery) | | | Granulomatous diseases |
| | | Direct trauma from nasal sprays | | | Vasculitis |
| | | Environmental toxins | | | Escaped blood from GI bleed, hemoptysis, etc |
| | | Illicit intranasal drugs (cocaine) | | | |

*No neurologic causes of epistaxis.

begins at or after puberty), intracranial hemorrhage (neurologic symptoms), hematemesis, pulmonary ateriovenous malformations
- <u>Rx</u>: repeated endoscopic laser or cautery ablation of telangiectasias, embolization, septoplasty or **septodermoplasty** (**Saunder's dermoplasty**; remove telangiectatic mucosa and replace with split-thickness skin, amniotic, or myocutaneous graft); systematic therapies include tamoxifen, estrogens, and anti-angiogenesis agents (eg, bevacizumab)

## Acute Management

### Acute Medical Management

- correct hypovolemia if needed (**3:1 rule**: for every 100 mL of blood loss, replace with 300 mL of crystalloid fluid)
- vigilant hypertension control (antihypertensive agents)
- address coagulopathy (fresh frozen plasma, platelets, cryoprecipitate)
- apply vasoconstrictive agents (phenylephrine, oxymetazoline)
- may apply digital pressure over anterior cartilaginous portion of nose (just superoposterior to alae) as temporizing measure

### Cauterization

- includes chemical (silver nitrate, chromic acid pearls), thermal, or electric cautery
- laser cauterization may be considered for vascular malformations
- <u>Indications</u>: minor bleeding, observable bleeding point, easily visualized regions (Kiesselbach's plexus)
- operative endoscopic instrumentation may be used for posterior and difficult to visualize bleeding
- <u>Advantages</u>: simple, quick, minimal tissue damage, potential to avoid packing
- <u>Disadvantages</u>: allows for coagulation of superficial vessel only, high rate of rebleeding; risk of perichondrial exposure, septal perforation (avoid cauterization of both sides of the septum at similar points), cartilage injury

### Topical Hemostatic Agents

- various resorbable hemostatic materials include gelatin (eg, Gelfoam), oxidized cellulose (eg, Surgicel), human-derived thrombin in gelatin matrix (eg, Floseal), fibrin glue (Tisseel), microfibrillar collagen (eg, Avitene, Davol)
- provides a procoagulant effect
- nasal saline spray for several days after placement to facilitate resorption

- <u>Indications</u>: mild observable bleeding point or irritated focal area suspicious for recent bleed
- <u>Advantages</u>: simple, quick, less damage than cautery, potential to avoid packing
- <u>Disadvantages</u>: may rebleed if no packing placed

### Anterior Nasal Packing

- **Nasal Tampons, Expandable Sponges, and Balloons**: various products that provide pressure against the nasal mucosa to tamponade bleeding; includes polyvinyl alcohol sponges that expand after saline instillation (eg, Merocel), inflatable balloon packs (eg, Rapid Rhino), and resorbable packing (eg, Nasopore)
- **Vaseline Strip-Gauze**: formal anterior packing placed to posterior choanae, controls most posterior bleeding
- keep packing in place for 3–5 days to allow vessel to develop a mature thrombus
- provide **antistaphylococcal antibiotics** to prevent toxic shock syndrome, rhinosinusitis, and otitis media
- may supplement with topical hemostatic agents (*see previous*)
- <u>Indications</u>: acute or recurrent epistaxis after conservative management or cauterization
- <u>Advantages</u>: controls most posterior bleeding; does not require inpatient monitoring
- <u>Disadvantages</u>: results in nasal obstruction; risk of pressure necrosis (nasal and septal cartilage), hypoxia, rhinosinusitis, bacteremia, and epiphora; requires prophylactic antibiotics

### Posterior Nasal Packing

- gauze, sponge pack, Foley catheter, pneumatic nasal catheter, or tonsillar packing is placed to close off the choana to prevent escape of bleeding into the nasopharynx
- requires subsequent formal (strip-gauze) anterior pack for stability and to convert the nasal cavity into a closed tamponaded space
- **Nasal Balloons**: catheter with two balloons (one placed in the nasopharynx and the other in the nasal cavity), designed for easier placement of a posterior pack, provides less trauma and is simple to adjust pressure
- keep packing in place for 2–4 days, provide **antistaphylococcal antibiotics** to prevent toxic shock syndrome
- <u>Indications</u>: failed anterior packing, skull base trauma, hemorrhage from a major branch of the sphenopalatine artery
- <u>Advantages</u>: may be inserted for severe bleed in the emergency room or office

- <u>Disadvantages</u>: risk of airway compromise (requires hospital monitoring, ICU if bilateral), requires patient cooperation (painful), may require intubation or general anesthesia, eustachian tube dysfunction (hearing loss), risk of alar necrosis where the anterior aspect of the pack is secured, other risks similar to anterior nasal packing

## *Operative Vascular Ligation*

- <u>Indications</u>: uncontrolled epistaxis (typically posterior bleed), identifiable bleeding site, recalcitrant recurrent epistaxis
- <u>Techniques</u>
  1. **Endoscopic Sphenopalatine Artery Ligation**: preferred operative approach for intractable **posterior** epistaxis; dissection of the posterior middle turbinate with ligation of the sphenopalatine artery
  2. **Endoscopic Anterior and Posterior Ethmoid Artery Ligation**: preferred operative approach for intractable **anterior** epistaxis; located at roof of ethmoid sinus
  3. **External Anterior and Posterior Ethmoidal Artery Ligation**: for anterior bleed; approach from a Lynch incision, anterior ethmoid artery is located **14–18 mm** posterior to frontoethmoid suture line, posterior ethmoid artery is located **10 mm** posterior to anterior ethmoid foramen, optic nerve is located **4–5 mm** posterior to the posterior ethmoid foramen
  4. **Transantral Maxillary Artery Ligation**: classic approach for intractable posterior epistaxis (rarely used today); pterygopalatine fossa contents exposed via a Caldwell-Luc (or transoral) approach allows ligation of the distal branches of the maxillary artery (ascending pharyngeal, sphenopalatine, posterior nasal)
  5. **External Carotid Artery Ligation**: severe uncontrolled, life-threatening bleeding; ligate above the origin of the lingual artery
- <u>Advantages</u>: decreases pressure gradient in nasal vessels to allow for natural clotting
- <u>Disadvantages</u>: periorbital ecchymosis; possible recurrence from collateral circulation; risk of retrobulbar hematoma, hemorrhage, optic nerve and infraorbital nerve injury; clip dislodging

## *Embolization*

- <u>Indications</u>: intractable nasal hemorrhage (usually for posterior origin), surgically inaccessible sites, nonoperative candidates
- typically embolize the distal maxillary or sphenopalatine artery
- <u>Advantages</u>: diagnostic (defines bleeding site) and therapeutic, may be repeated, can be done under local anesthesia

- <u>Disadvantages</u>: risk of embolic event (pulmonary emboli, stroke), requires active bleeding, facial pain, dependent on interventional radiology availability

## Preventive and Chronic Management

### Preventive and Chronic Medical Management

- **Nasal Hygiene**: moisture (gentle saline sprays, petroleum ointment, emollients, humidity, to reduce crusting and bleeding), avoid digital manipulation
- antimicrobial ointment to excoriated lesions
- long-term control of hypertension (consider medicine consult)
- avoid local trauma (digital manipulation, nose blowing, excess straining)
- when using intranasal sprays, do not touch or aim at the septum

### Preventive and Chronic Procedural Management

- **Cauterization**: consider if prominent vessels identified (*see previous*)
- **Operative Vascular Ligation**: for severe recurrent bleeds (*see previous*)
- **Embolization**: for severe recurrent bleeds (*see previous*)
- **Septoplasty**: reduces drying effect by decreasing turbulent airflow, fibrosis results in decreased vascularity
- **Saunder's Dermoplasty**: consider with Osler-Weber-Rendu syndrome, removes diseased mucosa and replaces with STSG (*see previous*)

### Educate Patient on Instructions for Acute Bleeds

- hold pressure over anterior cartilaginous part of nose (not over nasal bone) for 10–15 minutes continuously "without peeking"
- avoid placing tissue paper inside nose, which can cause trauma
- avoid swallowing blood
- oxymetazoline or phenylephrine spray may be used acutely

# ALLERGY AND RHINITIS
## Allergic Rhinitis
### The Allergic Response
#### Allergy Sensitization

- after initial antigen exposure **antigen-presenting cells** (macrophages, HLA class II) present processed peptides to **helper T-cells** (CD4+ cells) releasing interleukins (IL-4 and IL-13)

- IL-4 and IL-13 favor B-cell transformation to sensitized **plasma cells** with specific immunoglobulin E (**IgE**) production
- further exposure of the same antigen promotes differentiation of more plasma cells and T-cells and additional specific IgE production

### Primary Reaction Phase

- type I immediate hypersensitivity (*see* Table 1–4)
- occurs within 5 minutes of allergen exposure with maximum effect at 15 minutes
- allergen recognition by IgE antibodies attaching to mast cells and basophils (via the IgE Fc receptor)
- **degranulation** occurs after cross-linking of the IgE (via a calcium influx trigger) releasing preformed mediators (histamine, serotonin, and proteases) and newly generated mediators (arachidonic acid derivatives [leukotrienes, prostaglandins], TNF-$\alpha$)
- the net effect of the preformed inflammatory mediators causes **sneezing, clear rhinorrhea, congestion, and nasal pruritus**; rechallenged allergens stimulate mast cells more quickly and require less antigen load

### Secondary (Late) Reaction Phase

- occurs 4–6 hours after acute phase; prior to the late phase there is an asymptomatic phase in which inflammatory cells are being recruited and endothelial cells are being activated
- leukotrienes, cytokines (especially **IL-5**), and other mediators stimulate smooth muscles of the airway, increase migration and bone marrow proliferation of eosinophils, increase tissue edema, and stimulate airway secretions
- migration and infiltration of inflammatory cells (neutrophils and eosinophils) and continued activated basophils release a second phase of mediators (mast cells do not remain active)
- late phase reactions cause increased and persistent congestion, rhinorrhea, and sneezing
- **eosinophilia is the hallmark of an allergic response**

### Allergy and Asthma

- one-third of allergic rhinitis patients have asthma
- asthma and allergic rhinitis have similar inflammatory process (mast cells and eosinophils)
- nasal obstruction from allergic rhinitis results in less humidified and cooler inhaled breaths, which may stimulate a reactive airway
- **Nasal–Bronchial/Neural Reflex**: nasal provocation (histamine) increases lower airway resistance (*Curr Opin Pulm Med*.1999;5(1):35)

**TABLE 1–4.** Hypersensitivity Types

|      | Type | Mediators | Reaction |
|------|------|-----------|----------|
| I:   | Anaphylactic | IgE | • immediate, self-limiting<br>• IgE mediated, stimulates mast cells and basophils which release histamine and other inflammatory mediators |
| II:  | Cytotoxic | IgG, IgM | • IgG, IgM multivalent binding to phagocyte or complement<br>• eg, transfusion reactions, Goodpasture's syndrome, bullous pemphigoid |
| III: | Immune complex | IgG, IgM, IgA | • antibody and complement complexes cause increased blood viscosity<br>• removed by reticulo-endothelial system<br>• eg, renal deposition, arthritis, glomerulonephritis, serum sickness |
| IV:  | Cell-mediated | T-cells | • delayed-type hypersensitivity reaction (T-cell mediated)<br>• eg, graft rejection, contact dermatitis |
| V:   | Interference with receptor | Ig | • antibody "resembles" a ligand and thus blocks or stimulates the receptor<br>• pathophysiology of autoimmunity (eg, Hashimoto's thyroiditis, myasthenia gravis, Graves' disease) |

## Common Allergens

1. **Pollens**: trees and grass (spring, summer), ragweed and tumbleweed (fall)
2. **Noninsect Animals**: cats, dogs (allergens include skin, fur, feathers, saliva)
3. **Insects**: dust mites (allergen is feces), cockroaches, Asian ladybugs (central, Midwest, and southern United States)
4. **Molds**: perennial, but worse in humid and damp weather

# Diagnosis of Allergy

## History

- <u>Nasal SSx</u>: sneezing, congestion, watery rhinorrhea, itching, hyposmia
- <u>Ocular SSx</u>: redness, itching, epiphora, conjunctivitis, burning
- <u>Otologic SSx</u>: middle ear effusion, aural fullness (eustachian tube dysfunction)
- <u>Laryngeal SSx</u>: scratchiness, dry, irritated, cough
- <u>Oral SSx</u>: palatal itching, hypogeusia
- <u>Facial SSx</u>: frontal or periorbital headaches
- <u>Other SSx</u>: food hypersensitivity, fatigue
- <u>Timing</u>: seasonal (more associated with irritative symptoms such as sneezing and itching; eg, pollen, *see previous*) versus perennial (more associated with nasal obstruction and rhinorrhea; eg, dust, animals, insects)
- <u>Associated Disorders</u>: chronic rhinosinusitis (obstruction from mucosal edema), nasal polyps, asthma, otitis media with effusion

## Physical Exam

- <u>Eyes</u>: periorbital puffiness, darkening of skin under eyes ("allergic shiners," from venous congestion), fine creases in eyelids ("Dennie's lines"), conjunctival injection
- <u>Ears</u>: otitis media with effusion, tuning forks (conductive hearing loss)
- <u>Nose</u>: clear rhinorrhea, congested gray/blue turbinates, nasal tip transverse crease ("allergic salute," from chronic nose wiping), nasal twitching (from itching), observe for septal deformity; spray topical decongestant and examine for response (allergic obstruction should be reversible)
- <u>Mouth</u>: open-mouthed breathing ("adenoid facies"), secondary malocclusion (controversial)
- <u>Pharynx</u>: prominent pharyngeal lymphoid tissue (cobblestoning)
- <u>Lung</u>: auscultate for wheezing

## Adjunctive Testing

- <u>Nasal Endoscopy</u>: evaluate for nasal polyps, ostiomeatal unit obstruction, adenoid hyperplasia
- <u>Labs</u>: total serum eosinophils and IgE (not always accurate or cost-effective)
- **Nasal Smear**: obtained from inferior turbinate mucosa, >25% eosinophils on nasal smear suggests allergy (neutrophils suggest infection), questionable utility

- **Nasal Allergen Challenge**: increasing levels of antigen presented to nasal mucosa, observe for response, rarely performed

## *Skin Allergy Testing*

- considered best test for allergic rhinitis (most convenient, least expensive screening method)
- avoid antihistamines 48–72 hours prior to testing (increases false negatives)
- **Scratch Test**: scratch skin followed by application of allergen or scratch with allergen (epicutaneous, ie, into epidermis), not standardized, largely replaced by more objective and reliable techniques
- **Prick/Puncture Test**: drop of allergen is placed onto the skin surface (volar forearm or back) followed by insertion of a fine needle through the droplet into the skin (epicutaneous), positive "wheal-and-flare" reactions are compared to controls; rapid and safe test, risk of anaphylaxis, misses less sensitive allergy, grading is subjective
- **Intradermal Test**: similar to prick test except allergen is injected intradermally (percutaneously, ie, into dermis) with 26–27G needle creating a bleb; more sensitive than prick test; however, more time-consuming and painful; greater risk of anaphylaxis (more antigen introduced than with prick test), grading is subjective
- **Intradermal Dilutional Testing (Skin [Serial] Endpoint Titration)**: series of increasing concentrations of specific allergen are introduced intradermally to titrate to a positive response, useful for determining antigen concentrations for immunotherapy, highly sensitive and determines quantitative measurements, time-consuming
- Example of Preparation of Antigen Dilutions: begin with 1:100 weight/volume then dilute using 1 mL of concentrate with 4 mL of diluent will yield #1 dilution = 1:500, #2 = 1:2,500, #3 = 1:12,500, #4 = 1:62,500, #5 = 1:312,500, #6 = 1:562,500
- Determine Endpoint: **endpoint** is the concentration of antigen that causes an increase in the size of the wheal followed by confirmatory increase in wheal size

## *In Vitro Allergy Testing*

- **Radioallergosorbent Test (RAST)**: react serum with a series of known allergens, radiolabeled anti-IgE identifies specific antigen-IgE complexes (older technique)
- **Enzyme-Linked Immunosorbent Assay (ELISA)**: similar to RAST except fluorescing agents are used for markers of antigen–IgE complexes
- Indications: equivocal skin test results, high risk of anaphylaxis (severe asthma, prior history), skin disorders (eczema, dermatographia),

uncooperative patient (children and infants), failed immunotherapy; negative skin test is not an indication for *in vitro* allergy
testing

- Advantages: highly specific, no risk of anaphylaxis; no effect
  from skin color, skin conditions or medications (β-blockers,
  antihistamines, tricyclics)
- Disadvantages: **less sensitive**, requires up to 1–2 weeks for results,
  more expensive

## Management

### Anaphylaxis

- **ABCs**: establish airway (*see* pp. 628–630), breathing/oxygenation,
  and IV access
- inject up to 0.3 mL of **epinephrine** intramuscularly (IM)
- consider **dopamine** for hypotension
- add **diphenhydramine** 50 mg, **dexamethasone** 4 mg, and
  **cimetidine** 300 mg IV
- if needed **repeat** injection of up to 0.3 mL of epinephrine IM

### Avoidance

- Dust: dust mite-resistant mattress covers, foam pillows, plastic cases;
  low carpet or hardwood floors; frequent dusting and vacuuming;
  may apply benzyl benzoate to carpet to kill mites; consider synthetic
  carpets
- Molds: disinfect bathroom, clean furnace, reduce humidity (eg,
  dehumidify basement), clean refrigerator, avoid gardening, address
  potential sources of molds indoors (plants, old shoes, curtains)
- Pollens: air conditioning with filters, air cleaners, keep windows
  closed, avoid cutting grass
- Animals: keep out of bedroom, use special shampoos, or eliminate
  altogether
- high-efficiency particulate air (HEPA) filters (defined as removing
  99.97% of particles 0.3 microns in diameter) may be used for all
  airborne allergies
- home humidity (48–52%) prevents nasal dryness
- masks may be helpful in unavoidable allergy exposure

### Symptomatic Relief

- **Nasal Saline Irrigation**: removes nasal mucus and crusts, aids in
  mucociliary clearance, thins tenacious mucus

- **Nasal Antihistamines (H$_1$-Receptor Antagonists):** generally not very potent; <u>Examples</u>: azelastine (may be sedating if swallowed), olopatadine
- **First Generation Oral Antihistamines (H$_1$-Receptor Antagonists):** primarily for acute phase reactions, sneezing, itching, and rhinorrhea; side effects include sedation (several are also nonprescription sleeping pills), dryness, confusion, tolerance, and aggravation of prostate enlargement; <u>Examples</u>: diphenhydramine (Benadryl), chlorpheniramine, promethazine, hydroxyzine
- **Second Generation Oral Antihistamines (H$_1$-Receptor Antagonists):** lipophobic (do not cross blood–brain barrier) therefore less sedating, inhibit release of inflammatory mediators, several now available without prescription; <u>Examples</u>: fexofenadine, loratadine, certirizine
- **Nasal Decongestants:** α-adrenergic agonists, rapidly reduce nasal congestion through vasoconstriction of the nasal erectile mucosa; side effects include CNS stimulation (anxiety, anorexia); must **limit use to 3–5 days** to prevent rebound congestion, tolerance, and rhinitis medicamentosa (*see* p. 44); <u>Examples</u>: phenylephrine (Neo-Synephrine), oxymetazoline (Afrin)
- **Oral Decongestants:** same mechanism as nasal decongestants; reduced potency and more systemic adrenergic side effects compared to nasal decongestants (insomnia, anxiety, tremulousness, irritability, headache); however, avoids risk of rhinitis medicamentosa; many are synthetic precursors of methamphetamine and have been restricted; <u>Examples</u>: phenylephrine, pseudoephedrine (Sudafed)
- **Nasal Corticosteroids:** local reduction of inflammatory cells in nasal mucosa, decreased capillary permeability, reduced edema; **single most effective maintenance therapy for allergic rhinitis**; unlike nasal decongestants, take >1 week for maximal effect; use regularly for maximal benefit; decrease both acute and late phase reactions; minimal side effects (epistaxis, candidiasis, nasal dryness); oral corticosteroids used only for more severe disease (*see following*); <u>Examples</u>: fluticasone, beclomethasone, flunisolide
- **Nasal Anticholinergics:** specifically useful for rhinorrhea component of rhinitis (also indicated for vasomotor rhinitis and viral rhinitis); <u>Example</u>: ipratropium bromide
- **Oral Antileukotrienes:** competitive inhibitor of leukotriene receptors found on smooth muscles throughout the airway, inhibits the late phase reaction decreasing eosinophil infiltration, may consider for combination therapy; <u>Examples</u>: montelukast, zafirlukast
- **Nasal Mast Cell Stabilizers:** stabilize mast cells, preventing release of mediators in acute and late phase reactions; effective only for prophylaxis (eg, known upcoming cat exposure); mild efficacy;

minimal side effects (sneezing, epistaxis, nasal irritation); <u>Examples</u>: cromolyn, nedocromil

## Management of Complicating Factors

- must evaluate and treat potential concurrent disorders that may mimic allergy before changing treatment regimens
- such disorders include vasomotor rhinitis (*see* p. 44), rhinosinusitis (*see* pp. 45–49), and rhinitis medicamentosa (*see* p. 44)

## Corticosteroids

- most potent medication for symptomatic relief of severe persistent allergic rhinitis
- may be given orally, as nasal spray, or via intraturbinal injections
- may attempt a short oral course of 3–7 days
- <u>Mechanism of Action</u>: decreases inflammatory migration, blocks arachidonic acid metabolites, decreases vascular permeability
- <u>Side Effects of Oral Corticosteroids</u>: increased gastric acid production (consider prophylactic concurrent $H_2$-blocker), hypertension, masks signs of infection, sodium retention, hypokalemia, posterior subcapsular cataracts, CNS stimulation (psychosis, seizures, insomnia), menstrual irregularities, aseptic necrosis of femoral head
- <u>Steroid Dose Equivalence</u>: prednisone 5 mg = cortisone 25 mg = hydrocortisone 20 mg = methylprednisone 4 mg = dexamethasone 0.75 mg

## Immunotherapy

- desensitization technique that utilizes a controlled dosing of specific allergens to reduce the symptoms of allergic rhinitis and the complication of allergies
- <u>Indications</u>: severe, persistent symptoms; allergens that cannot be avoided or otherwise easily treated; failed maximal medical management; patients who wish to avoid chronic medication; coexisting asthma
- <u>Advantages</u>: suppresses allergy, potential long-term control
- <u>Disadvantages</u>: patient must be reliable for multiple injections, requires a chronic regimen, requires identified and administrable allergen, risk of worsening symptoms and anaphylactic shock
- <u>Contraindications</u>: pregnancy (anaphylaxis risk of hypoxia to fetus), autoimmune disorders, immunocompromised patients, severe or unstable asthma, β-blockers (increases sensitivity to allergens), easily avoidable allergens, noncompliant patients

- <u>Mechanism of Action</u>: uncertain, immunotherapy has demonstrated a rise in allergen-specific $IgG_4$-mediated mechanism which prevents binding of IgE. IgE may also become "exhausted" (decreased allergen-specific IgE), increase in IgA- and IgM-specific antibodies (may benefit by preventing entrance of allergen at the mucosal level)
- **Subcutaneous Immunotherapy**: most common
- **Sublingual Immunotherapy**: higher concentration of allergen is administered sublingually, effectiveness under investigation
- **Specific Nasal Immunotherapy (SNIT)**: allergen administered intranasally, effectiveness under investigation
- **Anti-IgE Monoclonal Antibody (Omalizumab)**: may be considered if concurrent persistent asthma

## Churg-Strauss Syndrome (Allergic Granulomatosis Angiitis)

- <u>Pathophysiology</u>: unknown etiology, small vessel **necrotizing vasculitis** causes **angiitis** and **allergic granulomatosis**
- <u>Principal SSx</u>: asthma, eosinophilia (>10%), allergic rhinosinusitis, pulmonary infiltrates, vasculitis, mononeuritis or polyneuropathy
- <u>Other SSx</u>: nasal polyposis, nasal obstruction, septal lesions, lung lesions, myocardial infarction (secondary to coronary arteritis), sensorineural and conductive hearing loss, fever, weight loss
- <u>Dx</u>: presence of principal symptoms, nerve or muscle biopsy, serum IgE and eosinophils, CXR, CT of paranasal sinuses
- <u>Rx</u>: corticosteroids, cytotoxic agents (cylophosphamide) reserved for life-threatening conditions, symptomatic medications for nasal symptoms, polypectomy or sinus surgery as needed

# Nonallergic Rhinitis

## Infectious Rhinitis

### Viral Rhinitis (Coryza, Common Cold)

- <u>Pathogenesis</u>: spread via infected droplets
- <u>Common Viral Pathogens</u>: rhinovirus (most common, 30–50% of colds, >100 types), coronavirus (10–15% of colds), parainfluenza virus, respiratory syncytial virus, adenovirus, enterovirus
- SSx and Stages
  1. **Dry Prodromal (Initial) Stage**: nasal drying and irritation, low-grade fever, chills, general malaise, anorexia
  2. **Catarrhal (Second) Stage**: watery clear rhinorrhea, anosmia, congestion, lacrimation, worsening of constitutional symptoms

3. **Mucous Stage**: thickened rhinorrhea (greenish and foul smelling if secondarily infected), improved constitutional symptoms
- may progress to viral rhinosinusitis or become secondarily infected by bacteria
- <u>Dx</u>: H&P
- <u>Rx</u>: no cure for the common cold; antibiotics should be given for suspected bacterial infections only; symptomatic therapy includes decongestants (topical [limit use to 3–5 days] and systemic), antihistamines, ipratropium bromide spray, hydration, humidification, nasal saline irrigations, analgesics, mucolytic agents

### Bacterial Rhinitis

- typically secondarily infected viral rhinitis
- may be part of bacterial rhinosinusitis (*see* p. 46)
- <u>Pathogens</u>: *Streptoccoccus*, *H. influenzae*, *S. aureus*, *B. pertussis*, chlamydia, diphtheria
- <u>SSx and Stages</u>: similar to previous; however, rhinorrhea may be thickened, greenish, and foul smelling
- <u>Dx</u>: H&P, culture
- <u>Rx</u>: antibiotics, symptomatic therapy similar to viral rhinitis

### Rhinoscleroma

- <u>Pathogen</u>: **Klebsiella rhinoscleromatis** (Frisch's bacillus)
- <u>Risks</u>: endemic to eastern Europe, North Africa, South Asia, Latin America
- <u>SSx</u>: nasal obstruction (nasal polyps), rhinorrhea, anosmia, epistaxis, nasal deformity; may also involve laryngeal, tracheal, and bronchial airway
- <u>Stages</u> (each may last years)
  1. **Catarrhal**: persistent purulent rhinorrhea, nasal honeycomb-color crusting, last weeks
  2. **Granulomatous**: painless granulomatous masses in nose and upper respiratory tract (including glottis and subglottis), septal destruction (epistaxis), thickened soft palate
  3. **Fibrotic**: lesions heal with extensive scarring (dense fibrotic narrowing of nasal passage)
- <u>Dx</u>: biopsy, culture, serum antibodies
- <u>Histopathology</u>: **Mikulicz cell** (foamy histiocytes with intracellular bacilli that they are unable to digest, "moth-eaten" cytoplasm), **Russell bodies** (bloated plasma cells with birefringent inclusions), pseudoepitheliomatous hyperplasia

- <u>Rx</u>: long-term antibiotics dictated by culture and sensitivity (tetracycline, ciprofloxacin), debridement, consider laser excision or cryotherapy, bronchoscopy

### *Rhinosporidiosis*

- chronic granulomatous infection of the nose and external eye
- <u>Pathogen</u>: ***Rhinosporidium seebri*** (sporangium with a thick-walled cyst)
- <u>Risks</u>: endemic to Africa, Pakistan, India, Sri Lanka, spread from contaminated water (public bathing)
- <u>SSx</u>: slow growing, painless, friable, "strawberry"-colored/textured (vascular) polypoid nasal lesion (epistaxis, unilateral obstruction); infection of the palpebral conjunctivae
- <u>Dx</u>: culture and biopsy
- <u>Histopathology</u>: pseudoepitheliomatous hyperplasia, submucosal cysts, fungal sporangia with chitinous shells
- <u>Rx</u>: surgical excision with cauterization of the base, oral antifungals, corticosteroid injections, may consider dapsone

### *Rhinocerebral Mucormycosis* (*see* p. 50)

## Nonallergic Rhinitis with Eosinophilia Syndrome (NARES)

- nasal eosinophilia without allergy
- <u>SSx</u>: perennial rhinitis, sneezing attacks, watery rhinorrhea, nasal congestion, and pruritus
- <u>Dx</u>: allergic symptoms with negative allergic tests, eosinophils on nasal smears (10–20%)
- <u>Rx</u>: symptomatic relief similar to allergic rhinitis (nasal corticosteroids, antihistamines, decongestants)

## Hormonal Rhinitis

- **Rhinitis of Pregnancy:** most common hormonal rhinitis, unclear pathophysiology, may be multifactorial (cholinergic effects from increased estrogen may contribute), estrogens may increase hyaluronic acid in nasal mucosa; manifests near the end of the first trimester, resolves after delivery
- **Other Causes:** oral contraceptive, hypothyroidism, puberty
- <u>SSx</u>: rhinitis, congestion without sneezing, pale-blue mucosa, turbinate hypertrophy,

- <u>Rx</u>: refractory to most regimens, conservative management (nasal saline irrigations, avoidance of allergens, may consider nasal steroids although pregnancy class C), avoid decongestants (may place fetus at risk), consult obstetrician for treatment

## Rhinitis Sicca Anterior

- <u>Pathophysiology</u>: dry, raw nasal mucosa secondary to a variety of causes including changes in temperature and humidity, nose picking, dust, and other irritants
- <u>SSx</u>: dryness, nasal irritation, nasal crusting, epistaxis, septal perforation
- <u>Dx</u>: H&P
- <u>Rx</u>: saline irrigation, topical antibiotics, oil-based nasal ointments

## Atrophic Rhinitis (Empty Nose Syndrome, Ozena)

- <u>Pathophysiology</u>: mucosal glands and sensory nerve fibers degenerate, epithelium undergoes squamous metaplasia, destroyed mucociliary transport
- <u>Causes</u>: excess nasal surgery (turbinectomy), suspected genetic component (more common in East Asia, Egypt, Greece), endocrine abnormalities, nutritional deficiencies (vitamin A or D, iron deficiency), chronic bacterial infection (eg, ***Klebsiella ozaenae***), trauma, and irritant exposure
- <u>SSx</u>: paradoxical sensation of nasal obstruction, mucosal and turbinate atrophy, wide nasal cavity, nasal crusting, offensive odor, epistaxis, anosmia
- <u>Dx</u>: anterior rhinoscopy, history
- <u>Complications</u>: increased risk for secondary infection
- <u>Rx</u>: moisture (saline irrigation, oil-based ointment impregnated nasal tampons, humidity), vitamin A and D and iron supplements, systemic or topical antibiotics (for secondary infections), consider nasal vestibuloplasty, augmentation techniques, or periodic nostril closure for failed medical therapy

## Anhidrotic Ectodermal Dysplasia

- <u>Pathophysiology</u>: X-linked genetic disorder resulting in abnormal development of **ectodermal** structures (skin, hair, nails, teeth, sweat glands), scant mucus production, and atrophic rhinitis; other types of ectodermal dysplasias also exist
- <u>SSx</u>: atrophy of inferior and middle turbinates, fevers, recurrent otitis media, malodorous rhinorrhea, nasal crusting

- <u>Triad</u>: **anhidrosis**, **hypotrichosis**, **anodontia**
- <u>Rx</u>: pressure equalization tubes, saline irrigations, nasal hygiene, denture appliances

## Rhinitis Medicamentosa

- <u>Pathophysiology</u>: semi-ischemic state secondary to any **topical nasal decongestants** (eg, oxymetazoline [Afrin]), results in rebound congestion from decreased vasomotor tone, increased parasympathetic activity, increased vascular permeability (also results in decreased ciliary activity)
- may be irreversible if vagal tone becomes atonic
- <u>SSx</u>: mucosal edema, nasal obstruction, dryness, irritation
- <u>Rx</u>: discontinue topical decongestants, aggressive saline irrigation, oral decongestants, nasal steroid spray; may consider nasal stents, submucosal steroids, or short-term oral corticosteroids (for weaning); avoid by limiting topical decongestants to 3–5 days

## Vasomotor Rhinitis (Hyperreflexive Rhinopathy)

- changes in vascular tone and permeability of the nose and sinus resulting in chronic rhinitis, multiple triggers, more common in older adults
- <u>Pathophysiology</u>: rhinitis secondary to overactive parasympathetic activity, exact mechanism unknown
- <u>SSx</u>: similar to allergic rhinitis; clear watery rhinorrhea, morning rhinorrhea, congestion, alternating sides, pale nasal mucosa
- <u>Dx</u>: **diagnosis of exclusion**, negative allergy workup

### Triggers

- <u>Environmental</u>: humidity and temperature changes, dust, smoke, pollution
- <u>Endocrine and Metabolic</u>: pregnancy, oral contraceptives (estrogen inhibits anticholinesterases), hypothyroidism
- <u>Medications</u>: antihypertensives, antipsychotics, cocaine
- <u>Psychotropic</u>: anxiety, stress, exercise

### Management

- eliminate irritants and address causal factors if possible
- <u>Medical Management</u>
  1. anticholinergic nasal sprays (ipratropium bromide)
  2. corticosteroid nasal sprays
  3. hypertonic saline nasal sprays

4. may consider short course of oral and topical decongestants or antihistamines
- <u>Surgical Management</u>: indicated for refractory cases (*see following*)

### *Vidian Neurectomy*

- <u>Anatomy of the Nerve of the Pterygoid Canal (Vidian Nerve)</u>: formed from branches of the greater petrosal nerve and the deep petrosal nerve (**floor of the sphenoid sinus**) → pterygopalatine fossa → pterygopalatine ganglion (parasympathetic to nose, lacrimal gland, and palate)
- transecting the Vidian nerve results in decreased parasympathetic activity to nose, lacrimal gland, and palate by transecting **preganglionic parasympathetic fibers**
- may be performed endoscopically approaching through the sphenopalatine foramen and advancing posterolaterally until the funnel-shaped opening of the Vidian canal is visualized
- postoperatively may use the Schirmer's test to show decreased lacrimation on the operated side

# PARANASAL SINUS DISEASE
## Rhinosinusitis
## Introduction

### *Pathophysiology*

- often preceded by viral rhinitis/URI, which causes inflammation and obstruction of sinus outflow tracts
- associated factors include dysfunction of cilia motility, changes in quality of secretions, and formation of bacterial biofilms
- numerous anatomic, allergic, and immune factors may predispose to rhinosinusitis

### *Pathogens*

#### Acute

- <u>Viral</u>: (most common) rhinovirus, parainfluenza virus, respiratory syncytial virus, influenza virus, coronavirus
- <u>Bacterial</u>: *S. pneumoniae* (most common bacteria), *H. influenzae, M. catarrhalis, S. aureus, S. pyogenes*
- <u>Fulminant Fungal</u>: *Aspergillus*, phaeohyphomycosis, *Mucor, Rhizopus*

**Chronic**

- <u>Bacterial</u>: anaerobes, *S. aureus, H. influenzae*
- <u>Fungal</u>: in 1–2%

**Complicated Rhinosinusitis**

- <u>Cystic Fibrosis</u>: *P. aeruginosa, S. aureus*
- <u>Nosocomial</u>: *P. aeruginosa, Klebsiella, Enterobacter, Proteus*
- <u>Immunocompromised</u>: similar to nonimmunocompromised patients; however, also susceptible to *Aspergillus, Rhizopus, Fusarium, P. aeruginosa, S. aureus*

## Evaluation

### Symptoms and Physical Exam Findings

- <u>Acute Rhinosinusitis SSx</u>: facial pain and tenderness worse with straining or bending over, pressure headache (frontal and occipital headaches may arise from sphenoid sinusitis), nasal congestion, postnasal drip, nasal obstruction, nasal discharge (mucopurulent, serous, mucoid), cough, and halitosis (especially in pediatric patients)
- <u>Chronic Rhinosinusitis SSx</u>: presents with more subtle symptoms of nasal obstruction, less fever and pain complaints
- <u>Associated SSx</u>: anosmia, loss of taste (chronic rhinosinusitis), allergic components (sneezing, watery eyes), fever, malaise, lethargy, cough, eustachian tube dysfunction, dental pain
- <u>Physical Exam</u>: rhinoscopy/nasopharyngoscopy (ostiomeatal unit obstruction, nasal masses and obstruction, purulence, adenoid hyperplasia), decreased sinus transillumination (not reliable), frontal and maxillary tenderness (acute rhinosinusitis), polyps and edema (chronic rhinosinusitis), ophthalmic manifestations (conjunctival congestion, lacrimation)
- <u>DDx of Facial Pain</u>: rhinogenic versus migraines and other headaches, dental disease, TMJ dysfunction, neuralgias, ocular disease, tonsillitis, pharyngitis, otologic disease, intracranial pathologiy, hypertension, temporal arteritis

### Evaluate for Causes and Risk Factors

- <u>Anatomic</u>: deviated septum, mucosal edema (rhinitis, allergic), adenoid hyperplasia, nasal masses, nasal foreign bodies, nasogastric tubes, nasal packing, facial fractures, concha bullosa, lateral deviated uncinate process, paradoxical middle turbinate, uncinate hypoplasia, nasal polyposis
- <u>Ciliary Dysfunction</u>: Kartagener's syndrome (*see following*)

- <u>Immunologic</u>: allergy, immunocompromise (HIV, diabetes, malnutrition)
- <u>Local Causes</u>: apical dental infection (isolated maxillary sinusitis), trauma, barotrauma
- <u>Other</u>: cystic fibrosis (*see* pp. 51–52, 547–548), smoking, granulomatous disease, elderly, GERD

## *Imaging Studies*

### Plain Radiography

- <u>Indications</u>: screening study for acute rhinosinusitis
- evaluates presence of air–fluid levels, opacification, and bone destruction
- **high rate of false positives and false negatives** for chronic rhinosinusitis

### CT of Paranasal Sinuses

- <u>Indications</u>: severe acute rhinosinusitis, medical failure of chronic rhinosinusitis, suspicious epistaxis, nasal or sinus tumors, nasal polyps, CSF leak, trauma, preoperative evaluation
- <u>Basic CT Evaluation Checklist</u>
  1. examine distribution of mucosal disease (mucosal thickening, air–fluid levels suggest acute inflammatory process)
  2. inspect development of sinus (symmetry, aeration of sinus cavities); examine nasal structures, airway, and access
  3. evaluate for underlying causes of disease (ostiomeatal complex patency, paradoxical turbinates, nasal septal defects, concha bullosas)
  4. examine for anatomic variations and landmarks (cribriform plate, posterior ethmoidal height, thickness of skull base, optic nerve, orbital dehiscence, carotid artery)

### MRI of Paranasal Sinuses

- improved soft tissue detail, poor bone resolution
- <u>Indications</u>: complicated rhinosinusitis (intracranial and intraorbital extension), evaluation of soft tissue masses (neoplasms), fungal rhinosinusitis (hypodensity, low signal on T2-weighted sequences from the presence of metallic proteinaceous material, magnesium, iron, and calcium)

## *Ancillary Studies*

- sinus cultures (may be obtained with an endoscope) indicated for failed medical management, complicated rhinosinusitis (sepsis,

orbital infection, intracranial extension), immunocompromised patients
- immunologic profile (qualitative immunoglobulins including IgG subclasses) and ciliary biopsy (Kartagener's syndrome) may be considered for complicated cases
- allergy testing
- evaluation for cystic fibrosis

## Management

### *Acute Rhinosinusitis (<1 Month)*

- <u>Antibiotics</u>: if suspect bacterial cause, may treat empirically with first-line oral antibiotics with gram-positive and gram-negative coverage (amoxicillin, amoxicillin/clavulanate, trimethoprim/sulfamethoxazole, cefuroxime, azithromycin) for 10–14 days, consider changing antibiotics if no improvement after 2–3 days, if no improvement after 1 week may consider sinus culture and sensitivity
- <u>Improve Nasal Clearance</u>: regular nasal saline irrigations, oral and topical decongestants (limit use to 3–5 days), mucolytic agents, humidity
- <u>Symptomatic Medications</u>: analgesics, antipyretics
- <u>Address Risk Factors</u>: smoking cessation, septoplasty, remove nasogastric tube, antireflux regimen, etc

### *Acute Frontal Sinusitis*

- frontal sinusitis is treated more aggressively to avoid intracranial complications
- identified by frontal pain and tenderness and frontal sinus air–fluid levels on imaging
- parenteral antibiotics, observation for intracranial involvement (select patients may be followed with close follow-up on an outpatient basis)
- headache, confusion, and eyelid pain may suggest complicated frontal sinusitis
- consider **surgical management** (trephination or other approaches, *see following*) if no improvement after 24–48 hours of aggressive medical management

### *Chronic Rhinosinusitis (Persistent Infection >6 Weeks)*

- <u>Antibiotics</u>: 3–6-week regimen with broad spectrum agents (eg, amoxicillin/clavulanate, cefuroxime, ciprofloxacin, clarithromycin, cefpodoxime, cefprozil)
- <u>Steroids</u>: nasal corticosteroid sprays, oral steroid course (particularly if polyps present)

- <u>Improve Nasal Clearance</u>: regular nasal saline irrigations, oral decongestants, mucolytic agents
- allergy management (*see previous*)
- medical management may fail with chronic sinus disease requiring surgical management

**Surgical Management** (*see following for indications and techniques*)

## Pediatric Rhinosinusitis (*see* pp. 546–548)

# Complicated Rhinosinusitis

## Fungal Rhinosinusitis

### Fungus Ball (Mycetoma)

- <u>Pathophysiology</u>: noninvasive fungal infection (most commonly *Aspergillus*)
- <u>SSx</u>: chronic or recurrent sinusitis of **one sinus** (typically maxillary sinus), unilateral proptosis, facial hypesthesia
- <u>Dx</u>: CT/MRI of paranasal sinuses, biopsy with culture
- <u>Aspergillosis Histology</u>: **septated 45 degrees, Y-shaped** (Sabouraud's agar stain)
- <u>Rx</u>: adequate surgical removal (usually endoscopic), consider less toxic adjuvant antifungal medications

### Allergic Fungal Rhinosinusitis

- <u>Pathophysiology</u>: fungal infection, such as *Aspergillus* or dematiaceous molds (*Alternaria, Bipolaris, Curvularia, Exophilia, Fusarium*), becomes the antigen for an allergic response, forming fungal debris, nasal polyps, and chronic mucosal thickening
- <u>Risks</u>: atopic disease, young asthmatics
- <u>SSx</u>: chronic rhinosinusitis symptomatology with allergic component (sneezing, watery eyes, periorbital edema, etc), nasal polyposis
- <u>Dx</u>: allergic evaluation for molds/fungus (RAST, skin testing), **allergic mucin** (nasal eosinophilia, **Charcot-Leyden** crystals, most reliable indicator), tissue stains reveal fungal hyphae **without invasion**, characteristic CT/MRI of paranasal sinuses; controversy arises in regard to diagnosis, most consider acute fungal rhinosinusitis as an immunologic rather than an infectious disorder
- <u>Rx</u>: surgical debridement (usually endoscopic), topical and oral steroids, consider adjuvant antifungal medications or immunotherapy

### *Acute Fulminant Invasive Fungal Sinusitis (Mucormycosis, Rhinocerebral Phycomycosis)*

- <u>Pathophysiology</u>: pathogen rapidly invades soft tissue and bone; in mucormycosis, pathogen invades vessel walls causing local vascular occlusion, thrombosis, infarction, and tissue necrosis
- <u>Pathogens</u>: *Aspergillus* (most common), saprophytics (*Mucor, Rhizopus, Absida*)
- <u>Risks</u>: almost exclusively in **immunocompromised** hosts (diabetic ketoacidosis, chemotherapy, HIV, bone marrow transplant)
- 50% mortality with CNS or cavernous sinus involvement
- <u>SSx</u>: fever, local symptoms (orbital swelling, facial pain, nasal congestion), anesthetic regions; in **mucormycosis** may present with necrotic black turbinates and soft palate, epistaxis, cranial nerve involvement, progresses rapidly into obtundation and death
- <u>Dx</u>: physical exam (nasal, oral, cranial nerves), nasal endoscopy, biopsy and culture, CT/MRI of paranasal sinuses (enhancement in T2-weighted images from fungal elements)
- <u>Mucormycosis Histology</u>: **nonseptated, 90-degree broad-branching hyphae**
- <u>Rx</u>: hospitalization with urgent surgical debridement and antifungals (eg, long-term amphotericin B), address underlying derangements (eg, correct ketoacidosis)

### *Chronic Invasive Fungal Rhinosinusitis*

- rare, occurs in immunocompetent patients
- subtype includes chronic granulomatous fungal rhinosinusitis (caused by *Aspergillus flavus*)
- <u>Pathophysiology</u>: indolent invasion of soft tissue
- <u>Pathogens</u>: *Aspergillus*, saprophytics (*Mucor, Rhizopus, Absidia*)
- <u>SSx</u>: chronic rhinosinusitis with or without symptoms of local invasion (eg, blindness, cerebritis)
- <u>Dx</u>: same as acute invasive fungal sinusitis
- <u>Rx</u>: surgical debridement and long-term amphotericin B and itraconazole (1 year)

## Sinobronchial Syndrome

- association of chronic rhinosinusitis with asthma, bronchiectasis, recurrent pneumonia, and chronic bronchitis
- <u>Pathophysiology</u>: controversial, may be from two separate manifestations with same underlying entity versus postnasal drip with bronchial seeding, which may result in bronchospasm

- <u>SSx</u>: **chronic cough with normal lung auscultation**, nasal obstruction, rhinorrhea, irritability
- <u>Dx</u>: H&P, CT of the paranasal sinuses, must exclude other causes of sinobronchial pathologies (ciliary dyskinesia, cystic fibrosis)
- <u>Rx</u>: similar management for chronic rhinosinusitis, consider antibiotics for acute exacerbations

## Rhinosinusitis in HIV

- 75% of untreated HIV patients develop rhinosinusitis
- <u>Pathophysiology</u>: increased risk of rhinosinusitis secondary to impaired immunity, mucociliary dysfunction, and atopy
- <u>Pathogens</u>: for CD4 count >200, similar to nonimmunocompromised patients; for <200, high incidence of unusual and more virulent organisms (mucormycosis, CMV, *Pseudomonas,* mycobacteria)
- *Pneumocystis jirovecii* (formerly *carinii*), which usually occurs in the lungs, can also occur in the sinus
- must also consider facial pain in AIDS patients secondary to Kaposi's sarcoma, lymphoma, or other tumor

### *Management*

- CD4 count >200 managed similar to a immunocompetent patient
- may initially consider one course of empiric therapy (broad-spectrum antibiotics)
- typical sinus regimen (saline irrigations, mucolytics, decongestants, etc)
- aggressive early workup (CT/MRI of paranasal sinuses, nasal endoscopy)
- low threshold for sinus aspirate culture and sensitivity to avoid empiric therapy
- early surgical management

## Cystic Fibrosis and Rhinosinusitis (*see* pp. 547–548)

## Mucocele

- <u>Pathophysiology</u>: obstructed sinus that undergoes expansile growth from mucous secretion
- frequency of sinus involvement is frontal > ethmoid > maxillary > sphenoid
- <u>Types</u>
  1. **Primary**: arises de novo, mucous retention cyst (*see following*)
  2. **Secondary**: due to surgery, trauma, tumor (or other nasal mass)
- <u>Causes</u>: trauma, chronic rhinosinusitis, polyposis, sinus surgery, allergy, osteoma, hyperaeration of ethmoid

- <u>SSx</u>: asymptomatic, dull headache that localizes to involved sinus, periorbital swelling, ocular symptoms (proptosis, diplopia)
- <u>Dx</u>: CT of paranasal sinuses reveals expansion of sinus with opacification, rounded process of a sinus cavity or air cell, bone remodeling (thinned sinus walls)
- <u>Complications</u>: bacterial infection (mucopyocele), rupture (bacteremia), orbital and intracranial involvement, pituitary abnormalities, cosmetic deformity
- <u>Rx</u>: endoscopic sinus surgery, open procedures reserved for inaccessible lesions or lateral lesions in the frontal sinus

## Mucous Retention Cyst

- <u>Pathophysiology</u>: serous or mucinous submucosal collection of fluid secondary to blocked glands, may be infectious or allergic in origin
- <u>SSx</u>: typically asymptomatic, larger cysts may cause dental pain or symptoms from sinus obstruction
- <u>Dx</u>: CT of paranasal sinuses, sinus x-rays (**10% incidental finding**); most commonly found on floor of maxillary sinus
- <u>DDx</u>: dental radicular or follicular cysts
- <u>Rx</u>: observation if asymptomatic or nonobstructing, otherwise may consider surgical management

## Primary Ciliary Dyskinesia (Kartagener's Syndrome, Immotile Cilia Syndrome)

- <u>Pathophysiology</u>: genetic disorder resulting in deficient outer dynein arm causing primary ciliary dyskinesis (abnormal ciliary motion), results in impaired mucociliary clearance
- **Kartagener's Triad**: chronic rhinosinusitis, bronchiectasis, situs inversus (50% of patients)
- <u>Other SSx</u>: otitis media, **male infertility** (sperm dysmotility)
- <u>Dx</u>: ciliary biopsy with phase contrast or electron microscopy
- <u>Management</u>
  1. aggressive antimicrobial therapy, mucolytics, bronchodilators, and postural drainage for respiratory or sinonasal disease, consider prophylactic antibiotics
  2. endoscopic surgical management for persistent rhinosinusitis, "standard functional" antrostomies do not work since there is no normal mucociliary clearance; consider "gravity-dependent" surgical inferior antrostomies for refractory sinus disease
  3. pressure equalization tubes for chronic otitis media

**Sinonasal Polyposis** (*see previous*)

# Complications of Rhinosinusitis

## Orbital Complications

- Intraorbital Pathways: direct extension (especially through thin-walled lamina papyracea), thrombophlebitis (valveless veins), congenital dehiscence, trauma, direct lymphatics
- Pathogens: similar to rhinosinusitis
- Dx: CT/MRI of paranasal sinuses with contrast
- ophthalmology consultation for any orbital complication from rhinosinusitis
- urgent surgical intervention should be considered for orbital abscesses (or orbital cellulitis), changes in vision, progressive involvement of symptoms despite appropriate medical therapy, relapse, involvement of opposite eye
- concurrent aggressive rhinosinusitis regimen (parenteral antibiotics, decongestants, mucolytics, saline nasal irrigations) is indicated for any complication of rhinosinusitis

### *Chandler Classification of Orbital Complications and Management*

1. **Periorbital (Preseptal) Cellulitis**: infection confined **anterior to the orbital septum** (primary barrier), presents with unilateral eyelid edema, erythema, fever, and tenderness (no vision changes, chemosis, proptosis, or restriction of ocular muscles); Rx: parenteral antibiotics and concurrent aggressive rhinosinusitis regimen (decongestants, mucolytics, saline nasal irrigations), may consider oral antibiotics with mild symptoms and compliant patient
2. **Orbital Cellulitis**: infection **posterior to the orbital septum** into the orbit proper; presents with proptosis, chemosis, may cause vision changes, **afferent pupillary defect**, may limit extraocular muscles; Rx: parenteral antibiotics, vision acuity checks, aggressive rhinosinusitis regimen (*see previous*); consider endoscopic sinus surgery if no improvement within 24 hours, worsening symptoms, or worsening visual acuity
3. **Subperiosteal Abscess**: collection of pus between bone and periosteum; presents with chemosis, may displace globe (proptosis), restrict extraocular motion, and affect vision; Rx: urgent surgical decompression (ethmoidectomy, orbital rim approach) with postoperative parenteral antibiotics

4. **Orbital Abscess**: collection of pus in orbital soft tissue; presents with proptosis, chemosis, restricted extraocular motion, may have no light perception (may be reversible); <u>Rx</u>: urgent surgical decompression with postoperative parenteral antibiotics
5. **Cavernous Sinus Thrombosis** (*see the following*)

### *Cavernous Sinus and Venous Sinus Thrombophlebitis*

- <u>Pathophysiology</u>: paranasal sinus infection → orbital extension → mural thrombus forms in vessel wall (thrombophlebitis) → propagates centrally as clot softens and begins to seed
- <u>Pathogens</u>: *S. aureus* (most common), hemolytic *Streptococcus* and type III pneumococcus
- <u>SSx</u>: "picket fence" spiking fevers, toxemia, involvement of contra-lateral eye, papilledema, paralysis of extraocular muscles (CN III, IV, and VI), proptosis, chemosis, eyelid edema
- <u>Dx</u>: CT/MRI may show intraluminal enhancement, positive blood cultures, **Tobey-Ayer or Queckenstedt's test** (tests for obstruction; external compression of jugular vein does not cause an increase in CSF pressure but compression on nonobstructed side does increase CSF pressure), CSF may reveal high cell and protein count
- <u>Complications</u>: meningitis, septic metastasis (pulmonary, blood), death
- <u>Rx</u>: parenteral antibiotics, may require ligation of internal jugular vein if septic emboli suspected, anticoagulants (*controversial*), bed rest, sinus surgery once patient is stable

## Intracranial Complications

- <u>Intracranial Pathways</u>: congenital dehiscence, trauma, direct extension (osteomyelitis), lymphatics, olfactory nerve sheath, venous system, foramina of Breschet
- <u>Pathogens</u>: *S. aureus, Streptococcus, S. epidermidis, anaerobes, H. influenzae, E. coli, Pseudomonas, Proteus* (abscesses are often polymicrobial)
- <u>Dx</u>: CT/MRI of brain with contrast, lumbar puncture for cells and culture (if imaging does not show mass effect that may cause risk of herniation)

### *Meningitis*

- most common intracranial complication from rhinosinusitis
- highest risk from sphenoid and ethmoid sinusitis
- <u>SSx</u>: headache, lethargy, nuchal rigidity, fever, Kernig's sign (with hip in flexion, pain is elicited with leg extension), Brudzinski's sign (flexion at neck causes a reflexive flexion of the legs), seizures, photophobia

- <u>Rx</u>: parenteral antibiotics, sinus surgery with exposure of diseased dura (if present)

### *Epidural Abscess*

- pus collection between skull and dura (biconvex disk on CT/MRI, does not cross midline)
- highest risk from frontal sinusitis (direct extension)
- <u>SSx</u>: headaches, low-grade to spiking fevers, malaise, mental status changes (may be asymptomatic)
- <u>Rx</u>: parenteral antibiotics, neurosurgical consultation for possible drainage procedure, sinus drainage or obliteration procedure with wide exposure of dura until healthy tissue is exposed on all sides

### *Subdural Abscess*

- pus collection between dura and arachnoid membrane (crescent-shaped enhancement on CT/MRI, may cross midline)
- highest risk from frontal sinusitis
- <u>SSx</u>: more neurologic sequelae than extradural infections (seizures, delirium, hemiplegia, aphasia), mild increase in intracranial pressure (ICP) depending on the size
- <u>Rx</u>: high-dose parenteral antibiotics, neurosurgical consultation for possible drainage procedure

### *Brain Abscess*

- highest risk from frontal sinusitis
- <u>SSx</u>: fever, headache, vomiting, lethargy, seizure, focal neurologic symptoms
- <u>Stages</u>
  1. **Encephalitis**: (initial invasion) fevers, headache, nuchal rigidity
  2. **Latency**: (organization of abscess, liquification necrosis) minimal symptoms, may last weeks
  3. **Expanding Abscess**: intracranial hypertension, seizures, paralysis
  4. **Termination**: rupture of abscess, often fatal
- <u>Rx</u>: parenteral antibiotics, neurosurgical consultation for possible drainage procedure, concurrent sinus surgery

## Other Complications

- **Osteitis**: diagnose initially with technetium bone scan (osteoblastic activity) and gallium bone scan (inflammation), follow with gallium scans; <u>Rx</u>: parenteral antibiotics, surgical debridement, sinus surgery

- **Pott's Puffy Tumor**: osteomyelitis or subperiosteal abscess of the frontal bone with overlying soft tissue swelling caused by invasion through the diploic vein resulting in thrombophlebitis; presents as "doughy" swelling of the forehead; <u>Rx</u>: parenteral antibiotics, trephination, may require surgical debridement with removal of infected bone
- **Superior Orbital Fissure Syndrome**: fixed globe, dilated pupil (CN III, IV, VI), ptosis, hypesthesia of upper eyelid (CN $V_1$); <u>Rx</u>: urgent surgical decompression
- **Orbital Apex Syndrome**: similar to superior orbital fissure syndrome with added involvement of CN II (papilledema, vision changes)
- **Sinocutaneous Fistula**: usually begins as a frontal osteomyelitis

# SINUS SURGERY

## Procedures

### Functional Endoscopic Sinus Surgery (FESS)

- <u>Advantages</u>: superior visualization, better precision, preserves function (recognizes normal mucociliary flow pattern at the ostiomeatal complex), completeness, no external scar
- <u>Disadvantages</u>: one-handed technique, monocular vision (difficulty with depth perception)
- <u>Typical Steps of FESS for Rhinosinusitis</u>: visualize anatomy, medialize middle turbinate, excise uncinate process, maxillary antrostomy, anterior ethmoidectomy, posterior ethmoidectomy, sphenoidotomy, frontal recess exploration
- <u>Variations of Technique</u>: consider **stereotactic guidance systems** especially for severe polyposis and recurrent disease; **balloon catheterization techniques** (**sinuplasty**) widen the maxillary, frontal, and sphenoid sinus os without performing an uncinectomy, have been considered for recurrent sinus disease, minimal chronic sinusitis, pediatric patients, as well as for access to the frontal sinuses
- <u>Postoperative Care</u>: consider resorbable or nonresorbable packing, oral antibiotics for a minimum of 1 week, aggressive nasal hygiene to prevent adhesions (saline irrigations), oral or nasal steroids, follow-up sinonasal debridement

### *Indications for FESS*

- failed medical management for acute, recurrent-acute, or chronic rhinosinusitis
- complicated rhinosinusitis

- fungal rhinosinusitis
- obstructive nasal polyposis
- sinus mucoceles
- removal of foreign bodies
- tumor excision (transsphenoidal hypophysectomy)
- orbital and optic nerve decompression (Graves' ophthalmopathy)
- dacryocystorhinostomy
- choanal atresia repair
- CSF leak repair
- epistaxis control

## Ethmoid and Maxillary Open Sinus Procedures

### Caldwell-Luc

- intraoral approach to anterior maxillary wall from canine fossa above gum line, the diseased mucosa is removed from the maxillary sinus, also allows for a middle meatal antrostomy, and ethmoidectomy (transantral ethmoidectomy)
- <u>Indications</u>: sinus disease not accessible by endoscopic sinus surgery, inspissated secretions, neo-ossification, cystic fibrosis, prior Caldwell-Luc procedure
- <u>Advantages</u>: allows adequate exposure of inside of maxillary sinus, favorable intraoral incision
- <u>Disadvantages</u>: nonfunctional, damages mucosa (decreased cilia count, increased fibrosis and bone growth), risk of infraorbital nerve and dental injury (hypoesthesia to teeth and lip), transantral ethmoidectomy does not allow exposure anterior to the ethmoidal bulla

### Intranasal Ethmoidectomy (Without Endoscopy)

- requires medialization of middle turbinate to gain access to the ethmoid cells, diseased mucosa is removed by piecemeal forceps dissection
- <u>Indications</u>: largely been replaced by endoscopic sinus surgery
- <u>Advantages</u>: no external scar
- <u>Disadvantages</u>: poor visualization (increased risk of bleeding and CSF leak), poor precision, excess mucosal damage, no visualization of frontal sinus recess or inside maxillary sinus

### External Ethmoidectomy

- requires ligation of angular and anterior ethmoid arteries, access gained through lamina papyracea and lacrimal fossa

- <u>Indications</u>: inability to obtain transnasal exposure, subperiosteal abscess or orbital abscess
- <u>Advantages</u>: can access ethmoid sinus in all cases
- <u>Disadvantages</u>: poor visualization (especially anteriorly), poor precision, excess mucosal injury, external scar

## Frontal Sinus Surgery

### *Endoscopic Techniques*

- most common and preferred approach with modern techniques and image-guided systems
- <u>Advantages</u>: no external scar or deformity
- <u>Disadvantages</u>: technically more difficult, risk of orbital and intracranial complications
- <u>Contraindicated</u>: aplastic frontal sinus

#### Frontal Sinusotomy Types

- **Draf I**: exposes outflow tract, leaves roof of the agger nasi cell and superior-most suprabullar cell
- **Draf IIa**: removes roof of the agger nasi cell and superior-most suprabullar cell
- **Draf IIb**: also removes head of the middle turbinate (exposes lamina papyracea to septum)
- **Draf III (Modified Lothrop)**: remove entire floor of frontal sinus as well as anterosuperior nasal septum

### *Osteoplastic Flap with Frontal Sinus Obliteration*

- <u>Technique</u>: bicoronal flap for exposure (also midline forehead and brow incisions), "trapdoor" access to the frontal sinus via a periosteal and bone flap (requires a template patterned from a Caldwell view x-ray), remove mucosa, obliterate cavity, and occlude frontal recess (may use fat, muscle, or bone)
- <u>Indications</u>: chronic or recurrent rhinosinusitis, mucocele (pyocele), frontal bone osteomyelitis, benign tumors, frontal sinus fractures, orbital or intracranial complications
- <u>Advantages</u>: best view of entire frontal sinus and anterior base of skull, minimal deformity, direct approach, fail-safe method to eradicate frontal sinus disease (permanent and complete removal of diseased mucosa)
- <u>Disadvantages</u>: technically more difficult, time-consuming, requires hospitalization, risk of mucocele formation (typically years later) and chronic pain
- <u>Contraindicated</u>: aplastic frontal sinus

## Other Open Techniques

- **Frontal Sinus Trephination**: considered for acute purulent frontal sinusitis, sinusitis refractory to conservative management, and complications of frontal sinusitis; useful to relieve pain and obtain cultures for acute frontal sinusitis; access from the medial eyebrow and supraorbital rim
- **Lynch Procedure (Fronto-ethmoidectomy)**: removal of the frontal sinus floor, middle turbinate, and anterior ethmoids through a "gull wing" curvilinear incision above the lateral nasal bones, easiest and quickest technique, risk of recurrent mucocele formation from stenosis of frontal recess; uncommon with modern endoscopic techniques
- **Riedel Method**: consists of removal of the frontal sinus floor and anterior wall (disfiguring), allows for complete obliteration
- **Killian Method**: modification of the Riedel by preserving a bridge at the supraorbital rim to reduce deformity, useful with "tall" frontal sinuses, technically challenging

# Approaches to the Sphenoid

## Endoscopic Approaches

- <u>Indications</u>: common for chronic rhinosinusitis, transsphenoidal hypophysectomy (tumors), mucocele, CSF leak, biopsy, optic nerve decompression
- <u>Advantages</u>: no septal incisions, when approached lateral to superior turbinectomy via natural os allows for natural mucociliary clearance, transethmoid approach (lateral to superior turbinate) is more common but risks injury to lateral sphenoid structures including optic nerve and carotid artery
- <u>Disadvantages</u>: compromised 3D exposure

### Surgical Landmarks of the Sphenoid Ostium

- adjacent to posterior border of nasal septum
- 6–8 cm posterior to the anterior nasal spine
- 30° angle from floor of nose
- typically 1.5 cm above the choanal floor and 8 mm inferior to skull base
- superior to the superior turbinate posterior attachment

## Sublabial Transseptal Approach

- <u>Indications</u>: transphenoidal hypophysectomy (tumors), rhinosinusitis, and mucocele
- <u>Advantages</u>: wide midline exposure, no external scar

- <u>Disadvantages</u>: soft tissue trauma, sensory disturbances, difficult to displace distal lateral nasal mucosa with speculum, oral contamination

### *Transcolumellar Transseptal Approach (External Rhinoplasty)*

- <u>Indications</u>: transsphenoidal hypophysectomy (tumors), rhinosinusitis, and mucocele
- <u>Advantages</u>: wide midline exposure, shorter access distance, no manipulation of upper lip (shorter recovery time)
- <u>Disadvantages</u>: small external scar, disrupts medial crura (major tip support), narrower exposure

## Complications of Sinus Surgery

### Ocular and Orbital Complications

- **Blindness**: may be secondary to an indirect injury (eg, retrobulbar hematoma, *see following*) or direct injury to the optic nerve (superior lateral aspect of sphenoid sinus or posterior lateral aspect of an Onodi cell)
- **Intraoperative Orbital Fat Penetration**: from violation of the lamina papyracea, increases risk of retrobulbar hematoma, occurs more commonly on the right side (right-handed surgeon) because the ethmoids may appear more lateral; <u>Rx</u>: recognize orbital fat (orbital fat floats); avoid further trauma; may complete the FESS; avoid tight nasal packing; observe for vision changes, proptosis, or restricted ocular gaze
- **Retrobulbar or Preseptal Emphysema**: may occur from micro-fracturing of lamina papyracea or lateral nasal wall, may manifest postoperatively if patient blows nose or strains; <u>Rx</u>: observation, no nose blowing, sneeze with mouth open, typically resolves within a few days
- **Diplopia**: orbital muscle injury, most commonly from injury to the medial rectus or superior oblique muscles
- **Epiphora**: injury to lacrimal duct system, common injury but rarely manifests clinically, avoid operating anterior to the attachment of the uncinate; <u>Rx</u>: observation initially, if no resolution then dacryocystorhinostomy

### *Retrobulbar Hematoma*

- permanent blindness can occur within **60–90 minutes** if untreated
- <u>Pathophysiology</u>: most commonly from retraction injury of the anterior ethmoid artery which causes increased orbital pressure that

compresses the vascular supply to the optic nerve, also may occur from venous injury near the lamina papyracea

- <u>Prevention</u>: maintain orientation and operate under direct vision, examine CT for dehiscence, correct coagulopathies, keep eye uncovered
- <u>SSx</u>: ecchymosis, proptosis, conjunctival changes (chemosis), pupillary changes (afferent pupillary defect)

**Management**

- if noticed intraoperatively control hemorrhage and terminate case
- ophthalmology consult
- mannitol (1–2 g/kg), consider high-dose steroids
- orbital massage and place ice pack
- lateral canthotomy (*see* p. 650), medial external (Lynch) procedure, or orbital decompression

## Intracranial Complications

- **CSF Leak**: may occur anterior to the frontal recess, cribriform plate, and posterior ethmoid sinus (fovea ethmoidalis); avoid cribriform injury by staying lateral to middle turbinate; <u>Rx</u>: recognize leak (clear or swirling fluid), prepare site of leak, apply graft (mucosa, fascia, or muscle flap), stabilize graft (dissolvable hemostatic material), consider neurosurgical consult, consider lumbar puncture, bed rest, avoid straining (*see also* pp. 661–662)
- **Intracranial Infections**: meningitis, intracranial abscess
- **Intracranial Hemorrhage**: uncommon

## Major Hemorrhage

- <u>Risks</u>: coagulopathy, nasal polyposis, and extensive disease
- **Anterior Ethmoid Artery**: anterior superior region of the anterior ethmoid; <u>Rx</u>: typically easily cauterized unless retracts into the orbit (risk of retrobulbar hematoma)
- **Posterior Ethmoid Artery**: posterior ethmoid cells; <u>Rx</u>: more difficult to cauterize, may need packing
- **Sphenopalatine Artery**: injured during middle turbinectomy, enlarging the maxillary ostia, or posterior ethmoidectomy; <u>Rx</u>: cauterization or nasal packing
- **Carotid Artery**: immediately life-threatening, 20–25% have only a thin wall between sphenoid sinus and carotid artery; <u>Rx</u>: immediate packing, compression of carotid in the neck, neurosurgical consultation, intraoperative angiography or ligation of artery

## Synechia

- most common complication of endoscopic sinus surgery
- scarring most commonly occurs between middle turbinates and nasal wall
- <u>Rx</u>: lysis of adhesions (endoscopic approach), may consider spacers (Telfa, Merocel, Gelfilm); prevent by minimizing trauma, reduce concha bullosas and symptomatic polypoidal middle turbinates, and good postoperative care (nasal hygiene, endoscopic debridements)

## Other Complications

- residual disease
- aspiration of packing material
- toxic shock syndrome
- osteomyelitis
- paresthesias from injury to infraorbital, supraorbital, or supratrochlear nerves
- embossment (frontal sinus obliteration)
- anosmia from injury to the olfactory epithelium
- facial edema (especially from Caldwell–Luc procedure)
- tooth numbness and pain (Caldwell–Luc)

# IMMUNOLOGY

## Introduction

### Cell-Mediated Immunity

- **Antigen-Presenting Cells**: macrophages, dendritic cells, Langerhans cells; phagocytize antigens then present a fragment of the antigen to the surface via major histocompatibility complex (MHC) type II receptor and secrete IL-1
- **Helper T-cells**: recognize the antigen presented by the MHC Type II receptor complex and are activated by IL-1, resulting in secretion of IL-2 (IL-2 upregulates other T-cells including killer T-cells, macrophages, and natural-killer cells), CD4+
- **Killer (Cytotoxic) T-Cells**: attack the body's own cells that have been transformed from infection or malignancy via the MHC type I receptor, CD8+
- **Major Histocompatibility Complex (MHC)**: surface receptors for antigenic determinants of foreign matter
  1. **Type I**: found on all nucleated cells; encoded by gene complex human leukocyte antigen (HLA) A, B, and C

2. **Type II**: found on antigen-presenting cells and B-cells; encoded HLA DR, DQ, and DP

### Common Clusters of Differentiation (CD) Markers:

- **CD2** and **CD3**: all T-cells
- **CD4**: helper T-cells, associated with MHC Type II response, receptor for HIV
- **CD8**: killer T-cells, associated with MHC Type I response
- **CD56** and **CD16**: natural killer cells

## Humoral Immunity

- B-cells are produced in bone marrow, migrate to lymph nodes and spleen, bare multiple receptors similar to the immunoglobulins they secrete
- B-cells are positive for CD19, 20, and 22, and carry MHC class II on their surface
- B-Cell Activation Types
  1. **T-Cell Dependent Activation**: B-cell receptors internalize antigen, fraction of antigen presents on surface via MHC type II receptor, which recognizes helper T-cells, T-cell then stimulates B-cell (via IL-2 and IL-4) to mature to plasma cells, which secrete immunoglobulins
  2. **T-Cell Independent Activation**: large antigens (eg, carbohydrates on bacterial cell walls) bridge immunoglobulins on B-cell surfaces that activate the B-cell

### Immunoglobulins

- glycoproteins produced by plasma cells that participate in antigen recognition, complement fixation, opsonization, and promotion of phagocytosis
- composed of two heavy chains (determines class: μ, γ, α, ε, δ) and two light chains (κ and λ), both heavy and light chains have a variable and a constant region
- antigen binds to the variable portion of heavy and light chains
- **Fab Fragment**: antigen binding portion of the immunoglobulin
- **Fc Fragment**: crystalizable fragment portion of the immunoglobulin that initiates other functions such as complement fixation
- kill bacterium by complement fixation via C1q (IgG and IgM) or antibody-dependent cellular cytotoxicity (**ADCC**), which attaches Fc to a cytotoxic cell

- Types
  1. **IgG** (γ): **most abundant, 2° response** phase, involved in complement fixation and ADCC, may cross the placenta (provides protection in the newborn), binds complement, divided into four subclasses (G$_{1-4}$)
  2. **IgA** (α): predominantly found in **external secretions**, prevents bacterial attachment to mucus membranes, associated with dimeric "secretory piece" and a "J" chain
  3. **IgD** (δ): initial type of immunoglobulin secreted, trace amounts in serum, unclear function
  4. **IgM** (μ): predominant antibody in **1° response** phase (declines rapidly and replaced with IgG of same specificity), does not cross the placenta, binds complement, pentamer arrangement
  5. **IgE** (ε): major contributor in **allergy** (type I hypersensitivity), Fc fragment binds to mast cells and basophils

## Nonspecific Immunity

- **Natural Killer Cells**: granular lymphocytes that participate in killing tumor cells and virus-infected cells, do not depend on prior immunization, activated by interferon, involved in ADCC
- **Complement System**: system of plasma proteins that act with each other to cause lysis of cells and bacteria, stimulation of chemotaxis and cell activation, and opsonization; IgG and IgM fix complement
- **Monocytes and Macrophages**: produced in bone marrow, recognize and ingest foreign and damaged material; a macrophage found within tissue is sometimes called a **histiocyte**
- **Polymorphonuclear Cells (PMNs, Neutrophils)**: granulocytes that accumulate in acute infections and participate in phagocytosis
- **Eosinophils**: granulocyte, active in allergic response and parasitic infections
- **Basophils and Mast Cells**: granulocytes that release histamine and other substances released with exposure to an allergen, IgE presents on cell surface
- Others: skin and mucosal lining, lysozymes, saliva, gastric acid, etc

## Cytokines

- immunomodulatory peptides produced by mononuclear inflammatory cells that participate in paracrine cellular modulation
- *see* Table 1–5 lists cytokines and their actions

**TABLE 1–5.** Cytokines and Their Actions

| Cytokines | Source | Primary Action |
|-----------|--------|----------------|
| IL-1 | Mφ and any nucleated cells, usually from stimulation by antigen MHC class II | activates other cells and stimulates IL-2 secretion, pyrogen |
| IL-2 | activated T-cells | essential to stimulate T-cells, B-cells, and NK cells |
| IL-3 | T-cells | proliferation of early hematopoietic cells |
| IL-4 | T-cells | stimulates B-cells |
| IL-5 | T-cells, mast cells | eosinophil proliferation, IgA production |
| TNF-α & β | lymphocytes, Mφ, endothelium, keratinocytes | same as IL-1 but may be more cytotoxic to tumors |
| TGF-β | lymphocytes, Mφ, platelets | inhibits cells (immunosuppressive) |
| IFN-α | leukocytes | anti-viral and anti-tumor effects, increases MHC cell surface proteins |
| IFN-β | fibroblasts, epithelial cells | similar to IFN-α |
| IFN-γ | T-cells, NK cells | direct cytotoxic effects |

# Immunodeficiency

## B-Cell Disorders

- SSx: recurrent upper respiratory (sinonasal, otitis media) and pulmonary infections, conjunctivitis, dermatitis, malabsorption, pyogenic bacterial infections
- Dx: quantitative immunoglobulins and subclasses, Schick test, serum protein, immunoelectrophoresis, in vitro-specific antibody responses
- Rx: antibiotics, IVIG (intravenous immunoglobulin)
- **Common Variable Immunodeficiency**: most common (hence the name) form of hypogammaglobulinemia, failure of B-cell maturation, usually acquired, associated with T-cell deficiencies and other autoimmune disorders, manifests in early adulthood
- **X-linked Agammaglobulinemia of Bruton**: X-linked recessive disorder causing a defect in tyrosine kinase, prevents pre-B cell

maturation to B-cells (does not affect T-cells), does not manifest until 6 months of age (after maternal IgG declines), increased risk of leukemia and lymphoma, can survive into adulthood

- **Selective IgA Deficiency**: most common inherited B-cell defect; selective IgA B-cells do not mature to plasma cells; often asymptomatic; associated with allergies, transfusion anaphylaxis, autoimmune disorders, and IgG subclass deficiency; keep IgA content of blood products low (may cause anaphylaxis)
- **Selective IgG Hypogammaglobulinemia**: may affect one or more subtype ($G_1$–$G_4$):
  1. **IgG$_1$**: rare, IgG$_1$ composes majority of total serum IgG
  2. **IgG$_2$**: most common hypogammaglobulin deficiency in children, inability to mount an antibody response to polysaccharides (encapsulated bacteria)
  3. **IgG$_3$**: most common hypogammaglobulin deficiency in adults, reduced ability to generate an antibody response to viral infections, *M. catarrhalis*, and *S. pyogenes*
  4. **IgG$_4$**: common, usually asymptomatic (unclear clinical significance)

## T-Cell Disorders

- <u>SSx</u>: increased viral, fungal, protozoal, and bacterial infections; atrophic lymphoid tissue
- <u>Dx</u>: total lymphocyte count, T-cell count, skin tests (candidal, mumps controls, PPD), functional tests (proliferation to mitogens, alloantigen helper/suppresser function)
- **DiGeorge Syndrome (Thymic Aplasia)**: disorder of **third and fourth branchial pouch development**, thymic hypoplasia, also associated with hypoplastic parathyroids (hypocalcemia, tetany), aortic arch and facial abnormalities, 90% due to chromosome 22q11 deletion
- **Chronic Mucocutaneous Candidiasis**: T-cell dysfunction resulting in skin and mucous membrane *Candidal* infections, onset usually in childhood; <u>Rx</u>: antifungals
- **HIV/AIDS**: *see following*

## Combined B- and T-Cell Disorders

- **Severe Combined Immunodeficiency (SCID)**: multiple genetic forms resulting in lack of T- and B-cell immunity, severe infections (pneumonia, diarrhea, thrush), higher risk of malignancy, variant associated with adenosine deaminase (ADA) deficiency (accumulation of deoxyadenosine, toxic to lymphocytes), presents within first few months of life, fatal if untreated; Rx: bone marrow transplant, gene therapy is experimental

- **Wiskott-Aldrich Syndrome**: X-linked disorder of WASP gene associated with IgM deficiency; triad of thrombocytopenia (bleeding), eczema, and recurrent infections due to poor functional antibody response to polysaccharides (otitis media, pneumonia, and pyogenic organisms); associated autoimmune disease and increased risk of malignancy; Rx: bone marrow transplant, splenectomy, IVIG, antibiotic prophylaxis, gene therapy is experimental
- **Ataxia-Telangiectasia**: defect in DNA repair, IgA deficiency, cerebellar ataxia, telangiectasias, mean survival is 25 years; Rx: antibiotics, possibly IVIG

## Human Immunodeficiency Virus (HIV) and Acquired Immune Deficiency Syndrome (AIDS)

- *see* Table 1–6
- HIV infection results from inoculation of infected body fluid (blood, semen, saliva, etc)
- Pathophysiology: HIV is a **retrovirus** that attaches to the CD4+ cell marker of T-helper cells, macrophages, and other immunologic cells → becomes internalized → proviral DNA synthesized from **reverse transcriptase** → proviral DNA integrates into host DNA; results in decreased number of T-helper cells and impaired function of macrophages, neutrophils, B-lymphocytes, and complement activation
- also associated with abnormal immune regulation, atopy, autoimmune disease
- **Acquired Immune Deficiency Syndrome (AIDS)**: defined when an HIV patient develops an AIDS-defining illness (eg, esophageal or tracheal candidiasis, CMV disease, Kaposi's sarcoma, *Pneumocystis* pneumonia), or a CD4 count <**200** cells/µL, or CD4 percentage <**14%**
- prior to effective antiretroviral therapy, the cause of death for most AIDS patients was sepsis or disseminated neoplasms
- Risks: multiple sex partners, unprotected intercourse, IV drug use, racial/ethnic minority status, blood transfusions (extremely rare in United States with current screening methods), health care workers (rare); most common methods of acquisition vary widely depending on region (male homosexual intercourse and IV drug use in the United States, heterosexual intercourse in the developing world, IV drug use in Eastern Europe)

**TABLE 1–6.** Head and Neck Manifestations of HIV by Anatomic Location

<u>Oral and Pharynx</u>
- oral candidiasis
- oral hairy leukoplakia
- herpes stomatitis
- thrombocytopenic purpura
- recurrent aphthous ulcers
- bone loss (bacillary angiomatosis)
- gingivitis (acute necrotizing ulcerative gingivitis, necrotizing stomatitis)
- Kaposi's sarcoma, non-Hodgkin's lymphoma, squamous cell carcinoma

<u>Larynx</u>
- epiglottitis
- Kaposi's sarcoma, non-Hodgkin's lymphoma
- laryngitis (*Mycobacterium*, fungal, cytomegalovirus, EBV, bacterial)

<u>Neck</u>
- deep-space neck abscess
- infectious lymphadenopathy (*Mycobacterium, Pneumocystis,* cytomegalovirus, EBV, *Toxoplasmosis,* cat-scratch disease, bacterial)
- neoplastic lymphadenopathy (Hodgkin's and non-Hodgkin's lymphoma, metastatic disease, thyroid tumors)
- persistent generalized adenopathy

<u>Salivary Glands</u>
- lymphoepithelial cysts of the parotid gland
- parotitis
- salivary gland neoplasms

<u>Otologic</u>
- acute and chronic otitis media, otitis externa, mastoiditis (invasive *Aspergillosis, Pneumocystis, Mycobacterium*)
- necrotizing otitis externa
- sensorineural hearing loss (cryptococcal or mycobacterial meningitis, otosyphilis, toxoplasmosis, autoimmune demyelination of the cochlear nerve, cerebellopontine angle tumors)
- tympanic membrane perforations
- aural polyps
- facial nerve paralysis (herpes zoster, cytomegalovirus, EBV, HIV, autoimmune demyelination, necrotizing otitis externa, meningitis and encephalitis)
- temporal bone neoplasms (Hodgkin's and non-Hodgkin's lymphoma, Kaposi's sarcoma)

<u>Paranasal Sinus</u>
- rhinosinusitis (*Mucor, Aspergillosis, Pseudomonas*)
- nasal tumors (Kaposi's sarcoma, nasal lymphomas)

- <u>HIV Dx</u>: typically diagnosed first by screening with an enzyme-linked immunosorbent assay (ELISA) to detect anti-HIV antibodies then confirmed with Western blot (confirmation test), immunofluorescence assays are less common and highly accurate, CD4+ count, CD4+/CD8+ ratio
- <u>Rx</u>: combination antiviral medications, prophylaxis against opportunistic infections

## Other Immunologic Disorders

- **Complement Disorders**: associated with autoimmune diseases, abnormal opsonization, and capsular organism infections
- **Chronic Granulomatous Disease**: multiple genetic forms result in dysfunction of NADPH oxidase and intracellular hydrogen peroxide production → impaired intracellular killing of phagocytized organisms, susceptible to catalase-positive bacteria and fungus (*S. aureus, Aspergillus, Candida, Serratia*); <u>Dx</u>: neutrophil function tests; <u>Rx</u>: antimicrobial prophylaxis, aggressive treatment of infections, bone marrow transplant

# Vaccinations (see Appendix C)

# CHAPTER

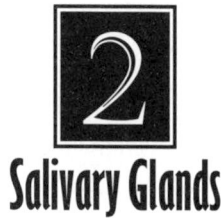

# Salivary Glands

Anthony J. Cornetta, Robert T. Sataloff, and Raza Pasha

# SALIVARY GLAND ANATOMY AND PHYSIOLOGY

## Anatomy

**Parotid Gland Anatomy** (*see* Figures 2–1 and 2–2)

- located between the ramus of the mandible and the external auditory canal and mastoid tip, overlies the masseter muscle (anteriorly) and sternocleidomastoid (SCM) muscle (posteriorly)
- facial nerve divides the parotid gland artificially into deep and superficial lobes
- the superficial layer of the deep cervical fascia forms the parotid gland fascia which incompletely surrounds the gland
- contains **lymphoid tissue** within the gland
- <u>Histologic Cell Type</u>: basophilic, **serous cells**
- **Stylomandibular Ligament**: formed by the fascial envelope between the styloid process and the mandible, separates the parotid gland from the submandibular gland
- **Stenson's Duct**: passes over masseter, through buccinator muscle, and opens opposite to the second upper molar (follows along plane from external auditory canal to columella and buccal branch of CN VII)

### Venous Drainage

- superficial temporal vein + maxillary vein → retromandibular vein
- retromandibular vein → passes deep to the facial nerve → anterior and posterior branches

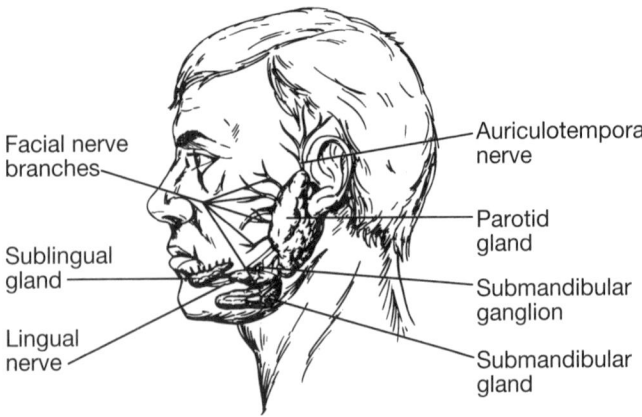

**FIGURE 2–1.** Positions of the major salivary glands and related nerves.

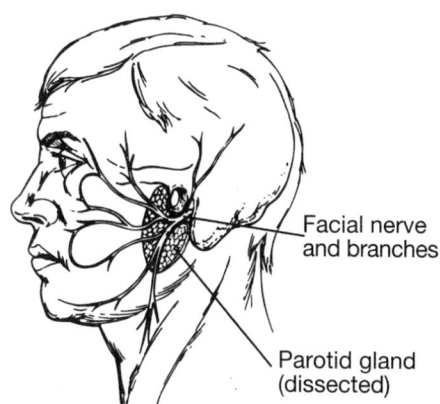

**FIGURE 2–2.** Position of the facial nerve, as illustrated following a superficial parotidectomy. The residual parotid gland pictured above is the deep lobe.

- anterior retromandibular vein + facial vein → common facial vein → internal jugular vein
- posterior retromandibular vein + posterior auricular vein (over SCM) → external jugular vein

## Submandibular Gland Anatomy

- within the submandibular triangle (inferior to mylohyoid muscle, superior to the digastrics)
- superficial layer of the deep cervical fascia envelops the gland and contains the marginal mandibular nerve
- hypoglossal nerve runs deep to the digastric tendon and medial to the deep layer of the deep cervical fascia
- facial artery arises from the external carotid artery and courses medial to the posterior digastric muscle then hooks over the muscle to enter the gland and exits into the facial notch of the inferior mandible
- lingual artery runs along the lateral aspect of the middle constrictors, deep to the digastrics, and anteriorly and medially to the hyoglossus
- <u>Histologic Cell Type</u>: **mixed cells** (serous and mucinous)
- **Wharton's Duct:** opens lateral to frenulum in the anterior portion of the floor of mouth, behind the incisors

## Minor Glands and Sublingual Gland Anatomy

- **Sublingual Gland:** located within the submucosal layer of the floor of mouth

- **Minor Salivary Glands:** several hundred glands within the submucosal layer of the oral cavity, oropharynx, nasopharynx, and hypopharynx
- <u>Histologic Cell Type</u>: **mucinous**
- **Ducts of Rivinus:** drain the sublingual gland at the sublingual fold or plica of the floor of mouth

## Histology (*see* Figure 2–3)

- <u>Secretory Unit</u>: **acini cells** (contain abundant endoplasmic reticulum, Golgi apparatus, and secretory granules; produce saliva) → **intercalated duct** → **striated duct** (contain abundant mitochondria for energy for water and electrolyte transport) → **excretory duct**
- **myoepithelial cells** surround acini and intercalated ducts

# Physiology

## Efferent Innervation of the Salivary Glands

### Parasympathetic Innervation

- **inferior salivatory nucleus** (medulla) → **glossopharyngeal nerve** (Jacobson's nerve) → lesser (superficial) petrosal nerve → **otic ganglion**) → *postganglionic parasympathetic fibers* → carried by auriculotemporal branch of CN $V_3$ → **parotid gland**
- **superior salivatory nucleus** (pons) → nervus intermedius → **chorda tympani** → carried on lingual nerve → **submandibular ganglion** → *postganglionic parasympathetic fibers* → **submandibular and sublingual glands**

### Sympathetic Innervation

- **superior thoracic nerves** → **superior cervical ganglion** → *postganglionic fibers via arterial plexus* → **submandibular and cutaneous vessels**

## Salivation

- 1–1.5 pints of saliva/day
- <u>Composition</u>: >99% water, salts (calcium phosphate, calcium carbonate), organic compounds and enzymes (amylase, albumin, lysozyme, immunoglobulin A, ptyalin initiates the first phase of starch digestion, others)

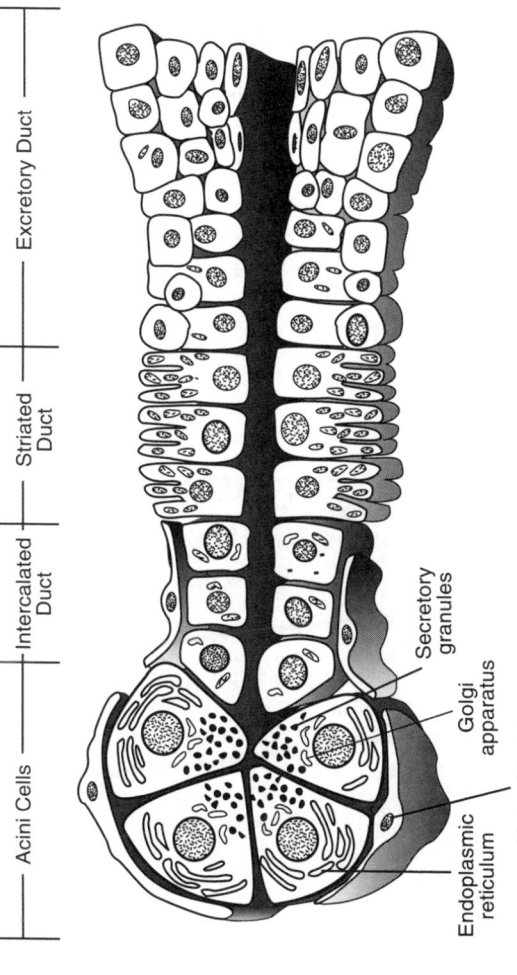

Acini Cells | Intercalated Duct | Striated Duct | Excretory Duct

Secretory granules

Golgi apparatus

Myoepithelial cell

Endoplasmic reticulum

**FIGURE 2-3.** Schematic drawing of the salivary gland duct system.

- <u>Function of Saliva</u>: antibacterial (contains "secretory piece" needed for IgA, ABO isohemagglutinogens, perioxidases, and other immunologic proteins), digestion (provides digestive enzymes and buffers), lubrication and moisturization, dental protection (prevents caries and promotes dental calcification), modulation of taste

## Salivary Gland Dysfunction

### Sialorrhea and Ptyalism (Drooling) (*see* pp. 568–569)

### Xerostomia

- <u>Causes</u>: central (rare), primary salivary disorders (Sjögren's disease, radiation sialadenosis), dehydration, medications (psychotropics, general anesthesia, β-blockers, chemotherapy agents), mouth breathing from nasal obstruction, stress, anxiety
- risk of dental caries, impaired taste, and malnutrition
- <u>Rx</u>: address underlying cause, artificial saliva, frequent small drinks, pilocarpine, aggressive dental care

# GENERAL SALIVARY GLAND PATHOLOGY

## Parotid Gland Masses

### Evaluation of the Parotid Gland Mass

#### *History and Physical Exam*

- <u>Character of Parotid Mass</u>: onset and duration, rapid (inflammatory) versus slow growing (neoplastic), diffuse versus discrete mass (tumor), unilateral versus bilateral (sialadenosis, mumps) involvement, associated pain, association with food ingestion (sialadenitis)
- <u>Contributing Factors</u>: exposure to radiation or toxins (lead or mercury); history of sarcoidosis, Sjögren's disease, tuberculosis, gout, amyloidosis; recent facial trauma, surgery, or dental work; immunization history (specifically measles, mumps, rubella [MMR] vaccine)
- <u>Associated SSx</u>: xerostomia, sialorrhea, weight loss, fever, trismus
- <u>Physical Exam</u>: palpation (mobility, size, consistency), bimanual intraoral palpation with duct inspection and saliva expression (or purulence), tenderness (inflammatory process), facial nerve function (malignancy), parapharyngeal space involvement (examine intraorally), cervical lymphadenopathy, complete H&N H&P

*Imaging and Ancillary Tests*

- **Fine Needle Aspirate (FNA):** indicated for discrete nodules of the parotid gland, widely practiced although controversial (may not change management); differentiates cysts, inflammatory processes, lymphoma, and other neoplasms
- **CT/MRI:** indicated if suspect a tumor or for preoperative evaluation (*see* Table 2–1), ultrasound (U/S) differentiates cystic lesions
- **Open Biopsy:** incisional biopsy (enucleation) without identifying facial nerve risks tumor seeding, recurrence, facial nerve injury, and violation of tumor margins, superficial/total parotidectomy (with facial nerve identification) typically required (*see below*)
- **Technetium-99m Isotope Scan:** rarely utilized, may differentiate a Warthin's tumor and oncocytoma from other salivary gland neoplasms
- **Sialography:** visualizes ductal anatomy, indicated for ductal calculi, trauma, fistulas, Sjögren's disease, contraindicated in acute infections
- <u>Labs</u>: may consider mumps titers, CBC, autoimmune and Sjögren's profile (SS-A, SS-B, ANA, ESR)

# Salivary Gland Enlargement

## Acute Sialadenitis

- <u>Pathophysiology</u>: salivary stasis or obstruction, retrograde migration of bacteria
- <u>Pathogen</u>: *S. aureus* (most common), *Streptococcus viridans, H. influenzae, S. pyogenes,* and *E. coli*; must also consider virus such as HIV, mumps, coxsackie, influenza
- <u>Risks</u>: dehydration, postsurgical (GI procedures), radiation and chemotherapy, Sjögren's syndrome
- <u>SSx</u>: erythema and tenderness over gland, warmth, purulence at ductal orifice, auricle may protrude (parotitis), trismus
- <u>Dx</u>: clinical history and exam, cultures (FNA not required)
- <u>Complication</u>: ductal fistula (cutaneous), abscess (toxemia), deep neck space invasion (**Ludwig's angina**)
- <u>Rx</u>: rehydration, warm compresses, antimicrobial therapy (may require parenteral antibiotics for severe cases), sialagogues, salivary gland massage, oral irrigations; if no resolution after 2–3 days then consider CT or U/S to evaluate for abscess (may require I&D)

## Salivary Calculi (Sialolithiasis)

- most common in **submandibular gland** (80%)
- **Sialolithiasis:** deposition of concretions within the ductal system of the gland

**TABLE 2–1.** Computed Tomography Versus Magnetic Resonance Imaging of the Parotid Gland

| Computed Tomography | Magnetic Resonance Imaging |
|---|---|
| • better for bone imaging | • better for soft tissue imaging (distinguish parotid tumors from parapharyngeal lesions, identifies capsule) |
| • less expensive | • multiplanar views |
| • quicker image | • no radiation required |
| • less sensitive to patient motion | • facial nerve or retromandibular vessels may be used to distinguish deep and superficial lobes |
| • may differentiate deep tumors by identifying a fat strip | • cannot be used with pacemakers and metallic implants (aneurysm clips, non-MRI safe cochlear implants) |
| • identifies calcific stones | • better determines involvement of the facial nerve and parapharyngeal masses |
| • distinguishes cystic nature of Warthin's tumors | • Note |
| • contrast allows differentiation of vascular channels and abnormal lymph nodes | $T_1$ weighted:  enhances fat, water appears dark, $T_R$ <1000, $T_E$ <25 ms |
| | $T_2$ weighted:  enhances water, fat appears dark, $T_R$ >1000, $T_E$ >40 ms |
| | Spin Density:  $T_R$ >1000, $T_E$ <25 ms |

- associated with gout (uric acid calculi)
- <u>Pathophysiology</u>: change in the viscosity of the saliva, injury to epithelial ductal system, salivary stagnation (dehydration) causes calcium phosphate and calcium carbonate precipitation resulting in obstruction
- <u>SSx</u>: recurrent pain, swelling, worse with meals (salivary colic)
- <u>Dx</u>: stone may be palpable, sialography (**90% of submandibular calculi are radiopaque, 90% of parotid calculi are radiolucent**, may be multiple), CT, U/S
- <u>Complications</u>: fistula, acute suppurative sialadenitis, ductal stricture
- <u>Rx</u>: gland massage, bimanual expression, transoral incision, sialodochoplasty (reconstruct duct), gland excision if recurrent or if stone is lodged within substance of the gland, (extracorporeal lithotripsy is *controversial*)

## Mumps (*see* pp. 569–570)

## Uveoparotid Fever (Heerfordt's Syndrome)

- more common in women
- <u>Pathophysiology</u>: extrapulmonary form of **sarcoidosis**, nerve dysfunction may occur secondary to local ischemia/infarct from granulomatous infiltration
- <u>SSx</u>: self-limited **uveitis, parotid enlargement, facial palsy** (50%), SNHL, malaise, fever
- <u>Dx</u>: based on clinical history and exam and evidence of sarcoidosis in salivary gland tissue
- <u>Rx</u>: corticosteroids, ocular care (artificial tears, ocular ointment at night, eye patch at night)

## Kuttner's Tumor (Chronic Sclerosing Sialadenitis)

- <u>Pathophysiology</u>: may be autoimmune mediated
- <u>SSx</u>: firm, enlargement of the submandibular gland (**mistaken as a malignancy**), may be painful
- <u>Dx</u>: biopsy (submandibular gland excision)
- <u>Histopathology</u>: chronic inflammation with destruction of acinar cells, sclerosis, "cirrhotic" changes
- <u>Rx</u>: submandibular excision for diagnosis and treatment

## Radiation Sialadenitis

- often permanent if exposed to **>40–50 Gy**
- <u>SSx</u>: xerostomia, hypogeusia, ageusia

- <u>Dx</u>: clinical exam and history of radiation exposure
- <u>Histopathology</u>: interstitial fibrosis
- <u>Rx</u>: symptomatic (pilocarpine drops, artificial saliva, frequent drinks), dental care (fluoride rinses)

## Sjögren's Syndrome (Myoepithelial Sialadenitis, Benign Lymphoepithelial Lesion)

- most common in middle-aged **women**
- <u>Pathophysiology</u>: systemic autoimmune lymphocytic infiltration of exocrine glands causing destruction
- associated with **non-Hodgkin's lymphoma**
- <u>Types</u>
  1. **Primary**: exocrine gland involvement only
  2. **Secondary**: associated with other connective tissue disorders (most commonly rheumatoid arthritis)
- <u>Other Siccalike Causes</u>: aging, medications (diuretics, anticholinergics, antihistamines, antidepressants), dehydration, hepatitis, other autoimmune disease
- <u>SSx</u>: **keratoconjunctiva sicca** (filamentary keratitis, sandy sensation in eyes), xerostomia (dental caries, dry mucosa), **intermittent bilateral parotid swelling** (atrophy at end stage of disease), fatigue, arthritis, achlorhydria, Raynaud's phenomenon, pancreatitis, myositis, anemia, glomerulonephritis, hepatosplenomegaly
- <u>Complications</u>: chronic keratoconjunctivitis, corneal ulcers, dental caries, candidal infections, dysphagia, and dysphonia
- <u>Rx</u>: artificial saliva, frequent small drinks, artificial tears, consider pilocarpine drops and oral corticosteroids for severe acute exacerbation

### Diagnosis

- <u>Clinical History  (Must Have 2 of 3)</u>: keratoconjunctiva sicca, xerostomia, or other connective tissue disease
- <u>Biopsy</u>: lip biopsy of minor salivary glands reveals lymphocytic infiltration with glandular atrophy, may consider parotid biopsy if high suspicion with negative lip biopsy
- <u>Serology</u>: ANA, RF, ESR, **SS-A**, and **SS-B** (antibodies specific for primary Sjögren's syndrome), decreased IgM (suggest higher risk of progression to malignancy)
- <u>Sialography</u>: globular, multiple contrast collections throughout gland ("pine tree" appearance)
- <u>Schirmer test</u>: evaluates tear production

## Other Causes of Salivary Gland Chronic Inflammation

- **Granulomatous Disease**: tuberculosis, atypical mycobacteria, actinomycosis (poor oral hygiene, dental caries), cat scratch fever, sarcoidosis (*see* pp. 243–244); Rx: address underlying cause
- **Secondary Chronic Inflammation**: secondary to acute sialadenitis; Rx: sialagogues, antibiotics, warm compress, massage, gland excision
- NOTE: *incisional biopsy should be avoided because of high risk of fistula formation (especially with mycobacterial infections)*

## Other Causes of Salivary Enlargement

- **Mikulicz's Syndrome**: nonautoimmune, recurrent parotid gland swelling due to nonspecific lymphocytic infiltration; common causes include amyloidosis, tuberculosis, bulimia, lymphadenitis, lead and mercury toxicity, chronic fatty infiltration from alcohol, and hypovitaminosis; Rx: address underlying cause
- **Sialadenosis**: recurrent, nontender, noninflammatory, nonneoplastic salivary gland swelling secondary to underlying **nutritional**, **endocrine**, or **metabolic** pathology (cirrhosis, diabetes, malnutrition, ovarian, thyroid, or pancreatic insufficiency) or **medications** (hypertensive medications, catecholamines, iodine-containing compounds); Rx: address underlying cause

# Salivary Gland Cysts and Minor Salivary Gland Lesions

## Benign Lymphoepithelial Cysts

- increased incidence with HIV
- may progress to pseudolymphoma
- SSx: multiple parotid cysts, asymptomatic, may be bilateral
- Dx: clinical history and exam, FNA
- Histopathology: lymphoreticular infiltrate, clusters of lymphoid tissue (germinal centers), acinar atrophy, ductal metaplasia
- Rx: aspiration (more common especially in HIV patients) or excision (superficial parotidectomy, less common), antiviral therapy in HIV may cause regression of the lesions, may also consider sclerosing agents (doxycycline)

## Mucous Retention Cysts, Mucoceles, and Ranulas

- Pathophysiology: obstruction of minor salivatory glands (may be from trauma)

- **Mucous Retention Cyst**: true cyst of the minor salivary glands (lined with epithelial layer)
- **Ranula**: mucous retention cyst of the floor of mouth, usually from the sublingual gland
- **Plunging Ranula**: ranula that extends into the cervical tissues (mylohyoid muscle) and may present as a neck mass
- **Mucocele**: not a true cyst, extravasation of mucus into soft tissue
- SSx: cystic mass on floor of mouth, lip, buccal mucosa, or minor salivary gland
- Dx: clinical history and exam, excisional biopsy
- Rx: excision or marsupialization

## Necrotizing Sialometaplasia

- **Necrotizing Sialometaplasia**: nonneoplastic, self-healing (inflammatory) process of unknown etiology of the salivary glands
- Pathophysiology: may be secondary to vascular ischemia
- SSx: asymptomatic mucosal ulceration or nodular lesion of the minor salivary glands (hard palate most common)
- Dx: excisional biopsy
- Histopathology: lobular necrosis, ductal and acinar squamous metaplasia, pseudoepitheliomatous hyperplasia may be present (**may be mistaken as a malignancy, eg, squamous cell carcinoma, or mucoepidermoid carcinoma**)
- Rx: self-limiting

# BENIGN SALIVARY GLAND TUMORS
## Introduction

- Risks: radiation (latency of 7–30 yrs); alcohol and smoking not associated with most salivary neoplasms (except Warthin's tumors)
- **Multicellular Theory**: neoplastic cells originate from their counterparts (eg, oncocytic tumors from striated duct, acinar tumors from acinar cells)
- **Bicellular Theory**: all neoplastic cells differentiate from basal cells found in excretory and intercalated ducts
- **80%** of **parotid** tumors are **benign**; **80%** of **salivary neoplasms** are located in the **parotid**
- in general, the smaller the gland the more likely malignant

## Pediatric Salivary Gland Tumors (*see* p. 608)

# Pleomorphic Adenoma
# (Benign Mixed Tumor)

## Introduction

- benign heterogeneous tumor composed of variable epithelial and myoepithelial components
- **most common salivary gland tumor** (may also be found in the respiratory tract and nasal cavity)
- slightly more common in women
- SSx: slow growing (over years), unilateral, painless, firm mass (usually toward the tail of the parotid); rarely progresses to dysphagia (pharyngeal extension), dyspnea, or hoarseness (laryngeal involvement), or facial nerve palsy; deep lobe (10%) involvement may present with intraoral swelling
- Recurrent SSx: multilobular nodules, not discrete; may arise in scar, subcutaneous tissue, deep lobe, or facial nerve sheath
- Complications: rare malignant transformation (carcinoma ex-pleomorphic adenoma and sarcoma) or "benign" metastasizing (*see* p. 89)
- Dx: clinical presentation, biopsy specimen, FNA
- Rx: surgical resection (eg, superficial or total parotidectomy [*see below*] or submandibular gland excision) with facial nerve preservation and wide margin for pseudopod extensions to prevent recurrence (>90% 10-year cure, approximately 30% recurrence rate for enucleation alone), radioresistant

## Histopathology

- Cellular Components
  1. **Myoepithelial Component**: spindle-shaped with hyperchromatic nuclei, may be more than one cell layer thick
  2. **Epithelial Component**: varied growth patterns (**trabecular, solid, cystic, papillary**)
  3. **Stromal Component**: product of myoepithelial cells (**myxoid, chondroid, fibroid, or osteoid** components)
- fibrous pseudocapsule (except minor glands)
- micropseudopod extensions

# Warthin's Tumor
# (Papillary Cystadenoma Lymphomatosum)

## Introduction

- <u>Pathophysiology</u>: entrapped lymphoid tissue (parotid is the last gland embryologically to be encapsulated), ectopic ductal epithelium that develops within intraparotid lymph nodes, or hypersensitivity disease resulting in metaplasia of the duct
- **second most common** salivary gland tumor
- almost exclusively found in **middle-aged to elderly men**, smoking association
- rarely presents outside parotid gland
- **10% bilateral** (synchronous or metachronous), **10% multicentric**
- rare malignant transformation
- <u>SSx</u>:  slow growing, painless, cystic, compressible mass
- <u>Dx</u>:  surgical biopsy (grossly multiple cystic mass with viscous fluid), FNA (thick, turbid fluid), radiosialography (concentrates technetium-99m due to the presence of high mitochondrial content of oncocytes)
- <u>Rx</u>:  superficial or deep parotidectomy with facial nerve preservation (*see below*)

## Histopathology

- <u>Biphasic Layers</u>
  1. **Epithelial Component**:  lines papillary projections; double lining of oncocytes; inner or luminal cells, nonciliated, tall columnar nuclei at luminal aspect; outer or basal cells are round, cuboidal with vesicular nuclei
  2. **Lymphoid Component**:  mature lymphocytes with germinal centers
  3. **Mucous-Secreting Cells**
- **Oncocytic Cell**:  metaplasia (cytoplasmic alteration) of myo- or epithelial cells

# Oncocytoma (Oxyphilic Adenoma)

- rare, benign tumor exclusively of oncocytic cells (1% of salivary gland tumors)
- rare "malignant" low-grade tumor transformation
- rarely presents outside parotid gland (rare in submandibular gland)
- <u>SSx</u>:  slow growing, painless mass
- <u>Dx</u>:  surgical biopsy, radiosialography (concentrates technetium-99m due to the presence of high mitochondrial content of oncocytes), FNA

- <u>Histopathology</u>: encapsulated with sheets of **oncocytic cells** (large, disctinctly bordered metaplastic myo- or epithelial cells with granular cytoplasm from large number of mitochondria)
- <u>Rx</u>: superficial or deep parotidectomy with facial nerve preservation (*see below*)

# Monomorphic Adenoma

## Introduction

- similar to pleomorphic except no mesenchymal stromal component: **predominantly an epithelial component** or (rarely) the myoepithelial component
- more common in the minor salivary glands (upper lip)
- 12% bilateral
- rare malignant potential
- <u>Dx</u>: surgical specimen
- <u>Rx</u>: surgical resection

### Types

- **Basal Cell Adenoma**: predominately basaloid cells with different subtypes (solid [most common], trabecular [ribbonlike pattern], tubular, and membranous)
- **Canalicular Adenoma**: more common in the minor salivary glands (upper lip), microscopically presents as single-layer columnar or cuboidal cells forming ductlike structures with a fibrous stroma
- **Myoepithelioma**: predominately myoepithelial cells, presents with three distinct patterns of growth (spindle cell [most common], plasmacytoid, and combination of both)
- **Clear Cell Adenoma**:  must evaluate for metastatic renal primary
- **Membranous Adenoma**
- **Glycogen-Rich Adenoma**

# Hemangioma

## Introduction

- benign tumor of endothelial origin
- usually discovered a few weeks after birth, enlarge for 6–12 months, but typically regress by second year of life
- 50% parotid hemangiomas are associated with cutaneous hemangiomas

- cutaneous hemangiomas may present anywhere in the head and neck, also common in the parotid, oral cavity (lip), and larynx
- <u>Complications of Head and Neck Hemangioma</u>: cosmetic deformity, ulceration, infection, bleeding, airway compromise (laryngeal), thrombocytopenia, and high output cardiac failure (rare)
- **Vascular Malformations:** differ from hemangiomas in that they are present at birth, enlarge proportionately with growth, rarely involute spontaneously, and become more apparent; common types include port wine stains, arterial malformations, and venous malformations

### Capillary Hemangioma

- more common
- constant shape, enlarges in proportion to growth of child
- <u>SSx</u>: lobulated, dark red and bluish mass overlying skin
- <u>Histology</u>: unencapsulated, capillary-sized vessels, may invade facial nerve (rare)
- <u>Rx</u>: typically observe (await regression), no universal treatment; may consider ablative or reduction management in select lesions that threaten function (airway compromise), cosmetic deformity, or can easily be removed; common treatment includes corticosteroids, laser photocoagulation (superficial or interstitial laser therapy), and surgical excision (with or without preoperative embolization); cryotherapy, sclerotherapy, and antifibrinolytic agents have been considered with variable efficacy

### Cavernous Hemangioma

- may enlarge rapidly
- less chance of regression than capillary hemangiomas (although 60% spontaneously resolve by 4–6 years old)
- <u>Rx</u>: similar to capillary hemangiomas; however, may be treated more aggressively as less likely to regress

# SALIVARY GLAND MALIGNANCY

## Introduction

- <u>SSx</u>: typically presents as a solitary nodule, malignancy suggested by facial nerve involvement, pain, trismus, fixed to soft tissue, and cervical lymphadenopathy
- <u>Dx</u>: preoperative FNA is often utilized to counsel patient of risk of facial nerve involvement and malignancy, confirmation must be determined by a superficial parotidectomy (incisional biopsies are

**contraindicated** due to the possibility of tumor seeding and violation of tumor margins)
- Poor Prognostic Indicators: submandibular gland involvement (parotid gland more favorable), parapharyngeal space involvement, high-grade tumors, larger size, facial nerve or skin involvement, pain, recurrence, regional lymph nodes, distant metastasis (more common in adenoid cystic and undifferentiated tumors)

# Malignant Salivary Gland Tumors

## Mucoepidermoid Carcinoma

- Features: **epidermoid** and **mucinous** components with intermediate cells, high- and low-grade tumors
- **most common salivary gland malignancy in children and adults** (adenoid cystic carcinoma is the most common in the submandibular gland)
- most commonly found in the parotid (also found commonly on the palate)
- commonly induced by radiation
- 30–70% overall regional metastatic potential

### *Types and Management*

#### Low-Grade (Well-Differentiated)

- Histopathology: **more mucinous cystic elements,** aggregates of mucoid cells with strands of epithelial cells, positive keratin staining
- approximately 70% 5-year survival
- Rx: salivary gland excision (superficial or total parotidectomy [deep lobe involvement], submandibular gland excision), neck dissection for clinically positive nodes only

#### High-Grade (Poorly-Differentiated)

- Histopathology: less mucinous elements, **more solid nests of cells,** requires mucin staining to differentiate from squamous cell carcinoma, positive keratin staining
- aggressive (<50% 5-year survival)
- Rx: salivary gland excision (superficial or total parotidectomy [deep lobe involvement], submandibular gland excision) with **elective neck dissection** (selective supraomohyoid neck dissection); neck dissection for clinically positive nodes; consider adjuvant radiation therapy for advanced tumors, regional disease, close or near surgical margins, or bone or neural involvement

## Adenoid Cystic Carcinoma (Cylindroma)

- <u>Features</u>:  high-grade tumor, aggressive, **insidious** growth (over several years), **perineural spread** (facial paralysis), local recurrence and distant metastasis (may present >5 years later)
- **most common submandibular and minor gland malignancy**
- <u>SSx</u>: solitary mass, however, tumor has a higher incidence of presenting with pain or facial nerve paralysis
- <u>Histopathology</u>: **low-grade** associated with **cribriform** (nests of cells with round spaces, "Swiss cheese" appearance) or **cylindromatous** (tubular pattern) pattern, **high-grade** associated with more **solid** pattern (dense cellular pattern with few spaces)
- <u>Prognosis</u>: high-grade associated with poor prognosis (<20% 5-year survival), low-grade up to 100% 5-year survival
- <u>Rx</u>: radical surgical resection (facial nerve resection may be considered), consider adjunctive radiation therapy (or neutron beam); long-term follow-up required because of indolent course and possible distant metastasis, elective neck dissection usually not indicated (rare cervical node involvement)

## Acinic Cell Carcinoma

- <u>Features</u>: **low-grade**, better prognosis (63–87% 10-year survival)
- second most common salivary gland cancer in pediatrics
- 3% bilateral
- most commonly found in the parotid (serous acinar cells)
- <u>Histopathology</u>: serous acinar cells or clear cytoplasm cells, several configurations (microcystic, papillary, solid, follicular), lymphoid infiltrate
- <u>Rx</u>: surgical excision with wide margins, neck dissection for positive nodes only, adjuvant radiation therapy may be considered for advanced disease

## Malignant Mixed Tumors

- <u>Features</u>:  high-grade tumor, aggressive, explosive growth rate, poor prognosis (<50% 5-year survival)
- <u>Rx</u>: surgical excision with postoperative radiation therapy, may consider elective neck dissection (supraomohyoid)

### Types

- **Carcinoma Ex-Pleomorphic Adenoma**: 2–3% malignant transformation from pleomorphic adenomas, **carcinoma components only** (arises from epithelial component)

- **Metastasizing Mixed Tumor**: distinct from carcinoma ex-pleomorphic, remains histologically benign
- **Carcinosarcoma**: contains components of both carcinomas and sarcomas
- **Noninvasive Carcinoma**: carcinoma in situ within a pleomorphic adenoma

## Other Salivary Gland Malignancy Types

- **Squamous Cell Carcinoma**: high-grade, aggressive, often not the primary (must evaluate for primary)
- **Lymphomas**: rare as a primary site although may arise from intraglandular lymphoid tissue (from embryonic development), associated with Sjögren's syndrome (*see* p. 80)
- **Adenocarcinoma**: high-grade, aggressive, originates from terminal tubules or intercalated ducts
- **Clear Cell Carcinoma (Glycogen-Rich Carcinoma)**: rare low-grade tumors that occur most frequently in the minor salivary glands of the palate or the parotid
- **Malignant Oncocytoma**: similar to the benign form with distant metastasis and local invasion
- **Epithelial-Myoepithelial Carcinoma**: low-grade tumor, mostly in parotid
- **Salivary Duct Carcinoma**: high-grade, similar to ductal carcinoma of the breast
- **Undifferentiated Carcinoma**: highly aggressive, worst prognosis, predominantly "small cell"

# PAROTIDECTOMY

## Superficial Parotidectomy

- <u>Indication</u>: diagnostic and therapeutic excision of benign or malignant tumors that involve the superficial lobe of the parotid only
- typically preserves facial nerve
- resects majority of parotid gland lateral to facial nerve (controversy on amount of parotid required for removal)

### Facial Nerve Markers

1. **Tragal Pointer**: the facial nerve may be located 1 cm anterior, inferior, and deep from tragal cartilage
2. **Tympanomastoid Suture Line**: the facial nerve is 6–8 mm deep to the inferior end of the tympanomastoid suture line

3. **Digastric Attachment to Digastric Ridge**: identifies the plane of the facial nerve
4. **Retrograde Dissection from Distal Branches**: may be required in select cases
5. **Stylomastoid Foramen**: may identify the main trunk
6. **Mastoidectomy**: for difficult cases (revisions), identify nerve from the vertical segment)

## Total Parotidectomy

- <u>Indications</u>: high-grade malignancy or deep lobe or facial nerve involvement
- excision of facial nerve may be indicated for malignant tumors (encasement or invasion of facial nerve)
- <u>Radical Parotidectomy</u>: includes possible mandibulectomy, petrosectomy, periglandular skin, or facial nerve, indicated for aggressive malignant disease

## Parotidectomy Complications

- **Facial Nerve Paresis/Paralysis**: iatrogenic injury should be repaired immediately (*see* pp. 431–433)
- **Hypesthesia of Greater Auricular Nerve**: usually resolves within 9 months if not deliberately transected
- **Salivary Fistula**: uncommon, usually spontaneously resolves in 2–3 weeks; <u>Rx</u>: probe wound to release fluid (aspiration), pressure dressing, surgical closure for prolonged drainage (may consider tympanic neurectomy)
- <u>Other Complications</u>: hematoma, infection, flap necrosis, trismus, seroma, and recurrence

### *Frey's Syndrome (Gustatory Sweating)*

- <u>Pathophysiology</u>: injury to the **auriculotemporal nerve** (sympathetic fibers) results in aberrant innervation of cutaneous sweat glands (which share the same neurotransmitter) by postganglionic parasympathetic fibers
- may occur up to 5 years postoperatively
- less incidence with the use of "thick" skin flaps or placement of dermal grafts or allograft under skin flap
- <u>SSx</u>: sweating and reddening of skin during meals
- <u>Management</u>
  1. **Medical Management**: antiperspirant and anticholinergic preparations (scopolamine, glycopyrrolate, diphemanil methylsulfate), Botox injections

2. **Surgical Management:** tympanic neuronectomy (Jacobson's nerve section via tympanotomy approach, *controversial*) high incidence of recurrence, interpose a sheet of fascia lata or dermis between skin and parotid gland

3. **Radiation Therapy:** reserved for failed management with severe symptoms

# CHAPTER

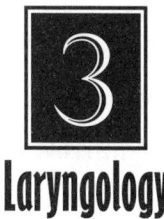

# Laryngology

Amanda Hu, James P. Dworkin, Robert J. Meleca, Robert J. Stachler,
Justin S. Golub, and Raza Pasha

# LARYNGEAL ANATOMY AND PHYSIOLOGY

## Embryology (see pp. 549–550)

## Anatomy

**Overview** (*see* Figure 7–3 *on* p. 295)

- Sites
    1. **Supraglottis**: epiglottis, aryepiglottic (A-E) folds, arytenoids, false vocal folds (vestibular or ventricular vocal folds)
    2. **Glottis**: true vocal folds
    3. **Subglottis**
- **Vestibule**: space between laryngeal inlet and false vocal folds (vestibular folds)
- **Ventricle**: space between false and true vocal folds

### Laryngeal Neuromuscular Anatomy (*see* Figure 3–1)

- Extrinsic Depressors: sternohyoid, sternothyroid, thyrohyoid, omohyoid (**strap [infrahyoid] muscles**; C1–C3)
- Extrinsic Elevators: geniohyoid (C1), digastric (CN V$_3$, VII), mylohyoid (CN V$_3$), stylohyoid (**suprahyoid muscles**; CN VII)
- **Posterior Cricoarytenoid (PCA)**: **only vocal fold ABductor** (RLN)
- **Lateral Cricoarytenoid (LCA)**: vocal fold ADductor (RLN)
- **Thyroarytenoid (TA)**: increases vocal fold tension, vocal fold ADductor, the medial aspect of the TA is called the **vocalis** (RLN)
- **Cricothyroid**: ADductor, increases vocal fold tension and length, **chief pitch-changing muscle** (**external branch of SLN**)
- **Interarytenoid**: only **unpaired** muscle, ADductor (RLN)

### Laryngeal Cartilages

- **Thyroid, Cricoid, Arytenoid**: **hyaline** cartilage (hyaline is the most common cartilage, found in most articular cartilage)
- **Epiglottis**: **fibroelastic** cartilage (less strength, has elastin), attaches to thyroid cartilage
- **Corniculate**: **fibroelastic** cartilage, **above** arytenoid cartilage, provides rigidity to A-E folds
- **Cuneiform**: **fibroelastic** cartilage, **within** A-E folds, provides rigidity
- **Triticeous**: sometimes found in **thyrohyoid ligament**, may be mistaken on x-ray as a foreign body when calcified

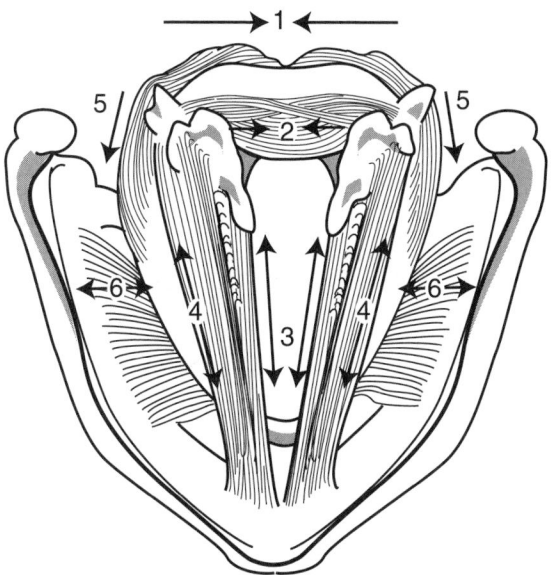

**FIGURE 3–1**. The intrinsic laryngeal muscles and their vector action: (1) posterior cricoarytenoid; (2) interarytenoid; (3) vocalis (medial aspect of thyroarytenoid); (4) thyroarytenoid; (5) lateral cricoarytenoid; (6) cricothyroid. (Adapted with permission, Icon Learning Systems, Netter Collection of Medical Illustrations, © 2005.)

## Laryngeal Joints

- **Cricothyroid Joint**: synovial, rocks (hinge)
- **Cricoarytenoid Joint**: synovial, rocks (anteromedially for vocal fold ADduction and posterolaterally for vocal fold ABduction)

## Vocal Fold Layers (*see* Figure 3–2)

- Layers from Superficial to Deep
  1. **Squamous Epithelium**: stratified, nonkeratinizing
  2. **Superficial Lamina Propria (SLP, Reinke's Space)**: loose fibrous matrix (few fibroblasts), gelatinous consistency permits fluency of vocal fold vibration (mucosal wave)
  3. **Intermediate Lamina Propria**: elastin (some fibroblasts)
  4. **Deep Lamina Propria**: fibroblasts and collagen (dense)
  5. **Thyroarytenoid Muscle Complex**: thyromuscular bundle (thyroarytenoid muscle) and thyrovocalis bundle (vocalis muscle)
- **Vocal Fold Cover**: epithelium + superficial lamina propria

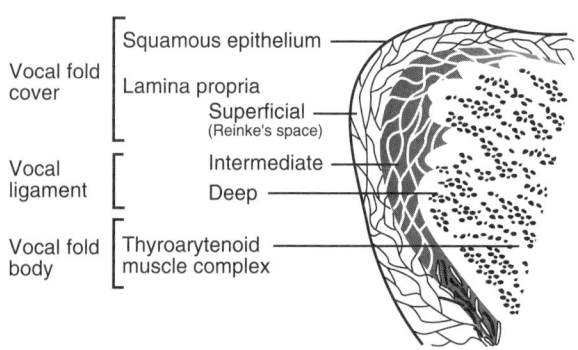

**FIGURE 3-2.** Histologic layers of the true vocal fold.

- **Vocal Ligament**: intermediate + deep lamina propria **(transition zone)**
- **Vocal Fold Body**: thyroarytenoid muscle complex
- gelatinous SLP consistency allows for fluency of vibration of the cover over the body during voicing (cover-body concept of vocal fold vibration), this vibratory activity can be visualized with stroboscopy and is referred to as the **mucosal wave**

# Physiology

## Zones of Laryngeal Airway Protection

1. **Epiglottis and A-E Folds**
2. **False Vocal Folds**
3. **True Vocal Folds**: most significant

## Laryngeal Sensory Innervation

- **Internal Branch of the SLN**: innervates laryngeal mucosa superior to the glottis
- **RLN**: innervates laryngeal mucosa inferior to the glottis
- **Negative Pressure Receptors**: SLN, maintains patency of airway during inspiration
- **Airflow Receptors**: cold receptors, stimulated from moving air
- **Drive Receptors**: proprioception
- **Laryngospasm**: exaggerated ADduction reflex caused by laryngeal irritation (reflux, foreign bodies, extubation, mucus); may be driven by the CNS, mediated by the SLN
- **Cardiovascular Collapse**: bradycardia and hypotension caused by laryngeal irritation (intubation); uncertain mechanism

# Voice Production

- **Requirements for Sound Production:** source of energy (ie, airflow from lungs) and source of vibration (ie, true vocal folds, neoglottis, articulator constrictions)
- **Myoelastic–Aerodynamic Theory:** true vocal folds are ADducted and tensed, subglottic pressure increases until level of pressure induces vocal fold vibration, which opens the glottis from an inferior to superior direction and closes from an inferior to superior direction
- **Bernoulli's Effect:** forced air across a constricted zone produces negative pressure, allowing the true vocal folds to be "sucked" back together
- normal vocal fold vibration occurs vertically from inferior to superior (not readily seen with stroboscopy), and horizontally along the superior surface of the vocal fold from medial to lateral (seen with stroboscopy)

## Components of Speech

- **Phonation:** production of voice; determined by vocal fold position, expiratory force, vibratory capacity of vocal folds, vocal fold length and tension
- **Resonation:** oral/nasal speech balance; determined by velopharyngeal musculature valving and by structure of the chest, nasopharynx, nasal cavity, and oral cavity
- **Articulation:** production of speech sounds; determined by actions of the lips, tongue, and jaw musculature activity
- **Respiration:** production of source of energy (airflow dynamics) for verbal speech; determined by inhalation/exhalation respiratory muscular activity
- **Prosody:** production of syllable stress, emphasis, and inflection patterns to provide affective speech tone; influenced by phonatory, articulatory, and respiratory forces

## Voice Parameters

- **Pitch** (Hz): perceptual term, related to **frequency** of vocal fold vibration (also Hz); determined by the length, tension, and speed of vibration of the vocal folds
- **Fundamental Frequency:** predominant pitch component of the speaking voice, **128 Hz** ("C" below middle "C" note) in males (long, thick vocal folds) and **256 Hz** (middle "C" note) in females (short, thin vocal folds)
- **Loudness** (dB): the intensity of the voice; determined by subglottic pressure, glottal resistance, airflow rate, amplitude of vocal fold vibration, and force of vocal contact

- **Quality (Timbre):** determined by the synchronicity of vocal fold vibration and glottal competence

# THE HOARSE (DYSPHONIC) PATIENT
## Evaluation

### History

- **Hoarseness (Dysphonia)**: altered vocal quality, pitch, loudness, or vocal effort that impairs communication or reduces voice-related quality of life; hoarseness is a symptom, dysphonia is a diagnosis (AAO-HNS Clinical Practice Guideline: Hoarseness. 2009.)
- Character of Hoarseness: onset and duration, time course (acute versus chronic), periodicity (morning hoarseness associated with LPR, evening hoarseness associated with vocal abuse)
- Contributing Factors: recent URI, sore throat, cough, congestion, vocal abuse, tobacco or alcohol, peripheral nerve or other neurologic disorder, LPR, hypothyroidism, psychological stressors, recent endotracheal intubation or laryngeal trauma, surgery involving the neck or RLN, radiation treatment to the neck, occupation as a high demand vocal user (singer, teacher) (AAO-HNS Clinical Practice Guideline: Hoarseness. 2009.)
- Medications That May Cause Hoarseness: warfarin, thrombolytics, phosphodiesterase-5-inhibitors (vocal fold hematoma); bisphosphonates (chemical laryngitis); ACE inhibitors (cough); danocrine, testosterone (hormonal); antipsychotics (dystonia); inhaled steroids (mucosa irritation, fungal laryngitis)
- Associated Symptoms: odynophagia, dysphagia, aspiration, weight loss, hearing loss, heartburn
- Think "KITTENS" for differential diagnosis (*see* Table 3–1)

### Physical Exam and Laryngeal Visualization

- H&N Exam: neck mass, thyroid mass, complete neurologic exam
- Assess Perceptual Quality of Voice: *see following*
- **Indirect Laryngoscopy**: visualization of the larynx through means other than a direct line of site (eg, mirrors and flexible scopes, *see following*), contrast to direct laryngoscopy (*see* p. 104); assess vocal fold mucosa for general health (color, edema, erythema, thickness, atrophy, etc), presence of masses/lesions, mechanical disturbances (immobility, hypomobility, tremor, spasmodic or muscle-tension disorders), glottis competence
- **Mirror Laryngoscopy**: angled mirror placed in oropharynx

**TABLE 3–1.** Differential Diagnosis of Dysphonia: KITTENS Method

| (K) Congenital | Infectious & Idiopathic | Toxins & Trauma | Tumor (Neoplasia) | Endocrine | Neurologic | Systemic |
|---|---|---|---|---|---|---|
| Congenital webs | Laryngitis (viral, bacterial, and fungal) | Laryngeal cysts, nodules, polyps, and ulcers | Recurrent respiratory papillomatosis | Hypothyroidism (laryngeal myxedema) | Spasmodic dysphonia | GERD |
| | Vocal fold immobility | Voice abuse | Laryngeal cancer | Adrenal, pituitary, and gonadal disorders | Tremor | Connective tissue disorders (rheumatoid arthritis, SLE) |
| | Muscle-tension disorders | Reinke's edema | Benign laryngeal masses (hemangiomas, lymphatic malformations) | Pubescence | Cerebral palsy | |
| | | Arytenoid dislocation | | | Multiple sclerosis | Psychogenic |
| | | Vocal fold granulomas | | | Extrapyramidal lesions (Parkinson's) | |
| | | Caustic inhalation injuries | | | Stroke | |
| | | | | | Guillain-Barré | |
| | | | | | Myasthenia gravis | |
| | | | | | Vocal fold paresis/paralysis | |
| | | | | | Other neurologic disorders | |

- **Flexible Nasolaryngoscopy**: traditional scopes carry image through fiber optics; newer devices (chip-tip or distal-chip) have a digital sensor (chip) on the tip of the flexible component and send the image digitally (without fiber optics) to a video display, allows for higher resolution images; also called flexible laryngoscopy, flexible nasopharyngoscopy, flexible nasopharyngolaryngoscopy
- **Stroboscopy (Videostroboscopy)**: performed through a flexible nasolaryngoscope or transoral angled rigid scope; frequency of strobe light is set near frequency of voice to produce a slow-motion effect for assessing vocal fold mucosal wave abnormalities
- **High-Speed Laryngeal Video**: captures thousands of frames (images) per second, video then played in slow motion to examine mucosal wave, newer and more expensive than stroboscopy
- AAO-HNS guideline recommends laryngoscopy when: (1) hoarseness does not resolve after 3 months of onset, or (2) if serious underlying cause is suspected (eg, tobacco or alcohol use, concomitant neck mass, trauma, hemoptysis, dysphagia, odynophagia, otalgia, airway compromise, accompanying neurologic symptoms, unexplained weight loss, worsening hoarseness, immunocompromise, possible aspiration of foreign body, neonatal hoarseness, after intubation or neck surgery) (AAO-HNS Clinical Practice Guideline: Hoarseness. 2009)

### *Perceptual Voice Abnormalities*

- **Abnormally High Fundamental Frequency:** may be due to tension-producing vocal fold mass, muscle tension phenomenon, protracted pubescence
- **Abnormally Low Fundamental Frequency:** consider load-producing vocal fold mass (Reinke's edema, growths) or hypothyroidism (laryngeal myxedema)
- **Abnormally Loud Voice:** may be secondary to sensorineural hearing loss, hyperfunction (muscle tension dysphonia), excessive respiratory efforts, or psychogenic disorder
- **Abnormally Soft Voice:** may be secondary to conductive hearing loss, reduced respiratory effort, glottic incompetence, vocal fold mass, vocal fold immobility, vocal fold bowing defect, or psychogenic disorder
- **Dysphonia:** consider vocal fold mass, vocal fold immobility, vocal fold bowing defect, muscle-tension abnormalities, vocal fold swelling, or psychogenic
- **Diplophonia:** two simultaneous pitches, may be due to recruitment of false vocal folds during phonation or the presence of an asymmetric mass (eg, unilateral vocal fold polyp or cyst)
- **Harshness:** strained or strangled; may be from upper motor neuron dysarthria (spastic), adductor spasmodic dysphonia, psychogenic,

muscle-tension abnormalities, or a compensatory result from an underlying vocal fold mass

- **Tremor:** suggests organic vocal tremor (extrapyramidal system), spasmodic dysphonia, or psychogenic
- **Breathiness:** excessive airflow from a longer "open phase" or incomplete ADduction; may be from a glottal chink (mass effect), bowed deformity secondary to vocal fold immobility, presbylaryngis, glottic lesions, muscle-tension dysfunction, abductor spasmodic dysphonia, or a psychogenic disorder
- **Arrest of Phonation:** sudden stops; consider spasmodic dysphonia, load-bearing vocal fold mass, muscle-tension disorders, psychogenic
- **Aphonia:** complete absence of phonated sound; often a functional disorder (psychogenic), bilateral ADductor vocal fold immobility, mass that results in an open glottis
- **Stridor:** may be due to bilateral vocal fold immobility, obstructing vocal fold mass, laryngospasm, paradoxical vocal fold motion disorder, or psychogenic
- **Hypernasality:** suggests velopharyngeal incompetence (flaccid or spastic dysarthria, anatomic defects)
- **Hyponasality:** may be secondary to adenoid or tonsilar hyperplasia, sinonasal disease, nasal obstruction (septal deformities, nasal masses), or nasopharyngeal mass

## Ancillary Tests

- **Acoustic Analysis:** measures of fundamental frequency, **pitch** period fluctuations or **jitter** (normal = 0.40%), **amplitude** fluctuations or **shimmer** (normal = 0.50 dB), and harmonic-to-noise ratio (normal = 11 dB)
- **Speech Aerodynamic Studies:** measures of mean transglottal airflow rate (normal = 100 mL/sec), glottal resistance (normal = 30–50 cm $H_2O$/lps), subglottal pressure (normal = 6–8 cm $H_2O$)
- **Perceptual Testing**: rating of voice features by an expert listener, utilizes numeric scoring system
- Perceptual Tests
  1. **GRBAS**: individually rates **G**rade, **R**oughness, **B**reathiness, **A**sthenia, and **S**train (0 = normal to 3 = severe)
  2. **CAPE-V** (**C**onsensus **A**uditory-**P**erceptual **E**valuation of **V**oice): visual analog scale that individually rates overall severity, roughness, breathiness, strain, pitch, and loudness
- **Laryngeal EMG:** *see* p. 120
- **Glottography:** measures light transillumination during vibration and degree of vocal fold contact (eg, open quotient [duration vocal folds are open over the length of the glottic cycle], speed quotient

[duration of glottal opening over glottal closure], and shift quotient [time of peak opening over duration of glottal opening])
- **CT/MRI:** may reveal mass lesion in larynx or along course of recurrent or superior laryngeal nerve, AAO-HNS guideline recommends first visualizing the larynx before obtaining a CT or MRI to avoid unnecessary testing

## Treatment

- treat the underlying cause when discovered
- <u>AAO-HNS Guideline Statements for Treatment of Hoarseness</u> (AAO-HNS Clinical Practice Guideline: Hoarseness. 2009.)
  1. recommend against prescribing antireflux meds without signs/symptoms of acid reflux
  2. option of providing antireflux meds for hoarseness with signs of chronic laryngitis
  3. recommend against routinely prescribing oral corticosteroids
  4. strongly recommend against routinely prescribing antibiotics
  5. recommend laryngoscopy before prescribing voice therapy and document/communicate results to speech pathology
  6. strongly recommend voice therapy for reduced voice-related QOL
  7. recommend surgery for suspected laryngeal malignancy, benign laryngeal soft tissue lesions, glottic insufficiency
  8. option of education/counseling about control/preventive measures

# UPPER AIRWAY OBSTRUCTION

## Evaluation of Stridor

### Initial Management (ABCs)

- **Evaluate Airway:** quickly determine severity and stability of airway (acute versus chronic, progression of stridor, dyspnea at rest versus with exercise)
- **Establish Airway:** *see* pp. 628–629 for complete protocol in establishing an airway
- room air consists of 21% oxygen ($FiO_2$ = 0.21), 78% nitrogen, 1% other
- **Administer Oxygen:** masked ventilation may adequately improve oxygenation until able to secure airway; after establishing a secure airway, ease of ventilation and maintenance of oxygenation should be evaluated (*see* Table 3–2)

**TABLE 3–2.** Types of oxygen-delivery masks

| Device | Oxygen Flow (L/min) | FiO$_2$ |
|---|---|---|
| Room air | N/A | 0.21 |
| **Low Flow** | | |
| Nasal cannula | 1–6 | 0.24–0.44 |
| Simple face mask | 5–10 | 0.30–0.60 |
| Partial rebreather mask | 8–12 | 0.40–0.70 |
| Non-rebreather mask | 10–15 | 0.60–0.80 |
| **High Flow** | | |
| Venturi mask | 4–12 | 0.24–0.50 |

- **Heliox:** may be considered for short-term oxygenation for stable airway obstructions; 80% helium, 20% oxygen (may increase O2 concentration to 40%); helium has a lower molecular weight (decreased density) allowing passage past narrow obstruction
- consider humidification, corticosteroids, nebulized racemic epinephrine, and antibiotics

## History and Physical Exam

- <u>Character of Upper Airway Sounds</u>: determine respiratory phase of stridor versus stertor *(see following),* onset and duration, constant versus intermittent
- <u>Contributing Factors</u>: recent URI, fever, cough, sore throat, allergy; recent trauma, caustic ingestion, previous tracheotomy, intubations or airway manipulations, surgeries; medications (medicine allergies, ACE inhibitors); history of sarcoidosis, connective tissue disorders, granulomatous diseases (Wegener's, TB), asthma, cardiac and pulmonary problems
- <u>Associated Symptoms</u>: dysphagia, drooling, hoarseness, airway bleeding, weight loss, odynophagia, cough (barking cough), sleep pattern (snoring, daytime somnolence), choking (LPR, foreign body), feeding difficulties (regurgitation, worse with feeding)
- <u>Flexible Nasolaryngoscopy/Mirror Exam</u>: always have low threshold to scope; assess airway patency, vocal fold mobility, supraglottis; examine tracheal stoma if present (retroflex to access subglottis)
- <u>Nasal Exam</u>: nasal endoscopy, nasoseptal deformities, nasal masses, nasal congestion, may attempt to pass #6 catheter through both nares to assess patency

- <u>Complete H&N PE</u>: oral cavity (macroglossia, tonsillar hyperplasia or infection), complete neurologic exam (cranial nerves), evaluate for external compression (trachea midline, goiter, palpable laryngeal fractures), cutaneous lesions (hemangiomas)
- cardiac and pulmonary H&P (wheezing, chest pain, retractions, cyanosis)
- think "KITTENS" for differential diagnosis (*see* Table 3–3)

### *Description of Upper Airway Sound by Site of Obstruction*

- <u>Nasopharyngeal</u>: **stertor** (snoring), no cough
- <u>Oropharynx</u>: gurgly
- <u>Supraglottic</u>: **inspiratory** stridor, throaty voice, **feeding problems**
- <u>Glottic</u>: **inspiratory** or **biphasic** stridor, hoarseness
- <u>Subglottic</u>: husky voice, **biphasic** stridor, **barking cough**
- <u>Tracheobronchial</u>: **expiratory** stridor, wheezing, suprasternal retractions indicate obstruction above thoracic inlet

## Endoscopy

- **Flexible Nasolaryngoscopy**: *see previous*
- **Direct Laryngoscopy (DL)**: evaluation and instrumentation of the glottis and supraglottis in the OR via a *direct line of site* (distinguishes from indirect laryngoscopy, *see* p. 98); addition of optical **rigid telescopes (rigid endoscope, rod lens, Hopkins rod)** allows magnified view and assessment of subglottis and trachea; addition of **microscope** allows 3D view and two-handed operating; **suspension** refers to spatial fixation of the hollow metal laryngoscope; terms may be combined in a variety of ways, such as suspension microlaryngoscopy (SML) or microdirect laryngoscopy (MDL)
- **Bronchoscopy**: **flexible bronchoscopy** allows identification of severity and location of stenosis, **rigid bronchoscopy** allows instrumentation and management of an emergency airway crisis

## Ancillary Tests

- **CXR and Neck X-rays:** screening for laryngotracheal structural defects, intrinsic lung and mediastinal disease
- **CT/MRI Neck:** evaluate location, extent, or compression of stenosis; also evaluates destruction of local laryngeal structures
- **Modified Barium Swallow (MBS, MBSS, Videofluoroscopic Swallow Study, VFSS) and Esophagram:** examine esophageal pathology, LPR, aspiration, and vascular abnormalities
- **Pulmonary Function Tests and Flow-Volume Loops:** identify level of obstruction and assess for intrinsic lung disease

**TABLE 3–3.** Differential Diagnosis of Upper Airway Obstruction: KITTENS Method

| | (K) Congenital | Infectious & Idiopathic | Toxins & Trauma | Tumor (Neoplasia) | Endocrine | Neurologic | Systemic/Psychiatric |
|---|---|---|---|---|---|---|---|
| **Above Larynx** | Micrognathia Macroglossia Choanal atresia Lingual thyroid Nasoseptal deformity | Retropharyngeal abscess Peritonsillar abscess Mononucleosis Diphtheria | Facial fracture Retropharyngeal hematoma | Juvenile nasopharyngeal angiofibroma Neurogenic nasal tumors | Myxedema | Posteriorly displaced tongue Central sleep apnea | Allergic rhinitis Granulomatosis with polyangiitis (Wegener's) Obesity (obstructive sleep apnea) |
| **Supraglottic** | Laryngomalacia | Epiglottitis | Intubation trauma | Squamous cell carcinoma | | | Sarcoidosis |
| **Glottic** | Glottic web Laryngeal atresia Vocal fold immobility | TB laryngitis Laryngeal diphtheria | Laryngeal fracture Foreign body | Respiratory papillomatosis Squamous cell carcinoma | | Vocal fold paralysis | Hereditary angioedema |
| **Subglottic** | Vascular ring and aortic arch anomalies Tracheoesophageal fistula Subglottic stenosis | LTB (Croup) | Subglottic stenosis Thyroid or neck masses (extrinsic compression) | Subglottic hemangioma | | Respiratory muscle paralysis (eg, Guillain-Barré syndrome) | Granulomatosis with polyangiitis (Wegener's) |
| **Tracheobronchial** | Tracheomalacia Vascular rings | Tracheitis Bronchitis | Foreign body | Mediastinal, tracheal, or bronchial tumors | | | External compression (goiter) Asthma |

- **Airway Fluoroscopy:** dynamic evaluation of airway, assess vocal fold motion
- **Arteriography:** if vascular abnormalities are suspected
- **Labs:** ABG, CBC, electrolytes

# Tracheotomy

## Introduction

- *see pp. 551–552 for pediatric tracheotomy*

### Terminology

- **Tracheotomy:** the incision (cut) in the trachea
- **Tracheostomy:** the opening between the trachea and the external world, derived from the Greek "stoma" (mouthlike opening), some reserve this for a more permanent opening
- these two terms have been used interchangeably in the literature
- **Tracheostomy Tube:** the tube placed through the tracheal opening
- **Trach**: colloquial term for all the above related terms
- **Cricothyroidotomy:** an incision in the cricothyroid membrane (typically employed during an airway emergency)

### Tracheotomy Indications

- bypass upper airway obstruction (eg, sleep apnea, tumor)
- prevent complications from prolonged intubation (eg, mucosal ulceration, laryngeal stenosis, granulomas) and allow mechanical ventilation long term
- assist with tracheal–bronchial suctioning (pulmonary hygiene/toilet)
- provide protection from gross aspiration
- eliminate dead space (eg, to promote weaning from a ventilator, in neuromuscular disorders)

### Tracheotomy Complications

- <u>Intraoperative Complications</u>: vessel injury (hemorrhage), pneumothorax, pneumomediastinum, damage to the tracheoesophageal common wall
- <u>Immediate Postoperative Complications</u>: postoperative pulmonary edema from release of pressure (<u>Rx</u>: positive pressure ventilation), acute obstruction (mucus plug, blood clot), tracheostomy tube displacement (airway loss can occur if tube not secured well), infection
- <u>Long-Term Complications</u>: tracheal/subglottic stenosis, granulation tissue, tracheal-innominate artery fistula, tracheitis

## Tracheotomy Management

- (based on AAO-HNS Clinical Consensus Statement: Tracheostomy Care. 2012)

### Tracheotomy Care

- **Prevent Tube Dislodgement:** especially for first several days to prevent accidental airway loss; suture tube to neck skin, tight tracheostomy tube ties (unless free flap)
- **Tube Replacement:** all supplies to replace accidentally dislodged tube should always be at bedside (obdurator, spare tube, suction, etc); replace dislodged tube with same size or smaller, if not possible then endotracheal tube, if still not possible and airway lost then orally intubate; first planned tube change is typically performed by otolaryngology and after no fewer than 3–5 days to allow tract maturation
- **Prevent Tube Plugging: humidity** prevents tracheal crusting and mucus plugs, initially saline should also be dropped into tube every 3–4 hours, regularly clean inner cannula
- **Acute Tube Occlusion:** most likely due to mucus plug, obstructing granuloma, or tube in a false passage
- **Pulmonary Hygiene/Toilet:** tracheotomy tubes disrupt ciliary function, decrease subglottic pressure required for an adequate cough, and increase risk of microaspiration; requires regular **aseptic technique suctioning** of the tracheal airway, especially for the first few days
- **Skin Care:** consider dressings to prevent skin breakdown
- **Patient/Caregiver Education:** important pre- and postprocedure; if patient is being discharged home with tracheostomy tube, assess competency and arrange appropriate supplies

### Cuffs, Caps, Feeding, and Speaking

- **Cuff Pressure:** should be less than capillary pressure (<25 cm $H_2O$) to prevent pressure necrosis (subglottic stenosis, tracheal-innominate artery erosion, tracheomalacia), see manufacturer instructions whether to inflate with air, water, or saline
- **Cuff Deflation:** keep cuff inflated for at least one day to reduce aspiration in event of bleeding, deflate when no longer mechanically ventilated or aspirating, suction just prior to deflation
- **Tube Capping:** placement of an occlusive cap prevents air flow through the tube and requires breathing around tube through mouth/nose, **never cap with inflated cuff** (no airway), consider change to cuffless tube before capping to prevent accidental capping with inflated cuff, patient must know how to self-remove cap

- **Feeding and Speaking:** feeding (especially solids) difficult while cuff inflated, capping tube (with cap or finger) or speaking valve facilitates speech and swallowing
- **Speaking/Swallowing Valve**: eg, Passy-Muir; one-way valve allows airflow through trach tube during inspiration only; during expiration valve closes and air flows through vocal folds; never use with inflated cuff

### Decannulation

- tracheostomy tubes should be removed (decannulated) as soon as possible (especially in children) to prevent long-term sequelae such as tracheal ulceration, subglottic stenosis, tracheomalacia
- prior to decannulation patient should undergo tracheostomy tube downsizing and a trial of capping (24 hours for 3–4 consecutive days without respiratory difficulties)
- original indication for tracheotomy must be resolved
- consider flexible nasolaryngoscopy (evaluate patency proximal to the tracheotomy) and tracheoscopy (through the tracheostomy, evaluate trachea to carina and evaluate subglottis via retroflexion)
- place airtight dressing to seal stoma after removal of tracheotomy tube, remind patient to apply pressure when talking/coughing

## Percutaneous Dilational Tracheotomy (PDT)

- alternative technique to conventional open tracheotomy for intubated ICU patients
- Steps: small skin incision over anterior trachea, dissect down to tracheal wall, under bronchoscopic guidance insert needle into tracheal lumen, through needle cannulate trachea with flexible wire; using Seldinger technique pass serial dilators over wire, place tracheostomy tube
- Indications: easily palpable anterior neck anatomy, intubated patient, ability to extend neck
- Contraindications: difficult or emergent airway, inability to palpate cricoid cartilage and trachea, obesity, nonintubated patient, children, inability to extend neck, spine disease, neck immobilization, neck mass, recent neck surgery, neck soft tissue infection, superior vena cava syndrome, uncorrectable coagulopathy, hemodynamic instability, high peak airway pressure (>20 cm $H_2O$)

# BENIGN LARYNGEAL PATHOLOGY
## Congenital Laryngeal Defects (see pp. 554–559)

## Laryngitis
### Acute Viral Laryngitis
- <u>Pathogens</u>: **rhinovirus** (most common), parainfluenza, respiratory syncytial virus, adenovirus, influenza virus, pertussis
- <u>SSx</u>: dysphonia, low-grade fever, hoarseness, cough, rhinitis, postnasal drip
- <u>Dx</u>: H&P
- <u>Rx</u>: conservative management (hydration, antipyretics, voice rest, decongestants, humidification, smoking cessation), antibiotics not indicated unless suspect secondary bacterial infection

### Pediatric Epiglottitis (*see* p. 562)

### Adult Supraglottitis (Adult Epiglottitis)
- <u>Pathophysiology</u>: typically secondary to purulent rhinosinusitis or tracheobronchitis
- <u>Common Pathogens</u>: *H. influenzae* (classic pediatric disease), *S. pneumoniae, S. aureus,* ß-hemolytic *Streptococcus*
- <u>SSx</u>: fever, muffled voice, dysphagia, stridor (inspiratory), **obstructive symptoms may progress within hours**
- <u>Dx</u>: lateral neck x-ray, mirror laryngoscopy or flexible nasolaryngoscopy
- <u>Rx</u>
  1. evaluate airway, severe and progressive symptoms may require intubation over a flexible scope versus an urgent surgical airway
  2. humidification, hydration, corticosteroids, antireflux medications
  3. parenteral antibiotics

### Laryngotracheobronchitis (Croup) (*see* pp. 560–561)

### Bacterial Tracheitis (Membranous Laryngotracheobronchitis, MLTB) (*see* pp. 561–562)

# Diphtheria (*see* p. 562)

# Laryngopharyngeal Reflux (LPR)

- *see also* pp. 194–196
- Pathophysiology: inflammatory response of laryngeal mucosa from **laryngopharyngeal acid reflux** and, less commonly, nonacid reflux
- SSx: hoarseness (worse in the morning), choking spells at night, regurgitation, bitter taste in mouth, globus sensation, cough, chronic throat clearing, postprandial heartburn (seen <50% of the time in LPR)
- Laryngeal Findings: erythema and edema of the posterior commissure, arytenoids, superior surface of the vocal folds, and laryngeal surface of the epiglottis; diffuse supraglottic edema; laryngeal pachydermia (interarytenoid); granulomas of the vocal process
- for diagnosis and management *see* pp. 195–196
- validated clinical tools include the **Reflux Symptom Index (RSI)**, a self-administered symptom questionnaire, and the **Reflux Finding Score (RFS)** based on laryngoscopy findings (*see* Table 3–4)

# Chronic Laryngitis

- Common Etiologies: smoking, pollution, vocal abuse, sinusitis, rhinitis, LPR
- SSx: hoarseness, pain, edema, dysphagia, respiratory compromise
- Dx: flexible nasolaryngoscopy (thick erythematous vocal folds), stroboscopy, direct laryngoscopy with biopsy to rule out malignancy
- Rx: address etiology (stop smoking, voice rehabilitation, treat rhinosinusitis, reflux regimen), humidification, mucolytics, consider short course of corticosteroids

## *Tuberculous Laryngitis*

- *see also* pp. 245–246
- typically secondary to pulmonary TB
- Histopathology: cellular inflammation, granuloma in subepithelium, perichondritis
- Lesion: granulation and ulcerative tissue in **posterior glottis** (posterior interarytenoids most common, laryngeal surface of epiglottis, vocal folds)
- Rx: isoniazid, rifampin, voice rest, narcotics for pain

TABLE 3–4. Validated Clinical Tools for Assessing Laryngopharyngeal Reflux (LPR)

**Reflux Symptom Index (RSI)**
**Belafsky et al, *J Voice*, 2002)**

9-item self-administered questionnaire regarding *symptoms* in past month
Each item graded from 0=no problem to 5=severe problem
Score ranges from 0 to 45, >13 is abnormal

1. Hoarseness or a problem with your voice
2. Clearing your throat
3. Excess throat mucus or postnasal drip
4. Difficulty swallowing food, liquids, or pills
5. Coughing after you ate or after lying down
6. Breathing difficulties or choking episodes
7. Troublesome or annoying cough
8. Sensations of something sticking in your throat or a lump in your throat
9. Heartburn, chest pain, indigestion, or stomach acid coming up

**Reflux Finding Score (RFS)**
**Belafsky et al, *Laryngoscope*, 2001)**

8-item clinical severity scale based on *flexible laryngoscopy findings*
Scale ranges from 0 to 26, >7 is abnormal

| | |
|---|---|
| 1. Subglottic edema | 0=absent, 2=present |
| 2. Ventricular obliteration | 2=partial, 4=complete |
| 3. Erythema/hyperemia | 2=arytenoids only, 4=diffuse |
| 4. Vocal fold edema | 1=mild, 2=moderate, 3=severe, 4=polypoid |
| 5. Diffuse laryngeal edema | 1=mild, 2=moderate, 3=severe, 4=obstructing |
| 6. Posterior commissure hypertrophy | 1=mild, 2=moderate, 3=severe, 4=obstructing |
| 7. Granuloma/granulation tissue | 0=absent, 2=present |
| 8. Thick endolaryngeal mucus | 0=absent, 2=present |

## Syphilitic Laryngitis

- *see also* pp. 244–245
- rare manifestation of oropharyngeal syphilis
- <u>Secondary Stage SSx</u>: temporary mild edema, **painless**
- <u>Tertiary Stage SSx</u>: **gummas** may break down cartilage
- <u>Rx</u>: penicillin, tetracycline, erythromycin

## Rhinoscleroma (Scleroma) of Larynx

- *see also* pp. 41–42
- <u>Pathogen</u>: *Klebsiella rhinoscleromatis*
- <u>Histopathology</u>: pseudoepitheliomatous hyperplasia of the larynx (similar to blastomycosis)
- <u>Rx</u>: long-term antibiotics as dictated by culture and sensitivity

### *Leprosy (Hansen's Disease)*

- *see also* p. 247
- <u>Pathogen</u>: *Mycobacterium leprae*
- <u>Lesion</u>: ulcerative lesions in the supraglottis
- <u>Dx</u>: biopsy (foamy leprous cells containing the bacillus), nasal smear
- <u>Rx</u>: dapsone (diaminodiphenylsulfone), corticosteroids

## Chondritis/Perichondritis of Larynx

- <u>Causes</u>: infection (TB, syphilis, septic laryngitis), trauma, tracheotomy, radiation effect (can have **chondronecrosis**), malignancy, autoimmune (**relapsing polychondritis**, has 50% laryngeal involvement, *see* p. 386)
- most commonly involves the thyroid cartilage, rarely involves epiglottis since fibroelastic cartilage (adherent perichondrium) protects from infection
- <u>SSx</u>: insidious onset, fever, odynophagia, tenderness, hoarseness, cough, dyspnea
- <u>Dx</u>: endoscopy reveals pale mucosal edema, CT neck
- <u>Complication</u>: subperichondrial abscess, stenosis (respiratory compromise)
- <u>Rx</u>: establish airway, aggressive antibiotic regimen, I&D if abscess, consider surgical debridement of necrotic or exposed cartilage

## Fungal Laryngitis

- <u>Risks</u>: immunocompromise (diabetes, HIV, chronic corticosteroids, posttransplant, etc), radiation, poor nutrition, debilitating illnesses, long-term antibiotics
- <u>SSx</u>: odynophagia, mucositis, dysphonia, cough, dyspnea, aspiration
- <u>Dx</u>: endoscopy and biopsy (may be confused with malignancy)
- <u>Rx</u>: establish airway, antifungal regimen

### *Pathogens*

- **Candidiasis** (**Moniliasis**): adherent, friable, cheesy, white plaques; spread from oral cavity (*see also* p. 208)
- **Aspergillosis**: allergic, noninvasive, or invasive forms (*see also* pp. 49–50)
- **Blastomycosis**: **red laryngeal ulcers** or **miliary nodules on vocal fold** (*see also* p. 246)
- **Histoplasmosis**: ulcerative lesions in larynx (anterior larynx and epiglottis) (*see also* p. 246)
- **Coccidiomycosis**: nodular laryngeal mass (*see also* p. 247)

# Benign Laryngeal Tumors

## Recurrent Respiratory Papillomatosis (RRP)
(*see* pp. 563–564)

## Chondroma

- more common in men
- Pathophysiology: most commonly arises from internal **posterior cricoid cartilage** (hyaline cartilage); may also arise from thyroid, arytenoid, epiglottic cartilage (fibroelastic cartilage)
- SSx: insidious hoarseness from vocal fold restriction, dyspnea from subglottic lesions, dysphagia from posterior cricoid lesions, globus sensation
- Lesion: smooth, firm, fixed tumor, normal mucosa
- Dx: endoscopic wedge biopsy, CT neck (calcification)
- Rx: complete excision via endoscopic or external approach (depending on the size of lesion)

## Granular Cell Tumor (Granular Cell Myoblastoma)

- 3% risk of malignant degeneration
- Pathophysiology: arise from Schwann cells in the posterior aspect of true vocal fold or arytenoids (originally believed to arise from myoblasts); may also be found on tongue, skin, breast, and subcutaneous tissue
- SSx: insidious hoarseness
- Lesion: small, sessile, gray mass
- Dx: endoscopy with biopsy
- Histopathology: may induce **pseudoepitheliomatous hyperplasia** near epithelial borders (often **confused with squamous cell carcinoma**), polygonal uniform cells with vesicular nucleus, coarsely cytoplasmic eosinophilic granules, PAS and S-100 positive
- Rx: complete excision via endoscopic or external approach (depending on size of lesion)

## Vascular Malformations and Vascular Tumors
(*see* pp. 535–540)

# Systemic Diseases Affecting the Larynx

## Sarcoidosis

- *see also* pp. 243–244
- <u>Laryngeal SSx</u>: supraglottic submucosal mass (epiglottis most common), dysphonia, globus sensation, dyspnea
- <u>Rx</u>: endoscopic removal for symptomatic lesions (hoarseness or airway obstruction), consider corticosteroids for significant exacerbations

## Granulomatosis with Polyangiitis (GPA, Wegener's Granulomatosis)

- *see also* pp. 249–250
- most commonly involves subglottis
- <u>Laryngeal SSx</u>: subglottic mass, dyspnea, biphasic stridor
- <u>Rx</u>: endoscopic removal for symptomatic lesions, medical management

## Amyloidosis

- *see also* pp. 212–213
- <u>Laryngeal SSx</u>: anterior subglottic mass (polypoid covered with smooth mucosa)
- <u>Rx</u>: endoscopic removal for symptomatic lesions (hoarseness or airway obstruction)

## Arthritis of Cricoarytenoid Joint

- cricoarytenoid joint mostly commonly affected
- rheumatoid arthritis most common etiology
- <u>SSx</u>: hoarseness, stridor, dysphagia, pain with swallowing
- <u>Rx</u>: corticosteroids, antireflux regimen

# Laryngeal Stenosis
## (see pp. 554–560)

# Other Laryngeal Lesions

## Laryngeal Edema

### Angioedema

- Types
  1. **Acquired Angioedema**: histamine-mediated inflammation (urticaria) secondary to a variety of substances
  2. **Congenital (Hereditary) Angioedema**: deficiency in **C1 esterase inhibitor** (controls the complement pathway)
- Common Causes of Acquired Angioedema: medications (**ACE inhibitors**, ASA, antibiotics, NSAIDs), food allergies (eggs, peanuts), insect bites, transfusions, infections (hepatitis B, viral), emotional, other allergens
- SSx: rapid onset of facial, oropharyngeal, or laryngeal edema, "hot potato voice," stertor or stridor, pruritus, hoarseness
- Dx: history, exam, flexible nasolaryngoscopy, C1 esterase inhibitor serum levels
- Rx
  1. evaluate airway, severe and progressive symptoms may require prompt intubation over flexible bronchoscope versus an urgent surgical airway
  2. epinephrine, parenteral corticosteroids, H1 and H2 blockers
  3. stop inciting medications
  4. for hereditary angioedema, C1 or kallikrein inhibitors, bradykinin receptor antagonist, FFP; danazol prophylaxis older option

### Reinke's Edema (Polypoid Degeneration, Polypoid Corditis)

- **Reinke's Space**: superficial layer of the lamina propria (SLP), loose connective tissue (susceptible to fluid accumulation)
- Risks: LPR, smoking, hypothyroidism, vocal abuse, chronic throat clearing, chronic cough
- not associated with increased risk of laryngeal cancer
- Dx: mirror laryngoscopy, flexible nasolaryngoscopy, direct laryngoscopy, stroboscopy
- Rx
  1. manage underlying conditions (hypothyroidism, LPR)
  2. voice rest
  3. smoking cessation
  4. consider microlaryngoscopy with removal of gelatinous material in Reinke's space

## Other Causes of Laryngeal Edema

- infection (*see* pp. 109–112)
- trauma (intubation)
- venous or lymphatic obstruction
- hypoproteinemia
- increased permeability secondary to connective tissue disorders, leukemia, hypothyroid myxedema

# Laryngeal Cysts

- **Vocal Fold Cyst**: subepithelial cyst, may open to free margin of vocal fold resulting in a sulcus, associated with reactive changes of opposite vocal fold; Rx: voice therapy (usually does not resolve), microflap excision (opposite vocal fold reactive changes typically resolve after removal of cyst)
- **Mucus Retention Cyst**: minor salivary gland cyst, **supraglottic lesion**, may be obstructive (especially in children); Rx: endoscopic laser excision or marsupialization
- **Branchial Cleft Cyst**: *see* pp. 599–600
- **Ventricular Prolapse**: not a cyst, laryngeal ventricle protrudes between true and false vocal folds, associated with chronic bronchitis; Rx: endoscopic excision

## Acquired Subglottic Cysts

- Pathophysiology: obstruction of mucous glands by endotracheal tube (requires less trauma than intubation granuloma)
- SSx: **postextubation stridor occurring after short-term intubation**, cyst in lateral subglottis
- Dx: flexible nasolaryngoscopy, stroboscopy, direct laryngoscopy
- Rx: endoscopic excision (laser)

## Laryngocele and Saccular Cyst

- **Laryngocele**: air-filled dilation of the appendix of the ventricle, communicates with laryngeal lumen
- **Laryngopyocele**: infected pus-filled laryngocele
- **Saccular Cyst**: fluid-filled dilation of the saccule (blind sac in ventricle) without communication with the laryngeal lumen
- Pathophysiology: congenital or acquired expansion from increased intraglottic pressure of laryngeal saccule
- Laryngocele Types
  1. **External**: laryngocele sac protrudes through thyrohyoid membrane presenting as a neck mass

2. **Internal**: laryngocele sac remains within thyroid cartilage, less common
3. **Combined**
- SSx: lateral compressible mass that increases in size with intralaryngeal pressure (external), or cough and hoarseness (internal)
- Dx: mirror laryngoscopy, flexible nasolaryngoscopy, stroboscopy, direct laryngoscopy, CT neck
- Complications: secondary infection, malignant potential, airway obstruction
- Rx: marsupialization, complete endoscopic removal (laser) for internal laryngoceles, open approach for external laryngoceles

## Presbylaryngis

- Pathophysiology: aging results in ossification of the laryngeal skeleton, arthritis of the cricoarytenoid and cricothyroid joints, degeneration of the vocal fold layers (resulting in a **bowing defect**)
- Causes: screaming, coughing, throat clearing, toxic fumes, smoking, LPR, endotracheal tube, allergy, rhinosinusitis, laryngitis
- SSx: hoarse–breathy voice, higher than normal pitch, voice fatigue, may have voice tremors, potential risk of aspiration
- Dx: mirror laryngoscopy, flexible nasolaryngoscopy, stroboscopy
- Rx: voice therapy, address aspiration if present, conservative vocal fold injection for bowing

## Vocal Fold Lesions Secondary to Vocal Abuse and Trauma

- Pathophysiology: trauma-induced dilation of vessels on superior surface of vocal folds results in reactive changes (hyperemia, edema, submucosal hemorrhage, possible scarring)
- Causes: screaming, coughing, throat clearing, toxic fumes, smoking, LPR, endotracheal tube, allergy, rhinosinusitis, laryngitis
- SSx: hoarseness, odynophagia, odynophonia
- Dx: mirror laryngoscopy, flexible nasolaryngoscopy, stroboscopy
- Rx: conservative management (speech therapy, humidification, antireflux regimen, smoking cessation, occasionally voice rest)

### Vocal Fold Contact Ulcer and Vocal Fold Granuloma

- ulceration or granulation tissue posteriorly on the **medial arytenoid near the vocal process**

- results from injury and exuberant healing process (eg, **intubation granulomas** from endotracheal intubation)
- typically self-limiting
- <u>Rx</u>: antireflux regimen, antibiotics, speech therapy, consider corticosteroids, prevent with smaller sized or earlier removal of endotracheal tube, rarely endoscopic removal (consider if symptomatic and pedunculated, avoid removal of sessile lesions)

### Vocal Fold Nodules

- colloquially called singer's nodules
- more common in young women and children
- **bilateral by definition**, thus a unilateral "vocal fold nodule" is incorrect terminology
- bilateral symmetric inflammatory tissue at **junction of anterior and middle third of vocal fold** (the middle portion of the membranous vocal fold has the greatest amplitude in the mucosal wave making it susceptible to injury with voice abuse)
- <u>Types</u>
  1. **Acute**: edematous, soft, erythematous, vascular vocal fold lesions
  2. **Chronic**: more organized fibrosis, hard, white, thickened vocal fold lesions
- <u>Rx</u>: conservative management (*as previous*), rarely endoscopic excision for failed voice therapy (avoid excision in children, high recurrence rate)

### Vocal Fold Polyp

- typically unilateral, middle, and anterior vocal folds at **free edge**
- <u>Types</u>
  1. **Mucoid**: translucent, broad-based lesion, stems from inflammation in Reinke's space
  2. **Angiomatous**: hemorrhagic (erythematous), protuberant, multinodular lesions
- <u>Rx</u>: conservative management (*as previous*), microflap excision for symptomatic lesions

## Sulcus Vocalis (Glottis Sulcus)

- more common in vocal overusers
- epithelium-lined depression (ie, sulcus) parallel to the free edge of the vocal fold
- voice often worse than expected from laryngoscopy, stroboscopy shows reduced vibration and mucosal wave, microdirect laryngoscopy may be needed to diagnose because lesion may be subtle

- <u>Types</u>
  1. **Congenital**
  2. **Acquired**: may have evolved from an epithelial cyst that spontaneously emptied, leaving a collapsed depression
- <u>Rx</u>: conservative management (*as previous*), surgical management is difficult as it may significantly disrupt the vocal fold mucosa, excising removes the whole invaginated mucosal pocket without damaging the underlying vocal ligament

# NEUROGENIC AND OTHER VOCAL PATHOLOGIES

## Vocal Fold Immobility (Paralysis)

### Evaluation of Vocal Fold Immobility

#### *Terminology*

- **Immobility**: nonmovement of vocal fold from *any cause* (eg, neurologic or mechanical)
- **Hypomobility**: *partial* nonmovement of vocal fold from *any cause* (eg, neurologic or mechanical)
- **Paralysis**: nonmovement of vocal fold from *neurologic* cause (eg, RLN injury)
- **Paresis**: *partial* nonmovement of vocal fold from *neurologic* cause (eg, RLN injury)

#### *History and Physical Exam*

- <u>Unilateral Vocal Fold Immobility SSx</u>: hoarse–breathy dysphonia, aspiration, stridor in children, dysphagia, limited phonation time, vocal fatigue, may be asymptomatic
- <u>Bilateral Vocal Fold Immobility SSx</u>: inspiratory or biphasic stridor, weak cry, aspiration, hoarseness (voice may be normal)
- <u>Contributing Factors</u>: recent URI, cough; previous neck trauma, toxin exposure, surgery (cardiothoracic, thyroid), or airway manipulation; history of tobacco or alcohol abuse; history of cancer, cardiopulmonary disease, peripheral nerve disease and other neurologic disorders, diabetes; neonatal history (complications, birth trauma, maternal infections, congenital defects)
- <u>Physical Exam</u>: neck mass (eg, thyroid), complete neurologic exam
- <u>Mirror Laryngoscopy or Flexible Nasolaryngoscopy</u>: evaluate vocal fold movement, positioning during phonation, symmetry, pooling of secretions, movement of the arytenoids, **PPP rule** (**P**osterior

commissure **P**oints to **P**aralyzed side in unilateral superior laryngeal nerve paralysis)

### Ancillary Tests

- **Direct Laryngoscopy**: allows for arytenoid palpation to differentiate paralysis from mechanical fixation
- **Stroboscopy**: mucosal wave characteristics
- **CXR**: evaluates thoracic etiology
- **CT from Base of Skull to Aortic Triangle**: evaluates lesions along course of vagus nerve
- **Modified Barium Swallow (MBS, MBSS, Videofluoroscopic Swallow Study, VFSS) and Esophagram**: evaluates for aspiration, esophageal lesions, vascular abnormalities
- **Laryngeal Electromyography**: determines vocal fold paralysis versus fixation, superior laryngeal nerve versus RLN injury, myopathy (normal frequency, lower amplitude), neuropathy (lower frequency, normal amplitude), and prognosis for recovery, ie, **denervation** (**fibrillations** after 3 weeks indicating unlikely recovery) versus **reinnervation** (**polyphasic** potentials indicating possible recovery)
- **Labs**: CBC, trepemonal studies (FTA-ABS), Lyme titers, thyroid function tests, toxin screen (lead and arsenic levels), fasting blood sugar

### Vocal Fold Positioning

- vocal fold position does not necessarily predict site of lesion
- **RLN Paralysis**: **paramedian vocal folds**, preserves partial ADduction from the action of the cricothyroid muscle (the only intrinsic muscle innervated by the SLN)
- **SLN Paralysis**: loss of cricothyroid innervation results in loss of vocal fold tension (lowers pitch of voice), bowing deformity, and loss of laryngeal sensory innervation (increased risk of aspiration); selective SLN injuries are rare (except thyroid surgery)
- **RLN and SLN Paralysis**: "**cadaveric**," intermediate vocal folds
- **Bilateral Vocal Fold Paralysis**: typically near midline (stridor, dyspnea, near normal voice) or abducted (breathy dysphonia, vocal fatigue, limited phonation time)

### Causes of Vocal Fold Immobility in Adults

- **Neoplastic**: lung, esophageal, other mediastinal, skull base, laryngeal, and thyroid tumors
- **Iatrogenic Injury**: thyroidectomy, neck surgery, cardiothoracic, vascular, and neurosurgical procedures; postintubation neuropraxia

(increased risk with cuff placed in proximal subglottis resulting in a pressure-induced neuropraxia of RLN)

- **Idiopathic**: usually self-limiting (may take up to 12 months to resolve)
- **Trauma**
- **Neurologic**: multiple etiologies that affect nucleus ambiguus in the medulla including poliomyelitis, pseudobulbar palsy, myasthenia gravis, amyotrophic lateral sclerosis, brainstem stroke, multiple sclerosis, **Wallenberg syndrome** (infarct of the posterior inferior cerebellar artery [PICA] affecting the lateral medulla)
- **Infectious**: Lyme disease, syphilis, EBV, TB, viral
- **Systemic Diseases**: sarcoidosis, diabetes, cardiomegaly
- **Toxins**: lead, arsenic, quinine, streptomycin
- left-sided paralysis more common in adults because left RLN is longer (greater risk of injury); however, right RLN has more oblique course increasing exposure to injury in thyroidectomy
- congenital anomalies affect the right RLN more because of its shorter length (more susceptible to traction forces)

### *Causes of Vocal Fold Immobility in Pediatrics*
(*see* pp. 555–556, 560)

## Unilateral Vocal Fold Immobility (Paralysis) Management

- must determine if self-limiting or permanent paralysis
- may not require surgical management if other vocal fold compensates to provide adequate voice quality and no aspiration (observation with voice therapy)
- goal of unilateral surgical procedures is to **medialize** vocal fold without compromising the airway

### *Vocal Fold Injection Medialization*

- <u>Indications</u>: vocal fold immobility, glottic insufficiency, may be used as a temporizing procedure
- <u>Advantages</u>: easy, immediate improvement, may be completed in the office or under general anesthesia in the operating room
- <u>Disadvantages</u>: irreversible if Teflon used, changes mucosal wave, does not correct large posterior defects, contraindicated if vocal folds are not at the same level
- <u>Complications</u>: granuloma formation (with superficial injections or migration of Teflon), under- or overinjection (risk of airway compromise), acute hypersensitivity
- <u>Injection Materials</u>

1. **Gelfoam**: 30% overcorrection to compensate for saline resorption, lasts 4–6 weeks (use if recovery expected, eg, neuropraxia)
2. **Fat**: no foreign body reaction, donor site morbidity, 40% overcorrection to compensate for resorption, ≤50% resorption at 6 months
3. **Collagen**: human or bovine collagen (risk of host reaction), eventually resorbed and replaced with host tissue, lasts 4–9 months
4. **Calcium Hydroxyapatite (Radiesse Voice)**: permanent, does not resorb
5. **Radiesse Voice Gel**: carrier from Radiesse Voice only, no calcium hydroxyapatite, lasts 1–2 months
6. **Hyaluronic Acid (Restylane):** lasts 6–8 months
7. **Micronized Alloderm (Cymetra):** lasts 6 months
8. **Teflon (PTFE) Paste**: largely replaced due to risk of granuloma formation, migration, stiffening of mucosal wave, difficulty with removal

- Approaches
  1. **Flexible Nasolaryngoscopy (Office)**: transoral (curved needle), transcricothyroid membrane, transthyrohyoid membrane, transthyroid cartilage (straight or bent needle)
  2. **Direct Laryngoscopy (OR)**: transoral under suspension and magnification, straight needle injection

## Thyroplasty

- **Type I (Medialization) Thyroplasty:** medializes vocal fold by inward compression with an implant (Silastic, Gore-Tex, hydroxyapatite) placed via a window in the thyroid cartilage
- Advantages: reversible, preserves mucosal wave, immediate results, may be done under local anesthesia to allow for voice and visual feedback
- Disadvantages: requires neck incision, technically more difficult, may not be adequate for posterior defects
- Complications: morbidity from neck incision (hematoma, wound infection, bleeding), under or overcompensation (risk of airway compromise), implant extrusion or migration
- Other Thyroplasty Types: less often used, include **type II** (*lateralizes* vocal fold via thyroid cartilage split with graft to anteriorly widen), **type III** (lowers vocal pitch or addresses ADductor spasmodic dysphonia by *shortening* and relaxing vocal folds), **type IV** (raises vocal pitch by *lengthening* and tensing vocal folds)

## *Arytenoid Adduction*

- <u>Indications</u>: large posterior glottic chinks (triangular defects) or uneven vocal folds
- <u>Advantages</u>: may be used in combination with type I thyroplasty
- <u>Disadvantages</u>: irreversible
- <u>Complications</u>: hematoma, airway compromise, slipped sutures, pharyngocutaneous fistula

## *Reinnervation Procedures*

- <u>Indications</u>: unilateral permanent vocal fold paralysis
- <u>Advantages</u>: maintains muscle tone, no foreign body reaction, best preservation of mucosal wave, most physiologic
- <u>Disadvantage</u>: does not result in active ADduction and ABduction, long operative time, delayed results (≤6 months), high technical skill, consider short acting injection medialization until reinnervation becomes effective
- ansa cervicalis nerve has similar fiber composition (myelinated versus unmyelinated) to the RLN making it compatible for RLN grafting
- <u>Types</u>
  1. end-to-end anastomosis of RLN
  2. ansa cervicalis to main trunk of RLN
  3. anastomosis of ansa cervicalis to ADductor branch of RLN
  4. ansa cervicalis neuromusclar pedicle (omohyoid) to TA muscle
  5. vagus, ansa, or phrenic nerve fibers or motor end plate insertion into TA muscle

## *Tracheotomy*

- indicated for respiratory distress or chronic aspiration (for pulmonary hygiene/toilet)
- *see also* pp. 106–108

# Bilateral Vocal Fold Immobility (Paralysis) Management

- goal is to **lateralize** vocal fold for airway improvement without compromising voice and causing aspiration
- **Tracheotomy**: gold standard for stabilizing airway, must undergo lateralizing procedure (at least 4 mm) before decannulation
- **Cordotomy (Laser)**: transect between vocal process and vocal fold
- **External or Endoscopic Arytenoidectomy**: arytenoid excised (total or partial), risk of posterior glottic scarring, may use laser with endoscopy

- **Arytenoidopexy**: lateralize vocal fold by plicating vocal process to external laryngeal architecture
- **Reinnervation Procedures**: attach neuromusclar pedicle to PCA muscle for ABduction (*see previous*)

# Other Neurogenic Voice Pathologies

## Adductor Spasmodic Dysphonia

- more common than ABductor spasmodic dysphonia
- <u>Pathophysiology</u>: focal laryngeal dystonia, causes vocal fold **hyper-ADduction** (phonation against a closed glottis), exacerbated by stress, better with alcohol
- <u>SSx</u>: strained or strangled voice, glottic stammering (phonation breaks); may be associated with other dystonias, tremors, or difficulty in breathing
- typically patients are able to whisper, sing, or speak in a character voice normally
- <u>Dx</u>: H&P, flexible nasolaryngoscopy, voice profile (difficulty with voiced sounds, especially words that begin with vowels; classic sentences to elicit: counting from 80 to 90, "we eat eggs every day")
- <u>Rx</u>: voice therapy, **botulinum toxin (Botox) injections of TA and LCA** muscles (lasts ~3 months, recommended by AAO-HNS clinical practice guideline on hoarseness)

## Abductor Spasmodic Dysphonia

- <u>Pathophysiology</u>: focal laryngeal dystonia, causes vocal fold **hyper-ABduction** during voicing; exacerbated by stress, better with alcohol
- <u>SSx</u>: abnormal whispered or breathy breaks during phonation, especially during voice onset
- <u>Dx</u>: H&P, flexible nasolaryngoscopy, voice profile (difficulty with voiceless speech sounds, especially vowels following a voiceless consonant; classic sentences to elicit: counting from 60 to 70, "the puppy bit the tape")
- <u>Rx</u>: voice therapy, **botulinum toxin to PCA** muscles (lasts ~3 months, recommended by AAO-HNS clinical practice guideline on hoarseness)

## Mixed Spasmodic Dysphonia

- affects both ABductors and ADductors
- <u>SSx</u>: include those of both ABductor and ADductor spasmodic dysphonia

## Spastic Dysarthria

- <u>Pathophysiology</u>: bilateral pyramidal tract disorder resulting in weakness, paresis, hypertonicity, and hyper-ADduction of vocal folds
- <u>SSx</u>: strained–strangled voice, periodic arrests of phonation
- <u>Dx</u>: mirror laryngoscopy, flexible nasolaryngoscopy
- <u>Rx</u>: voice therapy

## Flaccid Dysarthria (*see* Vocal Fold Immobility, pp. 119–124)

## Hypokinetic Dysarthria

- <u>Pathophysiology</u>: degenerative disease of the upper brainstem (**Parkinson's disease**) results in hypertonicity and rigidity of laryngeal muscles
- <u>SSx</u>: hoarse–harsh voice, limited volume and pitch
- <u>Dx</u>: mirror laryngoscopy, flexible nasolaryngoscopy
- <u>Rx</u>: voice therapy

## Hyperkinetic Dysarthria

- *see also* Spasmodic Dysphonia (*previous*)
- <u>Pathophysiology</u>: disorder of the extrapyramidal system resulting in an organic voice tremor
- <u>SSx</u>: tremorous voice
- <u>Dx</u>: mirror laryngoscopy, flexible nasolaryngoscopy
- <u>Rx</u>: voice therapy or botulinum toxin injections of TA muscle

## Ataxic Dysarthria

- <u>Pathophysiology</u>: cerebellar disorder resulting in incoordinated, clumsy, tremulous laryngeal muscular contraction during voicing (**not at rest**)
- <u>SSx</u>: uncontrolled loudness and pitch outbursts, mild hoarseness
- <u>Dx</u>: mirror laryngoscopy, flexible nasolaryngoscopy
- <u>Rx</u>: voice therapy

# Other Voice Disorders

## Puberphonia

- <u>Pathophysiology</u>: occurs during puberty, difficulty adjusting to the larger, more mature larynx
- <u>SSx</u>: recurrent "cracked," shrill, high-pitched voice

- <u>Dx</u>: clinical exam, history, and voice profile
- <u>Rx</u>: voice therapy

## Paradoxical Vocal Fold Motion Disorder (PVFD; Vocal Cord Dysfunction, VCD)

- attacks of stridor during which true vocal folds paradoxically ADduct during inspiration
- often seen in young females, exacerbated by stress, functional but involuntary
- <u>Dx</u>: flexible nasolaryngoscopy during attack to document paradoxical motion, otherwise easily misdiagnosed
- <u>Rx</u>: lorazepam to break attack, rarely need to intubate (however, patient may be intubated before consultation), speech therapy for breathing exercises, rarely tracheotomy

## Other Disorders

- **Conversion Disorders**: usually breathy–hoarse dysphonia with a normal laryngeal exam, not under voluntary control, secondary psychologic need; <u>Rx</u>: voice therapy, psychologic counseling
- **Plica Ventricularis**: faulty use of false vocal folds (hyper-ADduction), represents a form of **muscle tension dysphonia**, must rule out organic etiology; <u>Rx</u>: voice therapy

# CHAPTER

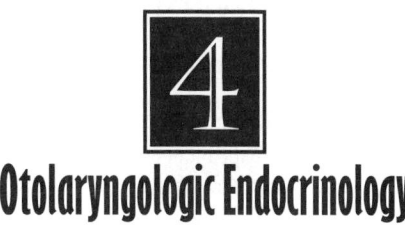

# Otolaryngologic Endocrinology

Raza Pasha

# THYROID

## Anatomy and Physiology

### Anatomy

- **Thyroid Gland**: two pear-shaped lobes, isthmus (connects the left and right lobes), and a pyramidal lobe (may present as a superior extension of the embryologic thyroid duct)
- the normal thyroid gland weighs approximately 20 g
- **Berry's Ligament (Posterior Suspensory Ligament)**: attaches thyroid lobes to the trachea
- **C-cells (Parafollicular Cells)**: cells within thyroid gland that secrete calcitonin
- Embryology: *see* p. 598

### *Vasculature*

- external carotid artery → superior thyroid artery → superior pole of the thyroid
- subclavian artery → thyrocervical trunk → inferior thyroid artery → lateral lobes of the thyroid and the **inferior and superior parathyroid arteries** (superior parathyroid arteries may also arise from superior thyroid artery)
- aortic arch or innominate artery → **thyroidea ima artery** → thyroid isthmus
- venous drainage from the superior, middle, inferior (largest) veins into the internal jugular and innominate veins
- lymphatic drainage of the isthmus and median lateral lobes → upward to the **Delphian** (prelaryngeal) and digastric nodes; inferior lateral lobes → pretracheal and cervical nodes

### *Nerves*

- **Superior Laryngeal Nerve (SLN)**: the **external branch** (motor fibers) parallels the superior thyroid artery and descends to innervate the **cricothyroid muscle**; the **internal branch** parallels the superior thyroid artery then pierces the thyrohyoid membrane (may anastomose with the sensory branch of the RLN to form the **loop of Galen**)
- **Recurrent Laryngeal Nerve (RLN)**: ascends 1 cm lateral to the tracheoesophageal groove, closely associates with the inferior thyroid artery, near the middle 1/3 of the gland the nerve crosses **posteriorly** or **superficially** to the inferior thyroid artery, continues superiorly and medially along the posterior thyroid capsule, then enters the larynx between the cricoid cartilage and the inferior cornu of the thyroid cartilage (just posterior to the articulation); **left** RLN loops

around **arch** of aorta and has straighter course, **right** RLN loops
around **subclavian** and has more oblique course

# Thyroid Hormone Physiology

## *Thyroid Hormone (TH) Synthesis and Release*

- anterior pituitary secretes TSH → increases thyroid iodide uptake
  (stored in lumen)
- iodination of thyroglobulin forms monoiodotyrosine (**MIT**) and
  diiodotyrosine (**DIT**) molecules (organification)
- MIT and DIT molecules link together to form **triiodothyronine**
  ($T_3$) **or thyroxine** ($T_4$), stored within the "colloid"
- released into blood after endocytosis and fusion with lysosome to
  release $T_3$ and $T_4$ ($T_4$ **is 90% of thyroid output**)
- <u>Thyroid Hormone Transport</u>: **thyroxine-binding globulin** (**TBG**,
  made from the liver, increased with increased estrogen and
  pregnancy, binds 75% of $T_4$); transthyretin (thyroxine-binding pre
  albumin, binds 15% of $T_4$); and albumin (binds 5% of $T_4$)
- liver, kidneys, muscle, and anterior pituitary convert $T_4$ to $T_3$ via 5′
  monodeiodinase ($T_3$ **is four times more active than** $T_4$ **and binds
  with higher affinity to TBG**) and reverse $T_3$ (**inactive form**)

## *Regulation*

- **Thyrotropin-Releasing Hormone (TRH)**: released from supraoptic
  and paraventricular nuclei of hypothalamus (not affected by TH)
- **Thyroid-Stimulating Hormone (TSH)**: secreted by anterior pituitary,
  stimulates iodide trapping, increases release of thyroid hormone, activates growth of thyroid gland (inhibited by TH for negative feedback)
- **Wolff-Chaikoff Effect**: excess iodine inhibits thyroid hormone
  (usually temporary)

## *Thyroid Hormone Effects*

- elevates metabolic rate (thermogenesis, increases oxygen consumption)
- essential for normal neural and skeletal development (stimulates
  chondrocytes, bone reabsorption, growth of neuronal tissue)
- increases sympathetic activity (increases heart rate and contractility)
- releases steroid hormones
- stimulates erythropoiesis

## *Pharmacology*

- **Levothyroxine**: (Synthroid) titrate to TSH levels (0.1-0.2 mIU/mL)
- **Liothyronine** (Cytomel): synthetic $T_3$, shorter half life, use
  immediately post-thyroidectomy if radioactive iodine is planned

- **Thioamides: propylthiouracil** (PTU), **methimazole** (Tapazole), inhibits $T_4$ conversion and the oxidation and organification of iodine; may cause hepatitis, agranulocytosis, parotitis; may be contraindicated in pregnancy
- **Iodine, Lugol's Solution**: excess iodine inhibits thyroid hormone (Wolff-Chaikoff Effect); contraindicated in rheumatoid arthritis
- **Glucocorticoids**: suppress the hypothalamic–pituitary–thyroid axis
- **Lithium**: inhibits thyroid hormone release; contraindicated in renal failure and cardiovascular disease
- **Propanolol, Metoprolol (β-blockers)**: used to control the peripheral manifestation of sympathetic overactivity (inhibits thyrotoxicosis)

### *Thyroid Function Tests* (TFTs, *see* Table 4–1)

- **Total $T_4$**: radioimmunoassay measures free and bound $T_4$
- **Free $T_4$**: measures unbound $T_4$, **more specific** for hypo- and hyperthyroidism
- **TSH**: radioimmunoassay measures TSH, **most sensitive** test for primary hypo- and hyperthyroidism
- **Total $T_3$**: radioimmunoassay measures free and bound $T_3$, useful for toxic nodules and toxic multinodular goiters (higher increase in $T_3$ than $T_4$)
- **TRH Stimulation Test**: measures TSH after infusion of TRH, tests pituitary secretion of TSH and hypothalamic response
- **Radioactive Iodide Uptake (RAIU)**: measures the percentage of radiolabeled iodine taken up by the thyroid, assesses metabolic status
- **Calcitonin**: elevated in medullary thyroid carcinoma
- **Resin $T_3$ Uptake ($RT_3U$)**: measures the binding capacity of existing TBG, indirect measurement of TBG, an increased $RT_3U$ suggests a decreased total TBG (pregnancy or estrogen from oral contraceptives increases TBG and therefore increases total $T_4$, however, will have a normal euthyroid state, ie, normal free $T_4$)

**TABLE 4–1.** Thyroid Function Test Results

| Condition | TBG | Total $T_4$ | $RT_3U$ | Free $T_4$ |
|---|---|---|---|---|
| Normal | Normal | Normal | Normal | Normal |
| Pregnant | ↑ | ↑ | ↓ | Normal |
| Liver/Renal Disease | ↓ | ↓ | ↑ | Normal |
| Hyperthyroid | Normal | ↑ | ↑ | ↑ |
| Hypothyroid | Normal | ↓ | ↓ | ↓ |

# Thyroid Nodules and Cysts

## Evaluation of the Thyroid Nodule

### *History and Physical Exam*

- Associated Symptoms: rate of growth of nodule, hoarseness, pain, dysphagia, symptoms of hypo- or hyperthyroidism (*see below*)
- Contributing Factors: radiation exposure, family history of thyroid disorders
- Physical Exam: palpation of nodule (consistency, mobility, size, tenderness), cervical adenopathy, vocal fold mobility (nasopharyngoscopy), stridor
- Factors That Favor Malignancy; males, <20 years old or >70 years old, neural involvement (hoarseness), family history, cervical adenopathy, radiation exposure

### *Fine Needle Aspiration (FNA)*

- may be considered the initial step in assessment of thyroid nodule
- Indications: to identify benign nodules, malignant nodules, metastasis, and lymphoma
- 1–10% false-negative, depending on size of needle, experience of pathologist and technician
- fine needle biopsies are preferred over large-bore needles to reduce the risk of malignant seeding and to allow for multiple biopsies
- larger needle biopsies may be considered for failed fine needle aspiration
- requires adequate specimen and a well-trained pathologist; cysts tend to reduce after aspiration (may be cystic degeneration in malignancy)

#### Interpretation and Management

- **Benign:** consider observation with consideration of repeat FNA after 6–12 months (especially with change in size)
- **Uniform Follicular Epithelium and Abundant Colloid:** suggest nodular or adenomatous goiters
- **Inflammatory Cells:** suggest thyroiditis
- **Papillary Cells (psammoma bodies, giant cells):** suggest papillary carcinoma because papillary adenoma is exceedingly rare
- **Follicular Cells:** may be **benign or carcinoma**, requires a hemithyroidectomy to examine architecture for differentiation (extracapsular spread, vascular invasion, metastasis indicate carcinoma)
- **Hürthle Cells:** may be **benign or malignant** (similar to follicular cells), also associated with **Hashimoto's thyroiditis**
- **Amyloid Deposits (stained with Congo red):** suggest medullary carcinoma

- **Undifferentiated, Bizarre Cells**: suggest anaplastic carcinoma
- **Indeterminate**: may consider repeat FNA, if second FNA is indeterminate consider lobectomy (possible total thyroidectomy)

### *Thyroid Radionucleotide Studies/Scintigraphy*

- Indications: to determine function of thyroid gland or nodule, identify ectopic thyroid tissue (including retrosternal goiter, lingual thyroid, and metastasis), determine size, shape, and symmetry of gland

#### Radionucleotides

- **$^{99m}$Tc Pertechnetate**: trapped by follicular cells, does not measure uptake, low-dose radiation, less expensive, image obtained in single visit within 30 minutes
- **$^{131}$I**: high radiation burden, results available in 48–72 hours, tracer of choice to evaluate **metastasis**, also used for **ablation** for hyperthyroidism, residual disease
- **$^{123}$I**: expensive, must be delivered daily, testing requires 2 visits at 4 and 24 hours (shorter half-life)

#### Interpretation and Management

- **Hypofunctioning/Nonfunctioning ("Cold") Nodule**: 5–20% **malignancy rate**, consider lobectomy and isthmusectomy, decision of completion of thyroidectomy based on accuracy of pathology (may consider a frozen section)
- **Hyperfunctioning or Autonomous Functioning ("Hot") nodule**: may be observed, if associated with decreased TSH levels may need iodine radioactive therapy versus surgery, 4% **malignancy rate**
- **Normal Functioning**: suggests normal thyroid function

### *Other Tests*

- Screening Thyroid Function Tests: TSH, free $T_4$
- Ultrasound: indicated to distinguish cysts, guide FNAs, and identify nonpalpable lesions
- CT/MRI: evaluates substernal goiter, nodal involvement, airway and vascular displacement, tumor invasion
- CXR: metastasis workup, tracheal displacement

## Thyroid Cysts

- Pathophysiology: typically arises from degenerated nodules, may result from cystic degeneration of malignancy

- SSx: smooth, round mass
- Dx: FNA, ultrasound, CT
- Rx: may observe for regression, FNA relieves pain and acquires cells for cytology, may consider lobectomy for recurrent cysts that are recalcitrant to drainage or bloody aspirates

# Thyroid Neoplasia

## Introduction

- High Risk Criteria (**AMES**, *Surgery*. 1988;104:951)
  1. Age: males ≥41 years old, females ≥51 years old
  2. Metastasis: presence of metastasis suggests malignancy
  3. Extent: extrathyroidal, major capsular involvement
  4. Size: nodule ≥5 cm
  5. Other: radiation therapy, autoimmune thyroiditis, more common in women (children and males have a higher risk of malignancy if presents with a thyroid nodule)
- **Well-Differentiated Thyroid Carcinoma (WDTC)**: includes papillary and follicular carcinoma

## Benign Adenoma

- 70% of solitary nodules
- SSx: painless, slow-growing solitary nodule
- Dx: FNA (typically reduces size) or imaging
- **follicular adenoma** is most common
- papillary adenoma is exceedingly rare
- Rx: observation, diagnostic FNA typically reduces cysts

## Papillary Carcinoma

- **most common thyroid cancer** (70-80%)
- more common in young females
- Risks: radiation exposure, **Gardner's syndrome**, may have an association with Hashimoto's thyroiditis
- 15–30% palpable regional nodes (70% occult nodes), 5–10% distant metastasis (lungs or bones)
- SSx: painless, slow-growing solitary nodule, often asymptomatic, may have hoarseness or dysphagia with larger tumors
- Dx: FNA (*see above*)
- Histopathology: unencapsulated neoplastic cells (ground glass appearance, pseudoinclusions) with fibrovascular stalks, **psammoma bodies** (calcific), intranuclear vacuoles ("Orphan Annie" eyes), **multicentric**

- <u>Prognosis</u>: **95%** 5-year survival; poor prognostic indicators include tumors >1.5 cm or extracapsular spread (cervical metastases have increased cervical recurrence rates without affecting survival)
- **Papillary/Follicular Carcinoma**: variant of papillary thyroid carcinoma (behaves more papillary than follicular)

### *Management*

- total or near total thyroidectomy, may consider lobectomy and isthmusectomy for limited disease (<1.0 cm in younger patients, controversial)
- modified neck dissection (MND) for palpable nodes only (no improvement in survival with elective neck dissections)
- follow-up in 6 weeks for radioactive iodine uptake (RAIU) study and thyroid radionucleotide scan (must be hypothyroid state) followed by radioactive ablation therapy ([131]Iodine, must be in hypothyroid state TSH >50 mIU/L) for residual or metastatic disease and thyroid hormone suppression therapy (typically titrated to maintain TSH to 0.1 mIU/L)
- monitor with whole body radioactive scans (6–12 months then ~2 years) and serum thyroglobulin levels for recurrence
- external beam radiation therapy or chemotherapy (doxorubicin) may be considered for radioactive iodine insensitive tumors, inoperable recurrence, and for palliative care

## Follicular Carcinoma

- **second most common thyroid cancer (~10%)**
- more common in the elderly and in females
- 20–50% **hematogenous** spread with distant metastasis (lymphatic spread rare)
- <u>SSx</u>: painless, slow-growing solitary nodule, often asymptomatic, may have hoarseness or dysphagia
- <u>Dx</u>: requires open biopsy (unable to distinguish adenoma from carcinoma by FNA)
- <u>Histopathology</u>: **unifocal**; neoplastic follicular cells (less distinct from malignant papillary cells), **malignancy differentiated by the presence of extracapsular spread, invasion of vasculature, or metastasis**; solid, trabecular, or follicular growth patterns
- <u>Prognosis</u>: **70–85%** 5-year survival (20% with distant metastasis), worse prognosis for angioinvasion, extracapsular spread
- <u>Rx</u>: surgical and medical management similar to papillary carcinoma (*see above*)

## Hürthle Cell Carcinoma (Oncocytic Carcinoma)

- variation of follicular carcinoma (Hürthle cells predominate)
- more aggressive than follicular carcinoma
- SSx: similar to follicular and papillary carcinoma
- Dx: requires open biopsy (unable to distinguish adenoma from carcinoma from FNA)
- Histopathology: predominately (75–100%) Hürthle cells (large granular eosinophilic cells); similar to follicular carcinoma; **malignancy differentiated by the presence of extracapsular spread, invasion of lymphatics or vasculature, or metastasis**
- Prognosis: **50%** 5-year survival
- Rx: more aggressive surgical management, Hürthle cell carcinomas do not take up radioactive iodine (less sensitive to thyroid suppression and to diagnostic and therapeutic radioactive iodine therapy)

## Medullary Thyroid Carcinoma

- Pathophysiology: derived from neuroendocrine parafollicular or C-cells (produce calcitonin)
- Types
    1. **Familial:** 20–25%, multiple endocrine neoplasia (MEN) 2a/b (*see* Table 4–2), familial medullary thyroid carcinoma (FMTC), **multicentric, bilateral**
    2. **Sporadic:** 75–80%, unifocal, unilateral, worse prognosis
- 50–60% lymph node involvement (late vascular involvement), approximately 8% distant metastasis
- secretory granules of malignant C-cells release calcitonin and also secrete gastrin, adrenocorticotropic hormone (ACTH), substance P, carcinoembryonic antigen (CEA), and others
- SSx: sporadic forms present similar to follicular and papillary carcinoma
- Dx: presence of ***Ret-3* oncogene mutation** (chromosome 10), FNA or biopsy, elevated serum calcitonin (consider IV pentagastrin to increase sensitivity), elevated CEA
- Histopathology: varied cells (small round, polygonal, or spindle-shaped neoplastic cells), amyloid stroma, may have peripheral C-cell hyperplasia
- Prognosis: 50–80% survival; worse prognosis if unilateral, sporadic type, younger patient, or with metastasis

### Management

- patient and family should be screened for MEN syndromes with assays for germline RET mutations (*see* Table 4–2), examine for mucosal neuromas, marfanoid habitus, serum calcium levels, urine catecholamines and metabolites (vanillylmandelic acid, metanephrine)

**TABLE 4-2.** Multiple Endocrine Neoplasms

| MEN 1 (I) (Werner's Syndrome) | MEN 2a (II) (Sipple Syndrome) | MEN 2b (III) |
|---|---|---|
| Parathyroid hyperplasia | Medullary thyroid carcinoma | Medullary thyroid carcinoma |
| Pancreatic tumors (insulinoma, gastrinoma) | Pheochromocytoma | Pheochromocytoma |
| Parathyroid hyperplasia | Mucosal neuroma | |
| Pituitary adenoma | | Marfanoid habitus |

- **total** thyroidectomy with **elective** modified neck dissection
- screen with yearly pentagastrin-stimulated calcitonin levels to monitor for recurrence
- **Prophylactic Thyroidectomy:** should be considered in childhood with positive germline RET mutations
- *NOTE:* radioactive iodine ($^{131}$I) is not effective because parafollicular cells do not take up $^{131}$I
- new targeted chemotherapy agents (eg, cabozantinib, vandetanib; *see* pp. 269–270)

## Anaplastic Carcinoma

- most commonly seen in the elderly
- <u>Pathophysiology</u>: may be from transformation of a well-differentiated carcinoma (may find coexistent follicular or papillary carcinoma)
- **uniformly fatal** (2–6 month median), often found with metastasis
- <u>SSx</u>: fast-growing firm thyroid mass, 50% with hoarseness (local invasion)
- <u>Dx</u>: FNA (as above)
- <u>Histopathology</u>: giant and spindle cell variation with high mitotic activity, large areas of necrosis, and significant infiltration; undifferentiated "**bizarre cells**"
- <u>Rx</u>: no adequate therapy, tracheotomy (protect airway), consider radiation and chemotherapy, surgical resection may be considered (*controversial*)

## Primary Lymphoma of the Thyroid

- most commonly **non-Hodgkin B-cell tumors**
- associated with **Hashimoto's thyroiditis**
- <u>Dx</u>: difficult to distinguish lymphoma from Hashimoto's thyroiditis by FNA alone, therefore a conformational open biopsy is required along with lymphoma staging workup (*see* Lymphoma, pp. 327–330)
- <u>Rx</u>: chemotherapy and radiation, surgery is usually not indicated

# Thyroidectomy

## Introduction

- preferable for patient to be euthyroid at time of surgery to avoid thyroid storm (*see below*)
- may consider preoperative potassium iodine (**Lugol's solution**) to reduce vascularity of thyroid gland

## Indications

- suspicion of malignancy
- compression symptoms (airway compromise, dysphagia)
- extension into mediastinum
- cosmesis
- failed medical management for Graves' disease or hyperthyroidism
- pregnancy in Graves' disease or Hashimoto's thyroiditis
- indication for transaxillary robotic approach is primarily cosmetic

## Postoperative Complications

- **Hematoma**: may present as respiratory compromise from compressive effect; <u>Rx</u>: for respiratory distress **immediately remove sutures** and open wound, for large hematomas control bleeding in operating room and place suction drains; for smaller hematomas may be observed (place on antibiotics) and aspirate contents after liquification (7–10 days)
- **Vocal Fold Paralysis**: RLN or SLN injury (SLN injury more common), prevent by identifying nerve; <u>Rx</u>: if discovered interoperatively may consider primary anastamosis (*see also* pp. 121–124 for further management)
- **Transient or Permanent Hypocalcemia**: if parathyroid is removed intraoperatively, cut into fragments and replace into adjacent muscle bed (sternocleidomastoid or brachioradialis muscles), prevent by identifying glands; <u>Rx</u>: persistent hypocalcemia requires chronic calcium supplementation
- **Thoracic Duct Injury**: rare, results in chyle leak or fistula (*see* p. 281 for management)

### *Thyroid Storm*

- **Thyroid Storm**: acute extreme state of thyrotoxicosis (life-threatening)
- <u>Etiology</u>: surgery (thyroidectomy), trauma, childbirth, infection, untreated hyperthyroidism, radioactive iodine treatment, diabetic ketoacidosis, vigorous palpation of thyroid gland
- **20–50% mortality**
- <u>SSx</u>: sudden fever, profuse sweating, tachycardia, nausea, abdominal pain, tremors, restlessness, psychosis, coma, stupor
- <u>Dx</u>: history and exam
- <u>Rx</u>
  1. immediate administration of **iodine, propylthiouracil, propanolol, and corticosteroids**

2. supportive measures (glucose-containing IV fluids, cooling blanket, supplemental oxygen, antipyretics)
3. ICU admission (cardiac monitoring)

# Thyroid Goiter

## Introduction

- <u>Causes</u>: iodine deficiency, thyroiditis (autoimmune, infectious), malignancy, benign cysts and adenomas, goitrogens (cabbage, turnips, Brussels sprouts, rutabagas), excess iodine (Wolff-Chaikoff effect), lithium, granulomatous disease, thyroid hormone resistance
- <u>SSx</u>: thyroid fullness, compression effects (hoarseness, dysphagia, respiratory distress), may have signs of hypo- or hyperthyroidism (*see below*), may be tender (thyroiditis)
- <u>Initial Workup</u>: consider CT (especially if substernal or in the presence of compressive symptoms) or U/S, for palpable nodules (*see workup above*), screening TSH and free $T_4$
- <u>Ancillary Tests</u>: consider thyroid-stimulating autoantibodies, ESR, calcitonin, and antithyroid peroxidase (antimicrosomal antibodies); barium swallow to evaluate esophageal obstruction, spirometry for airway obstruction

## Diffuse Colloid Goiter (Adenomatous Goiter, Multinodular Colloid Goiter)

- more common in women
- <u>Pathophysiology</u>: iodine deficiency → ↑TSH → chronic thyroid hyperplasia and involution → multinodularity
- **Toxic Nodular Goiter (Plummer's Disease)**: variation of diffuse colloid goiter in which one nodule is hyperfunctional resulting in hyperthyroidism
- <u>Types</u>
    1. **Endemic Goiter**: iodine deficiency, extrinsic goitrogens (soybeans, lithium, iodides, etc)
    2. **Sporadic**: uncertain etiology
- <u>SSx</u>: multiple nodules of varying size, may present with compressive symptoms (stridor, dysphagia)
- <u>Dx</u>: *as above*
- <u>Rx</u>: hormonal suppression may be considered for small goiters (requires careful monitoring with serum TSH to avoid hyperthyroidism, arrhythmias and osteoporosis); iodine replacement if deficient will reverse goiter; radioactive iodine therapy or surgical excision (subtotal thyroidectomy) may be considered for cosmesis, decompression, concern of malignancy, or toxicosis

## Mediastinal (Substernal) Goiter

- <u>Pathophysiology</u>: intrathoracic extension of thyroid gland (inferior extension is the path of least resistance)
- <u>SSx</u>: dyspnea, stridor, dysphagia, choking, superior vena cava syndrome
- <u>Dx</u>: CT/MRI of neck and chest, radionuclide scanning
- <u>Rx</u>: surgical excision, often able to access with finger dissection from a standard incision although a sternotomy may be required (cardiothoracic surgery consult)

# Hyperthyroid Disease

## Symptoms

- <u>Elevated Metabolic Rate</u>: weight loss, fatigue, sweating, heat intolerance
- <u>Increased Sympathetic Activity</u>: palpitations, tachycardia, tremor
- <u>Increased Protein Degradation</u>: weakness, fine hair
- <u>Neurologic Effects</u>: increased deep tendon reflex, nervousness
- <u>Reproductive Effects</u>: abnormal menstrual cycle, decreased libido

## Most Common Causes

- Graves' disease
- multinodular toxic goiter
- subacute thyroiditis
- exogenous from medications, iodine induced
- uninodular toxic goiter
- thyroid cancer
- pituitary tumors

## Graves' Disease

- <u>Pathophysiology</u>: thyroid-stimulating immunoglobulins (TSIs) → stimulate glandular hyperplasia via **TSH receptor** → goiter and increased $T_3$ and $T_4$ secretion
- <u>Risks</u>: radiation exposure, **women** (adolescence or 30–40-year olds), genetic disposition
- <u>Histopathology</u>: hyperplasia, increased colloid material, papillary projections
- <u>SSx</u>: diffuse goiter, hyperthyroid symptoms (*see above*), infiltrative dermopathy, **exophthalmos** (autoimmune → extraocular muscle deposition), blindness from optic neuropathy, pretibial myxedema, acropachy (clubbing of fingers from osteoarthropathy)

- <u>Complications</u>: secondary effects of hyperthyroidism (osteoporosis, heart failure, arrythmias, thyroid storm), vision loss
- <u>Dx</u>: thyroid-stimulating immunoglobulin levels; elevated $T_3$, $T_4$, RAIU, and thyroglobulin; decreased serum TSH; radioactive iodine scan reveals diffuse uptake

### Treatment

- **Radioactive Iodine** (131I): most common therapy, risk of hypothyroidism, contraindicated in pregnancy
- **Propylthiouracil and Methimazole:** (*see above*) may be considered for small goiter and mild disease
- **Propanolol:** (*see above*) may be supplemented for severe symptoms
- **Subtotal Thyroidectomy:** indicated for failed medical therapy, pregnancy (especially in second trimester), noncompliance, suspicious nonfunctioning ("cold") nodule, compressive symptoms

### Management for Exophthalmos and Optic Neuropathy

- ophthalmology evaluation
- artificial tears, taping retracted lids, protective eyewear
- if optic neuropathy persists despite medical therapy, a trial of corticosteroids is used for 2 weeks, if no improvement then surgical decompression
- if exophthalmos persists after 6 months despite adequate therapy, radiation therapy or surgical correction (orbital decompression, eyelid retraction release, strabismus surgery) is performed
- surgical decompression includes transnasal endoscopic approaches

# Hypothyroid Disease

## Symptoms

- **Reduced Metabolic Rate:** weight gain, cold intolerance, lethargy
- **Decreased Sympathetic Activity:** bradycardia, constipation
- **Decreased Protein Degradation:** weakness, coarse hair, hoarseness
- **Decreased Neurologic Response:** slowed deep tendon reflex, depression
- **Myxedema:** nonpitting edema
- **Cretinism**: hypothyroidism in children; mental retardation, impaired physical growth, macroglossia, protuberant abdomen
- **Myxedema Coma:** severe hypothyroidism; hypothermia, hypoglycemia, hypoventilation, ileus, death; <u>Rx</u>: parenteral levothyroxine, corticosteroids

## Causes

- radiation therapy
- idiopathic atrophy
- Hashimoto's thyroiditis
- other thyroiditis
- surgical or radioiodine ablation therapies
- secondary hypothyroidism (pituitary or hypothalamic dysfunction)
- iodine deficiency
- **Congenital Hypothyroidism**: from maternal iodine expectorants, antithyroid medications, and antithyroid antibodies

# Thyroiditis (see Table 4–3)

## Subacute Granulomatous Thyroiditis (de Quervain's)

- most common cause of painful thyroid
- <u>Pathophysiology</u>: may be viral (mumps, coxsackievirus) or postviral inflammatory response
- <u>SSx</u>: **painful**, mildly enlarged thyroid, self-limiting, malaise, may have flulike symptoms prior to thyroid tenderness
- <u>Dx</u>: history, TFT (may be transiently hyperthyroid initially, and transiently hypothyroid in the recovery phase)
- <u>Rx</u>: anti-inflammatory agents (NSAIDs), may consider corticosteroids, observation

## Hashimoto's (Chronic Autoimmune, Chronic Lymphocytic) Thyroiditis

- most common cause of hypothyroidism in the United States
- associated with lymphoma, neoplasms, other autoimmune disease (SLE, Sjögren syndrome, scleroderma)
- <u>Pathophysiology</u>: antithyroglobulin and antimicrosomal Ab → anti-TSH receptor → transient hyperthyroid then hypothyroidism
- <u>Risks</u>: women, genetic susceptibility (HLA-DR3), Sjögren's, DM, pernicious anemia
- <u>Histopathology</u>: fibrosis, lymphocytic infiltration
- <u>SSx</u>: slowly enlarging goiter, painless, symptoms of hypothyroidism (myxedema, weight gain, constipation) although may be subclinical
- <u>Dx</u>: **antithyroid peroxidase (antimicrosomal antibodies and anti-Tg)**, ESR, TFT (may have elevated, normal, or low serum levels of $T_4$ and TSH), FNA only for prominent nodules suspicious of carcinoma or lymphoma that do not resolve with medical therapy

| Condition | Subacute | Hashimoto's | Riedel's | Suppurative |
|---|---|---|---|---|
| Incidence | common | common | rare | rare |
| Thyroid hormone status | hyper- then hypothyroid | hyper- then hypothyroid | hypothyroid | — |
| Onset | acute | gradual | gradual | rapid |
| Pain | common | none | rare | common |
| Goiter | rare | common | hard gland | rare |

**TABLE 4–3.** Clinical Differences Between Thyroiditis Conditions

- <u>Rx</u>: long-term thyroxine therapy with TFT monitoring; surgical excision for compressive symptoms, suspicious nonfunctioning ("cold") nodule, and pregnancy

## Other Thyroiditis

- **Painless Thyroiditis**: like subacute (self-limiting hyperthyroid) but painless, common in women postpartum
- **Riedel's Thyroiditis**: thyroid fibrosis of unknown origin, "rock-hard" thyroid, produces local pressure and hypothyroidism; <u>Rx</u>: hormone replacement, may consider surgical release at isthmus
- **Acute Suppurative Thyroiditis**: uncommon; <u>Rx</u>: systemic antibiotics, consider drainage for abscess formation

# PARATHYROIDS
## Anatomy and Physiology

### Anatomy

- **Superior Parathyroids**: most commonly located in the posterolateral aspect of the superior pole, 1 cm above the intersection of the recurrent laryngeal nerve and the inferior thyroid artery
- **Inferior Parathyroids: more variable** location, most commonly located 1–2 cm from the entrance of the inferior thyroid artery into the lower thyroid pole (may also be associated with the superior thymus)
- each parathyroid weighs 20–40 mg
- <u>Embryology</u>: *see* p. 598
- <u>Vasculature</u>: inferior thyroid artery → inferior and superior parathyroid arteries (superior parathyroid arteries may also arise from superior thyroid artery)

### Calcium Physiology

- serum calcium is 46% ionized and 46% bound to albumin ($H^+$ competes with protein binding of calcium, therefore acidosis increases more ionized calcium)
- 99% of calcium is stored in bone
- **Vitamin D**: precursors formed in the skin after exposure of ultraviolet light to form vitamin $D_3$ (cholecalciferol), activation occurs after 25-hydroxylation in the liver and 1-hydroxylation in the kidneys (stimulated by PTH); stimulates calcium and phosphate

absorption in the intestine (minor effect of bone reabsorption and kidney reabsorption)
- **Parathyroid Hormone (PTH)**: formed in the parathyroid glands initially from preproparathyroid hormone → cleaved to proparathyroid hormone → cleaved to mature PTH; regulated by negative feedback loop from increased serum calcium; **increases** serum calcium and **decreases** serum phosphate by stimulating osteoclastic reabsorption of bone (↑Ca), increasing calcium absorption in the kidney (↑Ca), activating 25-hydroxyvitamin D to 1,25-dihydroxyvitamin D (↑Ca), and increasing phosphate excretion (↓$PO_4$)
- **Calcitonin**: produced by parafollicular cells (C-cells), inhibits calcium reabsorption from bone and increases kidney clearance of calcium and phosphate

# Hyperparathyroidism and Hypercalcemia

## Hypercalcemia

- <u>Causes</u>: hyperparathyroidism and think "**CHIMPANZEES**" for other causes of hypercalcemia (*see* Table 4–4)

### Signs and Symptoms

- "**Stones, Bones, Groans, Psychiatric Overtones:**" nephrolithiasis, osteitis fibrosa cystica, cholelithiasis, confusion
- <u>Renal</u>: polyuria, nephrolithiasis, nephrocalcinosis
- <u>Gastrointestinal</u>: constipation, dyspepsia, pancreatitis
- <u>Musculoskeletal</u>: muscle weakness, bone and joint pain (osteitis fibrosa cystica, calcific tendonitis)
- <u>Central Nervous System</u>: slow mentation, fatigue, depression, poor memory, psychosis
- <u>Cardiovascular</u>: shortened Q-T interval, heart block, hypertension

### Medical Management of Hypercalcemia

- **Saline Diuresis**: restores extracellular fluid volume and promotes calcium excretion, loop diuretics can also be given (thiazides impair calcium excretion)
- **Biphosphonates**: inhibit bone resorption, calcium serum levels decrease over several days
- **Plicamycin (Mithramycin)**: (discontinued in 2000) inhibits bone resorption; toxic side effects include thrombocytopenia, hepatic dysfunction, renal failure; was therefore used only for malignant hypercalcemia

| TABLE 4–4. Causes of Hypercalcemia: CHIMPANZEES Method |
| --- |
| **C**alcium: exogenous |
| **H**yperparathyroidism |
| **I**mmobility |
| **M**etastasis to bone |
| **P**aget's disease |
| **A**ddison's disease |
| **N**eoplasms: typically solid tumors (prostate, lung, colon, breast cancers) |
| **Z**ollinger-Ellison syndrome (hypergastrinemia) |
| **E**xcess: vitamin A or D, thiazides, lithium, estrogens, milk-alkali syndrome |
| **E**ndocrine disorders: familial hypocalciuric hypercalcemia, hyperthyroidism, pheochromocytoma |
| **S**arcoidosis: also other granulomatous diseases (tuberculosis and berylliosis) |

- **Calcitonin**: rapid onset (serum calcium falls within hours)
- **Glucocorticoids**: inhibit calcium intestinal absorption, may be effective for hypercalcemia secondary to malignancy
- **Gallium Nitrate**: inhibits bone resorption, used for parathyroid carcinoma
- **Hemodialysis**: indicated for life-threatening conditions

## Types of Hyperparathyroidism

### Primary Hyperparathyroidism

- elevated serum PTH causing hypercalcemia
- **Benign Adenoma**: most common (~85%), single adenomatous gland; <u>Rx</u>: medical management for hypercalcemia and parathyroidectomy (*see below*)
- **Parathyroid Hyperplasia**: associated with MEN 1 & 2a (*see* Table 4–2), familial hypocalciuric hypercalcemia (FHH, autosomal dominant, abnormally high PTH from impaired calcium serum detection, increased renal calcium absorption; detected by calcium-to-creatinine clearance ratio <0.010; surgery not indicated), familial hyperparathyroidism; <u>Rx</u>: medical management for hypercalcemia and parathyroidectomy (*see below*)
- **Carcinoma of the Parathyroid Gland**: rare tumor, suspect with a palpable, gray mass, vocal fold paralysis, or severe hypercalcemia;

Rx: en bloc resection including thyroid lobectomy, monitor for recurrence with serial serum calcium levels

### Secondary Hyperparathyroidism

- elevated serum PTH with **hypocalcemia**
- compensatory parathyroid hyperplasia causing peripheral resistance to PTH secondary to malfunction of another organ system
- Causes: **chronic renal disease** (most common), osteogenesis imperfecta, Paget's disease, multiple myeloma, bone metastasis, pituitary adenomas
- Rx: address underlying cause, cinacalcet

### Tertiary Hyperparathyroidism

- persistent elevated serum PTH (may have normal or low calcium)
- autonomous or irrepressible PTH production (parathyroid hyperplasia from secondary parathyroidism, persistent hyperfunction despite correction)
- Rx: consider parathyroidectomy

## Evaluation

- Contributing Factors: family history of MEN disorders, radiation exposure
- Serum Electrolytes: ionized calcium (should be elevated at 3 different times), magnesium (typically low), chloride (usually elevated from PTH-induced bicarburia), and phosphate (typically low)
- Intact PTH levels: immunoradiometric assay, "intact" PTH allows differentiation of primary hyperparathyroidism from hypercalcemia of malignancy (tumors secrete a larger protein)
- Plain Films: brown tumors (osteitis fibrosis cystica), loss of lamina, resorption of terminal phalanges, soft-tissue calcification, CXR (granulomatous diseases or metastasis), abdominal film (renal calculi)
- Others Labs: alkaline phosphatase (suggests bone disease), BUN/creatinine (renal function), 24-hour urine calcium (allows calculation of calcium-creatinine clearance to distinguish primary hyperparathyroidism from FHH), TFT, ACE levels (sarcoidosis), serum prolactin and gastrin and urine catecholamines and metabolites (evaluate for MEN syndromes)

### Localization

- **Thallium-Technetium Subtraction (Sestamibi Scan)**: thallium uptake by thyroid and parathyroid, technetium uptake by thyroid gland only, parathyroid glands identified by computer subtraction;

up to 90% sensitivity (less accurate for gland hyperplasia, associated thyroid disease, or small glands)
- **High-Resolution Ultrasound**: cannot locate mediastinal, retrotracheal, retroesophageal, or small nodes
- **Selective Venous Catheterization for PTH**: reserved after exploration has failed
- **CT/MRI**: poor resolution, MRI more useful in identification of glands

### Surgical Management

- surgery is the only definitive cure for parathyroid adenomas, avoids long-term complications of nephrocalcinosis and bone demineralization
- parathyroidectomy is indicated for **symptomatic** (bone pain, pathologic fractures, ectopic calcifications, intractable itching, etc) or **persistently elevated serum calcium**
- <u>Surgical Theory</u>: must first remove pathologic gland (adenoma), hyperplasia versus adenoma cannot be distinguished grossly, therefore, must identify one "normal" gland to evaluate hyperplasia, if other gland is also hyperplastic then assume parathyroid hyperplasia and perform a subtotal (3½ glands) or total parathyroidectomy with autotransplantation, if gland is normal may either assume adenoma and terminate case or further biopsy other contralateral glands (*controversial*)
- autotransplantation requires 20 mg of morcellized parathyroid tissue into muscle bed (usually to forearm)
- **Radioguided Parathyroidectomy**: increasing popularity, may be considered for an adenoma identified on a sestamibi scan, repeat tracer is injected 1.5–3 hours prior to surgery, a gamma probe is utilized to identify abnormal gland

#### Complications

- **Persistent Hypercalcemia**: most commonly from missed adenoma (the most commonly missed location is the posterior mediastinum), also from supernumerary gland, second adenoma, failed recognition of parathyroid hyperplasia, incorrect diagnosis, and residual adenoma
- **Postoperative Hypocalcemia and Hypomagnesemia**: usually temporary until replacement of low bone-calcium stores (increased risk with elevated alkaline phosphatase); <u>Rx</u>: if persistent may require long-term calcium and vitamin D supplementation
- **Nerve Injury and Hematoma**: *see above*

# Hypoparathyroidism and Hypocalcemia

## Hypocalcemia

- <u>Causes</u>: hypoparathyroidism (*see below*), vitamin D deficiency (renal failure, impaired GI absorption, pancreatic disease), hypomagnesemia, medications (calcitonin, furosemide, ketoconazole)

### Signs and Symptoms

- <u>Neuromuscular</u>: increased neuromuscular excitability or **tetany**, numbness and tingling (perioral, fingers, toes), muscle cramps
- <u>Central Nervous System</u>: mental changes, irritability, seizures,
- <u>Other</u>: cataracts, poor dentition, heart failure, brittle nails and hair
- **Chvostek's Sign**: facial twitch elicited by tapping the jaw
- **Trousseau's Sign**: carpal spasm after 3 minutes of inflation of a pressure cuff >20 mm Hg above patient's systolic pressure

## Hypoparathyroidism

- uncommon acquired disease
- most common cause is iatrogenic (thyroid or parathyroid surgery)
- **DiGeorge syndrome**: congenital abnormality of the **third and fourth** branchial pouches, causes agenesis of the parathyroid glands (may also be associated with athymia)
- **Pseudohypoparathyroidism**: caused by end-organ resistance to the effects of PTH
- <u>Rx</u>: calcium and vitamin D supplementation

# CHAPTER

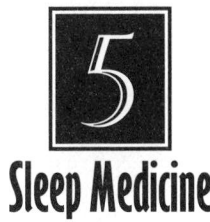

# Sleep Medicine

Raza Pasha, Mas Takashima, and Justin S. Golub

# SLEEP PHYSIOLOGY

## Sleep Wake Cycles

- **Homeostatic Drive (Process S)**: promotes **sleep**, increases while awake, decrease with NREM sleep
- **Circadian Rhythm (Process C)**: promotes **wakefulness**, two peaks at **late morning** (4–8 hours after minimal core temperature, during **warming**) and **early evening** (maximal core temperature); adjusted daily through entrainment (*see following*)
- **Zeitgeber**: a recurrent environmental cue or cycle that is capable of entraining a circadian rhythm (**light–dark cycle** is the most common) in a **constant condition in humans ≈24.2 hours** ("free running")
- **Entrainment**: coupling of a biological rhythm to a zeitgeber
- Circadian Physiology: **retinal ganglion cells** are stimulated by light (blue, green), contain **melanopsin** → **suprachiasmatic nucleus (SCN)** which is the principal coordinating pacemaker → hypothalamus → output hormones (**cortisol** and **TSH**; melatonin)
- Core Body Temperature: synchronized to **circadian rhythms**, wakefulness promoted during **warming** (core body temperature minimum [$CBT_{min}$] occurs 2 hours before waking, typically 4–5 AM, promoting wakefulness while the body warms) and **sleep** onset occurs with **cooling** (highest core temperature occurs 6–8 PM, promoting sleep as the body cools)
- **Dim Light Melatonin Onset**: time when melatonin levels start to rise, 2–3 hours before habitual bedtime

## Sleep Neuroanatomy and Neurotransmitters
(*see* Table 5–1)

### *Wake/Arousal Areas*

- **Reticular Activating System (RAS)**: ascending tract regulates arousal system via the thalamus, hypothalamus, and basal forebrain
- **Locus Ceruleus (LC)**: **dorsal pons**, releases **norepinephrine (NE)**, maintains **wakefulness** as discharged as a tonic tone, gradually reduces its firing rate during sleep (allows for a gradual sleep)
- **Pons**: **acetylcholine (ACh)** initiates and regulates **REM sleep** as well as **wakefulness**
- **Basal Forebrain:** ACh promotes wakefulness **and** REM sleep directly to cortex
- **Posterior (Dorsal) Hypothalamus**: promotes **wakefulness** through **histamine, hypocretin/orexin**, and dopamine
- **Dorsal Raphe Nuclei**: located in the core of the brainstem, produces **serotonin (5-HT)**, promotes **wakefulness**

| Neurotransmitter | Location | Wake | NREM | REM | Comments |
|---|---|---|---|---|---|
| Norepinephrine | Locus Ceruleus | ↑↑↑ | ↑ | - | |
| Serotonin | Dorsal Raphe Nuclei | ↑↑↑ | ↑ | - | Depressed patients with low 5-HT hypersomnic |
| Histamine | Post. Hypothalamus | ↑↑↑ | ↑ | - | $H_1$-blockers promote sleep |
| Dopamine | Substantia Nigra, Ventral Tegmental Region, Post Hypo. | ↑↑↑ | ↑ | - | Amphetamines promote wake by blocking DA reuptake |
| Hypocretin/Orexin | Post Hypothalamus | ↑↑↑ | ↑ | ? | Narcolepsy with cataplexy has undetectable CSF orexin, stimulates hunger |
| Acetylcholine | Pons, Basal Forebrain | ↑↑ | - | ↑↑↑ | ACh hypersensitivity may be related to narcolepsy |
| Glutamate | Medial Medulla | ↑↑ | → | ↑↑↑ | Promotes REM atonia in the medial medulla (main CNS excitatory neurotransmitter) |
| Glycine | Spinal Anterior Horn Cells | - | - | ↑↑↑ | Causes atonia during REM |
| GABA | Ant. Hypothalamus (VLPO), Basal Forebrain | - | ↑↑ | ↑ | Benzodiazepines and barbiturates act on $GABA_A$ |
| Galanin | Ant. Hypothalamus (VLPO) | - | ↑↑ | ↑ | |
| Adenosine | Basal Forebrain | - | ↑↑ | | Main homeostatic driver, inhibited by **methylxanthines** |

- **Substantia Nigra and Ventral Tegmental Region**: produces **dopamine (DA)**, which promotes **wakefulness**

### Sleep Promoting Areas

- **Anterior (Ventral) Hypothalamus**: specifically in the **Ventrolateral Preoptic (VLPO) area** produces **gamma-aminobutyric acid (GABA)** and **galanin** that promotes **NREM sleep** by inhibiting arousal systems
- **Basal Forebrain**: **adenosine** is an inhibitor in the basal forebrain that promotes sleep and activates the VLPO
- REM activation is promoted primarily by the **PPT/LDT (pons) releasing of ACh** in the thalamus

## Endocrine Function

- <u>Strongly Circadian Modulated</u>: cortisol and thyroid stimulating hormone (TSH)
- <u>Strongly Sleep Modulated</u>: growth hormone, prolactin, TSH, LH/FSH, and testosterone
- <u>First Half of Sleep</u>: ↑GH, ↓cortisol/ACTH, ↑TSH, ↑prolactin
- <u>Second Half of Sleep</u>: ↓GH, ↑cortisol/ACTH, ↓TSH, ↑↑prolactin
- **Growth Hormone (GH)**: large burst first half of sleep, N3 (1.5–3.5 hours after sleep) then less during the second half of sleep, GH causes ↑slow wave and ↑REM sleep; sleep deprivation causes ↓GH (**sleep modulated**)
- **Adrenocorticotropic Hormone (ACTH) and Cortisol**: initially cortisol levels decline then rise with sleep, peak at midmorning (8 AM) then decline with a nadir near sleep onset, sleep fragmentation causes ↑**cortisol** (**circadian modulated**); however, sleep deprivation has a ↓peak level and ↑nadir
- **Thyroid Stimulating Hormone**: peak after onset of sleep then decreases with sleep, stays low during the day; sleep deprivation and awakenings causes ↑TSH (**circadian modulated**), **but** NREM sleep inhibits the secretion of TSH (**sleep modulated**); hypothyroidism associated with OSAS, CSA, and sleepiness (although not a significant predictor of OSAS and does not require routine TSH levels)
- **Prolactin**: increases with sleep (**sleep modulated**) with increased levels during the second half of sleep; sleep fragmentation and sleep deprivation causes ↓prolactin while hypnotics and benzodiazapines cause ↑prolactin; hyperprolactinemia causes ↑slow wave sleep
- **LH/FSH**: no secretory sleep pattern in adult women, but in adolescence and in men LH rises during sleep (**sleep modulated**); LH may decline in sleep during the follicular phase of the menstrual cycle

- **Glucose/Insulin**: sleep ↑serum glucose and insulin (stabilizes glucose during sleep when not eating), sleep restriction ↓insulin response (insulin resistance)
- **Hypocretins/Orexins**: promote wakefulness, stimulate hunger
- **Leptin**: ↓hunger, proportional to body fat (released from adipocytes), signals adiposity ("fat burner," rises after food), sleep restriction causes ↓leptin, (weight gain), obesity has high levels but may be resistant to leptin, narcoleptics have lower leptin ("L" = "leptin, lean, lipocytes")
- **Ghrelin**: ↑hunger (rises before meal times), circadian regulated, increases at night, sleep restriction ↑ghrelin (weight gain)
- **Melatonin**: "hormone of darkness," produced in the pineal gland (tryptophan → serotonin → melatonin), synthesized during dark phase but then decreases through the night (**circadian modulated**, *NOTE*: β-blockers may interfere with melatonin production causing insomnia)
- **Renin**: increases during NREM (to prevent nocturia, along with antidiuretic hormone) and decreases during REM
- **Testosterone**: sleep modulated, peaks after sleep onset

## Effects of Sleep Deprivation

### *Acute Sleep Deprivation*

- most important consequence is sleepiness causing mood disorders, safety issues, hyperactivity in children, poor attention and cognition (↓learning), errors of omission (lapsing), **errors of commission** (false reports, "psychosis")
- slows cerebral glucose metabolism, slurred speech, tremors, hyperactive deep tendon reflexes (although sluggish corneal reflexes)
- ↑**Sympathetic Activation**: ↑**cortisol in the late afternoon and evening** (at the nadir, normally peaks in the morning) and ghrelin (weight gain) and insulin resistance
- **Hormonal Changes**: ↓GH, ↑evening cortisol, ↑TSH, ↓prolactin, ↓leptin (weight gain), ↓insulin
- ↑**Proinflammatory Markers**: IL-1, IL-6, TNF-α
- **EEG Changes**: ↓alpha activity, ↑delta and theta waves (can be present in wake), no changes in beta
- <u>Recovery Sleep PSG Findings</u>
  1. **Day 1**: ↑slow wave sleep, ↓sleep latency, unchanged or ↓REM duration, ↓alpha activity
  2. **Day 2**: ↑REM sleep
  3. **Day 3**: normal sleep architecture
- may reduce immunological function

- *NOTE*: lack of REM sleep does not distinctly cause symptomatic sleepiness

## *Chronic Sleep Restriction (<4–6 hours/night)*

- <u>PSG</u>: ↓sleep latency, ↓**REM** (may be absent), ↓N2 **but** only slight increase in slow wave sleep (unlike acute sleep deprivation), "microsleeps" (N1 interrupts sleep)
- <u>Recovery PSG</u>: requires >3 nights of restorative to recover, ↑**REM** (eg, ↑REM after placing OSAS patient on CPAP)
- ↓oculomotor responses, ↓psychomotor vigilance testing (although there is significant individual variability)
- ↑BMI from ↓glucose intolerance, ↑ghrelin, and ↓leptin
- <u>Endocrine/Inflammation</u>: **similar to acute phase**
- elderly have less effect from sleep deprivation

## *Sleep Fragmentation*

- frequent brief arousals (even in the absence of EEG changes) cause daytime sleepiness
- sleepiness is more related to sleep fragmentation than to sleep stages
- if the arousals are >10 minutes then the effect is less (**therefore restorative sleep requires ≥10 minutes**)

# POLYSOMNOGRAPHY (PSG)

(based on the *AASM Manual for Scoring Sleep, 2007*)

## Introduction

- typically 2–3 EEG derivations are required to monitor activity from the frontal, central, and occipital regions (individual electrode impedance <5 kΩ)
- EEG measures postsynaptic potentials from the gigantic pyramidal cells
- EOG measures left and right eye movement (cornea = positive charge, retina = negative charge)
- submental EMG records chin movement (used to determine phasic REM)
- airflow may be determined by changes in temperature, pressure, end tidal $CO_2$, or an algorithm from efforts signals
- apnea is best measured by an **oronasal thermosensor**
- hyponea is better measured by **nasal air pressure transducer**

- respiratory effort is measured by esophageal manometry (**best**), intracostal EMG, or **respiratory inductive plethysmograph** (**RIP**, indirect measure of airflow, calculated by the **sum** of changes in the thoracic and abdominal cross-section area)
- Filters: typically not adjusted routinely, high-pass filters (low-frequency filter) block low frequencies (used with EMG and snore channels), low-pass filters (high-frequency filters) block high frequencies (used with respiratory channels); midrange used for EEG and EOG
- Amplifiers: AC (alternating current) amplifies high frequencies such as EEG, ECG, EOG, EMG; DC (direct current) amplifies low frequencies such as pulse oximeter, respiratory channels
- Impedance: measures the contact of the electrode with the skin (should be <5kΩ)
- **Home (Portable) PSG**: may be considered if suspect a moderate to severe OSAS without comorbidities, suspicion of central events, or symptoms of other sleep-related disorders (eg, narcolepsy); **not** to be used as a screener for asymptomatic patients
- Types of PSG
  I. attended, all channels, in lab
  II. unattended, all channels in the home (typically impractical)
  III. unattended, 4-channels (airflow, abdomen/chest movement, pulse oximeter, ECG/pulse), standard "home sleep study"
  IV. unattended, 1-2-channel (not used)

## Stages of Sleep (*see* Figures 5–1 through 5–5 and Table 5–2)

- **Epoch**: typically 30 seconds of sleep, stage is assigned to each epoch
- **Sleep Onset**: first epoch staged other than stage W (typically first stage N1)
- **Stage W (Wakefulness/Drowsiness)**: primarily **alpha waves** in occipital leads
- **Stage N1 (NREM1)**: primarily low amplitude, mixed frequency (**LAMF**), and **slow eye movements**, may also have **vertex** sharp waves, ~<**5% of sleep, transitional sleep** ("drifting off," easily awakened)
- **Stage N2 (NREM2)**: presence of a spontaneous **K-complex** (without an arousal occurring within 1 second of the end of the K-complex) or **sleep spindle** in the first half of the epoch; ~**50% of sleep**
- **Stage N3 (NREM3)**: >20% (6 seconds) of **slow wave activity** (0.5 Hz–2 Hz, >75 µV amplitude), typically minimal eye movements ~**10% of sleep**, deepest, restorative sleep, occurs mainly in first half of the night

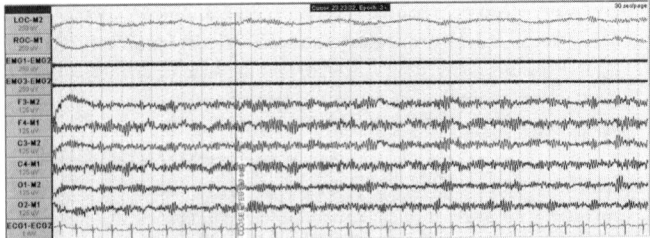

**FIGURE 5–1.** One epoch of wakefulness (W) with representative alpha waves in all of the EEG leads.

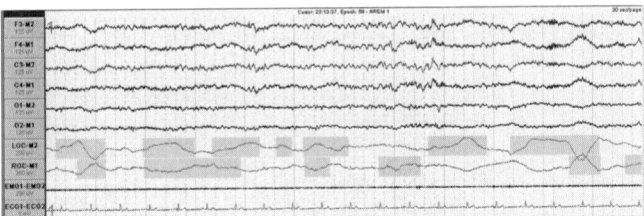

**FIGURE 5–2.** One epoch of Stage N1 with low amplitude, mixed frequency waves in the EEG leads as well as the beginning of slow eye movements in the EOG leads.

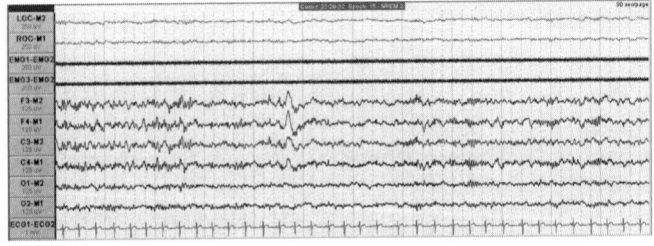

**FIGURE 5–3.** One epoch of classic Stage N2 with both K-complexes and sleep spindles more prominent in the frontal EEG leads.

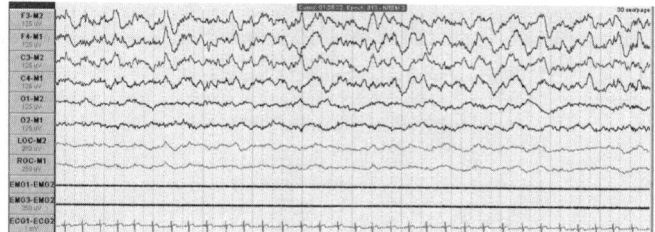

**FIGURE 5–4.** One epoch of Stage N3 with characteristic delta (slow-wave) activity in the EEG leads.

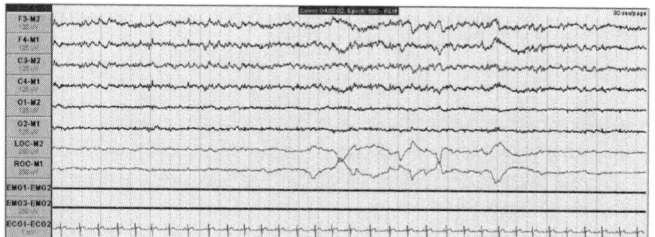

**FIGURE 5–5.** One epoch of phasic REM stage sleep with the presence of rapid eye movements in the EOG leads, decreased tone in the EMG chin leads, and a background low amplitude, mixed frequency EEG (similar to N1).

- **Stage R (REM)**: low EMG tone (chin), REM, low amplitude, mixed frequency (similar to N1) may have saw tooth waves (**phasic REM** includes REM, **tonic REM** does not have REM); **~25% of sleep,** occurs more often and with greater length with more sleep time
- *NOTE*: if a major body movement occurs (movement that obscures the EEG for **more than half the epoch**), stage as W if alpha waves are present or if stage W appears before or after the epoch, otherwise stage as the same stage that **follows** the epoch
- *NOTE*: if a major body movement is followed by low amplitude, mixed frequency (LAMF) without a K-complex or spindles, stage the sleep based on the presence of **slow eye movement** (N1) or **no** slow eye movement (N2)

## Waves and Rhythms

- **Beta Rhythm**: frequency EEG waves (13–30 Hz, seen in **active** wakefulness)

**TABLE 5–2.** Key Characteristics of Sleep Stages

| Stage | PSG Characteristics | Clinical Characteristics | % of Sleep |
|-------|---------------------|--------------------------|------------|
| W | β-waves and α-waves in relaxed state | wake and drowsiness | - |
| N1 | LAMF, θ-waves, slow eye movements | transitional sleep, drifting off, easily awakened | <5% |
| N2 | K-complexes and spindle waves | intermediate sleep, awakened by sound | ~50% |
| N3 | >20% slow wave (δ-waves) | deep sleep, restorative sleep | ~10% |
| R | ↓EMG tone, ±REM, LAMF (N1 like) | easily awakened | ~25% |

- **Alpha Rhythm**: EEG sinusoidal waves (**8–12 Hz**) maximal over the **occipital** region (seen in **relaxed, eyes closed** wakefulness, W)
- **Theta Rhythm**: EEG waves (4–8 Hz, N1, N2), predominant background of sleep
- **Delta Rhythm**: EEG waves (1–4 Hz, N3), **>75-μV amplitude**
- **Low Amplitude, Mixed Frequency Activity (LAMF)**: waves with low amplitude with frequencies typically from theta waves 4–7 Hz (N1, REM)
- **Vertex Sharp Waves (V waves)**: sharp negative EEG wave <0.5 seconds, maximal over the **central/vertex** region (N1)
- **K-Complex**: **triphasic wave** (sharp negative, upward, then positive, downward, then negative) lasting ≥0.5 seconds (N2) maximal over the **frontal** region (*NOTE*: commonly seen before an arousal but not counted in staging)
- **Sleep Spindle**: series of rapid frequencies (11–16 Hz) lasting ≥0.5 Hz (N2) maximal in **central/vertex** region, produced in the reticular nucleus of the thalamus; **pseudo-spindles (drug spindles),** which are longer in duration and a higher frequency, may be seen in N2 with benzodiazepines and antidepressants
- **Slow Wave Activity**: EEG waves with slow frequency 0.5–2.0 Hz and peak-to-peak amplitude **>75 μV** maximal over the **frontal region** (N3)
- **Sawtooth Waves**: triangular waves 2–6 Hz, maximal over the **central** region (R)
- **Positive Occipital Sharp Transient of Sleep Wave (POSTS)**: normal downward spike found in the occipital channels
- **Epileptiform Discharges**: initial "**spike and wave**" sharp wave followed by a slow wave

- **Interictal Spikes**: associated with focal epilepsy, may appear like an electrode pop artifact
- **Alpha Intrusions**: alpha seen in nonwake sleep or REM, may be from chronic pain, rheumatoid arthritis, postsurgical; may represent nonrestorative sleep
- **Disorganized Sleep**: sleep pattern appears awake, seen with opioids

## Eye Movements

- **Eye Blinks**: sharp vertical eye movements with eyes open or closed (W)
- **Reading Eye Movements**: conjugate slow eye movement followed by a rapid opposite eye movement (W)
- **Slow Eye Movement (SEM)**: conjugate, regular sinusoidal eye movements (lasts >0.5 seconds) (N1)
- **Rapid Eye Movement (REM)**: conjugate sharply peaked eye movements lasting <0.5 seconds (R but may also be seen in wakefulness when scanning)
- **Rolling (Prozac) Eyes**: rolling eye movements seen in all stages with SSRIs

## Respiratory Scoring Data

- **Apnea**: drop in oronasal thermal sensor ≥90% of baseline lasting >10 seconds (**no** oxygen desaturation or arousals required)
- **Hyponea**: nasal air pressure decrease by ≥30% of baseline lasting >10 seconds, associated with a ≥4% oxygen desaturation, **no** arousal required (**"30-4" criteria**); alternative definition requires ≥50% of baseline lasting >10 seconds, associated with a ≥3% oxygen desaturation **or** an arousal, similar criteria for pediatrics, (**"50-3/ arousal" criteria**)
- **Respiratory Effort-Related Arousal (RERA)**: an arousal that is preceded by a respiratory effort but does not meet criteria for an apnea or hyponea lasting ≥10 seconds
- **Obstructive Apnea**: apneic event associated with increase in respiratory effort throughout event
- **Central Apnea**: apneas without associated respiratory effort
- **Mixed Apnea**: apneic event that begins with an absent respiratory effort (central apnea) but effort resumes in the last portion of the event
- Indices
  1. **Apnea Index (AI)** measures apneas/hour only
  2. **Apnea Hyponea Index (AHI)** measures apneas and hyponeas/hour
  3. **Respiratory Distress Index (RDI)**: measures apneas, hyponeas, and RERAs/hour

- **Cheyne-Stokes Breathing**: 3 cycles of crescendo and decrescendo breathing amplitude lasting 10 minutes or associated with ≥5 central apneas or hyponeas
- **Sleep-Related Hypoventilation**: ≥10 mm Hg increase in $PaCO_2$, (not related to hypoxemia)

## Movement Scoring Data

- **Leg Movement**: increase in the anterior tibialis EMG lasting between 0.5–10 seconds (**not scored if during an apneic episode**)
- **Periodic Leg Movement** (**PLM**): **4** leg movements occurring within **5–90 seconds** of each other (not scored if before or after 0.5 seconds of a respiratory event)
- **Alternate Leg Muscle Activation** (**ALMA**): >4 bursts of activity from alternating legs (not commonly measured)
- **Hypnagogic Foot Tremor** (**HFT**): bursts of foot activity (not commonly measured), occurs during sleep initiation
- **Excessive Fragmentary Myoclonus** (**EFM**): benign single bursts of movement (not commonly measured)
- **Sleep-Related Bruxism**: may be sustained (tonic) or phasic, measured by elevation of chin EMG for >2 sec (2× background EMG), best measured by **masseter muscle**
- **Sustained Muscle Activity in REM Sleep**: tonic increase in chin EMG during REM sleep (>50% of the epoch), seen in REM sleep behavior disorders
- **Excessive Transient Muscle Activity in REM Sleep**: bursts of phasic increase in chin EMG during REM sleep, seen in REM sleep behavior disorders

## Other Scoring Data

- **Arousal**: abrupt shift of EEG >16 Hz lasting **at least 3 seconds** (arousal during REM must have an increase in chin EMG ≥1 second), must be preceded by **10 seconds** of sleep
- **Cardiac Parameters**: bradycardia <**40** BPM, tachycardia >**90** BPM (different than awake), asystole >3 second pause, wide complex tachycardia >100 BPM (**seek help**) and QRS duration ≥120 milliseconds (requires 3 consecutive beats), narrow complex tachycardia QRS duration <120 milliseconds
- **Sleep Efficiency**: time asleep/recording time

## Artifacts and Troubleshooting

- **Artifacts**: extraneous signals that represent activity not intended for that channel (physiological or from instrumentations and environment)

- **60-Hz Artifact**: electrical interference "fast" artifact caused by loose leads or electrodes, regular high frequency pattern, most common ("felt tipped marker pattern"); <u>Rx</u>: check electrodes, remove interference electronics (nonshielded power cords, cell phones), may consider a 60-Hz filter ("notch" filter)
- **Muscle Artifact**: **mixed** "fast" artifact caused by EEG or EOG or localized muscle activity near a lead, **irregular** high frequency wave ("fuzzy lines"), differentiated from 60 Hz by the presence of mixed frequencies; <u>Rx</u>: **often resolves with sleep**
- **ECG Artifact**: activity lines with the ECG lead; <u>Rx</u>: move mastoid lead away from the neck, check impedance levels, consider double references
- **Slow Artifacts (Respiration and Sweat Artifacts)**: seen in EEG and EOG channels from increased impedance or "sweat," appears as a motion/respiratory pattern; <u>Rx</u>: reposition patient, cool room, change reference leads, place electrodes on bony areas, may consider increasing high pass (low frequency) filter
- **Electrode Pop**: K-complex-like artifact that is found in one electrode and not consistent in other derivations; <u>Rx</u>: fix electrode
- **Mixed Frequency Artifact**: combination of signal interferences from poor application or broken wire; <u>Rx</u>: check connections and wires
- may correct for artifacts by re-referencing (choosing a different electrode), reapplying electrodes, and use of filters (severe sweating)
- <u>Other Artifacts</u>: bruxism, movements, DC artifact (improper calibration), high frequency interference from other electrical equipment, oximeter artifact, pacemaker

## Pediatric Sleep Scoring (>2 months to 13–18 years old)

- **Stage N**: occurs when NREM sleep without ever going into definable N2–N3 stages (no sleep spindles/K complexes or <20%/epoch slow wave sleep)
- **Dominant Posterior Rhythm (DPR)**: EEG pattern occurs in occipital region in children during drowsy wakefulness (replaced later by alpha rhythm), frequency 3.5–4.5 Hz at 3–4 months then 7.5–9.5 Hz by 3 years old
- **Rhythmic Anterior Theta Activity**: pattern of 5–7 Hz theta activity in the frontal region found in children indicating Stage N1
- **Hypnagogic (Theta) Synchronicity**: theta waves (high amplitude, low frequency) found in the onset of sleep in children/adolescence (N1)
- **Tracé Discontinue (TD)**: <37 conceptional age (premature), bursts of high voltage sleep waves (0.5–3 Hz) with interburst interval activity of long and low amplitude waves, occurs in **quiet** sleep

- **Tracé Alternant (TA)**: >37 conceptional age, similar to TD with **shorter interburst** interval (4–5 seconds) with interburst higher amplitude, also occurs in **quiet** sleep
- **Low Voltage Irregular (LVI)**: low voltage (14–35 µV, occurs in **active/REM sleep**)
- **Delta Brush**: bursts of alpha-like activity during TA/TD, detected at 26 weeks post-conceptual age
- **Apneic Events**: do not need to last 10 seconds but rather the duration of 2 baseline breaths
- *NOTE*: central apnea in pediatrics is similar to adults; however, the event must last ≥20 seconds **or** 2 missed breaths with an arousal/ awakening or with a ≥3% desaturation
- **Hyponea Events**: nasal air pressure decreases by ≥50% lasting the duration of 2 breaths and must be associated with a ≥3% oxygen desaturation or an arousal/awakening
- **RERAs**: nasal air pressure flattens and decreases in amplitude but **not** ≥50% and is associated with snoring, noisy breathing, increased work of breathing, or elevation of end-tidal or transcutaneous $PCO_2$
- **Sleep-Related Hypoventilation**: >25% of total sleep time is spent with $CO_2$ >50 mm Hg

## Multiple Sleep Latency Test (MSLT)

- measures the physiological tendency to fall asleep
- <u>Indications</u>: narcolepsy, daytime sleepiness
- <u>Protocol</u>: patient **asked to nap 4–5** times, allow for **20** minutes to sleep at **2**-hour intervals (stay awake in between naps, minimum 4 naps), first nap 1.5–3 hours after morning awakening or end of PSG, allow patient to sleep for 15 minutes after sleep onset
- conducted after PSG (at least 6 hours of total sleep time to rule out sleep disordered breathing)
- should have 1–2 weeks of regular sleep prior without stimulants
- measure **sleep latency** ("lights out" to sleep) and **REM latency** (sleep onset to REM)
- sleep defined as >15 cumulative seconds of any stage of sleep in one epoch (some protocols may require 3 consecutive N1 or any one epoch of another stage)
- if sleep is achieved allow 15 minutes of sleep to relieve REM burden
- **≥2 sleep onset REM** (**SOREM**, any REM during a nap) and **mean sleep latency < 8 minutes suggests narcolepsy**

## Maintenance of Wakefulness Test (MWT)

- measures a person's ability to **maintain wakefulness** in quiet, reclined position, dimly lit room

- <u>Indications</u>: assess treatment or for occupational requirements (drivers, pilots), treatment efficacy
- previous PSG not required
- <u>Protocol</u>: patient **asked to stay awake** for 4 trials for **40** minutes at **2** hour intervals in a calm, dimly lit room, wake patient if any sleep (sleep defined as >15 cumulative seconds of any sleep, some protocols may require 3 consecutive N1 or any one epoch of another stage)
- **mean sleep latency determines level of impaired ability** (may require subjective decision)

# SLEEP-DISORDERED BREATHING (SDB)
## Pulmonary Sleep Physiology

- <u>Overview</u>: cortex (conscious breathing), pons (determines rate), medulla (controls rhythm)
- <u>Ventilation Control</u>: peripheral chemoreceptors (carotid body, aortic body), central chemoreceptors (medulla, slow responding), stretch receptors, irritant receptors, and proprioreceptors; hypoxia is the least sensitive trigger to cause an arousal, hypercapnia is a brisk trigger to an arousal; $PaCO_2 = VCO_2$ ($CO_2$ production)/$V_A$; $\uparrow$alveolar ventilation causes $\downarrow PaCO_2$
- <u>NREM</u>: **no change in respiratory rate** $\downarrow$metabolic and hypercapnic sensitivity (pH, $PaO_2$, $PaCO_2$); $\downarrow$tidal volume, $\downarrow$FRC, $\downarrow$minute ventilation, $\uparrow$upper airway resistance
- <u>REM</u>: irregular respiratory pattern (periodic breathing may occur during phasic REM), $\downarrow\downarrow$metabolic and hypercapnic sensitivity ($\downarrow PaO_2$ by 2–12 mmHg, $\downarrow SaO_2$ by 2%, $\uparrow PaCO_2$ by 2–8 mmHg), $\uparrow\uparrow$upper airway resistance

## Obstructive Sleep Apnea Syndrome (OSAS)
### Introduction

- <u>Diagnostic Criteria</u> (*ICSD-2*): ≥5/hour respiratory events (apnea, hyponea, or RERA) with respiratory effort with symptoms (eg, daytime somnolence, snoring, fatigue, insomnia, witnessed apneic events) **or** ≥15/hour respiratory events with respiratory effort **without** symptoms
- **1.5–4%** prevalence of OSAS

- <u>Pathophysiology</u>: multiple etiologies including anatomical (upper airway collapse, inability for airway dilators to respond), neurogenic (sensitivity of chemoreceptors, ↓central drive, defective ventilatory receptors), and **high loop gain** (ventilatory control)
- respiratory effort is the strongest stimulus to an arousal (more than hypoxia or hypercapnia)
- <u>Risks</u>: obesity, family history, anatomical considerations, elderly (soft tissue laxity), South Asians, Marfan's syndrome, myopathies, neural disease, allergies, ApoE4 allele, males except **postmenopausal females equal males in risk of OSAS** (↓risk in postmenopausal women who use hormonal replacement therapy, women also have lower survival than men with similar AHI), **left ventricular heart failure** (independent risk factor)
- <u>Stroke</u>: OSAS and snoring increases risk of stroke and stroke leads to OSAS (may also have CSA)
- <u>OSAS in the Elderly</u>: elderly have less daytime somnolence, snoring, and associated obesity; less risk of cardiopulmonary complications; more common in males, however, increase prevalence in postmenopausal women
- <u>SSx</u>: daytime somnolence, snoring, witnessed apneic events, morning headache (nocturnal $CO_2$ retention), mouth breathing, weight gain, abnormal motor activity, bruxism, depression, irritability, insomnia, enuresis (children), sexual dysfunction, nocturnal motor activity

## Anatomical Evaluation

- **velopharynx most common location of collapse** (normal >11 mm)
- **2/3** incidence of multiple airway collapse at the **retropalatal and retrolingual airway**
- collapse occurs at the **end of expiration** (abnormal if >50% collapse)
- <u>Muscles that Maintain Patency</u>: tensor palantini, pterygoids, genioglossus, genihyoid, sternohyoid
- **Modified Müller Maneuver**: look retropalatal and retrolingual and measure collapse at the end of expiration (1+ <25%, 2+ 26–50%, 3+ 51–75%, 4+ 76–100%), abnormal if >50% collapse
- **Modified Mallampati Score**: performed with tongue extruded; Class I normal, Class II uvula/tonsils partly visible, Class III base of uvula only visible/tonsils not visible, Class IV soft palate not visible
- **Friedman Scale**: same as Mallampati except Friedman does not extrude the tongue
- **Fujita Classification**: Type I oropharyngeal collapse, Type II oropharyngeal and hypopharyngeal collapse, Type III hypopharyngeal collapse
- **Cricomental Distance**: >15 mm

- **Neck Circumference**: ≥17 inches (male) and ≥15.5 inches (female); **most predictive indicator of OSAS**
- **Waste/Hip Ratio**: >0.9 men and >0.85 in women
- <u>Nasal Disorders</u>: septal deflection, obstructing turbinates, allergies
- <u>Other</u>: kyphosis, micro/retro-gnathia, high arched palate, flat maxilla, tracheo/laryngo-malacia, enlarged tongue (Down's), hypertrophic parapharyngeal fat pad
- **Lateral Cephalometric Analysis**: x-ray of the head studying the relationships of the bony and soft tissue landmarks
- **Sleep Endoscopy**: flexible laryngoscopy performed under drug-induced sleep, allowing for a more physiological assessment of upper airway collapse (ie, velopharyngeal collapse, base of tongue collapse, retroflexed epiglottis); various indications including complicated or severe OSAS, revisions, suspect hypopharyngeal involvement

## Effects of Untreated OSAS

- <u>Mortality</u>: 2.5× risk of driving accident, 3–6× risk of sudden cardiac death **at night** (may not have an effect in overall risk especially during the day), higher mortality from **heart failure**
- <u>Morbidity</u>: 3× risk of hypertension (AHI > 15, although a direct correlation of causality has not been proved), pulmonary hypertension (independent of cardiopulmonary disease, although mild) stroke, insulin resistance, arrhythmias, ischemic heart disease
- 75–100% have gastroesophageal reflux disease (GERD) or laryngophargeal reflux (LPR) from ↓intrathoracic pressure (improves with CPAP)
- many physiological effects are independent of symptoms of sleepiness (**important to treat "asymptomatic" sleep apneic patients AHI>30**)
- <u>Physiological CV Effects in OSAS</u>: ↑sympathetic tone, ↓R-R interval (bradycardia), ↑BP variability (↑afterload, ↑endothelin), arrhythmias (**sinus arrhythmias most common,** also sinus pauses, bradycardia, PVCs, ventricular tachycardia, AV block), ↑monocyte adhesion index (causes endothelial injury), ↑transmural pressure from ↑negative chest pressure (↑wall stress, ↑atrial sizes, ↑aortic aneurysm, ↑aortic dissection)
- <u>Physiological Endocrine Effects in OSAS</u>: ↑C-reactive protein, ↑serum amyloid, ↑cortisol, ↓GH, ↓prolactin
- <u>Immunity</u>: ↑other proinflammatory cytokines (↑IL-6, CRP, TNF), which improves with CPAP; ↓IL-10
- <u>Pathophysiology of Increased Cardiac Risk</u>: reoxygenation of hypoxic tissues → free radicals → altered gene expression → ↑proinflammatory cells (TNF, IL-6, IL-8) and ↑adhesion molecules → endothelial dysfunction

- mortality from OSAS in the elderly is less (compensation), although will have sleepiness, nocturia, and disruptions (improved with CPAP)

## Other Types of Obstruction Disorders

- **Overlap Syndrome**: OSA with COPD, ↓baseline $PaO_2$ and ↓VQ mismatch causes exaggerated desaturations during apneas, ↑pulmonary hypertension, ↑mortality than COPD alone
- **Obesity–Hypoventilation**: daytime hypoventilation (hypercapnia, $PaCO_2$ >45 mmHg) **not** secondary to respiratory or neuromuscular disorder, severe obesity (BMI > 40 kg/m$^2$); <u>Rx</u>: requires BiPAP (to improve ventilation)
- **Primary Snorer**: snoring without significant apneas or hyponeas
- **Upper Airway Resistance Syndrome**: daytime somnolence secondary to arousals (RERAs) during upper airway resistance **without** apneas/hyponeas
- **Complex Sleep Apnea**: combination of OSA and CSA, usually noted after overtitrating CPAP for OSAS or with opiate use

# Medical Management of Obstructive Sleep Apnea

## Management Overview

- **treat comprehensively taking into consideration all therapeutic options, management of subjective symptoms, and possibility of complex OSAS** (*see* Figure 5–6)
- <u>Behavior Modifications</u>: weight loss, abstain from sedatives and alcohol, positional therapy, safety precautions (avoid driving, heights, machinery when tired)
- <u>CPAP/BiPAP</u>: *see following*
- <u>Mandibular Repositioning Device</u>: indicated for snorers and mild to moderate OSAS; custom devices most effective with ↓BMI, ↓AHI, positional sleep apnea, and significant mandibular protrusion by the device; risk of temporomandibular joint disease and teeth shifting, may cause excess salivation; shown to improve Epworth score, high blood pressure, and heart rate variability
- <u>Surgical</u>: *see following*
- modafinil (Provigil) may be considered for residual sleepiness after therapy

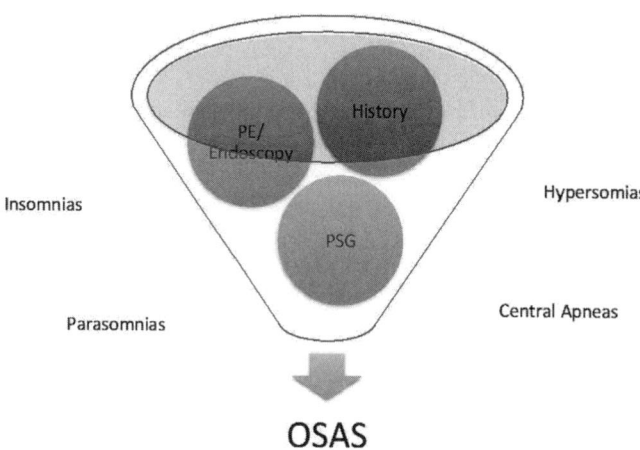

**FIGURE 5–6.** Treat obstructive sleep apnea comprehensively taking into account history, physical findings, confounding sleep-related issues, and objective data in determining a treatment plan.

## Continuous and Bi-Level Positive Airway Pressure (CPAP/Bi-PAP)

- **CPAP**: provides positive airway pressure, same level during both inspiration and expiration, applied via a nasal or oronasal mask to maintain airway patency
- <u>CPAP-Compliant Improved Cardiovascular and Pulmonary Physiological Effects</u>: ↑oxygen saturation, ↓pulmonary HTN, ↑functional residual capacity, ↓work of breathing, ↓**nocturnal recurrent atrial fibrillation and ventricular arrhythmias (PVCs)**, ↓cyclic heart rate variations, ↓preload, ↓afterload, ↓mortality from ischemic heart disease, ↓atherosclerosis, ↓nocturnal angina, ↑injection fraction; improvements in hypertension of 10 mm Hg occur with **severe OSAS patients** and require "all night" CPAP use independent of sleepiness (improvements within a few weeks); despite improvement in CV function CPAP does not improve survivability of heart failure patients unless it suppresses CSA
- <u>Other Improved CPAP-Compliant Effects</u>: GERD, erectile dysfunction, nocturia, depression, marginal improvement in insulin sensitivity
- <u>Titration Parameters</u>: remove apneas, RERAs, hyponeas, PLMs, hypoventilation, Cheyne–Stokes respiration
- **~50% noncompliance rate**, compliance more with daytime sleepiness symptoms, AHI does **not** correlate with compliance

- <u>Increase CPAP Compliance</u>: add humidity, consider a hypnotic (eg, **eszopiclone**), treat nasal congestion/obstruction (septoplasty, turbinate reduction), desensitization techniques for claustrophobia, **minimal compliance improvement by changing mask, APAP, BiPAP, or using C-Flex** (expiratory pressure relief)
- **BiPAP**: provides independent inspiratory positive airway pressure (**IPAP**) and expiratory positive airway pressures (**EPAP**); set EPAP (lower number) to adjust for the closed-airway apneas (similar to CPAP level); IPAP (higher number) set for ventilatory support and hyponeas, RERAs, and snoring; some modes may set a minimum rate (ideal for hypoventilatory patients)
- <u>BiPAP Indications</u>: pressure support for obesity–hypoventilatory patients, hypoxemic patients, respiratory muscle (myopathies) and neurological dysfunction, potential of barotraumas, or poor compliance with CPAP (although data does not show an increase in compliance)
- <u>CPAP/BiPAP Contraindications</u>: no respiratory drive, risk of aspiration, hypotension, CSF leak (cribriform plate injury), bullous lung disease, pneumocephalus, pneumothorax
- **Auto CPAP (APAP)**: most commonly uses flow sensors to manage each breath; mean pressure generally lower but peak airway pressures may be higher, contraindicated with CHF, COPD, obesity–hypoventilation, nonsnorers, and patients who are expected to desaturate due to conditions other than OSAS
- supplementary oxygen may be considered for comorbidities (CHF, COPD) and uncorrected desaturations after CPAP/BiPAP
- *NOTE*: in treating severe sleep OSAS, placing a patient on CPAP may inhibit the respiratory drive, which is stimulated by the respiratory effort (not hypoxia or hypercapnia), therefore you may have apnea with severe hypoxia

# Surgical Management of Obstructive Sleep Apnea

## Overview

- <u>Indications</u>: improve quality of life and health, failed CPAP trial (claustrophobia, pulling mask off at night, air leak around mask, unwilling), CPAP not practical (traveler, patient noncompliance), surgically correctable significant focal anatomic upper airway obstruction with high chance of "cure" (eg, 3+ obstructing tonsils with significant soft palate redundancy in a normal weight young adult), address snoring

**TABLE 5–3.** Assessment of Favorable Versus Unfavorable Surgically Correctable Anatomy

| Favorable | Unfavorable |
|---|---|
| Tonsillar Hyperplasia | Obesity |
| Adenoid Hyperplasia | Jowling or "Rounded Face" |
| Hyperplastic Lingual Tonsils | (Parapharyngeal Fat, Masseter Muscle |
| Elongated Soft Palate | Hypertrophy, East Asians) |
| Nasal Septal Deformities | Retrognathia/Micrognathia |
| Velopharynx > 11 mm | Macroglossia |
| Uvular Hypertrophy | Nasopharyngeal Stenosis or Collapse |
| Isolated Velopharyngeal Collapse | Bulky Base of Tongue |
| | Large Neck Circumference |
| | Lateral/Posterior Pharyngeal Wall Collapse |
| | High Arched Palate |

- Relative Contraindications: severe obesity, severe cardiopulmonary disease, substance abuse, aged, unrealistic outcomes, unfavorable anatomy (*see following*)
- surgical management usually requires a multimodality approach including weight loss program, follow-up sleep testing, **staged** surgical procedures, and possible continued CPAP use
- surgical considerations include the presence of surgically correctable anatomy (favorable) versus more difficult anatomical findings (unfavorable), *see* Table 5–3
- *NOTE*: surgical "success" is exceedingly controversial and variable due to arbitrary definitions of success, difficulty in stratifying preoperative conditions and postoperative measures, use of multiple procedures, overemphasis of AHI, no standard follow-up, and challenges in achieving statistical power; standardization of outcomes data are required

## Nasal Surgery

- Types: septoplasty, turbinate reduction, polypectomy, nasal valve reconstruction, functional rhinoplasty
- Indications: improve nasal airway, decrease mouth breathing, nasopharyngeal snoring, **improve CPAP compliance by decreasing pressure requirements**
- Advantages: simple procedures with easier recovery, best surgical method to improve CPAP compliance
- Disadvantages: does not address OSAS directly
- Risks: bleeding, septal perforation, atrophic rhinitis, crusting, cosmetic deformity

## Nasopharyngeal Surgery

- <u>Types</u>
  1. **Adenoidectomy**: most common
  2. **Transpalatal Advancement Pharyngoplasty**: requires removal of palatal bone segment with advancement of soft tissue to gain superior nasopharyngeal space
  3. **Maxillary Advancement**: technically difficult, *see following*
- <u>Indications</u>: significant nasopharyngeal stenosis or collapse
- <u>Risks</u>: bleeding, nasopharyngeal stenosis, oral/nasal fistula (transpalatal advancement)

## Oropharyngeal and Velopharyngeal Surgery

- <u>Types</u>
  1. **Adenotonsillectomy**: primary treatment for OSAS in children
  2. **Palatal Reconstruction Techniques, Uvulopalatopharyngoplasty (UP3, UPPP)**: various techniques that reconstruct and reduce the posterior edge of the soft palate and uvula, often combined with a tonsillectomy, variations include uvulopalatal flap and palatal advancement flaps
  3. **Lateral Pharyngoplasty**: techniques that expand the lateral diameter
  4. **Palatal Stiffening Procedures**: includes implants, sclerosing injections, and radiofrequency ablation procedures; may be combined with a uvulectomy; may be completed in the office; **limited benefit** for significant sleep apnea, may address primary snoring with favorable anatomy (nonobstructing tonsils, limited oropharyngeal and hypopharyngeal collapse, normal weight)
- <u>Indications</u>: significant oropharyngeal (velopalatine) crowding, adenotonsillectomy treatment of choice in children over CPAP, snoring
- <u>Advantages</u>: common procedures with multiple surgical techniques, addresses snoring directly
- <u>Disadvantages</u>: **reduction of the soft palate and uvula carries risk of air leaks with CPAP which can worsen compliance**; long-term results are unfavorable possibly due to multiple sites of obstruction, painful recovery, globus sensation
- <u>Risks</u>: bleeding, scar formation (oropharyngeal/nasopharyngeal stenosis), flash pulmonary edema (<u>Rx</u>: positive airway pressure, possible overnight intubation), voice changes, velopharyngeal insufficiency, worsening of TMJ, tooth injury, extrusion of implants

## Hypopharyngeal Surgery

- <u>Types</u>
  1. **Tongue Base Reduction, Lingual Tonsillectomy**: various en bloc resection and reduction techniques to address the retrolingual space including the use of coblation, radiofrequency, cautery; also may consider transoral robotic surgery (TORS, *see following*); risk of dysgeusia, injury to the lingual artery, lingual hematoma
  2. **Midline Glossectomy**: various techniques to reduce midline soft tissue medial to the neurovascular bundle; risk of injury to lingual neurovascular bundle, dysgeusia, and hematoma
  3. **Genioglossal Advancement**: repositions the tongue anteriorly by advancing a segment of mandible with the genioglossus attached, does not move the teeth; limited anterior advancement; risk of relaxation of tongue base, infection, extrusion of hardware, osteitis, necrosis of bone segment, sublingual hematoma
  4. **Genioglossal Suspension**: tongue base is suspended anteriorly to mandible using various material including sutures, simple technique; limited anterior advancement; risk of breakage and relaxation of tongue base
  5. **Hyoid Myotomy and Suspension**: hyoid bone is repositioned anteriorly by releasing infrahyoid muscles and suspending to the lingual surface of the mandible or to the thyroid cartilage; risk of breakage, infection, mental nerve injury, and hyoid injury
  6. **Epiglottoplasty, Hyoepiglottoplasty**: debulks or stabilizes the epiglottis, may require neck incision, risk of aspiration
  7. **Transoral Robotic Surgery (TORS)**: utilizes advances in robotic instrumentation to access the hypopharynx to address lingual tonsils, tongue base, and epiglottis; excellent visualization (*see also* pp. 333–334)
- <u>Indications</u>: significant hypopharyngeal obstruction, relative macroglossia, base of tongue obstruction, retroflexed epiglottis
- <u>Advantages</u>: may be coupled with an oropharyngeal procedure

## Mandibular and Midface Advancement Techniques

- <u>Types</u>: includes various maxillomandibular advancement (MMA) techniques such as LeFort I and mandibular osteotomies, requires multidisciplinary approach (oro-maxillofacial surgery)
- <u>Indications</u>: obstruction involving the retrolingual and retropalatal airway
- <u>Advantages</u>: considered more effective in addressing the retrolingual/palatal airway than soft tissue oropharyngeal and hypopharyngeal techniques, may be performed in 1 stage

- <u>Disadvantages</u>: requires osteotomies, prolonged recovery, may change facial appearance, requires maxillomandibular fixation, may change occlusion (requiring orthodontics), technically difficult
- <u>Risks</u>: bony nonunion, unacceptable facial deformity, occlusion disorders, TMJ, tooth injury, nerve injury (paresthesia), swelling

## Tracheotomy

- <u>Indications</u>: noncompliant CPAP use with severe OSAS, obese patients, cor pulmonale
- <u>Advantages</u>: most effective surgical treatment for sleep apnea
- <u>Disadvantages</u>: requires postoperative care, presence of a stoma
- <u>Risks</u>: bleeding, infection, pneumothorax, dislodgement, tracheal stenosis

# Central Sleep Apnea (CSA)

## Introduction

- <u>SSx</u>: similar to OSAS except milder snoring, awaken with **choking** sensation, obesity is less common
- marked variations in $PaCO_2$ but fewer changes in $O_2$
- fewer associations with pulmonary and cardiac complications
- <u>Rx</u>: **treat underlying disorder**, CPAP (may increase $PCO_2$), may consider adaptive seroventilator (ASV) for Cheyne-Stokes, nasal oxygen helps in heart failure (helps but does not eliminate CSA) and for high-altitude periodic breathing
- <u>Pharmacological Treatment for CSA</u>: acetazolamide for high-altitude periodic breathing, respiratory stimulants, short-acting benzodiazepine decreases arousals
- **Adaptive Servo-Ventilation (ASV)**: BiPAP that reacts to **hypo**- and **hyper**-ventilatory phases (set IPAP, variable EPAP), indicated for Cheyne-Stokes breathing and when CPAP does not eliminate central apneas, provides maximal support during apneas and minimal support during hyperventilation (**not** indicated for hypoventilation patients), used in pain patients on opioids (variable increase in central apneas)
- may occur normally when titrating CPAP (as a "sigh") and during wake–sleep transitions

## Central Sleep Apnea Mechanisms

- **Hypercapnic CSA**: secondary to **obesity/hypoventilation syndrome, congenital central apnea, central alveolar**

**hypoventilation, and neuromuscular disease**; ↓ventilatory response to hypercapnia causes eventual hyperventilation → ↓$PaCO_2$ → **hypocapnia reaches apneic threshold** ($PCO_2$ level in which a CSA occurs, during NREM) → apneic event→ ↑$PaCO_2$ **but also causes** ↓$O_2$ → hyperventilation → vicious cycle; associated with daytime hypoventilation (waking ↑$PaCO_2$)

- **Normocapnic Mechanisms**: transient instability of the drive, ↑ventilatory response to hypercapnia (**heart failure, stroke, renal failure, high-altitude CSA**) → ↑circulatory time → ↑feedback delay or ↑chemoreflex loop gain (*see previous*); associated with normal waking $PaCO_2$

## Types of Central Sleep Apnea

- **Primary CSA**: idiopathic, >5 CSA/hour
- **Cheyne-Stokes Breathing Pattern**: waxing and waning tidal volume pattern of hyperpnea and apneas; may be **asymptomatic**; associated with CHF, stroke, and renal failure; presents most commonly in **N1** and **N2**, longer cycle time than primary CSA, arousal may occur when tidal volume is at the **maximum**
- **High-Altitude CSA**: normal response with ascent >4,000 meters, at high levels hyperventilation from hypoxia causes a ↓**PCO₂** suppressing ventilatory drive, cycle length of CSA 15–30 seconds; Rx: descent, oxygen therapy, acetazolamide
- **CSA Due to Medical Condition/Drug or Substance: opioids** (CSA is chaotic and slow pattern)
- **Central Apnea Induced by CPAP**: temporary response to initiating CPAP

## Hypoventilation Syndrome

- abnormal increase in $PaCO_2$ during sleep resulting in hypoxia **without apneas/hyponeas**
- SSx: fatigue, daytime somnolence, erythrocytosis, pulmonary hypertension
- Pathophysiology: hypoxemia caused by lung parenchymal or pulmonary vascular disease
- Causes: **lower airway obstruction** (emphysema, chronic bronchitis, nocturnal asthma), **upper airway obstruction** (neuromuscular and chest wall disorders), obesity, interstitial lung disease, pulmonary hypertension, sickle cell anemia, myxedema (hypothyroid), central drive disorders
- Complications: nocturnal hypoxemia, pulmonary hypertension, cor pulmonale

- <u>Dx</u>: PFTs, pulmonary artery catheterization, echocardiogram
- <u>PSG</u>: **sustained long desaturation** (SpO$_2$ <90% for 5 minutes, nadir ≤85%) **without** apneas/hyponeas, airflow limitations, or snoring, may have a **PaCO$_2$ > 45 mm Hg** (depends on baseline PaCO$_2$), **worse during REM**
- <u>Rx</u>: treat underlying cause, CPAP although **BiPAP** may be better with possible nocturnal oxygen and backup rate (titrate EPAP for **upper airway patency** and IPAP as **pressure support**), weight loss, tracheotomy
- **Central Alveolar Hypoventilation Syndrome**: sleep hypoventilation (secondary to obesity or neuromuscular disorder) causes hypercapneia, an idiopathic form may be secondary to a ventilatory chemoreceptor defect in the medulla
- **Obesity Hypoventilation Syndrome (OHS, Pickwickian)**: associated with daytime hypercapnia and hypoxemia, cor pulmonale, HTN, morning headaches, and red eyes; sleep ↑PCO$_2$ > 10 torr and with **persistent desaturations** (OSAS usually normalizes between apneas), obesity by itself causes a decrease in expiratory reserve volume and a functional residual capacity (FRC), but OHS results in a further decrease in FRC as well as total lung capacity

# OTHER SLEEP-RELATED DISORDERS
## Sleep-Related Movement Disorders

### Restless Leg Syndrome (RLS)

- <u>Pathophysiology</u>: possibly from ↓**CNS iron** causing cell death in the substantia nigra (↓**dopamine**)
- <u>Criteria</u>: 1. urge to move, 2. worse with rest, 3. relief with movement, 4. worse at night
- <u>SSx</u>: irresistible urge to move during sleep or inactivity causing discomfort (paraesthesia, restlessness, pain, "creepiness"), may disturb sleep, **relieved with movement**, insomnia
- more common in women (2×), family history (>90%, autosomal dominant)
- **BTBD9 gene** (broad complex-tramtrack bric-a-brac–domain 9): chromosome 6, may interfere with iron homeostasis, more associated with PLMs rather than specific to RLS
- <u>Dx</u>: primarily clinical, consider PSG (suspect OSAS), consider lab work-up (serum ferritin, renal function, glucose, anemia, thyroid, B$_{12}$, Mg, ANA, RF), **CSF transferrin levels** (most sensitive)

- <u>Types</u>
  1. **Primary Type**: onset in youth, familial, more gradual onset
  2. **Secondary Type**: iron-deficiency (Fe <50 mcg/L), renal failure, **20–25%** of pregnancy, medication withdrawal, **medications (SSRIs, TCAs, lithium**, antihistamines, antipsychotics, **lithium**, dopamine antagonists); rheumatoid arthritis, multiple sclerosis, pain disorders, psychiatric and neurological disorders
  3. **Idiopathic**: most common
- <u>PSG</u>: **80%** of RLS have PLMs, PLMs are **not** necessary for diagnosis
- <u>DDx</u>: nocturnal leg cramps (actual brief spasm), frontal lobe complex partial seizures, neuropathies, pain syndrome, myoclonus, vascular disease, hypnagogic jerks

## Treatment

- <u>Address Secondary Cause</u>: supplemental iron (with Vitamin C for absorption) or $B_{12}$; remove RLS-inducing medications (see *previous*)
- <u>Behavior Modification</u>: change sleep phase, stretching, exercise, massage, avoid EtOH/caffeine

  ### Dopamine Agonists

  - **Pramipexole and Ropinirole**: first-line, requires titration and renal dosing
  - <u>Side Effects</u>: impulse behavior (gambling, hypersexuality), **sleep attacks**, hypersomnia, nausea (**most common side effect**), chorea and hallucinations are rare
  - **Carbidopa–levadopa**: does need to be titrated (may be used as needed), may cause tardive dyskinesia and high risk of augmentation (80%)
  - **Rebound**: RLS symptoms worsen at the end of the drug's half-life (4–6 hours)
  - **Augmentation**: side effect of dopamine agonists in which RLS symptoms begin to occur progressively **earlier,** ↑frequency, ↑intensity, ↑body parts, **or** ↑duration; **must be distinguished** from natural progression of RLS (occurs slowly over years), tolerance (requires higher dosing but symptoms are not worse than baseline), and rebound; if augmentation occurs add an earlier dose or discontinue for weeks

- <u>Second-Line Agents</u>: benzodiazapines (clonazapam), anticonvulsants (gabapentin), opioids (codeine); may consider adding **buproprion** (an antidepressant) because of dopaminergic effects

# Insomnia

## Introduction

- <u>Types</u>: 1. difficulty initiating sleep; 2. difficulty maintaining sleep; 3. waking up too early; 4. nonrestorative sleep
- most common sleep complaint, **10–15%** of general population and **35–50% of elderly**
- <u>Associations</u>: **90% of insomnia is associated with a comorbidity**; **36%** of insomniacs have a mental disorder (20–30% **anxiety**, 10–25% **depression**), >70% chronic pain, cardiovascular disease, postmenopausal women, smoking, prescription drug use
- <u>Rx</u>: cognitive behavior treatment (CBT, *see following*), address secondary causes, medication considered after addressing secondary causes and CBT

## Workup

- <u>History</u>: severity, duration, sleep patterns, napping, awakenings, parasomnias, sleep environment
- <u>Medications/Substance Abuse</u>: alcohol, caffeine, stimulants, over-the-counter drugs
- <u>Circadian Factors</u>: sleep late, cannot wake early, shift work
- <u>Psychiatric Disorders</u>: depression, anxiety about sleep (psychophysiological insomnia), acute stressors (adjustment insomnia)
- <u>Medical and Neurological Factors</u>: hyperthyroidism, hypertension, Parkinson's
- <u>PSG</u>: considered for primary sleep disorders (periodic limb movement disorder, parasomnias, and SDB)
- <u>Sleep Diary</u>: kept for 1 week and after therapy
- <u>Actigraphy</u>: wrist device that measures activity and total sleep time but not reliability for sleep onset

## Types

- **Adjustment Insomnia**: temporary insomnia associated with an identifiable stressor, **<3 months;** <u>Rx</u>: focus on CBT (sleep restriction techniques)
- **Psychophysiological Insomnia**: conditioned sleep difficulty (>1 month) associated with anxiety about sleep, somatized tension during the desired bedtime, "racing mind," **relieved when sleep at another location** (eg, normal sleep at a sleep lab) or when not intending to sleep; <u>Rx</u>: CBT (stimulus control and relaxation techniques), may consider meds

- **Idiopathic Insomnia**: chronic course with insidious onset during childhood or infancy (**lifetime disorder**), no periods of remission, independent of emotional adaptation, naps are **unrefreshing**; <u>Rx</u>: may be recalcitrant to CBT and meds, may emphasize sleep consolidation
- **Paradoxical Insomnia (Sleep State Misperception)**: perceives themselves as insomniacs but have adequate sleep, overestimate their sleep latency, and underestimate their total sleep time; <u>Rx</u>: CBT (stimulus control, relaxation, sleep hygiene, and education techniques)
- **Secondary Insomnia**: due to mental disorder, medical condition, drug or substance abuse, or poor sleep hygiene
- **Fatal Familial Insomnia**: autosomal dominant and spontaneous forms, mutation in prion protein gene causing **autonomic hyperactivity** (sweating, tachycardia), loss of circardian regulation and spindle fibers, bronchopulmonary infections, **oneiric stupor** (dream like enactment similar to REM behavior disorders), ataxia, myoclonus, leads to insomniac death; occurs in the elderly
- **Delayed Sleep Phase Disorder**: circadian rhythm disorder, young (teenagers), difficult to wake and tired all day except at night, genetic component; <u>Rx</u>: chronobiotic treatment (bright light in the AM melatonin in PM), address social issues
- **Advanced Sleep Phase Disorder**: circadian rhythm disorder, elderly, difficulty staying awake at conventional times, early morning awakening; may be caused by ↓sensitivity to light or ↓homeostatic drive; strong genetic component; <u>Rx</u>: chronobiotic treatment (bright light in the PM for 20–60 minutes, melatonin in AM)

## Cognitive Behavior Treatment (CBT)

- **Sleep Hygiene**: regularize sleep times, comfortable bed, lighting, remove stimulants (TV, children), avoid late evening caffeine and alcohol, avoid clock watching, regular exercise (except before sleep, the cooling after exercise takes awhile), hot bath before sleep (the cooling induces sleep)
- **Stimulus Control: most effective**, get out of bed if you are not sleepy, go to sleep only when sleepy, limit bed activity to sleep and sex
- **Sleep Restriction**: limit time in bed to average sleep time and avoid naps (increases homeostatic sleep drive), calculate time in bed to keep sleep efficiency **> 85%** (time asleep in bed/total time in bed)
- **Relaxation Based Biofeedback**: must be practiced, good to address "racing thoughts"
- **Paradoxical Intention**: patient instructed to try to stay awake ("reverse psychology"), removes the stressor of trying to fall asleep

- **Cognitive Restructuring**: address thoughts and beliefs that interfere with sleep, suggest "worry-time"
- <u>Outcome</u>: improves **sleep onset latency**, improves wake after sleep onset (WASO), **less effect to total sleep time (medications are better for ↑total sleep time**, but **CBT is better in ↓sleep onset latency)**; combined therapy with hypnotics is **not** better than with CBT alone for the short- and long-term (except in the initial stages)

## Hypnotic Medications

- use the lowest dose with shortest half-life, prefer as-needed dosing
- all hypnotics cause sleep disturbances upon discontinuation, therefore taper short-acting agents for a few days
- **Benzodiazepines**: enhances the inhibitory effect of GABA at the GABA$_A$ receptors (opens chloride channels); ↓sleep latency, ↓awakenings, ↑sleep duration (↑N2), **powerful ↓slow wave sleep** (↓N3), ↑**sleep spindles**, ↓**PLMs**, all benzodiazepines cause mild respiratory depression and impaired **episodic anterograde amnesia** (ability to remember **new** information)
- **Non-Benzodiazepine Benzodiazepine Receptor Agonists (Zolpidem, Zaleplon, Eszopiclone)**: binds to the BZ subunit ($\alpha$-1 **subunit**) of the GABA$_A$ receptor; less anxiolytic effect and reducing slow wave sleep and potential abuse than benzodiazepines
- **Ramelteon**: selective **melatonin** agonist, good for sleep onset insomnia only, more potent than melatonin, **no respiratory depression** (may be used in COPD)
- **Trazodone**: antidepressant that **sedates** with less effect on sleep architecture, 8-hour half-life may cause daytime sedation; risk of priapism, arrhythmias, and orthostatic hypotension, low abuse potential
- **Tertiary Tricyclic Antidepressants** (amitriptyline, doxepin, clomipramine, imipramine): more unfavorable side effects, anticholinergic effects (arrhythmias, constipation, urinary retention), **potent REM suppression**
- **Haloperidol**: antipsychotic, risk of extrapyramidal symptoms, hypotension, weight gain, and tardive dyskinesia
- **Diphenhydramine**: H$_1$-receptor antihistamine, improves total sleep time and efficiency

# Hypersomnia and Narcolepsy

## Hypersomnia

- <u>SSx</u>: fatigue, impairment of attention, napping, emotional lability, drooping of eyelids, miosis, may present as paradoxical hyperactivity in children
- <u>Causes</u>: chronic sleep deprivation (**most common**), sleep-related breathing disorders, substance abuse, medicine, environmental causes, movement-related disorders (if associated with arousals), circadian rhythm abnormalities (**delayed phase type most common cause in adolescence**), medical and psychological causes, parasomnias
- <u>Dx</u>: Epworth Sleepiness Scale (ESS), Stanford Sleepiness Scale (SSS), MSLT, MWT, sleep diary, consider work-up for medical causes (thyroid tests, CBC, blood glucose, urine analysis), consider MRI
- <u>Workup</u>: assess sleep diary for sufficient sleep and sleep environment, detailed sleep history to assess secondary causes (medication, medical/psychological, parasomnias), consider PSG if suspect SDB or PLMD, PSG/MSLT if suspect narcolepsy

## Narcolepsy

- <u>Pathogenesis</u>: REM-related phenomena (sleep paralysis) of unknown cause, may be **decreased hypocretin neuropeptide** (released during wakefulness)
- <u>Tetrad SSx</u>: **daytime sleepiness** (relief with naps, first symptom, may be mild), **cataplexy** (~50%), **sleep paralysis**, **hypnagogic hallucination** (while falling asleep), may also be **hypnopompic** (while awakening)
- <u>Secondary SSx</u>: sleep attacks, micro-sleeps (amnesic episode associated with an autonomic behavior), memory loss, visual disturbance, driving risk, REM behavior disorder, obesity, nocturnal sleep disruption, psychosocial effects
- **Cataplexy**: sudden loss of **bilateral** muscle tone with an emotional trigger, usually **positive** emotion, **preserved consciousness** in the beginning of the attack, may lose deep tendon reflexes and papillary light response
- <u>Dx</u>: clinical history, MSLT/PSG, may consider **CSF hypocretin-1 levels** (<110 pg/ml, 5% false positive, **usually positive only if with cataplexy**)
- <u>Risks</u>: more common in males, genetic predisposition, DM type 2, sarcoidosis, multiple sclerosis, Niemann-Pick, degenerative neurologic disease
- <u>PSG</u>: short sleep latency <10 minutes, sleep onset REM <20–30 minutes (**highly specific**)

- <u>MSLT</u>: 5 naps, **2 or more sleep onset REMs, sleep latency <8 minutes**

## Management

- <u>Behavior Modification</u>: structured **sleep naps**, sleep hygiene, support/safety issues (driving, work)
- **Modafinil**, **Armodofinil**: inhibits the dopamine and norepinephrine transporter, expensive, **headache** common side effect (10–15%, increase dose as usually resolves), less abuse potential; approved also for **shift work** and **OSAS** after CPAP optimization; does **not** change sleep architecture
- **Methylphenidate**, **D-amphetamines**: **short-acting** amphetamine-like, blocks **dopamine** reuptake, can produce rebound, **D-isomers is the active form**, side effects include anxiety, irritability, weight loss, psychosis, and palpitations; may be added before lunch
- <u>Cataplexy Medications</u>: antidepressants (clomipramine, venlafaxine, and atomoxetine), **gamma-hydroxybutyrate (GHB)/sodium oxybate** (requires night time dosing, abuse potential, short acting)

## Other Causes of Hypersomnia

- **Idiopathic Hypersomnia**: daytime sleepiness **not relieved by naps** (unlike narcolepsy), **prolonged nocturnal sleep** (>10 hours), >3-month duration, may have autonomic nervous system dysfunction (orthostatic hypotension, headaches), no REM-related events; PSG reveals shortened sleep latency, major sleep period >10 hours, confirm MSLT to rule out narcolepsy; <u>Rx</u>: modafanil/armodofinil but is less effective than narceptics
- **Secondary Hypersomnia**: due to medical condition (**Parkinson's**), poor hygiene, insufficient sleep, posttraumatic
- **Kleine-Levin Syndrome (Recurrent Hypersomnia)**: rare condition, presents in early adolescence males, causes recurrent episodes of hypersomnia lasting few days to several weeks, occurs 1–10× year, cognitive and behavior abnormalities (confusion, hallucinations, **hypersexuality**, **aggressiveness**, **hyperphagia**), normal behavior in between episodes; <u>Rx</u>: may consider mood stabilizer (lithium) and antiepileptic (carbamazepine)
- **Sleeping Sickness**: from *Trypanosoma brucei* via the tsetse fly; causes an initial hemolytic phase with fever, adenopathy, arrythmias, then progresses to a terminal (meningoencephalitic) stage with hypersomnia leading to death; <u>Rx</u>: antiparasitic medications

# Parasomnias

## Introduction

- **Parasomnia**: undesirable physical experience that occurs in sleep
- <u>NREM Associated</u>: confusion on arousal, sleep walking, sleep terrors, dreams are more realistic
- <u>REM Associated</u>: REM sleep behavior disorder, recurrent isolated sleep paralysis, nightmare disorder with recollection, dreams are complex and irrational
- **Nocturnal Frontal Lobe Epilepsy**: mimics parasomnias (requires EEG to differentiate), various similar periodic episodes **throughout the night** (unlike parasomnias)

## Disorders of Arousals (NREM)

- <u>SSx</u>: occurs in early sleep (**slow wave sleep**), confused, impaired cognition, antero/retrograde insomnia
- worsens with factors that cause deep sleep (sleep deprivation, hypnotics, fever) or arousals (OSAS, stress, pain, pregnancy, PLMs, GERD), **no** increased risk with alcohol
- **Confusional Arousals**: recurrent mental confusion behavior occurs during an arousal from nocturnal sleep or daytime, more common in children ("stares into space")
- **Sexsomnia**: "sleep sex," subtype of confusional arousal, may be violent
- **Sleep Terrors**: arousal from slow wave sleep with intense fear (cry, loud), amnesia to event (nightmares occur during REM sleep with recollection), may be associated with dangerous activity, associated with a family history
- **Sleep Walking**: ambulation during sleep, confusion, amnesia, difficult to arouse, may demonstrate complex behavior (cooking, urinating), strong family history
- <u>DDx</u>: frontal lobe epilepsy (better recollection, less ambulation, shorter but multiple attacks, more symmetrical movements), REM sleep behavior disorder (**if awakened out of NREM** you are **confused and easy to fall asleep; if in REM** you are **awake, alert, can recollect, and more difficult to return to sleep**), malingering
- <u>Dx</u>: PSG with video
- <u>Rx</u>: safety issues (alarms, padding, sleep on floor), sleep hygiene, in prepubertal patient may consider waking the child up after 30 minutes of sleep onset, increase sleep time, reduce stress, not recommended to wake child during episode (may prolong event); consider benzodiazepine or TCAs for severe cases; treat conditions that cause arousals (OSAS, RLS)

## REM Sleep Behavior Disorder (RBD)

- <u>Pathophysiology</u>: dysfunction of systemic maintenance of atonia in REM
- <u>SSx</u>: occurs later in sleep (more REM and sympathetic tone), dream recollection, easy to awaken, more difficult to return to sleep, dreams may be more confrontational with dream enactment (gestures, talking, kicking), may cause sleep-related injury
- **Isomorphism**: dream action corresponding to observed sleep behavior
- <u>Risks and Secondary Causes</u>: men, elderly, narcolepsy, use of antidepressants (venlafaxine common cause, fluoxetine), depression, substance abuse, **50–75% of men <50 years old with RBD will develop Parkinson's**, **RBD common initial symptom in young women with multiple sclerosis**, neurodegenerative disorders, caffeine and alcohol withdrawal
- <u>Dx</u>: PSG with video shows dream-enacting behavior
- <u>PSG</u>: sustained **tonic activity during** REM (50% chin tone in one epoch) **or** bursts of **phasic activity** in REM (sequential 3-second periods in 50% of one epoch) without significant movement
- <u>Rx</u>: similar to NREM sleep behavior disorder, **clonazapam** most common treatment, remove medications that may aggravate (antidepressants), consider melatonin

## Other REM Disorders

- **Recurrent Isolated Sleep Paralysis**: inability to move at sleep onset or awakening, 40–50% of normals, genetic disposition
- **Nightmare Disorder**: differs from sleep terror in that there is dream recollection, less fear, easy arousal, occurs later in night, and is more common, associated with posttraumatic stress disorder (PTSD); <u>Rx</u>: reassurance, REM suppressing TCAs or SSRIs; **prazosin** (an α-blocker to treat hypertension) has been used for PTSD

# CHAPTER

# General Otolaryngology

Robert J. Stachler, Terry Y. Shibuya, Justin S. Golub, and Raza Pasha

*continued*

# ESOPHAGEAL AND SWALLOWING DISORDERS

## Swallowing Phases

### Oral (Preparatory) Phase

- under voluntary control
- Components
  1. solid mastication or liquid bolus contol (lip closure is key for oral competency)
  2. saliva mixes with food bolus, tongue, and facial muscles prevent bolus from falling into lateral sulci
  3. food bolus molded by tongue and teeth (ends preparatory phase) and forced to the dorsum of the tongue
  4. anterior tongue and base of tongue elevate to contact palate, posterior pharyngeal wall, and floor of mouth contract; hyoid bone slowly elevates
  5. food bolus propelled into oropharynx (up to vallecula in some cases)

### Pharyngeal Phase

- under reflexive control (posterior pharyngeal wall receptors, CN IX and CN X)
- transient time <1 second in normal subjects
- includes fast anterior, superior motion of the hyoid bone
- Components
  1. **Nasopharynx (Velopharyngeus) Closure**
     - levator veli palatini muscle lifts the soft palate
     - palatopharyngeus (posterior pillar) muscle tightens and raises the pharynx and narrows the oropharyngeal inlet
     - superior pharyngeal constrictor (Passavant's pad) contracts to meet the soft palate and posterior pharyngeal walls

2. **Base of Tongue Propels Bolus Past Vallecula Through Pharynx**
   - base of tongue squeezes against posterior pharynx
   - glossectomy patients have difficulty with bolus propulsion
3. **Laryngeal Elevation and Closure**
   - larynx elevates up to 2 cm
   - <u>Three Sphincters for Laryngeal Closure</u>
     1. **Laryngeal Inlet**: epiglottis, aryepiglottic folds, arytenoids
     2. **False Vocal Folds**
     3. **True Vocal Folds**: most effective
   - **Laryngeal Adductor Reflex (LAR) or Glottic Closure Reflex**: an airway protective reflex (mediated principally by superior laryngeal nerve) stimulated by the laryngeal mucosa, which causes a rapid adduction of the true vocal folds to prevent aspiration (excess stimulation causes **laryngospasm**)
4. **Pharynx Shortens**
   - pharynx shortens up to 2 cm
   - pharyngeal constrictors push bolus while epiglottis directs food to piriform sinus, posterior pharyngeal wall contracts (pharyngeal weakness results in pooling of saliva and food bolus retention in the lateral gutters [piriform sinuses])
5. **Upper Esophageal Sphincter (Cricopharyngeus) Opens**
   - relaxation of the muscle and anterior displacement of the hypolaryngeal complex opens the sphincter
   - food bolus enters the cervical esophagus
   - inefficient relaxation of the cricopharyngeus results in a cricopharyngeal bar with a narrowing of the esophagus

## Esophageal Phase

- fluid movement is passive, solid movement is active
- *see* Esophageal Anatomy and Physiology *following*

# Dysphagia and Aspiration

## Introduction

- <u>Causes of Dysphagia</u>: obstruction, misdirection (retrograde [nasopharynx] and anterograde [aspiration]), fragmentation of the bolus
- oropharyngeal secretions most common aspirated substance (gastric contents are second most common)

## Evaluation of Dysphagia and Aspiration

### History and Physical Exam

- <u>Character of Dysphagia</u>: solid dysphagia (obstructive) versus liquid dysphagia (neurologic), progressive (tumor, scleroderma, achalasia), odynophagia (suggests acute process, foreign body, pharyngitis, laryngitis), regurgitation (nasal or gastric regurgitation, timing), type of regurgitated food (digested or undigested), aspiration (cough after ingestion, recurrent pneumonia, gagging, choking), difficulty with mastication or oral competence (drooling)
- <u>Contributing Factors</u>: history of GERD; history of recent caustic or foreign body ingestion or trauma; risk factors for malignancy (recent weight loss, family history of cancer, hoarseness, odynophagia, otalgia, tobacco, smoking, alcohol abuse); history of neurologic, connective tissue, or autoimmune disorders; recent dietary changes
- <u>Associated Symptoms</u>: voice changes (laryngeal involvement), heartburn (reflux esophagitis), hypothyroidism (fatigue, hair loss, depression, weight gain), neurologic changes (weakness, paresthesias, diplopia, vertigo, mental status changes)
- <u>Physical Exam</u>: full neurologic exam (cranial nerves and peripheral exam), indirect laryngeal exam or nasopharyngeal scope (pooling of secretions, vocal fold mobility, masses, sensation), complete H&N exam with high suspicion for malignancy (palpate base of tongue, indirect mirror exam for lesions, evaluate nasopharynx, palpate thyroid)
- think "KITTENS" for differential diagnosis (*see* Table 6–1)

### Modified Barium Swallow (MBS) or Videofluoroscopic Swallow Study (VFSS)

- <u>Indications</u>: determines oral and pharyngeal motility, laryngotracheal elevation, laryngeal penetration or aspiration, and safety of oral feeding
- may be combined with an esophagram (*see following*)
- <u>Technique</u>: uses radiographic videofluoroscopy to visualize oral and pharyngeal phases of swallowing using varying bolus amounts and consistencies (typically reviewed with a swallowing therapist)

### Functional (Flexible) Endoscopic Evaluation of Swallowing (FEES)

- allows bedside evaluation of swallowing function
- FEESST (FEES with sensory testing) adds sensation testing
- <u>Indications</u>: assesses aspiration risk (penetration), laryngeal function, dietary tolerance, swallowing management techniques,

**TABLE 6–1.** Differential Diagnosis of Dysphagia and Aspiration: KITTENS Method

| (K) Congenital | Infectious & Idiopathic | Toxins & Trauma | Tumor (Neoplasia) | Endocrine | Neurologic | Systemic |
|---|---|---|---|---|---|---|
| Tracheoesophageal fistulas | Laryngitis | Caustic ingestion | CNS tumors | Hypothyroidism | Altered mental status (alcohol, sedatives, head injury) | Gastrointestinal disorders (Zenker's diverticulum, GERD, achalasia, esophageal diverticulum, cricopharyngeal spasm, Plummer-Vinson syndrome, etc.) |
| Dysphagia lusoria | Pharyngitis | Foreign body ingestion | Esophageal tumors | | Degenerative diseases (Parkinson's disease, multiple sclerosis) | |
| Congenital esophageal webs | Esophagitis | Mallory-Weiss syndrome | Extrinsic compression of esophagus | | Motor neuron disease (amyotrophic lateral sclerosis) | |
| Cleft palate | Chagas' disease | | | | | |
| | Tracheotomy, endotracheal, intubation | | | | Stroke | Myopathies (muscular dystrophy, metabolic myopathies, polymyositis) |
| | Postsurgical head and neck resection | | | | Encephalopathies | |
| | | | | | Guillain-Barré | |
| | Radiation | | | | Myasthenia gravis | |
| | | | | | Bulbar and pseudobulbar palsy | Connective tissue disorders (progressive systemic sclerosis) |
| | Recurrent laryngeal nerve injury | | | | Dementia | |
| | | | | | Vocal fold paralysis | Globus hystericus |

hypopharyngeal sensitivity (sensory defects), and handling of
secretions (does not evaluate esophageal dysfunction)
- <u>Technique</u>: nasopharyngoscope placed initially to visualize the
function of the larynx, laryngeal adductor reflex (LAR) is evaluated
using pulses of air to stimulate reflex (FEESST), swallowing phases
are evaluated using varying consistencies of food (may be assisted by
a swallowing therapist)

### Other Ancillary Tests

- **Esophagram (Barium Swallow)**: evaluates esophageal phase of
swallowing (motility), luminal integrity (large ulcers, intrinsic/
extrinsic masses, strictures, webs), reflux
- **Water Soluble (Gastrografin) Swallow**: used in lieu of barium
when suspicious of an esophageal perforation, often followed by
barium swallow if negative
- **Manometry**: measures duration, amplitude, and velocity of
peristaltic waves
- **CXR**: reveals pneumonitis, pneumonia, masses, or a displaced airway
- **Direct Laryngoscopy and Esophagoscopy**: indicated if suspect
malignancy, for uncertain etiology, to evaluate esophagus, to remove
foreign bodies, and to biopsy a mass or lesion
- **Dyed Food**: indirect evaluation of aspiration in the presence of a
tracheotomy, oral feeds are dyed (eg, methylene blue), tracheotomy is
suctioned to evaluate for the presence of stained aspirates
- **GERD/LPR Evaluation**: (*see following*)
- **Videostroboscopy**: evaluates vocal fold motion, pooled secretions,
and anatomic defects (masses, glottal chinks, etc)
- **Scintigraphy**: can quantify the amount of aspirated material
(infrequently employed)
- **Manofluorography**: quantitative analysis of pressure generation
at tongue, palate, larynx, and pharyngeal walls (labor intensive,
primarily for research)
- **CT/MRI**: may be considered to evaluate endolaryngeal masses or
suspected malignancy

## Management

### Medical Management

- if possible address underlying cause (eg, iron supplementation for
Plummer-Vinson, pyridostigmine for myasthenia gravis, benztropine
for Parkinson's disease, antibiotics for acute bacterial pharyngitis)
- use an alternative temporary route of nutrition (nasogastric tube
feeds, parenteral nutrition)

- begin a reflux regimen (*see following*)
- aggressively address aspiration pneumonia (hold oral feeds, antibiotic regimen, and aggressive pulmonary toilet)
- **Botulinum Toxin Injections**: may be considered for cricopharyngeal spasms, inject toxin into cricopharyngeus muscle

## Swallowing Rehabilitation

- change food consistencies (pureed diet easier to tolerate initially, liquids are more difficult to manage)
- posture techniques (chin tuck, head turn to the poorer functioning side), palatal prostheses, muscle-strengthening exercises
- **Supraglottic Swallow**: patient voluntarily closes airway at vocal folds by holding breath before swallow, voluntary cough after swallow, follow with an additional swallow for residual bolus in pharynx or piriform
- **Mendelsohn Maneuver**: voluntarily elevates and anteriorly displaces larynx to prolong UES opening
- **Masako Technique**: tongue holding between the teeth during the swallow, increases bolus transit through pharynx by increasing the pharyngeal pressure
- **Effortful Swallow**: hard swallow to help clear the pharynx, designed to improve tongue base contact to the posterior pharyngeal wall during the swallow; patient squeezes all throat and neck muscles during the swallow

## Surgical Management

- **Esophageal Dilation**: may be considered for achalasia (LES spasm), pharyngeal or esophageal strictures, webs, postoperative scarring, and postradiation strictures
- **Cricopharyngeal Myotomy**: may be considered for cricopharyngeal spasms (incomplete UES relaxation) or abnormal muscular contraction during relaxation (*controversial*), theoretically relaxes pharyngoesophageal segment and results in anterior elevation of larynx; complete myotomy includes part of the lower inferior constrictor, cricopharyngeus muscle, and part of the upper cervical esophagus
- **Gastric or Jejunal Feeding Tube**: temporary or permanent enteric feeding
- **Vocal Fold Medialization**: for unilateral vocal fold immobility, *see* pp. 121–123
- **Tracheotomy (Cuffed)**: indicated for severe pulmonary complications, prevents aspiration pneumonia by allowing easier pulmonary toilet and preventing gross aspiration (does not prevent

microaspiration); however, increases risk of aspiration by inhibiting laryngeal elevation, interfering with ciliary motion, and preventing production of subglottic pressure for an adequate cough

- **Laryngeal Stenting**: for short-term use
- **Laryngeal Closure Techniques**: requires a permanent tracheostomy; glottic closure may be considered for bilateral vocal fold immobility; epiglottopexy allows voicing, improves aspiration, and is potentially reversible
- **Laryngeal Suspension**: indicated for severe aspiration from supraglottic and pharyngeal dysfunction (may be considered after supraglottic resection), suspends larynx anteriorly by positioning thyroid cartilage under mandible, may improve voicing and swallowing
- **Laryngeal Diversion (Lindeman Procedure) or Separation**: indicated for severe aspiration, creates a permanent tracheostomy with the proximal tracheal segment diverted back to the esophagus; a variation of Lindeman's method creates a blind pouch from the proximal tracheal segment; potentially reversible
- **Laryngectomy**: indicated for life-threatening complications, gold standard for definitive therapy

# Esophageal Anatomy and Physiology

## Anatomy

- Esophageal Layers
  1. **Mucosa**: epithelium, lamina propria, muscularis mucosa
  2. **Inner Circular Muscle**
  3. **Submucosa**
  4. **Outer Longitudinal Muscle**: no serosa layer, therefore minimal barrier to infection and tumor infiltration
- Three Physiologic Narrowings
  1. **Upper Esophageal Sphincter**: *see following*
  2. **Crossing of the Aortic Arch and Left Main Bronchus**: anatomic narrowing about 27 cm from incisor opening
  3. **Lower Esophageal Sphincter**: *see following*
- Embryology: *see* p. 550
- Vasculature: segmented from inferior thyroid artery (upper 1/3), thoracic aorta (middle 1/3), and left gastric and inferior phrenic arteries (lower 1/3)
- Histology: stratified squamous epithelium except distal 1–3 cm (columnar epithelium)

- <u>Innervation</u>: mixed somatic innervation from CN IX and CN X (left CN X passes anteriorly and the right CN X passes posteriorly to form the esophageal plexus)
- <u>Auerbach's Plexus</u>: myenteric plexus, between muscle layers, parasympathetic
- <u>Meissner's Plexus</u>: submucosal plexus

### *Upper Esophageal Sphincter (UES)*

- UES is composed of the **cricopharyngeus muscle** (about 16 cm from incisor opening)
- tonic contracture prevents air reflux, aspiration, and regurgitation
- relaxes during the pharyngeal phase

### *Lower Esophageal Sphincter (LES)*

- normal tone: **10–40 mmHg** (achalasia: **>40**; scleroderma: <10)
- normally positioned below diaphragm (hiatal hernias result in LES positioned above diaphragm)
- physiologic sphincter (not a true anatomic sphincter), aided by the crura of the diaphragm (vagal innervation)
- <u>Agents That Increase LES Pressure</u>: proteins, acid, gastrin, vasopressin, α-adrenergics
- <u>Agents That Decrease LES Pressure</u>: secretin, nitrates, calcium channel blockers, glucagon, chocolate, fat, β-adrenergics, alcohol, mints, nicotine

## Physiology

- minimal secretion and absorption
- upper 1/3 is composed of voluntary striated muscle (1 second of esophageal phase)
- lower 2/3 is composed of involuntary smooth muscle (3 seconds of esophageal phase)

### *Peristalsis Types*

- **Primary Peristalsis**: initiated by food bolus, contracts proximally to distally
- **Secondary Peristalsis**: initiated by esophageal distention (residual food bolus) and reflux
- **Tertiary Contractions**: nonperistaltic, spontaneous contractions, may propel bolus in a retrograde direction to proximal esophagus

# Gastroesophageal Reflux Disease and Laryngopharyngeal Reflux

## Introduction

- *see also* pp. 110–111
- **Gastroesophageal Reflux Disease (GERD)**: abnormal amount of gastric secretions that reflux into the esophagus causing symptoms
- **Laryngopharyngeal Reflux (LPR)**: supraesophageal chronic symptoms from reflux of gastric acid
- 50% of the U.S. population experiences chronic heartburn
- Pathophysiology
  1. LES (GERD) or UES (LPR) incompetence or transient relaxation
  2. delayed esophageal clearance
  3. delayed gastric emptying (may increase gastric volume)
- Risks: obesity, alcohol abuse, hiatal hernia, pregnancy, scleroderma, feeding tube
- GERD SSx: **postprandial** heartburn, **supine reflux**, choking spells at night, regurgitation, hoarseness (worse in the morning), esophagitis, abnormal esophageal pH monitoring, abnormal esophageal acid clearance/motility
- LPR SSx: chronic hoarseness (worse in the morning), globus sensation (often the primary symptom), dysphagia, daytime (**upright**) reflux, mouth burning, halitosis, dry or itchy throat discomfort, throat clearing, chronic cough, recurrent respiratory
- disease, laryngospasm, otalgia, torticollis (**Sandifer syndrome**: distinctive neck posture in children that protects against acid reflux)
- LPR typically does not present with heartburn (<50%) or esophageal peptic injuries (esophagitis)
- Laryngeal Findings: erythema and edema of the posterior commissure, arytenoids, superior surface of the vocal folds, and laryngeal surface of the epiglottis; diffuse supraglottic edema; laryngeal pachydermia (interarytenoid); granulomas of the vocal fold process; subglottic stenosis
- Complications: reflux esophagitis, Barrett's esophagus (gastric metaplasia of the distal esophagus), esophageal stricture, gastric and esophageal ulcerations, globus pharyngis, chronic cough, aspiration pneumonia, laryngeal granulomas, failure to thrive, sudden infant death syndrome (SIDS), possibly laryngeal carcinoma

## Diagnosis

- H&P (*as previous*)
- **Response to Therapeutic Trial**: may begin empiric reflux regimen (typically proton-pump inhibitors, *see following*) based on history;

consider ancillary testing after failed empiric management, atypical symptoms, recurrent symptoms, or complications (weight loss, dysphagia)

- **Nasolaryngoscopy**: allows for visualization of characteristic findings (*as previous*) as well as complications (vocal fold granulomas)
- **Barium Swallow**: good initial screening test for demonstrating esophageal anatomy, **high false-negative rate** (especially LPR), identifies hiatal hernias and strictures
- **24-hour Dual-pH Probe**: most sensitive, "gold standard," distal probe 5 cm above LES and proximal probe 2 cm above UES, allows differentiation of GERD and LPR; triple probe monitoring adds a nasopharyngeal probe
- **Esophagoscopy (Transnasal or Oral)**: evaluates for esophagitis and esophageal strictures, allows histologic confirmation of Barrett's esophagus or esophagitis
- **Gastroesophageal Scintiscan**: uses swallowed radiolabeled technetium, allows evaluation of gastric emptying and reflux; used primarily in children to detect aspiration and delayed emptying
- **Impedance Testing**: generally combined with pH probe, can determine whether reflux is gaseous or liquid as well as direction of flow
- **Pepsin Assays** (investigational)

## Management

1. <u>Behavior Management</u>
   - smoking cessation
   - elevate head of bed at night
   - avoid tight-fitting clothing
   - avoid overeating, eating before sleep
   - abstain from caffeine, fatty foods, alcohol, mints, chocolate, and other reflux-inducing foods
   - avoid aspirin, nitrates, and calcium channel blockers
2. <u>Medical Management</u>
   - **Proton-Pump Inhibitors (PPI**; omeprazole, pantoprazole): **indicated as first-line agents for complicated GERD and LPR** or failed first-line regimens, blocks the "proton pump" responsible for acid secretion; recurrence of symptoms is common in patients who require PPI therapy for initial treatment; if effectiveness of acid suppressive therapy is uncertain may consider 24-hour pH probe while on PPIs to assess; **typically, GERD requires single-dose PPI and LPR requires double-dose PPI,** take 1 hour before meals, avoid taking with calcium

- **H₂-blockers** (cimetidine, famotidine, ranitidine): may be considered for uncomplicated GERD, blocks histamine interaction with its receptor; side effects include constipation, diarrhea, confusion, and elevated liver enzymes
- **Prokinetic Agents** (metoclopramide): indicated for delayed gastric emptying, also increases LES pressure; side effects include tardive dyskinesia, drowsiness, depression, and confusion
- **Liquid Antacids** (calcium carbonate, hydroxides of aluminum and magnesium, sodium bicarbonate): may be considered as first-line therapy for mild GERD, take after meals and before sleep, overuse may result in acid–base and other metabolic disturbances
- **Sucralfate**: nonsystemic oral medication, covers and protects exposed ulcerated mucosal surfaces

3. <u>Surgical Management</u>
   - indicated for failed medical regimen or those who require continuous or increasing acid suppressive therapy (effectiveness of acid suppression therapy should be the major criteria for predicting successful outcome of fundoplication operation)
   - fundoplication procedures increase tone of distal esophagus (LES); minimally invasive laparoscopic approach has primarily replaced open approach
   - **Transoral Incisionless Fundoplication**: 270-degree stomach wrap endoscopically performed, limited to hiatal hernias < 2 cm

# Esophageal Disorders

## Achalasia (Megaesophagus)

- <u>Pathophysiology</u>: degeneration of Auerbach's plexus resulting in aperistalsis and increased LES pressure (LES does not relax with bolus)
- <u>SSx</u>: progressive dysphagia, vomiting, malodorous breath, chest pain, aspiration, weight loss
- <u>Dx</u>: esophagram (bird beak appearance, air-fluid levels, aperistalsis, failed LES relaxation), manometry (increased LES pressure), esophagoscopy to rule out mass (carcinoma) and esophagitis
- <u>Complications</u>: increased risk of esophageal carcinoma
- <u>Rx</u>: serial esophageal pneumatic dilation (1–5% perforation risk), "wash" meals down with fluids, esophagomyotomy (Heller procedure) with fundoplication, Botox to LES, may consider calcium channel blockers and nitrates to decrease LES pressure (*controversial*)

## Progressive Systemic Sclerosis (Scleroderma)

- <u>Pathophysiology</u>: autoimmune disease causes small vessel vasculitis, widespread collagen deposition, and **smooth muscle** atrophy (esophageal dysmotility is thus limited to the lower 2/3)
- associated with other connective tissue diseases
- <u>H&N SSx</u>: severe GERD, dysphagia, fixed facial appearance (tight skin, thin lips, sclerotic skin)
- <u>Systemic SSx</u>: initial edematous skin (later tight skin), pulmonary hypertension and fibrosis, pericarditis, microcytic anemia (hypertensive renal crisis), carpal tunnel syndrome, Raynaud's phenomenon, sclerodactyly, telangiectasia
- <u>Dx</u>: barium swallow (dilated, flaccid esophagus similar to achalasia, however, **patent LES**), manometry (normal UES pressure, loss of tone of LES, aperistalsis)
- **CREST Syndrome**: milder variant, **C**alcinosis (cutaneous), **R**aynaud's phenomenon, **E**sophageal dysmotility, **S**clerodactyly, **T**elangiectasia
- <u>Rx</u>: reflux regimen, calcium channel blockers for Raynaud's phenomenon, consider corticosteroids and NSAIDs

## Polymyositis and Dermatomyositis

- <u>Pathophysiology</u>: idiopathic inflammatory myopathy of **striated muscle**
- **Dermatomyositis**: variant with associated rashes, higher risk of malignancy
- associated with other connective tissue diseases, **malignancies**, hiatal hernia, reflux esophagitis, vasculitis
- <u>SSx</u>: proximal muscle (hip, shoulder, neck) weakness and wasting, dysphagia, aspiration, dysmotility in upper 1/3 of the esophagus and pharyngeal weakness (striated muscle), nasal regurgitation, dysrhythmias, periorbital heliotrope rash (dermatomyositis)
- <u>Dx</u>: EMG; muscle biopsy; increased serum creatine phosphokinase, liver enzymes, LDH
- <u>Rx</u>: antireflux regimen, corticosteroids, antimetabolites, immunosuppressives

## Esophageal Diverticulum

- <u>Pathophysiology</u>: pouch created by herniation of mucosa through mucosal wall

- Pathophysiologic Types
    1. **Pulsion Diverticulum**: created from elevated intraluminal pressure
    2. **Traction Diverticulum**: caused by "tugging" effect from inflammation (lymph nodes) and fibrotic adjacent tissue
- Upper Esophageal/Hypopharyngeal Areas of Weakness
    1. **Killian's Triangle**: superior to posterior cricopharyngeus, superior to cricothyroid muscles, below raphe of inferior constrictors
    2. **Killian-Jamieson Space**: laterally, between cricopharyngeus and esophagus muscle
    3. **Laimer-Haeckermann Space**: between cricopharyngeus superiorly and circular fibers inferiorly

## Zenker's Diverticulum (Pharyngoesophageal Diverticulum)

- Pathophysiology: **pulsion** diverticulum typically at Killian's triangle (*see previous*)
- **False Diverticulum**: contains mucosa and submucosa only
- SSx: insidious dysphagia, spontaneous regurgitation of undigested food, malodorous breath, aspiration, may become obstructive
- Complications: diverticulitis, fistula formation, perforation, bleeding
- Dx: esophagram and endoscopy (80–90% located on the left side)
- Rx: observe if small/asymptomatic; **endoscopic esophagodiverticulostomy** is now mainstay (common wall divided with an Endo GIA stapler); larger diverticuli may require open **transcervical diverticulectomy with cricopharyngeal myotomy** (must complete a cricopharyngeal myotomy to prevent recurrence); **diverticulopexy** (theoretically reduces risk of fistula); may also consider botulinum toxin injection into cricopharyngeus (*controversial*)

## Midesophageal Traction Diverticulum

- Pathophysiology: **traction** diverticulum typically in middle third of esophagus
- **True Diverticulum**: contains all layers of esophageal wall (including muscularis)
- SSx: dysphagia, usually asymptomatic
- Dx: esophagram and esophagoscopy (high risk of perforation)
- Rx: if symptomatic or complicated may undergo right thoracotomy with diverticulectomy

## Epiphrenic Diverticulum

- Pathophysiology: **pulsion** diverticulum in the lower esophagus often above an obstruction

- associated with GERD, hiatal hernia, esophageal spasm, esophageal carcinoma, and other esophageal disease
- <u>SSx</u>: dysphagia, regurgitation, obstruction
- <u>Dx</u>: esophagram and esophagoscopy
- <u>Rx</u>: if symptomatic or complicated may consider diverticulectomy, must address underlying cause

## Cricopharyngeal Dysfunction (Cricopharyngeal Spasm, Cricopharyngeal Dysphagia)

- <u>Pathophysiology</u>: abnormal coordination between pharynx and cricopharyngeus (UES), failure of cricopharyngeus relaxation with swallowing leading to dysphagia and possibly aspiration
- <u>Types</u>
  1. **Reflux-Induced**: most common
  2. **Idiopathic**: may be secondary to subclinical reflux
  3. **Neurologic**: secondary to neurologic process
- <u>SSx</u>: localized dysphagia to the cervical esophagus, globus sensation, choking
- <u>Dx</u>: esophagram may be normal or reveal cricopharyngeal bar with functional obstruction, manometry more accurate
- <u>Complications</u>: diverticulum formation, aspiration, pulmonary disease
- <u>Rx</u>: cricopharyngeal myotomy (open or endoscopic), botulinum toxin injections, reflux regimen

## Esophagitis

- **Reflux Esophagitis**: most common, secondary to gastric acid reflux, causes mucosal erosion of distal esophagus
- **Candidal Esophagitis**: white plaques with erythematous base, associated with odynophagia, increased risk with immunocompromised patients and long-term antibiotics; <u>Rx</u>: systemic antifungals
- **Herpes and CMV Esophagitis**: multiple ulcerations, increased risk with immunocompromised patients
- **Pill Esophagitis**: typically punctate ulcerations; common causes include tetracycline, potassium, quinidine, aspirin, and clindamycin pills; <u>Rx</u>: prevent by taking with sufficient fluid
- **Bullous Dermatoses**: pemphigoid, epidermolysis, and others
- **Radiation Esophagitis**: may be acute (during therapy) or chronic (scarring and stenosis may occur 6–18 months after radiation therapy)
- **Eosinophilic Esophagitis** (*see* p. 564)

## Esophageal Rupture and Perforation

- Causes: iatrogenic instrumentation (most common cause), blunt and penetrating trauma, neoplasm, inflammation, increased abdominal pressure
- Variants
  1. **Mallory-Weiss Syndrome**: incomplete tear of esophageal mucosa and laceration of submucosal arteries from increased abdominal pressure (emesis in alcoholics), presents as an upper GI bleed; Rx: fluids, usually self-limiting, may decompress (nasogastric tube), rarely requires endoscopic coagulation or open procedures
  2. **Boerhaave Syndrome**: increased abdominal pressure results in spontaneous rupture of all 3 layers of the esophagus (usually distal, posterior wall), severe symptoms (hematemesis, chest pain, dyspnea, hypovolemic shock)
- SSx: tachycardia (typically first), chest pain, fever, respiratory distress, dysphagia, subcutaneous emphysema, **Hamman's sign** (crunching sound over heart from subcutaneous emphysema)
- Dx: clinical exam, CXR (mediastinal widening, pneumothorax), water soluble (Gastrografin) esophagram
- Complications: chemical mediastinitis (saliva, bile, gastric acid), septic shock
- Rx: early surgical repair and drainage (thoracotomy), may consider medical therapy (antibiotics and observation) for small perforation in select patients

## Esophageal Foreign Bodies and Caustic Ingestion
(*see* pp. 564–568)

## Diffuse Esophageal Spasm

- Pathophysiology: simultaneous nonperistaltic contractions in esophageal smooth muscle (with otherwise normal peristalsis), contractions are of normal pressure (unlike **nutcracker esophagus**, in which contractions are of greater than normal pressure)
- SSx: odynophagia to solids and liquids, dysphagia, chest pain
- Dx: esophagram (corkscrew, normal LES relaxation), manometry
- Complications: diverticuli
- Rx: nitrates, calcium channel blockers, anticholinergics, may consider dilation and myotomy for severe symptoms, possibly Botox

## Dysphagia Lusoria (Bayford Syndrome)

- <u>Pathophysiology</u>: anomalous right subclavian artery from descending aorta (fourth branchial arch anomaly) has a retroesophageal course causing dysphagia from extrinsic compression of the esophagus
- associated with a right **non-recurrent laryngeal nerve**, aortic and subclavian aneurysms, diverticuli
- <u>SSx</u>: intermittent dysphagia (usually presents at middle age with loss of elasticity of vessels), weight loss
- <u>Dx</u>: barium swallow, arteriogram, esophagoscopy (pulsating horizontal bar at obstruction site)
- <u>Rx</u>: ligate and reanastomose to right common carotid for severe symptoms

## Eagle Syndrome (Styloid Process Syndrome)

- <u>Pathophysiology</u>: elongated styloid process or ossified stylohyoid ligament causes mechanical irritation of surrounding nerves
- <u>SSx</u>: odynophagia, unilateral tonsillar pain, pain behind mandibular angle, referred otalgia, palpation at site reproduces pain
- <u>Dx</u>: radiography
- <u>Rx</u>: excision from intraoral or external approach

## Plummer-Vinson Syndrome

- <u>Pathophysiology</u>: unclear etiology, may be secondary to nutritional deficiency (iron)
- more common in young to middle-aged women
- <u>Risks</u>: northern hemisphere (Scandinavians)
- <u>SSx</u>: dysphagia (degeneration of esophageal muscle), cervical (pharyngoesophageal) webs, **microcytic hypochromatic anemia** (iron deficiency), cheilitis (fissures at corners of lips), hypothyroidism, hiatal hernia, splenomegaly, achlorhydria
- <u>Dx</u>: clinical exam, iron levels, CBC, esophagram
- <u>Complications</u>: increased risk of upper esophageal and hypopharyngeal carcinoma
- <u>Rx</u>: iron supplements (improves most symptoms), esophageal dilation

## Esophageal Webs and Rings

- **Web**: asymmetric, thin, membranous projection into the lumen, covered by esophageal epithelium (composed of mucosa and submucosa only)
- **Ring**: thicker, composed of mucosa, submucosa, and muscularis

- **Schatzki Ring**: web-like narrowing at squamocolumnar junction (junction of esophageal and gastric mucosa), only 1/3 are symptomatic
- upper cervical webs may be associated with Plummer-Vinson syndrome
- <u>SSx</u>: usually asymptomatic, may cause dysphagia, weight loss
- <u>Dx</u>: esophagram or esophagoscopy
- <u>Rx</u>: surgical intervention rare, dilation, endoscopic excision (laser)

## Tracheoesophageal Fistulas (*see* p. 559)

## Effects of Other Systemic Diseases on the Esophagus

- **Presbyesophagus**: reduced peristalsis and decreased LES pressure in the elderly, likely neuropathic
- **Chagas Disease**: parasitic infection (*T. cruzi*), destroys Auerbach's plexus, results in achalasia-like symptomatology
- **Diffuse Idiopathic Skeletal Hyperostosis (DISH) (Forestier's Disease)**: paraspinous ligament calcification causes dysphagia from cervical osteophyte compression or periesophageal soft tissue inflammation; <u>Dx</u>: lateral neck x-ray, esophagram; <u>Rx</u>: surgical reduction for severe symptoms

# Esophageal Neoplasms

## Benign Tumors and Cysts

- **less common** than malignant tumors
- may be intraluminal, intramural, or periesophageal
- <u>SSx</u>: dysphagia, pressure behind the sternum, bleeding, weight loss
- <u>Dx</u>: barium swallow (highly sensitive), endoscopy (biopsy), CT/MRI, CXR (displacement of structures)
- <u>Rx</u>: typically requires endoscopic or open excision

### *Types*

- **Leiomyoma**: most common benign tumor of the esophagus, intramural, arises from muscularis (usually distal 2/3); <u>Rx</u>: excision if symptomatic
- **Polyps**: most common intraluminal lesion, usually in cervical esophagus; <u>Rx</u>: endoscopic removal
- <u>Others</u>: myoma, fibroma, neurofibroma, lipoma, adenoma, papilloma, hemangioma

## Malignant Tumors

- <u>SSx</u>: initial painless dysphagia develops later into odynophagia, hemoptysis, cough, hoarseness, weight loss, emesis
- <u>Dx</u>: barium swallow, endoscopy (biopsy), CT/MRI (evaluate extent, invasion, displacement of structures, regional metastasis), endoscopic ultrasonography (may determine depth of invasion)

### Types

- **Adenocarcinoma**: currently most common (incidence has risen dramatically), distal esophagus; <u>Risks</u>: **Barrett's esophagus**, GERD, radiation, tobacco, obesity, esophagitis, elderly white male
- **Squamous Cell Carcinoma**: usually middle third of esophagus; <u>Risks</u>: **tobacco and alcohol**, history of head and neck cancer, Plummer-Vinson syndrome, caustic injury, tylosis (nonepidermolytic palmoplantar keratoderma), achalasia, radiation, poverty, hot beverages, esophagitis, African American male
- <u>Others</u>: adenoid cystic carcinoma, mucoepidermoid carcinoma, small cell carcinoma, sarcoma

### Management

- absence of a serosa layer allows early transmural spread, overall a poor prognosis (<15% 5 year survival)
- involvement of the prevertebral fascia, trachea, carotids, or metastatic disease should be considered incurable
- high-grade Barrett's esophagus should undergo prophylactic excision
- <u>Rx</u>: surgical resection with adjunctive chemoradiation, may consider palliative chemotherapy and radiation
- <u>Reconstruction Methods</u>
  1. **Pectoralis/Deltopectoral Flaps**: may be tubed, bulky, poor speech, high fistula and stenosis rate
  2. **Colonic Interposition**: one-stage procedure, high infection rate
  3. **Gastric Pull-Up**: reliable, one-stage procedure, vagotomy and pyloroplasty required, single anastomosis (*see also* p. 294 for complications)
  4. **Jejunal Free Flap**: laryngeal preservation and replacement of cervical esophagus only (*see also* p. 457)

# ORAL AND OROPHARYNGEAL BENIGN DISORDERS
## Anatomy and Physiology

### Tongue and Palate Anatomy

#### Surface Anatomy

- **Fungiform Papillae**: small red structures found at tip and edge of anterior 2/3 of tongue
- **Foliate Papillae**: located at the posterolateral tongue base
- **Circumvallate Papillae**: raised circular structures, arranged in V-shape at junction of anterior 2/3 and posterior 1/3 of tongue
- **Filiform Papillae**: distributed throughout tongue, bumpy appearance, do not participate in taste
- **Sulcus Terminalis**: groove between anterior and posterior tongue
- **Foramen Cecum**: central point of the sulcus terminalis (origin of thyroid gland)

#### Muscular Anatomy

- <u>Tongue Extrinsics</u>: genioglossus, styloglossus, hyoglossus (CN XII); palatoglossus (CN X)
- <u>Tongue Intrinsics</u>: superior longitudinal, inferior longitudinal, vertical, transverse layers (CN XII)
- <u>Palatal Muscles</u>: palatoglossus (anterior pillar), palatopharyngeus (posterior pillar), musculus uvulae, levator veli palatini (CN X); tensor veli palatini (CN $V_3$)

#### Afferent Innervation

- <u>Anterior 2/3 of Tongue</u>
  1. **Taste**: taste receptors (fungiform and foliate papillae) → lingual nerve → chorda tympani nerve → **geniculate ganglion** (taste fiber cell bodies) → nervus intermedius (**CN VII**) → nucleus solitarius
  2. **Touch and Temperature**: lingual nerve → **CN $V_3$**
- <u>Posterior 1/3 of Tongue</u>
  1. **Taste**: taste receptors (foliate and circumvallate papillae, posterior oropharynx, vallecula, and base of tongue) → **CN IX** → inferior petrosal ganglion → nucleus solitarius
  2. **Touch and Temperature**: CN IX
- **Taste from Laryngeal Surface of Epiglottis**: superior laryngeal nerve → CN X → nucleus solitarius

# Evaluation of Disorders of Taste

## Introduction

- <u>Sensations of Taste</u>: salty, sweet, sour, and bitter (topographic mapping of taste does not exist, all sensations are perceived by each taste receptor)
- <u>Perception of Taste Components</u>: taste, smell, texture, and temperature
- taste buds are found in fungiform, foliate, and circumvallate papillae (not in filiform papillae) of the tongue; taste buds are also located on the hard palate, anterior pillar, tonsil, and posterior pharyngeal wall
- saliva is required for taste

## Classification of Taste Disorders

- **Ageusia**: no taste sensation (eg, congenital aplasia, toxins, cranial nerve injury)
- **Hypogeusia**: decreased sensitivity to taste (eg, radiation effect)
- **Hypergeusia**: increased sensitivity to taste (eg, glossopharyngeal neuralgia)
- **Dysgeusia/Parageusia**: foul or abnormal perception of taste (eg, infectious stomatitis, taste phantoms)

## Workup and Management

- <u>History and Associated Symptoms</u>: medications (*see following*); recent URI, toxin exposure; other neurologic symptoms (paresthesia, stroke, weakness, anosmia); history of diabetes, endocrine disorders, connective tissue disease, or depression
- <u>Physical Exam</u>: complete H&N exam including oral and oropharyngeal exam, otologic exam (chorda tympani), cranial nerve assessment, and other neurologic evaluation
- <u>Dx</u>: clinical exam, olfactory (eg, UPSIT; U Penn Smell Identification Test) and gustatory objective testing is largely limited to research/ academic settings
- <u>Rx</u>: address underlying cause and nasal obstruction, artificial saliva or salivary stimulants, advise to chew food well and change foods midmeal, simulated cooking odors may be considered

## Causes

- **80% of taste disorders are primary smell disorders**
- recent URI second most common cause

- **Mucositis/Stomatitis**: common causes include oral/oropharyngeal infections, radiation-induced mucositis, and other causes of inflammation that may involve taste buds or oral cavity (Sjögren syndrome, lichen planus, geographic tongue)
- **Poor Oral Hygiene**: may cause dysgeusia and parageusia
- **Chorda Tympani Nerve Injury**: iatrogenic injury usually causes only temporary dysgeusias because of bilateral innervation
- Medications: antibacterial mouthwash, anticholinergics, aspirin, anti-Parkinson drugs, acetazolamide, lithium, penicillamine
- Neurologic: rare for selective lesions of gustatory nerves, may also occur in multiple sclerosis, stroke, and facial paralysis
- Other Causes: neoplasms, aging effects, surgical resections (laryngectomy, glossectomy), nutritional deficiencies (zinc), endocrine disorders (diabetes, hypothyroidism, pregnancy), renal disease, hereditary taste disorders (may result in aplasia of taste buds)

# Evaluation of Oral and Oropharyngeal Lesions

## Introduction

- **5–20%** of leukoplakia is malignant or premalignant
- erythroplakia has higher risk of malignancy (25%)

## History and Physical Exam

- History of Lesion: onset, duration, and progression of lesion; painful
- Contributing Factors: trauma (gum biting, poor fitting dentures) or caustic ingestion; risk factors for malignancy (weight loss, smoking, alcohol abuse, family history, etc); history of connective tissue diseases, autoimmune disorders, immunodeficiency, diabetes, radiation therapy, other malignancies
- Associated Symptoms: taste disturbances, persistent sore throat (>3 weeks), odynophagia, dysphagia, halitosis, hoarseness, trismus, fever, malaise, persistent otalgia (referred pain with normal otologic exam)
- Physical Evaluation of Lesion: describe lesion (eg, macular, papular, ulcerative, vesicular), color (leukoplakia, erythroplakia, *see* Table 6–2), adherency, induration, tenderness
- Type of Leukoplakia
  1. **Keratotic**: adherent, insidious development, protracted course, nonerosive surface (**higher risk of carcinoma**)
  2. **Nonkeratotic**: nonadherent, acute onset, erosive and ulcerative features (associated more with **acute infections**)

**TABLE 6–2.** Differential Diagnosis of Benign Pigmented Oral Lesions

| Color | Causes |
|---|---|
| Generalized pale mucosa | Anemia, thalassemia |
| Black/brown discolorization | Bismuth and arsenic intoxication |
| Blue-gray gingival margin (Burton's Line) | Lead intoxication |
| Generalized redness | Polycythemia vera, hepatic insufficiency |
| Perioral melanotic macules | Puetz-Jeghers syndrome (GI hamartomatous polyps) |
| Small yellow spots | Fordyce's disease (sebaceous gland histology) |
| Black-hair tongue | Elongated (hyperplastic) filiform papillae |
| Telangiectasia | Osler-Weber-Rendu syndrome |
| Diffuse hyperpigmentation of mucosa | Addison's disease |

- <u>Oral and Oropharyngeal Exam</u>: visually inspect all areas of oral and oropharyngeal cavity (indirect mirror exam) for masses and lesions (ulceration, leukoplakia, erythroplakia), palpate floor of mouth and base of tongue, assess mobility of tongue and any involvement of mandible, inspect dentition (quality of teeth, occlusion), assess surface and consistency of the tongue, palpate salivary glands and Stenson's duct
- <u>Other Physical Exam</u>: complete H&N exam (signs of underlying malignancy, cervical adenopathy), associated cutaneous lesions

## Diagnostic Testing

### Biopsy

- **all chronic leukoplakia or ulcerative lesions that fail to heal after 1–2 weeks should undergo excisional biopsy (must keep a high suspicion for malignancy)**
- biopsy specimen should include a clear margin
- consider direct and indirect immunofluorescence staining

### Other Ancillary Tests

- <u>Culture and Sensitivity</u>: consider culture of oral/oropharyngeal mucosa or lesion if suspect infection (eg, fever, tender cervical adenopathy); must evaluate for aerobic, anaerobic, and fungal organisms
- <u>CT/MRI</u>: indicated if suspect tumor, evaluates size and involvement of adjacent structures; aids in staging and determining nodal status
- <u>Labs</u>: CBC with differential, autoimmune, and connective tissue profiles (eg, ANA, SS-A, SS-B, ESR, Rh factor, LE cell), ACE level

## Infectious Stomatitis

### Herpetic Gingivostomatitis

- <u>Pathophysiology</u>: primary infection or reactivation of herpes simplex virus (HSV) type 1; HSV-2 more associated with genital lesions, although may be found in oral lesions as well
- <u>Types</u>
  1. **Primary**: most common in seronegative children, associated with fever, malaise, cervical lymphadenopathy
  2. **Secondary**: recurrence of dormant virus in the trigeminal ganglion (migrates along axonal sheath); triggered by stress, trauma, immunosuppression, UV light
- <u>SSx</u>: small painful vesicles that ulcerate leaving an erythematous base with a gray cover, heals without scar, odynophagia, fever, malaise,

cervical adenopathy, usually resolves in 1–2 weeks; secondary
reactivation often occurs at mucocutaneous junction of lips (herpes
labialis) and may be preceded by prodrome of burning, itching,
tingling
- <u>Dx</u>: H&P, viral culture in early stages, monoclonal antibodies, DNA
hybridization
- <u>Rx</u>: oral acyclovir for infections or prophylaxis (eg,
immunocompromised), topical acyclovir for labial lesions

## Acute Necrotizing Ulcerative Gingivitis (Trench Mouth, Vincent's Gingivitis)

- <u>Pathophysiology</u>: mucosa infected by multiple synergistic pathogens
including spirochetes (***Borrelia vincentii***), fusiform rods, and
anaerobic bacteria
- <u>Risks</u>: malnutrition, degenerative diseases, immunocompromised,
debilitating diseases
- <u>SSx</u>: ulcerative ("punched out") craters of the interdental papilla,
gray pseudomembranous cover, malaise, fever, cervical adenopathy,
halitosis
- <u>Dx</u>: culture, H&P
- <u>Rx</u>: oral hygiene, antibiotics

## Oral Candidiasis (Thrush)

- <u>Pathophysiology</u>: opportunistic infection, typically *Candida albicans*
(*Aspergillus* may also be cultured)
- <u>Risks</u>: long-term antibiotics, infants, elderly, immunosuppression
(corticosteroids, poorly controlled diabetes), poor nutrition status,
radiation and chemotherapy, local irritation (poor oral hygiene, ill-
fitting dentures)
- <u>SSx</u>: friable, white (cheesy) plaques that scrape off leaving an
erythematous base, pseudomembranous erythematous plaques,
odynophagia, taste disturbances
- <u>Dx</u>: H&P, culture **(fungal stain reveals 90°, pseudohyphae yeast)**
- <u>Rx</u>: topical antifungals (eg, nystatin swish and swallow), systemic
antifungals for severe forms, oral hygiene

## Actinomycosis

- <u>Pathophysiology</u>: *Actinomyces israelii*, present within normal teeth,
invades tissue through an extraction site or damaged tooth
- <u>Risks</u>: oral mucosal trauma, poor oral hygiene, dental infections,
immunocompromised

- <u>SSx</u>: may occur almost anywhere in head/neck, usually presents as a palpable mass, may have a purplish discoloration of overlying skin
- <u>Dx</u>: culture (requires 1–2 weeks for growth)
- <u>Histopathology</u>: branching anaerobic gram-negative **bacteria**, **sulfur granules**
- <u>Rx</u>: surgical debridement and long-term antibiotics (penicillin, tetracycline, erythromycin)

## Syphilis (*see* pp. 244–245)

# Noninfectious Stomatitis

## Erythema Multiforme

- <u>Pathophysiology</u>: antigen–antibody complex deposit in small vessels of the dermis and submucosa, may occur spontaneously (50%) or in association with a **hypersensitivity reaction** (medication or infection)
- <u>SSx</u>: oral or cutaneous target lesion with concentric erythematous rings, explosive presentation, self-limited fever, regional adenopathy
- <u>Dx</u>: positive direct and indirect immunofluorescence (nonspecific presentation)
- <u>Rx</u>: supportive, corticosteroids

### *Stevens-Johnson Syndrome and Toxic Epidermal Necrolysis*

- severe life-threatening forms of erythema multiforme
- <u>SSx</u>: Stevens-Johnson Syndrome includes widespread lesions (mouth, eyes, genitalia, respiratory tract), photophobia, blindness, fever; TEN hallmark is full thickness epithelial detachment and necrosis
- <u>Rx</u>: supportive (hydration, analgesics, antipyretics), airway management, high-dose corticosteroids, topical creams

## Pemphigus Vulgaris

- <u>Pathophysiology</u>: autoantibodies against desmosome-tonofilament complexes (intracellular bridges) result in acantholysis (loss of cellular cohesiveness) and **intraepithelial** blistering
- <u>Risks</u>: Ashkenazi Jews, Mediterranean region, other connective tissue disorders
- <u>SSx</u>: painful blisters in oral or pharyngeal mucosa, desquamative gingivitis, **Nikolsky's sign** (rubbing or trauma of uninvolved mucosa produces an ulcer)

- <u>Histopathology</u>: intraepithelial cell splitting (**suprabasilar**), attached rows of basal cells to lamina propria (row of tombstones), **Tzanck cells** (free squamous cells, more spherical from loss of intracellular attachment)
- <u>Dx</u>: direct immunofluorescence of intracellular substance (intraepithelial blistering), **positive** serum antibodies (indirect immunofluorescence)
- <u>Rx</u>: oral corticosteroids, may consider immunosuppressives; often fatal if untreated

## Cicatricial Pemphigoid (Ocular Pemphigus, Benign Mucous Membrane Pemphigoid, Mucosal Pemphigoid)

- <u>Pathophysiology</u>: autoantibodies result in **subepidermal** blistering
- <u>SSx</u>: occurs in **mucus membranes (cutaneous lesions rare)**, subepithelial bullae or desquamative gingivitis primarily involving attached gingiva, **Nikolsky's sign** (*see* Pemphigus Vulgaris), **ocular lesions** (50–70% incidence; conjunctivitis, blindness, symblepharon, entropion); presents in 4th–5th decade in females > males, often recurs
- <u>Dx</u>: direct immunofluorescence in **basement membrane (subepithelial clefting), negative** indirect immunofluorescence (too localized)
- <u>Rx</u>: topical, intralesional, and oral corticosteroids, may consider immunosuppressives and antimalarials

## Bullous Pemphigoid

- <u>Pathophysiology</u>: autoantibodies result in **subepidermal** blistering
- <u>SSx</u>: similar to cicatricial pemphigoid; however, bullous pemphigoid has **cutaneous lesions (oral lesions rare)**, subepithelial bullae of flexor surfaces, groin, and abdomen; presents in 7th–8th decade in males/females equally, self-limited
- <u>Dx</u>: direct immunofluorescence in **basement membrane (subepithelial clefting), positive** serum indirect immunofluorescence (70%)
- <u>Rx</u>: oral corticosteroids, may consider immunosuppressives

## Lichen Planus

- <u>Pathophysiology</u>: autoimmune disease in which the basal layer is destroyed by activated lymphocytes, may be familial, may be induced by medication (eg, penicillamine, methyldopa, phenothiazide, antimalarials)

- Types
  1. **Reticular**: lacy white lines (**Wickham's striae**), most commonly occurs on buccal mucosa (may also be found on palate, lips, and tongue)
  2. **Plaque**: appears like leukoplakia
  3. **Atrophic**: atrophy in the center of the papule, painful
  4. **Erosive and Bullous**: painful, ulcerative lesions, common on buccal mucosa and dorsum of tongue
  5. **Ulcerative**: may involve buccal mucosa (more common on the feet and toes), painful
  6. **Annular**: more common on the lips (may also be found on the penis), ringed edges composed of small papules
- SSx: recurrent "purple, polygonal, pruritic papules" of various features (depending on type) with a predilection for the flexor surfaces and trunk; however, 60–70% may present on the lips, oral mucosa, or eyelids; oral lesions tend to be chronic
- Dx: clinical exam, biopsy
- **Kobner Isomorphic Phenomenon**: lesions may be provoked by physical trauma (eg, itching, scratching)
- Histopathology: vacuolar alteration of the basal cell layer resulting in **Civatte bodies** (degenerative eosinophilic ovoid keratinocytes), "sawtooth" pattern of epidermal hyperplasia, lymphocytic infiltration of lamina propria
- Complications: 1–4% risk of malignant transformation (higher risk with ulcerative lesions)

### Management

- **no cure**, treat painful, erythematous, and erosive lesions; closely follow suspicious lesions
- Identify Reversible Contributing Factors: medications, dental restoration, improve oral hygiene (frequent teeth cleaning), avoid tobacco, alcohol, and smoking abuse
- Medical Therapy: may consider oral or topical corticosteroids and retinoids; may also consider cryotherapy, UV light, and laser surgery

## Aphthous Ulcers

- most common oral ulcer
- Pathophysiology: idiopathic, may be immunologic, infectious, hormonal, stress-induced, traumatic, or nutritional
- Types
  1. **Minor**: most common, burning and tingling before ulcer formation, <1 cm in diameter, painful, lasts 7–10 days

   2. **Major**: more painful and larger (1–3 cm in diameter), multiple
      (1–10), risk of scar formation, lasts >1 month
   3. **Herpetiform**: numerous small ulcers 1–3 mm in diameter, risk of
      scar formation, lasts >1 month
- **Sutton's Disease**: recurrent aphthous ulcers (major type)
- <u>SSx</u>: painful, white ulcerations on the keratinized gingiva surrounded
  by a border of erythematous mucosa, may be multiple
- <u>Dx</u>: H&P
- <u>Rx</u>: observation (self-limited), consider anti-inflammatory agents,
  antibiotics, antivirals, oral and topical corticosteroids, cauterization
  (silver nitrate), *Lactobacillus* capsules

## Behçet's Disease

- <u>Pathophysiology</u>: idiopathic vasculitis
- <u>SSx</u>
   1. recurrent painful **aphthous ulcers** of the **upper respiratory tract
      and genitalia**
   2. ocular inflammation (uveitis, iritis, papilledema, blindness)
   3. cutaneous vasculitis
   4. progressive SNHL, tinnitus, vertigo
   5. systemic involvement (CNS, GI tract, large vessel vasculitis)
- <u>Dx</u>: clinical symptomatology
- <u>Rx</u>: no proven cure, may consider immunosuppressives,
  corticosteroids, IVIG

# Other Oral Lesions

## Amyloidosis

- <u>Pathophysiology</u>: abnormal deposition of fibrillar protein and
  polysaccharide complexes
- <u>Types</u>
   1. **Primary Systemic** (>50%): cardiac, tongue, and GI involvement
   2. **Secondary Systemic** (<10%): associated with other chronic
      diseases
   3. **Localized** (<10%)
   4. **Multiple Myeloma Associated** (25%)
   5. **Hereditary–Familial** (1%)
- more common in African Americans and Puerto Ricans, 3rd–4th
  decade (rare <15 years old)
- <u>H&N SSx</u>: 10–15% present in the H&N, macroglossia (tongue
  most common H&N site, 50%), true vocal fold deposition, anterior
  subglottic mass, orbital deposition

- <u>Dx</u>: biopsy and stain with Congo red (**apple-green birefringence under polarized light**)
- <u>Rx</u>: conservative surgical excision for symptomatic lesions

## Primary Leukoplakia

- <u>Pathophysiology</u>: many potential etiologies including chronic irritation (dentures, teeth), smoking, and infection
- <u>SSx</u>: white patch that cannot be removed by rubbing (keratotic)
- <u>Dx</u>: excisional biopsy (must rule out malignancy)
- <u>Histopathology</u>: hyperkeratosis, acanthosis, atypia
- <u>Complications</u>: 10–30% malignant potential
- <u>Rx</u>: excision (usually at time of biopsy)

## Hairy Leukoplakia

- <u>Pathophysiology</u>: benign mucosal hyperplasia associated with EBV
- strongly associated with HIV patients
- <u>SSx</u>: painless, lateral tongue lesions
- <u>Dx</u>: H&P, biopsy
- <u>Histopathology</u>: hyperkeratosis, acanthosis, atypia
- <u>Rx</u>: observation, may consider high-dose acyclovir

## Squamous Papilloma

- most common benign tumor of oral cavity and pharynx
- <u>Pathophysiology</u>: benign lesion associated with the human papilloma virus (HPV)
- <u>SSx</u>: well-demarcated papillary lesion, painless
- <u>Dx</u>: excisional biopsy
- <u>Rx</u>: excision

## Salivary Gland Cyst and Mucocele (*see* pp. 81–82)

# Pharyngitis

## Acute Pharyngitis

- <u>Pathogenesis</u>: primarily infectious, may be secondary to sinonasal disease, caustic injury, chronic allergy, GERD, smoking, and endotracheal intubation
- <u>Pathogens</u>: viral (40–60%) > bacterial, secondary bacterial infections less common (streptococci, pneumococci, *H. influenzae*)

- <u>SSx</u>: sore throat, odynophagia, otalgia (referred), malaise, fever, erythema, cervical adenopathy
- <u>Dx</u>: clinical exam; consider throat cultures, GABHS rapid antigen test, antistreptolysin-O (ASO), Monospot test; viral smears rarely indicated
- <u>Rx</u>: assess airway, supportive care (bed rest, hydration, humidity, lozenges, anesthetic sprays [eg, benzocaine, lidocaine], iodine glyceride solutions, antipyretics, decongestants), antibiotics for suspected bacterial infections

## Viral Pharyngitis

- most common cause of pharyngitis
- viral infections tend to have lower grade fever, more indolent course, generalized adenopathy, and other associated symptoms of a URI (cough, sneezing, rhinorrhea)
- **Rhinovirus**: associated with URI symptoms (rhinorrhea, fever, cough)
- **Coronavirus**: similar to rhinovirus
- **Adenovirus**: associated with conjunctivitis (pharyngoconjunctival fever)
- **HSV**: associated with vesicular lesions
- **EBV**: *see* Infectious Mononucleosis *following*
- **Coxsackievirus**: hand-foot-mouth disease, herpangina (*see following*)
- <u>Others</u>: influenza, parainfluenza, HIV, CMV, enterovirus, mumps, rubella

## Group A β-Hemolytic Streptococcus (GABHS) Pharyngitis

- most common cause of bacterial pharyngitis ("Strep throat")
- <u>SSx</u>: more sudden onset than viral, headache, typically not associated with a cough or rhinorrhea, high-grade fever, tonsillar/palatal petechiae (also seen in mononucleosis), exudative tonsils, tender anterior cervical adenopathy
- <u>Dx</u>: clinical exam, GABHS rapid antigen test (70–90% sensitive, >95% specific), throat culture (90–95% sensitive), antistreptolysin-O (ASO)
- <u>Rx</u>: all GABHS should be treated to prevent rheumatic fever, antibiotics and supportive care as previous

### Rheumatic Fever

- <u>Pathophysiology</u>: local invasion causes release of extracellular toxins and proteases; bacterial **M proteins** are similar to myocardial sarcolemma antigens, results in inflammatory lesions of the connective tissue of the heart, joints, blood vessels, and subcutaneous tissue

- rare complication of untreated GABHS infection (more common in tropical and developing nations, Australia)
- typically resolves after 6 weeks
- <u>SSx and Dx</u>: based on American Heart Association Modified Jones Criteria, must have a previous streptococcal infection + 2 major Jones criteria or 1 major and 2 minor Jones criteria
- <u>Major Jones Criteria</u>: carditis (cardiomegaly, valvular disease, CHF), migratory polyarthritis (occurs 2–6 weeks after initial infection), subcutaneous nodules (**Aschoff bodies**), erythema marginatum (serpiginous rash), chorea
- <u>Minor Jones Criteria</u>: arthralgia, fever, elevated acute phase reactants (CRP, ESR), prolonged PR interval
- <u>Rx</u>: treat GABHS infection, NSAIDs and corticosteroids, may require cardiac medications as well as haloperidol for chorea

## Acute Poststreptococcal Glomerulonephritis

- <u>Pathophysiology</u>: may result from antibody–antigen complex deposition in glomeruli
- typically self-limiting after 3 months
- <u>SSx</u>: may be asymptomatic; 1–3-week latent period postinfection; generalized edema, hypertension, gross hematuria, general malaise, and fever
- <u>Dx</u>: positive streptococcal tests (cultures, antibodies), urine analysis (proteinuria, hematuria, and urinary casts), renal tests, reduced total hemolytic complement (decreased C3); renal biopsy rarely required
- <u>Rx</u>: supportive medical management (antihypertensives, diuretics, fluid restriction, nephrology consultation), antimicrobial management for GABHS

## Scarlet Fever

- <u>Pathophysiology</u>: secondary effect from exotoxin produced by GABHS
- <u>SSx</u>: skin erythema initially on trunk then becomes generalized, tonsils and pharynx deep red, strawberry tongue, perioral skin erythema and desquamation, dysphagia, malaise, severe cervical lymphadenopathy
- <u>Dx</u>: H&P, cultures and sensitivity, Dick test (involves injection of diluted erythrogenic toxin that elicits local erythema if positive)
- <u>Rx</u>: antibiotics and oral hygiene

### *Other Causes of Acute Pharyngitis*

- **Syphilis** (*Treponema pallidum*): spirochete infection, may present as a form of secondary syphilis 2–3 months after primary infection, presents as dark red papules on the tonsils or pharyngeal wall; <u>Rx</u>: penicillin, tetracycline, erythromycin
- **Pertussis** (*Bordetella pertussis*): gram-negative coccobacillus associated with paroxysmal coughing with loud inspiratory sound ("whooping" cough), affects tracheobronchial tree and pharyngeal/laryngeal mucosa, progresses in 3 stages (catarrhal, paroxysmal, convalescent); <u>Rx</u>: supportive care, typically self-limited, immunization (preventive)
- **Gonorrhea** (*Neisseria gonorrhea*): gram-negative diplococcus transmitted by sexual contact, typically asymptomatic although may present as a sore throat; PCR, gram stain, or culture on chocolate or Thayer-Martin agar for identification; <u>Rx</u>: high incidence of penicillin-resistant strains, consider ceftriaxone and doxycycline, also tetracycline, trimethroprim-sulfamethoxazole
- **Diphtheria** (*Corynebacterium diphtheriae*): rare since vaccine, presents with a pharyngeal grayish exudative membrane, lethargy, and swollen neck; <u>Rx</u>: airway management, diphtheria antitoxin, antibiotics (*see also* p. 562)
- **Infectious Mononucleosis**: *see* p. 526
- **Candidiasis**: *see* p. 208

## Herpangina

- <u>Pathogen</u>: coxsackie A virus
- <u>SSx</u>: **small oropharyngeal vesicular or ulcerative lesions** (anterior pillar, palate, and buccal mucosa), benign rapid course, high fevers, fatigue, anorexia, variable rash
- similar lesions may occur in **hand, foot, and mouth disease**
- <u>Dx</u>: H&P
- <u>Rx</u>: oral hygiene, observation (rapid self-limiting course), analgesics, hydration, bed rest

## Chronic Pharyngitis

- <u>Causes</u>: postnasal drip (chronic rhinosinusitis), irritants (dust, dry heat, chemicals, smoking, alcohol), LPR, chronic mouth breathing (adenoid hypertrophy), voice abuse, allergy, granulomatous diseases and connective tissue disorders, malignancy
- <u>SSx</u>: constant throat clearing, dry throat, odynophagia, thickened and granular pharyngeal wall, pharyngeal crusting

- <u>Dx</u>: H&P, culture and biopsy if failed empiric therapies
- <u>Rx</u>: address underlying etiology, avoidance of contributing factors (smoking, dust, dry environment, etc), symptomatic treatment similar to acute pharyngitis

**Adenotonsillar Pathology** (*see* pp. 523–526)

# ODONTOGENIC, JAW, AND BONE PATHOLOGY
## Evaluation of the Jaw Mass

### History and Physical Exam

#### *History*

- <u>Character of Jaw Mass</u>: onset, duration, and progression of growth, presence of pain (pain is typically associated with infected or malignant lesions)
- <u>Contributing Factors</u>: complete dental history including recent dental work and caries, history of other skin lesions (basal cell nevus syndrome), recent trauma, history of other congenital defects (cleft palate or lip)
- <u>Associated Symptoms</u>: fever, weight loss, malaise, TMJ pain

#### *Physical Exam*

- <u>Character of Jaw Mass</u>: size, distribution, tenderness, consistency, solitary versus multiple lesions
- <u>Dental Exam</u>: complete dental exam including percussion, presence of impacted teeth (follicular or dentigerous cysts) and nonviable teeth, malalignment (may result from divergent roots from compressive effects of underlying mass)

### Management

#### *Radiographs*

- <u>Intraoral Radiographs</u>: indicated for screening dental disease; provide excellent detail; available in dental offices; inadequate evaluation of ramus, condyle, and inferior aspect of the mandible
- <u>Panorex (Orthopantomogram)</u>: assesses entire mandible in a single view, inadequate visualization of symphyseal region
- <u>Mandibular Series</u>: multiple extraoral views, difficult to delineate small lesions

- <u>CT/MRI</u>: not cost-effective for screening; indicated for large, distorting lesions and preoperative planning for malignancy

### *Biopsy*

- <u>Fine Needle Aspiration (FNA)</u>: allows acquisition of cells with minimal morbidity, may aspirate cysts for culture and sensitivity (vascular lesions may be aspirated to avoid hemorrhage from open biopsies)
- <u>Excisional Biopsy</u>: indicated for small lesions with low suspicion for malignancy by radiographs
- <u>Incisional Biopsy</u>: indicated for larger, potentially malignant lesions to obtain diagnosis prior to definitive resection

# Jaw Cysts

## Introduction

- **Odontogenic Cysts**: epithelial-lined structures derived from odontogenic (tooth-forming) epithelium
- lesions are defined primarily by location of cyst and less from the histology

## Odontogenic Cysts

### *Periapical Cyst (Radicular Cyst)*

- **most common odontogenic cyst**
- <u>Pathophysiology</u>: **nonviable tooth** (dental decay) results in osteitis of periapical bone from dental canal, **epithelial cell rests of Malassez** proliferate from inflammatory stimulation in the periodontal membrane causing cyst formation
- typically located on anterior maxilla and posterior mandible
- **Lateral Periodontal Cyst**: less common variant found on lateral aspect of the tooth
- <u>SSx</u>: typically asymptomatic, may illicit pain with percussion or heat
- <u>Radiographic Findings</u>: radiolucency at root apex of tooth with associated dental caries or pulp injury
- <u>Histopathology</u>: stratified squamous epithelium lining
- <u>Complications</u>: local cellulitis; fascial plane infections; abscess formation; fistula to oral cavity, skin, or nasal cavity; sepsis; jugular vein thrombosis; osteomyelitis; orbital extension, rare malignant transformation
- <u>Rx</u>: antibiotics, drainage of abscess, and endodontic therapy (root canal to remove tooth)

## *Follicular Cyst (Dentigerous Cyst)*

- **second most common odontogenic cyst**
- <u>Pathophysiology</u>: disruption of late odontogenesis (associated with an **impacted tooth**, especially mandibular and maxillary third molar), cyst grows within the normal dental follicle
- <u>SSx</u>: initially asymptomatic, often diagnosed late with jaw deformity
- <u>Radiographic Findings</u>: radiolucency at crown of an unerupted tooth, may displace teeth
- <u>Histopathology</u>: outer thin connective tissue wall with a thin stratified squamous epithelium inner layer
- <u>Complications</u>: **risk of malignant transformation in cyst wall** (unicystic ameloblastoma, epidermoid carcinoma)
- <u>Rx</u>: enucleation and curettage

## *Primordial Cyst*

- <u>Pathophysiology</u>: degeneration of odontogenesis results in **cyst development where a tooth would normally develop**
- <u>SSx</u>: typically asymptomatic
- <u>Radiographic Findings</u>: ovoid, well-demarcated lesions, may be multiloculated
- <u>Complications</u>: may become secondarily infected, 50% are considered keratocystic odontogenic tumors
- <u>Rx</u>: enucleation and curettage, must consider keratocystic odontogenic tumor if recurs

## *Keratocystic Odontogenic Tumor (KCOT)*

- previously called **odontogenic keratocyst** (OKC)
- **more aggressive and more difficult to remove than other odontogenic cysts**
- <u>Pathophysiology</u>: similar to primordial cysts
- may be associated with a crown of unerupted tooth (follicular cyst) or tooth root (periapical cyst)
- most commonly found in the mandibular third molar and ramus
- <u>SSx</u>: usually asymptomatic
- <u>Dx</u>: based on histology, FNA (white keratin-containing aspirate)
- <u>Radiographic Findings</u>: similar to primordial cysts
- <u>Histopathology</u>: (determines diagnosis) thin stratified squamous epithelium, columnar, or cuboidal basal cell layer, both parakeratin or orthokeratin may be present, lumen may be filled with degenerated keratin
- <u>Complications</u>: local destruction, secondary infection, 10–60% recurrence

- **Basal Cell Nevus Syndrome**: autosomal dominant, **multiple KCOTs**, also basal cell carcinoma, bifid ribs, hypertelorism, mandibular prognathism, calcification of falx cerebri (85%), palmar pitting (65%), depressed midface, and frontal and parietal bossing
- <u>Rx</u>: enucleation and aggressive curettage (rotary bur) often **multilocular**, careful follow-up for recurrence, consider resection with 1 cm margins for recurrent KCOTs

### *Eruption Cyst*

- <u>Pathophysiology</u>: developmental cyst within the soft tissue
- <u>SSx</u>: bluish cyst overlying the alveolar ridge, typically resolves
- <u>Radiographic Findings</u>: translucent, dome-shaped cyst
- <u>Rx</u>: usually none, excise if symptomatic

## Nonodontogenic Cysts

- **Nasopalatine Duct Cyst (Incisive Canal Cyst)**: most common nonodontogenic cyst, derived from embryologic remnant of the nasopalatine duct, located between the maxillary central incisors (heart-shaped lucency, >10 mm); <u>Rx</u>: enucleation and curettage if symptomatic
- **Midpalatal Cyst of Infants**: arises from epithelium trapped between embryologic palatal shelves ("fissural"), midline palatal mass; <u>Rx</u>: enucleation and curettage
- **Nasolabial Cyst**: arise within the labial vestibule, present as a swelling of the upper lip or nasal floor; <u>Rx</u>: excision
- **Stafne Bone Cyst (Static Bone Cavity, Latent Bone Cyst)**: due to aberrant salivary gland tissue located in the posterior mandible, not actually a cyst; <u>Rx</u>: observation
- **Aneurysmal Bone Cyst**: more common in teenagers with a history of trauma to the mandible, painful, not a true cyst; <u>Rx</u>: rapid enucleation to avoid hemorrhage
- **Idiopathic Bone Cavity (Traumatic Bone Cyst)**: not a true cyst, may be secondary to a traumatic intramedullary hemorrhage with degeneration of the clot, resulting in an air-filled bony space; <u>Rx</u>: biopsy to rule out other lesions

# Odontogenic Tumors

## Epithelial Tumors

### *Ameloblastoma*

- **most common odontogenic epithelial tumor**

- <u>Pathophysiology</u>: benign neoplasm of uncertain origin, arises from dental lamina, locally invasive (thought of as the oral counterpart to basal cell carcinoma)
- peak occurrence 3rd–4th decade
- 80% mandibular
- rare malignant transformation (*see following*)
- <u>Types</u>
  1. **Central**: arises in bone (intraosseous)
  2. **Plexiform Unicystic**: more aggressive central variant, occurs in the lining of follicular cysts or impacted teeth
  3. **Peripheral**: arises in soft tissue around alveolar bone, much less aggressive, may be treated with local excision
- <u>SSx</u>: slow growing, painless, intrabony mandibular swelling, may resorb tooth roots
- <u>Radiographic Findings</u>: expansile radiolucent multiloculations ("soap bubbles" or "honeycombed")
- <u>Histopathology</u>: various histologic patterns, most common is the follicular pattern with islands of epithelium lined with columnar cells, central mass of loosely arranged cells (stellate reticulum), collagenous stroma
- <u>Rx</u>: wide excision with 1 cm bony margin and immediate reconstruction for central ameloblastomas, 3–5 cm margin for plexiform unicystic types)

### Malignant Ameloblastoma

- <u>Pathophysiology</u>: rare malignant degeneration from ameloblastoma resulting in metastasis
- <u>SSx</u>: regional or distant metastasis with aggressive local invasion
- <u>Radiographic Findings</u>: radiolucency with poorly defined margins
- <u>Dx</u>: biopsy of metastasis reveals similar histology to primary ameloblastoma with malignant features (atypical mitotic figures, invasion, pleomorphism)
- <u>Rx</u>: aggressive local resection, neck dissections for positive lymphadenopathy, consider postoperative radiation and/or chemotherapy

### Calcifying Epithelial Odontogenic Tumor (Pindborg Tumor)

- <u>Pathophysiology</u>: rare, benign infiltrating lesion, derived from the stratum intermedium
- associated with **impacted molars**
- <u>SSx</u>: slow growing, painless, intrabony mandibular swelling (similar to ameloblastoma), can be infiltrative and destructive

- <u>Radiographic Findings</u>: unilocular radiolucency with calcifications
- <u>Histopathology</u>: sheets or islands of epithelial cells with eosinophilic cytoplasm, may contain amyloid with concentric calcifications or psammoma-like bodies (**Liesegang rings**)
- <u>Rx</u>: similar to ameloblastoma

### Ameloblastic Fibroma

- <u>Pathophysiology</u>: true neoplasm with epithelial and mesenchymal elements, occurs in younger patients (5–20 years old)
- <u>SSx</u>: similar to ameloblastoma
- <u>Radiographic Findings</u>: similar to ameloblastoma
- <u>Histopathology</u>: islands of columnar or cuboidal epithelium with various arrangements (islands, cords, strands), central papilla-like connective tissue
- <u>Rx</u>: enucleation and curettage (does not require 1 cm margin as with ameloblastoma)

### Ameloblastic Odontoma

- <u>Pathophysiology</u>: hamartomatous (nonneoplastic) lesion derived from epithelial (enamel-secreting) and mesenchymal (dentin-secreting) elements
- associated with dentigerous cyst
- <u>SSx</u>: typically asymptomatic, may prevent tooth eruption
- <u>Radiographic Findings</u>: radiopaque mass surrounded by a thin radiolucency (may be associated with an unerupted tooth)
- <u>Histopathology</u>: presence of dentin and enamel (similar to a dental follicle), "ghost" cells
- <u>Rx</u>: enucleation and curettage (low risk of recurrence)

### Adenomatoid Odontogenic Tumor

- <u>Pathophysiology</u>: hamartomatous growth
- **"Two-Thirds Tumor"**: 2/3 occur in the anterior maxilla, 2/3 occur in females, 2/3 associated with an impacted tooth (**cuspids**); also occurs in 2nd and 3rd decades of life
- <u>SSx</u>: maxillary mass, typically anterior to the molars, slow progressive growth
- <u>Histopathology</u>: spheres of cuboidal and spindle cells, amyloid and dystrophic calcifications
- <u>Rx</u>: enucleation and curettage (low risk of recurrence since often degenerates)

### Calcifying Odontogenic Cyst (Gorlin's Cyst)

- <u>Pathophysiology</u>: derived from proliferating epithelium, necrotic degeneration forms cysts
- <u>SSx</u>: anterior mandibular asymptomatic swelling
- <u>Radiographic Findings</u>: well-circumscribed radiolucency with central calcifications
- <u>Histopathology</u>: cysts with solid forms, lined by eosinophilic cells and "ghost" cells, may cause giant-cell reaction
- <u>Rx</u>: enucleation and curettage (en bloc resection for rare neoplastic variants)

## Mesenchymal Tumors

### Cementomas

- class of benign tumors that secrete cementum
- <u>Types</u>
    1. **Periapical Cemental Dysplasia**: more common in black females, multiple lesions, develops through varying stages (osteolytic, cementoblastic, and maturation)
    2. **Cementoblastoma**: true benign tumor of cementoblasts of the tooth root, usually from first mandibular tooth
    3. **Cementifying Fibroma**: similar to ossifying fibroma (*see following*)
- <u>SSx</u>: asymptomatic mandibular bony mass
- <u>Rx</u>: observation for periapical cemental dysplasia, curettage with extraction for cementoblastomas

### Odontogenic Fibroma and Myxoma

- <u>Pathophysiology</u>: arise from periodontal ligament, dental papilla, or dental follicle
- <u>SSx</u>: slow growing, asymptomatic mandibular mass
- <u>Radiographic Findings</u>: smooth-bordered radiolucency, may occur around the crown of an unerupted tooth
- <u>Histopathology</u>: fibromas contain an abundance of collagen-producing fibroblasts, myxomas have fewer cells with a mucoid intracellular matrix
- <u>Rx</u>: fibromas require simple enucleation, myxomas are more difficult to excise and have a 25% recurrence rate

# Nonodontogenic Tumors

## Fibro-osseus Jaw Lesions

### Osseous Dysplasia

- <u>Pathophysiology</u>: **reactive disorder**
- more common in young African Americans
- <u>SSx</u>: alveolar bone mass, typically asymptomatic
- <u>Dx</u>: biopsy, Panorex or plain x-rays (multiple radiolucent/radiopaque intraosseous lesions, "cotton wool" appearance)
- <u>Rx</u>: observation, excision if symptomatic

### Ossifying Fibroma

- <u>Pathophysiology</u>: benign, nonodontogenic tumor of the mandible or maxilla
- more common in females
- <u>SSx</u>: painless, slow-growing mandibular mass, may displace teeth
- <u>Radiographic Findings</u>: well-demarcated, cannonball-like, homogeneous opacity
- <u>Histopathology</u>: abundant collagen with varying calcification
- <u>Rx</u>: enucleation with curettage, may consider en bloc resection for aggressive or recurrent lesions

### Fibrous Dysplasia

- <u>Pathophysiology</u>: **genetically based**, hamartomatous lesions of maxilla or mandible, medullary bone replaced by fibro-osseous tissue
- more common in middle-aged women
- <u>Types</u>
  1. **Monostotic**: one bone involved, **most common form**
  2. **Polyostotic**: more than one bone involved (**McCune-Albright Syndrome**: polyostotic fibrous dysplasia, precocious puberty, abnormal skin pigmented lesions)
  3. **Juvenile**: rapidly destructive, aggressive, destroys teeth, refractory to treatment
- <u>SSx</u>: slow growing, painless, well-circumscribed, marble-like mass, destroys bone, unilateral facial deformity (mass does not cross midline, developmental plates)
- <u>Dx</u>: biopsy; CT, Panorex, and plain x-rays (ground glass, "Chinese writing," irregular, multiloculated, diffuse margins, eggshell-thin cortex from destruction of cortical bone, may obliterate the sphenoid and frontal sinuses)
- <u>Rx</u>: excision and curettage of lesions if disfiguring, cosmetic shaping

## Other Nonodontogenic Lesions

### Torus Mandibularis and Palatinus

- <u>Pathophysiology</u>: developmental anomaly, enlargement of bone of the lingual surface of the mandible or the hard palate
- <u>SSx</u>: typically asymptomatic
- <u>Dx</u>: clinical exam
- <u>Rx</u>: observation, excision if symptomatic

### Cherubism

- <u>Pathophysiology</u>: autosomal dominant mutation, results in symmetric enlargement of mandibular body and ramus (rarely involves maxilla)
- <u>SSx</u>: painless, round "cherub" face (broad cheeks, enlarged jaw), regresses at puberty
- <u>Radiographic Findings</u>: multilocular cystic changes in the mandible and maxilla and often in the anterior ends of the ribs
- <u>Rx</u>: observation, may consider surgical options after puberty for persistence

### Paget's Disease (Osteitis Deformans)

- <u>Pathophysiology</u>: autosomal dominant, increased bone resorption and formation resulting in dense but fragile bone, involves the lumbosacral regions and skull
- <u>Phases</u>
  1. **Lytic**: replacement of bone with vascularized stroma, destructive phase
  2. **Mixed**: increased osteoclastic and osteoblastic activity, formation of Paget bone
  3. **Sclerotic**: decreased osteoclastic activity, increased hard, dense bone formation
- more common in patients >40 years old (fibrous dysplasia affects younger patients)
- <u>SSx</u>: bone pain, enlarged skull, dorsal kyphosis, bowed legs, nonunion fractures, hearing loss (SNHL and CHL), neurologic sequelae from compressive effects
- <u>Dx</u>: characteristic Panorex and plain x-rays (polyostotic, mosaic pattern of bone); bone scan (evaluate extent of disease); elevated serum alkaline phosphatase (used as a marker to monitor therapy), calcium, and urine hydroxyproline from increased bone turnover
- <u>Radiographic Findings</u>: **multiple**, multiloculated, well-defined radiolucencies (**lytic lesions**), thin cortex, sclerotic lesions in later phases

- Complications: hypercalcemia, polycythemia, cardiac failure, malignant transformation (osteosarcoma, giant cell tumor), neurologic compression, normal pressure hydrocephalus, pathologic fractures
- Rx: consider physical therapy (to increase muscle support) if asymptomatic and localized, medical management for symptomatic or complicated disease includes calcitonin, cytotoxic agents, etidronate, analgesics

# Temporomandibular Joint Disorders

## Temporomandibular Joint (TMJ) Anatomy
### (Figure 6–1)

- Vascular Supply: superficial temporal artery
- Sensory Innervations: auriculotemporal, masseteric, and deep posterior temporal nerves (CN $V_3$)
- **Diarthrodial Joint**: true synovial joint (freely mobile) with two modes of movement (gliding and hinging)
- **Glenoid Fossa**: socket within the temporal bone, lined with fibrocartilages
- **Articular Eminence**: anterior aspect of the glenoid fossa which articulates with the condyle

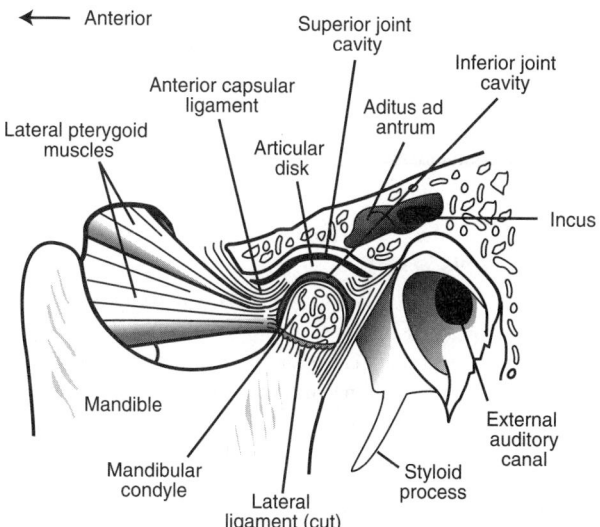

**FIGURE 6–1.** Components of the temporomandibular joint.

### *Fibrocartilaginous Articular Disk (Meniscus)*

- the articular disk is interposed between the articulating components (separates the superior and inferior synovial compartments)
- attaches to the condyloid process by the lateral and medial ligaments and by the inferior lamina of the meniscotemporomandibular frenum
- <u>Disk Bands</u>: anteriorly attaches to the lateral pterygoid muscle (2 mm disk thickness), intermediate region (thinnest zone, 1 mm disk thickness), posteriorly (thickest, 3-mm disk thickness)
- **Functions**: stability, allows rotational and translatory motions, absorbs shock forces

## Temporomandibular Joint Syndrome

- <u>Risks</u>: nocturnal **bruxism** (jaw clenching during sleep, associated with muscle strain), recent trauma or intubation, stress, psychiatric history
- <u>SSx</u>: jaw pain or referred otalgia (worse with movement or chewing), tender/warm TMJ (may have crepitus and clicking), reduced intraincisor opening (normal 40–50 mm), headaches, toothache, facial pain, trismus
- <u>Dx</u>: clinical exam, CT/MRI may be considered for select cases

### *Types*

- **Myofascial Pain Dysfunction Syndrome**: most common, no destructive changes of TMJ, commonly involves muscles of mastication, stress disorder, associated with bruxism
- **Internal Derangement**: from TMJ disk displacement (*see following*) or chronic dislocations

### *TMJ Disk Displacement*

- <u>Pathophysiology</u>: joint dislocation secondary to disruption of the ligamentous attachments
- <u>Causes</u>: hyperextension of jaw secondary to intubation, forceful teeth extraction (especially third molars), or retraction from tonsillectomy; chronic clenching, facial trauma
- <u>Types</u>
  1. **Reducing**: joint "clicks" back into alignment with jaw opening (**anterior displacement** most common due to vector force of the lateral pterygoid muscles)
  2. **Nonreducing**: joint "locks" with jaw opening

## *Medical Management*

- early management is key to preventing progression of joint degeneration
- <u>Behavior Modifications</u>: soft diet (may require liquid diet, smaller bites), avoid gum chewing, warm compresses
- <u>Physical Therapy</u>: reduction (may require sedation), repositioning, repetitive jaw stretching, active and passive mobilization
- <u>Medical Management</u>: analgesics and NSAIDs (narcotics should be avoided), muscle relaxants, antidepressants, benzodiazepines, may consider corticosteroid injections
- <u>Dental Management</u>: consult for malocclusion, carious teeth, poorly fitting dentures, possible orthognathic surgery
- <u>Prosthetic Devices</u>: occlusal splints (can reduce muscle pain associated with bruxism)

## *Surgical Management (Controversial)*

- effectiveness *controversial,* indicated for confirmed TMJ intracapsular derangements
- **Arthroscopy and Arthrotomy**: exploration of TMJ, removes debris, lyses adhesions
- **Discoplasty, Discectomy**: repositioning, plication, removal, or reduction of articular disc; indicated for fractured or malaligned discs

# Other Articular and Osteogenic Pathology

## *Congenital and Developmental Diseases*

- **Agenesis**: typically unilateral, associated with otologic abnormalities
- **Maxillomandibular Hypoplasia or Hyperplasia**: facial asymmetry, malocclusion (cross-bite), hypoplasia may be acquired (radiation effects, infection, trauma)

## *Arthritis*

- **Degenerative Arthritis**: occurs in the elderly, primarily a mechanical process, minimal inflammatory changes, destroys articular tissue; radiograph may reveal erosion of condyle; <u>Rx</u>: conservative management (*as previous*), rare surgical indications
- **Infectious Arthritis**: rare, unilateral lesion; <u>Rx</u>: antibiotics, restrict movement, consider aspiration or incision and drainage for suppurative infections
- **Rheumatoid Arthritis**: usually bilateral lesions, radiograph reveals bone destruction; <u>Rx</u>: medical management (eg, anti-inflammatory

agents, hydroxychloroquine, monoclonal antibodies), jaw exercises, consider surgery for ankylosis (*see* p. 249)
- **Traumatic Arthritis**: trauma-related edema, intraarticular hemorrhage, and disk injury; <u>Rx</u>: NSAIDs, heat compress, restrict jaw motion

### Other Causes

- **Mandible and Maxilla Fractures**: *see* pp. 635–646
- **Neoplasm**: rare benign and malignant tumors of bone and cartilage
- **Ankylosis**: most often from trauma or rheumatoid arthritis, typically unilateral, fibrous and bony types; <u>Rx</u>: surgical management (*see previous*), physical therapy

# NECK MASSES

## Anatomy of the Neck (Figures 6–2 and 6–3)

### Anterior Cervical Triangle

- <u>Boundaries</u>: midline of the neck, posterior border of SCM, inferior border of the mandible
- **Submandibular (Digastric) Triangle**: bordered by the inferior border of the mandible, and by the anterior and posterior digastric
- **Submental (Suprahyoid) Triangle**: bordered by the left and right anterior digastric and the hyoid bone (only unpaired triangle)
- **Carotid (Superior Carotid) Triangle**: bordered by the superior omohyoid, posterior digastric muscle, posterior border of SCM
- **Muscular (Inferior Carotid) Triangle**: bordered by the superior omohyoid, midline of the neck, posterior border of SCM

### Posterior Cervical Triangle

- <u>Boundaries</u>: clavicle, posterior border of SCM, anterior border of the trapezius muscle
- **Occipital Triangle**: bordered by the posterior border of SCM, anterior border of the trapezius, inferior omohyoid
- **Supraclavicular (Subclavian) Triangle**: bordered by the posterior border of SCM, clavicle, inferior omohyoid
- <u>Contents of the Posterior Triangle</u>: scalene, posterior cervical, and supraclavicular nodes; pleural apices; phrenic nerve, brachial plexus (trunks); subclavian artery and vein; anterior scalenes; thyrocervical trunk branches (dorsal scapular, transverse cervical, supraclavicular, and inferior thyroid arteries)

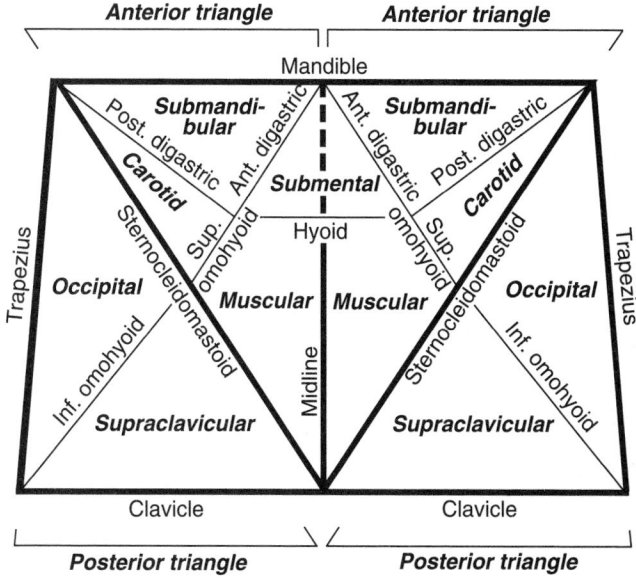

**FIGURE 6–2.** Schematic of cervical neck triangles and subtriangles.

# Evaluation of the Neck Mass

## History

- <u>Character of Neck Mass</u>: onset, duration, and progression of growth; pain
- <u>Contributing Factors</u>: recent URI, sinus infection, otitis media, or other H&N infection; exposure to pets and other animals; recent travel; exposure to TB; risk of malignancy (previous excision of skin or scalp lesions, smoking and alcohol abuse, radiation therapy, other malignancies, family history of cancer); recent trauma; immunodeficiency (risk of HIV, corticosteroids, uncontrolled diabetes); age (often infectious in children, higher risk of malignancy in adults)
- <u>Associated Symptoms</u>: fever, postnasal drip, rhinorrhea, sore throat, otalgia, night sweats, weight loss, malaise, dysphagia, hoarseness
- think "KITTENS" for differential diagnosis (*see* Table 6–3)

**TABLE 6-3.** Differential Diagnosis of the Neck Mass: KITTENS Method

| (K) Congenital | Infectious & Iatrogenic | Toxins & Trauma | Endocrine | Neoplasms | Systemic |
|---|---|---|---|---|---|
| Branchial cleft cyst | Bacterial or viral lymphadenitis | Hematoma | Thymic cyst | Metastatic or regional malignancy | Granulomatous disease |
| Lymphatic malformation | Tuberculosis | | Thyroid hyperplasia | | Laryngocele |
| Teratoma and dermoid cyst | Cat-scratch disease | | Aberrant thyroid tissue | Thyroid neoplasm | Plunging ranula |
| Thyroglossal duct cyst | Syphilis | | Parathyroid cyst | Lymphoma | Kawasaki disease |
| External laryngocele | Atypical mycobacteria | | | Hemangioma | |
| | Persistent generalized lymphadenopathy | | | Salivary gland tumor | |
| | Mononucleosis | | | Vascular tumor | |
| | Sebaceous cyst | | | Neurogenic tumor | |
| | Deep inflammation or abscess | | | Lipoma | |

## Physical Exam

- <u>Character of Neck Mass</u>: size (normal hyperplastic nodes rarely >2 cm), distribution, mobility, tenderness and fluctuance (infectious), consistency (firm, elastic, soft, compressible), solitary mass versus general cervical adenopathy, lesions and character of the overlying skin (eg, erythematous, blanching, vascular signs, fistulas, induration, radiodermatitis, necrotic)
- <u>Physical Exam</u>: thorough H&N exam for primary malignancies (attention to nasopharynx, oral cavity, base of tongue, tonsillar fossa, nasal cavity, EAC, scalp, thyroid, and salivary glands); palpate other lymphatic sites (eg, inguinal, axillary, supraclavicular); palpate thyroid gland, liver, and spleen (lymphoma, mononucleosis); auscultate for vascular abnormalities

## Ancillary Tests

- **CT/MRI of Neck**: provides greater differentiation of abscess, neoplasm, vascular lesion, hematoma, or congenital abnormality
- <u>Labs</u>: CBC with differential, Monospot, PPD, HIV testing, cat-scratch antigen titers, toxoplasmosis titers, EBV serology tests
- **Ultrasound**: identifies cystic masses, when combined with Doppler further defines vascular lesions
- **Fine Needle Aspiration (FNA)**: provides fluid for culture and sensitivity, indicated for nonresolving mass or if suspect malignancy (firm, large [>2 cm], nontender, asymmetric neck masses) **without** a known primary
- **Open Biopsy**: indicated for persistent idiopathic adenopathy or high suspicion of malignancy (if FNA is negative or indeterminate and complete workup does not reveal a primary site), prepare for possible completion of neck dissection if frozen section is positive
- **Angiography**: indicated if suspect a primary vascular disorder
- **Panendoscopy**: direct laryngoscopy, esophagoscopy, and bronchoscopy may be considered to evaluate for a primary site of malignancy

## Congenital Neck Masses (see pp. 599–604)

## Infectious Neck Masses

### Viral Cervical Lymphadenitis

- **most common cause of lymphadenitis**
- <u>Pathogens</u>: most commonly EBV, CMV, HSV, adenovirus, enterovirus, roseola, rubella, HIV

- <u>SSx</u>: similar to bacterial lymphadenitis (*see following*), tends to have lower grade fevers, more indolent course, posterior adenopathy (tender submandibular and submental nodes common with oral herpetic stomatitis)
- <u>Dx</u>: clinical exam
- <u>Rx</u>: supportive

## Bacterial Cervical Lymphadenitis

- <u>Pathogens</u>: most commonly group A streptococci and *S. aureus*
- <u>Pathophysiology</u>: draining infection results in migration and division of lymphocytes, plasma cells, monocytes, and histiocytes resulting in larger tender nodes
- <u>SSx</u>: acute development of tender, mobile cervical mass, associated with constitutional symptoms (malaise, fever), initially may present with a single discrete node before developing generalized lymphadenopathy
- <u>Dx</u>: clinical exam, aspiration for culture and sensitivity
- <u>Complications</u>: cellulitis, abscess, internal jugular thrombosis, mediastinitis, sepsis
- <u>Rx</u>: antibiotic regimen, incision and drainage for abscess formation

## Cat-Scratch Disease

- <u>Pathogen</u>: *Bartonella henselae*
- presents 2 weeks after a cat bite or scratch
- <u>SSx</u>: cutaneous papular lesions at primary site, tender cervical lymphadenopathy (later becomes painless, may last months), mild fever and malaise, pustulous lesions tend to ulcerate (risk of fistula formation)
- <u>Dx</u>: culture (Warthin-Starry stain), cat-scratch antigen test, history of cat exposure
- <u>Histopathology</u>: intracellular, gram-negative bacillus (**Warthin-Starry stain**); central area of avascular, granulomatous necrosis surrounded by lymphocytes
- **Parinaud Oculoglandular Syndrome**: unilateral conjunctivitis and regional lymphadenitis, inoculation may occur near eye or from eye rubbing
- <u>Rx</u>: observation with supportive care (self-limited) versus antibiotics (immunocompromised), avoid incision and drainage to prevent sinus formation (may consider aspiration)

## Atypical Mycobacteria

- <u>Pathogens</u>: *Mycobacterium avium* complex, *M. scrofulaceum, M. kansasii*

- typically less virulent than *M. tuberculosis*; however, less responsive to antituberculosis medications
- may colonize respiratory tract
- <u>Risks</u>: children (more common than TB), immunocompromised, history of foreign travel, may have history of surgery as port of entry
- <u>SSx</u>: unilateral cervical lymphadenopathy (**adhesive to overlying skin**), corneal ulceration (most common H&N manifestation)
- <u>Dx</u>: acid-fast stain, culture (requires 2–4 weeks for growth), tuberculin skin testing often negative
- <u>Rx</u>: complete excision (avoid incision and drainage), antituberculars (may consider rifampin to reduce the bulk of the infected node prior to excision)

## Other Causes of Lymphadenitis

- **Tuberculosis (TB)**: typically presents as a postprimary disease, lymphadenitis suggests hematogenous spread, pulmonary TB must be examined, less common than atypical mycobacteria in children (*see also* pp. 245–246)
- **Syphilis**: may present in primary or secondary disease (*see also* p. 245 for management)
- **Toxoplasmosis**: *Toxoplasma gondii* presents as an influenza-like illness in adults; congenital form presents with hydrocephalus, chorioretinitis, and intracerebral calcifications; diagnosed with serum titers and lymph node biopsy; <u>Rx</u>: antiprotozoals
- **Nonspecific Lymphadenitis**: reactive adenitis typically secondary to a nasopharyngeal infection, may occur from any infection of the H&N, primary infection may have resolved; <u>Rx</u>: consider trial of broad-spectrum antibiotics versus observation

# Other Head and Neck Masses

## Pilomatrixoma

- benign appendageal tumor with hair follicle differentiation
- bimodal presentation at 5–15 and 50–65 years old
- 50% occur in head/neck, usually ≤3 cm, firm
- <u>Rx</u>: wide local excision

## Kawasaki Disease (Mucocutaneous Lymph Node Syndrome) (*see* p. 603)

**Plunging Ranula** (*see* pp. 81–82)

**External Laryngocele** (*see* p. 116)

## Cervical Lymphadenopathy in HIV

### Introduction

- idiopathic follicular hyperplasia is the most common cause of cervical lymphadenopathy in HIV
- higher risk for lymphoma, carcinoma, atypical mycobacteria, TB
- open biopsy should be reserved for highly suspicious lesions (failed antibiotic trial, enlarging, mediastinal adenopathy, suspicious FNA, >2 cm nodes, asymmetric lesions)

### Persistent Generalized Lymphadenopathy (PGL)

- <u>Pathophysiology</u>: idiopathic lymphadenopathy, may be a direct effect of the HIV
- cervical lymphadenopathy is the third most common lymphatic site (axillary and inguinal more common)
- <u>SSx</u>: typically asymptomatic lymphadenopathy
- <u>Dx</u>: H&P, neoplastic and infectious causes must be ruled out, must have adenopathy of 2 or more sites (extrainguinal) for >3 months in HIV patient
- <u>Histopathology Patterns</u>: follicular hyperplasia, follicular involution (small follicles), lymphoid depleted (no follicles)
- <u>Rx</u>: observation

# NECK PLANES, SPACES, AND INFECTION

## Cervical Fascial Planes (see Figure 6–3)

### Superficial Cervical Fascia

- condensed sheath of connective tissue under skin from the zygomatic process to the thorax and axilla
- includes superficial musculoaponeurotic system (SMAS)
- <u>Contents</u>: platysma and facial muscles of expression

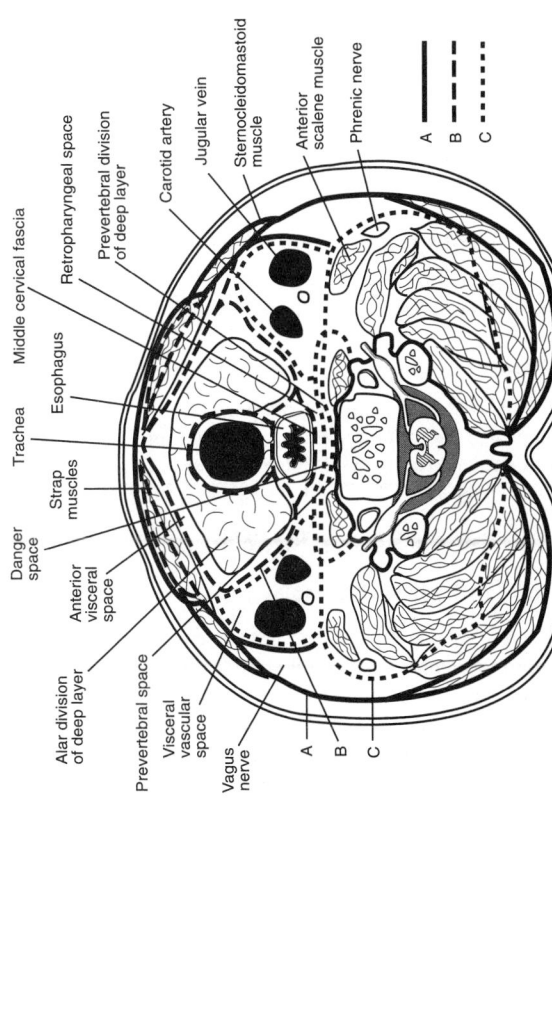

**FIGURE 6-3.** Cross-section anatomy of the neck demonstrating the cervical fascial planes. Adapted with permission from Rosse C., Gaddum-Rosse P. *Hollinshead's Textbook of Anatomy*, 5th ed, p. 710. Philadelphia, PA: Lippincott Williams & Wilkins; 1997.

## Deep Cervical Fascia

### Superficial (Investing) Layer of Deep Cervical Fascia

- forms stylomandibular ligament
- <u>Contents</u>: trapezius, SCM, masseter; submandibular and parotid glands

### Middle Layer of Deep Cervical Fascia (Pretracheal Fascia)

- forms midline raphe, pteryogomandibular raphe, and pretracheal fascia
- <u>Muscular Division Contents</u>: strap muscles
- <u>Visceral Division Contents</u>: pharynx, larynx, trachea, esophagus, thyroid, constrictor, and buccinator muscles (buccopharyngeal fascia)

### Deep Layer of Deep Cervical Fascia (Prevertebral Fascia)

- divided into prevertebral and alar layers
- <u>Contents</u>: paraspinus muscles and cervical vertebrae

### Carotid Sheath

- made up of all layers of deep cervical fascia
- attaches to jugular and carotid foramina at the base of skull
- <u>Contents</u>: carotid artery, internal jugular vein, vagus nerve

# Neck Space Infections

## Introduction and Management

- <u>Sources</u>: odontogenic (most common), tonsils (most common pediatric source), trauma, URI, salivary glands, IV drug injections, instrumentation (bronchoscopy, esophagoscopy), neck infections (adenitis, thyroiditis, branchial cleft cysts)
- <u>Pathogens</u>: usually wide array of organisms including aerobic and anaerobic, must also consider actinomycosis, which may cross fascial planes (*see* pp. 208–209)
- <u>SSx</u>: erythematous and tender neck, spiking fever, asymmetric neck lymphadenopathy, torticollis, trismus, cranial nerve involvement (hoarseness), dyspnea, stridor, dysphagia
- <u>Dx</u>: lateral and AP neck radiographs may be considered for screening (examine for soft tissue swelling in the posterior pharyngeal region, abnormal if space >50% the width of the vertebral body), CT/MRI of neck with contrast, CXR

- <u>Rx</u>: secure airway (consider tracheotomy), aggressive antibiotic therapy, local drainage (culture and sensitivity), extraction of tooth (if source), debridement of osteomyelitic bone

## Necrotizing Fasciitis (Necrotizing Soft Tissue Infection) of the Head and Neck

- <u>Pathophysiology</u>: aggressive polymicrobial infection invades the subcutaneous tissue and fascia causing local ischemia (vascular occlusion) and localized anesthesia (neural damage)
- <u>Risks</u>: immunocompromised (HIV, uncontrolled diabetes), IV drug users
- <u>Pathogens</u>: **Group A β-hemolytic streptococci** (exotoxins A, B, and C and streptococcal superantigen), staphylococci, and gram-negative rods (myonecrosis occurs from superinfections from anaerobes and other gram-negative organisms)
- <u>SSx</u>: rapid, severe necrosis of the skin, fascia, and soft tissues; may form crepitus, sepsis (fever spikes, hypotension, tachycardia)
- <u>Dx</u>: CT reveals subcutaneous emphysema, necrotic soft tissue; biopsy for culture and sensitivity; most important lab indicators are high CRP, high Cr, low Na, low Hb, high WBC, low glucose
- <u>Complications</u>: rapid spread to mediastinum and abdomen, systemic infection (sepsis), historically 25–70% mortality rate

### *Management*

- ICU admission
- daily aggressive surgical debridement and irrigation with viable tissue margins
- broad-spectrum parenteral antibiotics
- may consider hyperbaric oxygen (HBO) and IVIG
- control of diabetes

## Parapharyngeal Space (Lateral Pharyngeal Space, Pharyngomaxillary Space)

- <u>Boundaries</u>: cone-shaped with base at base of skull and apex at hyoid bone; bounded by pharynx, parotid, mandible, and pterygoid muscles
- <u>Compartments</u>
  1. **Prestyloid**: contains maxillary artery; fat; inferior alveolar, lingual, and auriculotemporal nerves
  2. **Poststyloid**: neurovascular bundle (carotid artery, internal jugular vein, sympathetic chain, CN IX, X, XI)

- <u>Sources of Infection</u>: odontogenic, tonsil, pharynx, nasopharynx, and parotid gland
- <u>SSx</u>: pronounced trismus, fever, muffled voice, intraoral bulge, dysphagia, drooling
- <u>Complications</u>: aspiration, airway compromise, cranial nerve palsies, septic thrombophlebitis, carotid blowout, endocarditis, extension into adjacent spaces
- <u>Rx</u>: external drainage, aggressive antibiotics, airway management

## Peritonsillar Space (*see* pp. 525–526)

## Pterygopalatine Fossa (Pterygomaxillary Space)

- <u>Boundaries</u>: pyramidal-shaped space below the apex of the orbit
- <u>Contents</u>: CN $V_2$, vidian nerve, sphenopalatine nerve, lesser and greater palatine nerves, sphenopalatine (ptergyopalatine) ganglion, maxillary artery
- <u>Sources of Infection</u>: maxillary teeth, osteomyelitis
- <u>SSx</u>: gingival edema, facial cellulitis, trismus, ocular manifestations, extension into infratemporal fossa
- <u>Rx</u>: drainage procedure from a Caldwell-Luc or alveobuccal sulcus approach, antibiotic regimen

## Masticator Space

- <u>Compartments</u>
  1. **Masseteric**: between masseter muscle and ramus of the mandible
  2. **Pterygoid**: between pterygoid muscles and ramus of the mandible
  3. **Superficial Temporal**: between superficial temporal fascia and temporalis muscle
  4. **Deep Temporal**: between temporal fascia and temporal bone
- <u>Contents</u>: muscles of mastication, maxillary artery, CN $V_3$
- <u>Sources of Infection</u>: molars (third molar most common)
- <u>SSx</u>: edema over posterior ramus, trismus
- <u>Complications</u>: osteomyelitis of the mandible, extension into neck spaces
- <u>Rx</u>: incision and drainage, antibiotics, airway management

## Submandibular and Sublingual Space

- <u>Compartments</u>
  1. **Sublingual**: between floor of mouth and mylohyoid muscle; contains sublingual gland, CN XII, Wharton's duct; communicates with opposite space and submental space

**2. Submandibular**: between body of mandible and mylohyoid, hyoglossus, and styloglossus; contains submandibular gland, lingual nerve, and facial artery; communicates with sublingual and pharyngeal spaces
- <u>Sources of Infection</u>: odontogenic, submandibular gland, paranasal, pharynx
- <u>SSx</u>: salivary gland tenderness, odynophagia
- <u>Complications</u>: Ludwig's angina (*see following*)
- <u>Rx</u>: external or internal drainage, aggressive antibiotics, airway management

### Ludwig's Angina

- <u>Pathophysiology</u>: bilateral cellulitis of **submandibular, sublingual, and submental** spaces
- <u>SSx</u>: "wooden" floor of mouth, neck swelling and induration, drooling, respiratory distress, swollen tongue, dysphagia, trismus, may rapidly progress to airway compromise
- <u>Complications</u>: rapid respiratory compromise, sepsis
- <u>Rx</u>: early tracheotomy under local anesthesia or awake fiberoptic nasotracheal intubation, external incision (usually straw-colored weeping but no true abscess fluid), aggressive antibiotic therapy

## Parotid Space

- formed by the splitting of the superficial layer of deep cervical fascia
- <u>Contents</u>: parotid gland, CN VII, posterior facial vein, lymphatics, external carotid artery
- <u>Sources of Infection</u>: parotid
- <u>SSx</u>: tenderness over parotid region
- <u>Complications</u>: extension into parapharyngeal space
- <u>Rx</u>: treat for parotitis (hydration, sialagogues, oral hygiene, antibiotics, warm compresses, massage), may require aspiration or I&D (risk of facial nerve injury)

## Buccal Space

- <u>Boundaries</u>: buccinator, cheek skin, pterygomandibular raphe, zygomatic arch, inferior mandible
- <u>Sources of Infection</u>: odontogenic
- <u>SSx</u>: buccal swelling that may extend up to eyelid (preseptal) and orbicularis oris
- <u>Complications</u>: cavernous sinus thrombosis (from angular vessels), intracranial infection, extension into orbit and other spaces
- <u>Rx</u>: urgent drainage (external approach), aggressive antibiotic regimen

## Carotid Sheath Space

- <u>Boundaries</u>: extends from base of skull to thoracic inlet
- <u>Contents</u>: carotid artery, internal jugular vein, CN X
- <u>Sources of Infection</u>: extension from adjacent fascial planes
- <u>SSx</u>: torticollis (toward uninvolved side)
- <u>Complications</u>: shock, carotid blowout, endocarditis, cavernous sinus thrombosis
- <u>Rx</u>: surgical drainage, aggressive antibiotic regimen

## Visceral Space

- <u>Boundaries</u>: pharyngeal constrictors muscles and alar fascia, extends from hyoid to mediastinum
- <u>Contents</u>: pharynx, esophagus, larynx, trachea, thyroid
- <u>Sources of Infection</u>: typically from perforations of the anterior esophageal wall (instrumentation, trauma)
- <u>SSx</u>: dysphagia, hoarseness, respiratory compromise, subcutaneous emphysema
- <u>Complications</u>: mediastinitis, sepsis, pneumonia, laryngeal edema
- <u>Rx</u>: nothing by mouth, external drainage, aggressive antibiotic regimen, possible tracheotomy

## Retropharyngeal Space (Retrovisceral Space)

- infection more common in children
- <u>Boundaries</u>: pharyngeal constrictor muscles and alar fascia, extends from skull base to **mediastinum**
- <u>Contents</u>: retropharyngeal lymphatics that drain nose, nasopharynx, paranasal sinuses, adenoids
- <u>SSx</u>: odynophagia, "hot potato" voice, drooling, stiff neck, stridor, spiking fevers
- <u>Sources of Infection</u>: tonsils, paranasal sinuses, and nasopharynx
- <u>Complications</u>: mediastinitis (50% mortality), respiratory distress, ruptured abscess (aspiration pneumonia), spread into danger and prevertebral space
- <u>Rx</u>: urgent drainage (external versus internal approach), aggressive antibiotic regimen

## Danger Space

- <u>Boundaries</u>: alar and prevertebral fascia, extends from skull base to **diaphragm**
- <u>Contents</u>: loose areolar tissue (spreads fast)

- <u>SSx</u>: same as retropharyngeal space infections
- <u>Complications</u>: same as retropharyngeal, although may spread into abdominal cavity
- <u>Rx</u>: same as retropharyngeal space infections

## Prevertebral Space

- <u>Boundaries</u>: prevertebral fascia and vertebral bodies, extends from skull base to **coccyx**
- <u>Contents</u>: longus colli muscle
- <u>SSx</u>: same as retropharyngeal and danger space infections
- **Pott's Abscess**: tuberculous osteomyelitis of the spine
- <u>Complications</u>: same as retropharyngeal and danger space infections, osteomyelitis of the spine
- <u>Rx</u>: same as retropharyngeal and danger space infections

# HEAD AND NECK MANIFESTATIONS OF SYSTEMIC DISEASES

## Noninfectious Granulomatous Diseases

### Langerhans Cell Histiocytosis (*see* pp. 608–609)

### Midline Destructive Syndromes

#### *Nasal Extranodal NK/T-Cell Lymphoma (Angiocentric T-Cell Lymphoma, Polymorphic Reticulosis, Lymphomatoid Granulomatosis, Lethal Midline Granuloma)*

- <u>Pathophysiology</u>: originates from natural killer or T-cells, form of **extranodal non-Hodgkin's lymphoma**, subtypes based on the β-chain of the T-cell receptor, forms perivascular infiltrates (angiocentric, **not a true vasculitis**)
- <u>SSx</u>: pansinusitis and nasal obstruction (most common initial finding); cutaneous involvement (maculopapular rash, ulcerative cutaneous lesions); may also involve the orbital, pulmonary, renal, GI, or CNS regions
- <u>Stages</u>
  1. **Prodromal**: clear rhinorrhea, nasal obstruction
  2. **Ulcerative (Active)**: purulent rhinorrhea, ulceration and septal perforations (epistaxis), destruction of osteocartilaginous tissue
  3. **Terminal**: malaise, fever, sloughed tissues, death

- <u>Dx</u>: biopsy, CT/MRI of paranasal sinuses
- <u>Histopathology</u>: sheets of atypical polymorphonuclear cells, no granuloma, no palisading histiocytes
- <u>Rx</u>: radiation therapy for local disease, cyclophosphamide and prednisone for multiregional disease

### *Idiopathic Midline Destructive Disease*

- <u>Pathophysiology</u>: nomenclature controversial, many cases may actually be due to granulomatosis with polyangiitis or sinonasal lymphoma, localized to H&N, **more aggressive**
- <u>SSx</u>: ulcerative lesions of the nose or sinus, pansinusitis, nasal obstruction
- <u>Dx</u>: biopsy, CT/MRI of paranasal sinuses
- <u>Histopathology</u>: sheets of typical polymorphonuclear cells, no granuloma, no vasculitis (pseudovasculitis)
- <u>Rx</u>: radiation therapy for local disease, cyclophosphamide and prednisone for multiregional disease

## Granulomatosis with Polyangiitis (Wegener's)
(*see* pp. 249–250)

## Sarcoidosis

- <u>Pathophysiology</u>: systemic granulomatous disease of unknown etiology, mononuclear cells accumulate in affected organs followed by formation of granulomas, may lead to irreversible fibrosis of tissue
- more common in **African American women** (less common in blacks of other nations)
- <u>H&N SSx</u>: cervical lymphadenopathy (25–50%, most common H&N presentation); **uveoparotid fever** (**Heerfordt's disease**; uveitis, facial palsy, SNHL, fever, and parotid enlargement; *see* p. 79); **supraglottic** submucosal mass (epiglottis most common), TVF immobility; nasal mass, orbital mass, nasal perforations
- <u>Systemic SSx</u>: 40% asymptomatic (incidental **hilar adenopathy** CXR finding, most common presentation); pulmonary involvement (88%, cough, dyspnea), cutaneous lesions (erythema nodosum, rashes), "**Darier-Roussey**" nodules (subcutaneous lesions), hepatic and renal involvement, splenomegaly, cardiac involvement (arrhythmias), bone lesions, neuropathies, fever, weight loss
- <u>Dx</u>: biopsy of lung or affected organ, CXR, anergy skin tests, serum ACE level, serum protein electrophoresis (hypergammaglobulinemia), electrolytes (hypercalcemia)

- <u>Histopathology</u>: **noncaseating granulomas**, accumulation of T-cells, mononuclear phagocytes, derangement of normal tissue architecture
- <u>Complications</u>: progressive interstitial lung disease, blindness (uveitis), airway obstruction (rare)
- <u>Rx</u>: corticosteroids for significant exacerbations (pulmonary), do not treat asymptomatic lesions, sinus lesions may be treated with topical and injectable corticosteroids, may require surgical excision of obstructing laryngeal lesions

## Pyogenic Granuloma (Lobular Capillary Hemangioma)

- <u>Risks</u>: young males, postpubescent females, pregnancy (hormonally related)
- <u>SSx</u>: painless, friable, ulcerated, or polypoid dark red lesion that intermittently bleeds; found on lips (40%), nasal cavity (30%, epistaxis), tongue (20%), oral mucosa (15%); difficult to distinguish from hemangioma
- <u>Dx</u>: biopsy
- <u>Histopathology</u>: circumscribed capillaries arranged in lobules
- <u>Rx</u>: surgical excision

## Necrotizing Sialometaplasia (*see* p. 82)

# Infectious Granulomatous Diseases

## Syphilis

- <u>Pathophysiology</u>: chronic infection caused by the spirochete *Treponema pallidum*, sexually transmitted or from maternal transmission
- **Primary**: initial stage, painless chancre at inoculation site (penis, cervix, anal canal), lymphadenopathy
- **Secondary**: "The Great Imitator," highly contagious, general malaise and fever, arthralgia, hepatosplenomegaly, genital condyloma lata, maculopapular rash, nephrotic syndrome, "mucous patches"
- <u>Late Stages</u>
  1. **Latent**: **asymptomatic** phase (may have return to mucocutaneous lesions)
  2. **Tertiary**: rare, may occur years after initial infection, slowly progressive, characterized by **gummas** (rubbery texture with a center of necrotic tissue), affects CNS (**neurosyphilis**) and cardiovascular system (aortic involvement)

3. **Resolution**

- H&N SSx: generalized cervical lymphadenopathy, laryngitis and vocal fold immobility, oral chancres, granulomatous infiltration of tongue and palate, abrupt profound **SNHL, Ménière's symptoms**, interstitial keratitis, Argyll-Robertson pupil (constricts with accommodation but not to light), TM perforation, saddle-nose deformity, rhinitis, osseous and cartilaginous destruction, septal perforation
- **Congenital Syphilis**: often fatal; **Hutchinson's Triad** (abnormal central incisors [Hutchinson's teeth], interstitial keratitis, deafness); cutaneous lesions, hepatosplenomegaly, lymphadenopathy, labyrinthitis, Clutton's joints (bilateral knee effusion), neurosyphilis, "mulberry molars," frontal bossing, mental retardation, saddle-nose deformity, epiphysitis
- Dx: nonspecific screening RPR or VDRL (Venereal Disease Research Laboratory), specific FTA-ABS (fluorescent treponemal antibody-absorption test), darkfield microscopy, Warthin-Starry stain
- Histopathology: mononuclear infiltrate, obliterative arteritis, hydrops, gummas, and osteolytic lesions in otic capsule
- Rx: penicillin, ampicillin, tetracycline, erythromycin, corticosteroids for otologic involvement; treat until serologic markers normalize

## Tuberculosis (TB)

- Pathophysiology: inhalation of acid-fast bacilli, *Mycobacterium tuberculosis*, into lungs resulting in latent or active disease (10–30%)
- Risks: immunocompromised (historically 50% of HIV population), health care workers, immigrants, elderly, poor
- Primary SSx: typically asymptomatic; lower lobe lesion, **Ghon complex** (calcified lung lesion and draining lymph node)
- Secondary SSx: reinfection; weight loss, fever, night sweats, nonproductive cough; endogenous, caseating granulomatous tubercles, apical lung involvement
- H&N SSx: usually secondary to pulmonary source; **cervical lymphadenopathy** (bilateral, most common H&N manifestation); granulation and ulcerative tissue in posterior **glottis** (posterior interarytenoids, laryngeal surface of epiglottis, vocal folds); painless, odorless, watery otorrhea and multiple TM perforations; diffuse salivary gland enlargement; ulcerative oral lesions; conjunctivitis and uveitis
- Dx
    1. Screening: tuberculin intradermal skin test using purified protein derivative (PPD); positive if induration **≥5 mm** in HIV or other immunosuppresion, recent contact with contagious case; **≥10 mm**

in health care workers, prisoners, homeless, age < 4 years, certain medical conditions and cancers; **≥15 mm** in low-risk population; immunocompromise may cause false-negative, BCG vaccination or nontuburculous mycobacteria may cause false-positive

2. <u>Diagnostic Tests</u>: sputum culture (Ziehl-Neelsen acid-fast bacilli stain), CXR, excisional biopsy, FNA with DNA amplification tests or culture; avoid incision and drainage

- <u>Rx</u>: isolate any patient with active disease until confirmed by 3 consecutive negative sputum cultures; multidrug antitubercular regimen; consider isoniazid (INH) prophylaxis for immunosuppressed patients with exposure or positive PPD, history of TB (without active disease) and without proper previous treatment, positive PPD with inactive disease, or household contacts of patients with active disease

## Fungal Granulomatous Disease

- **Aspergillosis**: allergic, noninvasive, or invasive forms (*see* p. 49)
- **Rhinosporidiosis**: fungal sporangium, paranasal involvement (*see* p. 42)
- **Phycomycosis (*Mucor/Rhizopus*)**: *see* p. 50

### Histoplasmosis

- <u>Pathophysiology</u>: airborne transmission of *Histoplasma capsulatum* (endemic to **Mississippi and Ohio River Valley**, found in bird feces) causes chronic pulmonary infection, may disseminate in immunocompromised
- <u>H&N SSx</u>: (in 25%–66% of disseminated disease) painful, ulcerative, granulomatous lesions (heaped edges) of pharynx, larynx, epiglottis, oral cavity (tongue, lip, oral mucosa)
- <u>Histopathology</u>: intracellular organisms, epithelioid granulomas, pseudoepitheliomatous hyperplasia
- <u>Dx</u>: culture on Sabouraud's agar, skin test, complement fixation test, latex agglutination
- <u>Rx</u>: antifungals (azoles, amphotericin B)

### Blastomycosis

- <u>Pathophysiology</u>: airborne transmission of *Blastomyces dermatitidis* (endemic to Central America and the Midwest) causes **chronic pulmonary infection**, may disseminate
- <u>H&N SSx</u>: (disseminated form) skin, oropharyngeal, and verrucous laryngeal lesions
- <u>Histopathology</u>: **pseudoepitheliomatous hyperplasia**, intraepithelial microabscess, **broad-based bud** ("figure 8" formation)

- <u>Dx</u>: culture on Sabouraud's medium, skin test
- <u>Rx</u>: antifungals (azoles, amphotericin B)

### Coccidiomycosis

- <u>Pathophysiology</u>: airborne transmission of *Coccidioides immitis* (desert, Southwest United States, Latin America, "**Valley Fever**")
- <u>H&N SSx</u>: nodules or erosions of skin (external ear), mucous membranes, epiglottis, thyroid, trachea, salivary glands
- <u>Histopathology</u>: "sac with bugs"
- <u>Dx</u>: skin test, complement fixation
- <u>Rx</u>: antifungals (azoles, amphotericin B)

### Cryptococcosis

- <u>Pathophysiology</u>: exposure to *Cryptococcus neoformans* from bird droppings
- <u>Risks</u>: immunocompromised, pigeon carriers
- <u>H&N SSx</u>: meningitis (SNHL), membranous nasopharyngitis, laryngitis
- <u>Dx</u>: culture on Sabouraud's agar (**capsule** seen with India ink stain), fluorescent antibody staining
- <u>Rx</u>: antifungals (azoles, amphotericin B)

## Other Bacterial Granulomatous Disease

- **Cat-Scratch Disease**: intracellular, pleomorphic, gram-negative bacilli, cervical and general adenopathy, cutaneous lesions (*see* p. 233)
- **Brucellosis**: aerobic, Gram-negative bacilli; acquired from products from butter, pigs, cattle, goats; presents with flu-like symptoms; <u>Dx</u>: serum titers; <u>Rx</u>: tetracycline
- **Rhinoscleroma**: *Klebsiella rhinoscleromatis*, affects paranasal sinuses (*see* pp. 41–42)
- **Leprosy (Hansen's Disease)**: *Mycobacterium leprae*, peripheral cutaneous lesions, may present with ulcerative lesions in the larynx and oral mucosa, nasal collapse, anesthetic plaques, lymphadenopathy; <u>Rx</u>: dapsone, rifampin, clofazimine, fluoroquinolones, consider corticosteroids
- **Atypical Mycobacteria**: presents most commonly with corneal ulceration and cervical adenopathy (*see* p. 603)
- **Actinomycosis**: branching anaerobic or microaerophilic Gram-negative bacteria, may present as a mass anywhere in the H&N (*see* pp. 208–209)
- **Nocardiosis**: similar to *Actinomyces*, soil saprophyte, primary lung disease with hematogenous spread, lymphocutaneous lesions, <u>Rx</u>: sulfa antibiotics, may require incision and drainage

# Connective Tissue Diseases

## Lupus Erythematosus

- <u>Pathophysiology</u>: idiopathic autoimmune multisystem vasculitis, causes damage by deposition of antibodies and immune complexes
- <u>Risks</u>: female (90%, especially childbearing age or pregnant), African American, genetic disposition (HLA DR2, DR3)
- <u>Complications</u>: severe systemic vasculitis (mononeuritis multiplex, mesenteric vasculitis), acute psychosis, organic brain syndrome, severe thrombocytopenia with a thrombotic thrombocytopenic purpura (TTP)-like syndrome, rapidly progressive glomerulonephritis, diffuse alveolar hemorrhage
- <u>Dx</u>: antinuclear antibodies (ANA, nonspecific, screen), anti-dsDNA (highly specific), anti-Sm (highly specific); other diagnostic tests include SS-A and SS-B, direct immunofluorescence, LE cell phenomenon (serum from patient is added to buffy coat of normal blood, reaction is a rosette of neutrophils surrounding a pale nuclear lymphocytic mass), and other ancillary tests depending on organ involvement (urine analysis, ECG, etc)
- <u>Rx</u>: medical regimen depends on severity; control of inflammation with oral and topical corticosteroids, NSAIDs, or salicylates; may consider immunosuppressives for severe disease; avoid sun; supportive care for oral lesions and xerostomia

### Types

1. **Discoid (DLE):** least aggressive, only affects superficial tissues, more common in middle-age women, oral lesions (20–25%) and cutaneous lesions (face in 85% of cases, elevated erythematous plaques, hypopigmented edges, alopecia, leaves a scar), no visceral involvement
2. **Subacute Cutaneous (SCLE):** mild systemic form, oral and cutaneous lesions (papulosquamous lesions, no scar)
3. **Systemic (SLE):** occasional oral lesions, butterfly rash, multiple visceral organs involvement

### Symptoms

- <u>H&N SSx</u>: malar rash, mucosal oral ulcerations with an erythematous halo, cutaneous lesions (*as previous*), ulcerated nasal septum (nasal perforation), hoarseness from thickened vocal folds and cricoarytenoid joint arthritis, acute parotid enlargement, cranial neuropathies, SNHL (autoimmune inner ear disease), nonspecific lymphadenopathy

- <u>Other SSx</u>: constitutional (fever, malaise, weight loss, nonerosive polyarthritis), pleuritis, proliferative glomerulonephritis, anemia, Raynaud's phenomenon, diffuse interstitial pulmonary fibrosis, pericarditis, endocarditis

## Rheumatoid Arthritis

- <u>Pathophysiology</u>: idiopathic autoimmune disease causing inflammation of synovial joints
- <u>H&N SSx</u>: involves TMJ (50%), cricoarytenoid joint (ankylosis causes hoarseness), ossicular joints (rare CHL), cervical spine; Sjögren's syndrome
- <u>Other SSx</u>: symmetric polyarthritis, rheumatoid nodules (subcutaneous nodules), visceral nodules, rheumatoid vasculitis
- <u>Dx</u>: history, rheumatoid factor (titer >1:64), CXR, ESR, complement levels, synovial fluid analysis
- <u>Rx</u>: ASA, NSAIDs, corticosteroids, methotrexate, hydroxychloroquine, immunologic monoclonal antibodies

## Mixed Connective Tissue Disease

- <u>Pathophysiology</u>: distinct syndrome of unknown etiology that combines features of SLE, RA, polymyositis, and scleroderma
- <u>SSx</u>: lupus erythematosus cutaneous and oral manifestations, esophageal dysmotility, polyarthralgia, Raynaud's phenomenon, visceral disease (pulmonary, renal, CNS)
- <u>Dx and Rx</u>: similar to SLE and scleroderma, hypogammaglobulinemia, high titer of ribonucleoprotein antibody (anti-U1 RNP)

## Other Connective Tissue Disorders

- **Scleroderma (Progressive Systemic Sclerosis)** (*see* p. 196)
- **Polymyositis and Dermatomyositis** (*see* p. 197)
- **Sjögren's Disease** (*see* p. 80)
- **Relapsing Polychondritis** (*see* p. 386)

# Vasculitis

## Granulomatosis with Polyangiitis (Wegener's)

- <u>Pathophysiology</u>: uncertain etiology causing idiopathic necrotizing granulomatous vasculitis of upper and lower respiratory tract with glomerulonephritis (may be autoimmune)

- <u>Types</u>: limited (no renal involvement), systemic (pulmonary and renal involvement)
- <u>Histopathology</u>: **necrotizing granulomas** (multinucleated giant cells) with vasculitis of upper and lower respiratory tract
- <u>Rx</u>: corticosteroids for initial control followed by cyclophosphamide, azathioprine, or methotrexate; may consider prophylaxis trimethroprim-sulfamethoxazole; nasal hypertonic saline irrigations and nasal debridement for local therapy

### Systemic Symptoms

- <u>Pulmonary</u>: most common (90%), hemoptysis, cough, dyspnea
- <u>Nonspecific Focal Glomerulonephritis</u>: hematuria, urine blood casts (renal involvement accounts for most deaths)
- <u>Other</u>: fever, various cutaneous lesions, nausea, malaise, night sweats, arthralgia, myalgia

### Head and Neck Symptoms

- <u>Sinonasal</u>: recurrent and chronic sinusitis (60–90%, most common H&N symptom), nasal deformity, septal perforation, nasal obstruction, epistaxis
- <u>Nasopharyngeal</u>: ulcerations (75%)
- <u>Laryngeal</u>: ulcerations (25%), subglottic stenosis (<20%)
- <u>Otologic</u>: CHL from serous otitis media (20–25%), SNHL
- <u>Ocular</u>: uveitis, keratitis (40%)
- <u>Oral</u>: gingival hyperplasia, gingivitis

### Evaluation

- **Antineutrophil Cytoplasmic Autoantibodies (cANCA and PR3)**: suggests active disease, (cANCA + neutrophil Ab = 86% specific)
- **Pulmonary or Nasal Biopsy**: pulmonary highest yield, nasal biopsy often obscured with acute inflammatory cells
- **Renal Biopsy**: glomerulonephritis
- <u>Other Studies</u>: CBC, ESR, SPEP, BUN, creatinine, VDRL, UA, CXR, autoimmune panel, smooth muscle and neutrophil cytoplasm antibodies; sinus imaging

# Giant Cell (Temporal) Arteritis

- most common systemic vasculitis
- <u>Pathophysiology</u>: focal granulomatous inflammation of medium and small arteries primarily of the H&N
- <u>Risks</u>: elderly white females

- <u>SSx</u>: headache (most common initial symptom), tenderness over scalp, jaw, and tongue claudication, fever, visual changes
- <u>Dx</u>: elevated ESR, **temporal artery biopsy** (2–5 cm, up to 40% false-negative rate because of skip lesions, if negative biopsy contralateral side)
- <u>Complications</u>: intracranial involvement resulting in blindness (1/3 of untreated patients), cranial nerve defects, psychosis, or vertebrobasilar insufficiency
- <u>Rx</u>: prompt corticosteroids (may be required long term), ophthalmology consult

## Behçet's Disease (*see* p. 212)

# CHAPTER

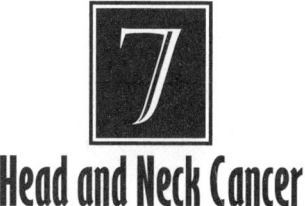

# 7

# Head and Neck Cancer

Richard Chan Woo Park, Vishad Nabili, George H. Yoo, Justin S. Golub, and Raza Pasha

## CANCER STAGING INDEX
(*See* Appendix A)

## INTRODUCTION TO HEAD AND NECK CANCER

### Evaluation of the Head and Neck Cancer Patient

#### History

- <u>Otologic</u>: persistent otalgia (referred pain with normal otologic exam), hearing loss, aural fullness, pulsatile tinnitus
- <u>Nasal/Paranasal/Nasopharynx</u>: recurrent epistaxis, unilateral nasal obstruction, persistent rhinorrhea or sinusitis

- <u>Oral/Pharyngeal</u>: persistent sore throat (>3 weeks), odynophagia, dysphagia, trismus, nonhealing ulcers, halitosis, numbness in lower teeth
- <u>Laryngeal</u>: persistent hoarseness and throat pain (>3 weeks), difficulty breathing
- <u>Neck</u>: character and duration of neck masses
- <u>Neurologic</u>: diplopia, cranial nerve palsies, mental status changes
- <u>Risk Factors</u>: pack-year history of smoking, alcohol use, other tobacco use, sun exposure, HPV exposure, previous cancers, family history of cancer, radiation exposure, exposure to wood dust or heavy metals
- <u>Constitutional Symptoms</u>: extent of weight loss, bone pain, hemoptysis, malaise, anorexia
- <u>Other History</u>: comorbid medical conditions including cardiac history, pulmonary disease, diabetes, hepatic dysfunction, previous stroke, and renal failure; psychological profile; previous skin lesion removal

## Physical Exam

- <u>Otologic</u>: assess for middle ear fluid, external auditory canal masses, and other lesions
- <u>Nasal/Paranasal/Nasopharynx</u>: rhinoscopy and endoscopic exam for masses including the nasopharynx (fossa of Rosenmüller)
- <u>Oral/Pharyngeal</u>: visually inspect all areas of oral and oropharyngeal cavity (mirror exam) for masses and lesions (ulceration, leukoplakia, erythroplakia); palpate floor of mouth and base of tongue; assess mobility of tongue and any involvement of mandible; evaluate airway; inspect dentition (quality of teeth, occlusion)
- <u>Laryngeal</u>: mirror or flexible laryngoscopy, examine all areas of larynx (vallecula, piriform sinus, postcricoid region, supraglottis, vocal folds), assess vocal fold motion
- <u>Neck</u>: palpate nodes (mobility, size, level), palpate salivary glands and thyroid
- <u>Ocular/Neurologic</u>: assess extraocular motility, visual acuity, and presence of proptosis; complete cranial nerve exam
- <u>Skin</u>: thoroughly examine skin including scalp, presence of jaundice
- <u>General Physical Exam</u>: complete physical exam to evaluate comorbidities and overall nutritional status

## Initial Evaluation

- typically an accurate H&P, endoscopy with biopsy, CXR, and CT of neck with contrast are all that is essential for an initial workup of most head and neck cancers; these and possible additional studies are listed below

### *Imaging and Ancillary Studies*

- **Fine Needle Aspiration (FNA)**: indicated for suspicious neck nodes if no primary identified and for any suspicious thyroid nodules
- **Excisional/Incisional Biopsy**: may be performed in the office for most oral, oropharyngeal, nasal, and skin tumors; difficult biopsy sites may be taken during endoscopy
- **CXR**: screening for pulmonary metastasis or primary pulmonary cancer
- **CT of Primary Site and Neck**: obtained with contrast, evaluates extent of primary tumor size and involvement of adjacent structures (carotid artery, base of skull, floor of neck, bone); aids in staging and determining nodal status (**radiographic criteria for nodal malignancy is lesions >1 cm and presence of central necrosis, CT up-stages 10–20% nodal disease**, however CT and MRI are not very good at predicting extracapsular spread); CT not indicated for the T1 N0 glottic cancer
- **MRI of Head and Neck**: consider for nasopharyngeal, infratemporal fossa, temporal bone, parotid, parapharyngeal, skull base, or intracranial involvement
- **PET/CT**: utilizes physiologic rather than anatomic parameters; PET defines tissues with increased metabolic rate (usually glucose uptake); indicated for evaluation of the neck in both pre- and postchemo/radiation therapy, defining therapy for advanced disease, monitoring of recurrent, and detection of unknown primary; can be used in the posttreatment setting as well but should be performed no earlier than 12 weeks
- **CT of Chest**: obtained with contrast, indicated for suspicious findings on CXR
- **CT of Abdomen**: indicated if abdominal metastasis or primary suspected (elevated hepatic transaminases, abdominal masses), lymphoma evaluation
- **Panorex (Orthopantomogram)**: indicated to evaluate dentition or tumor involvement, preoperative films for a mandibulotomy
- **Modified Barium Swallow (MBS/VFSS) with Esophagram**: evaluates aspiration and swallow, indicated for suspicion of esophageal carcinoma or lesions
- **Nuclear Medicine Studies**: consider in evaluating thyroid, parathyroid, mandible invasion, and metastatic bone disease; usually not indicated as a screening tool for head and neck cancer

## *Preoperative Labs and Studies*

- <u>Preoperative Evaluation</u>: depends on type of tumor but in general, coagulation studies (PT, PTT), CBC, electrolytes, BUN and serum creatinine, ECG, LFTs (albumin, transaminases, alkaline phosphatase)
- **Pulmonary Function Tests**: preoperative evaluation for pulmonary disease, preoperative assessment for consideration of partial laryngectomy

## *Diagnostic and Ancillary Procedures*

- **Tracheotomy**: low threshold for surgical airway management in anticipation of swelling due to radiation, postoperative effects, and tumor growth
- **Examination Under Anesthesia**: re-evaluate nodal disease (bimanual exam); palpate primary, base of tongue, and floor of mouth
- **Direct Laryngoscopy with Possible Biopsy**: evaluate oral cavity, soft palate, hard palate, tonsillar fossa, base of tongue, and larynx (vallecula, piriform sinus, postcricoid region, supraglottis, subglottis and vocal folds) for lesions
- **Esophagoscopy**: evaluate esophagus for abnormalities and second primaries
- **Bronchoscopy**: evaluate tracheobronchial tree for abnormalities and second primaries
- **Triple Endoscopy (Panendoscopy)**: direct laryngoscopy, esophagoscopy, and bronchoscopy; indicated when primary unknown; consider for routine screening of second primaries and other abnormalities (controversial for negative CXR and no signs or symptoms of esophageal or tracheobronchial involvement)
- **Videostroboscopy**: visualize vocal fold vibration and assess the viscoelastic properties of the phonatory mucosa by using a synchronized, flashing light with a flexible or rigid scope
- **Feeding Tube**: long-term (gastrostomy tube) or temporary (nasogastric tube), allows enteral feedings with lower risk of aspiration, may place with anticipation of radiation effects, postoperative effect, and tumor growth
- **DNA in Situ Hybridization**: tests for HPV DNA in tumors (gold standard)

## *Immunohistochemistry (IHC)*

- utilizes antigen–antibodies reactions that bind to specific cellular components that aid in the histologic diagnosis
- most markers are not tumor specific and not utilized on a routine basis (due to expense)

- useful for paranasal malignancy and poorly differentiated cancers (small- and large-cell tumors)
- squamous cell carcinoma typically is not difficult to distinguish, possible false positives include necrotizing sialometaplasia and mucoepidermoid carcinoma (especially high-grade variant)

### Common Immunohistochemical Markers

- **Lymphoma**: leukocyte common antigen (LCA), T-cell and B-cell markers
- **Carcinoma**: cytokeratin
- **Melanoma**: S-100 (high sensitivity, low specificity; also found in neural and cartilaginous tumors), HMB-45 (sensitive and specific, does not stain spindle cell type), Mitf and tyrosinase (sensitive and specific), MART-1 and melan-A (newer, sensitive, and specific for melanocytes)
- **Neuroendocrine**: chromogranin, neuron-specific enolase (NSE), synaptophysin
- **Sarcoma**: vimentin, desmin (smooth and skeletal muscle), myoglobin (skeletal muscle, rhabdomyosarcoma), actin (skeletal muscle), S-100
- **HPV Infection**: p16 can be a surrogate marker for HPV infection

## Classification of Malignant Neoplasms

- based on histologic specimen and evaluation of size and spread of primary tumor (tumor mapping)
- Grading: categorizes the histologic type of cancer according to the degree of differentiation; well-differentiated (**G1**), moderately well-differentiated (**G2**), poorly differentiated (**G3**), undifferentiated (**G4**); less related to prognosis
- TNM: categorizes size and spread of cancer
    1. **T**: primary tumor (**T0-4**); TX indicates the primary tumor is not fully assessed, T0 indicates no evidence of a primary tumor, Tis indicates carcinoma in situ, otherwise criteria vary for each type of cancer
    2. **N**: regional lymph node spread (**N0-3**); *see* p. 276
    3. **M**: distant metastasis (**M0-1**); M0 indicates no distant metastasis, M1 indicates distant metastasis
- Staging: grouped TNM classification used to guide treatment plan and apply statistical data such as prognosis and treatment effectiveness, *see* Figure 7–1

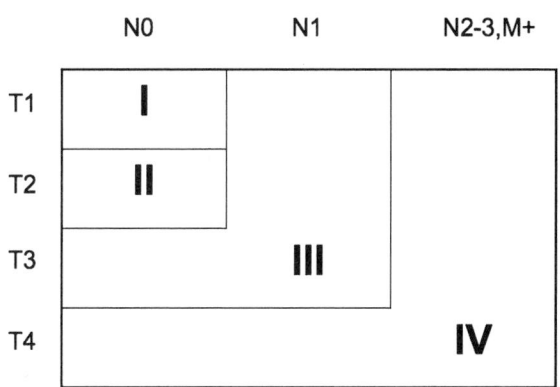

**FIGURE 7–1.** General staging criteria for head and neck cancer (excludes naso-pharyngeal, salivary, and thyroid). Note that M1 (M+) is always stage IV. (With permission from Lee KJ. *Essential Otolaryngology: Head and Neck Surgery*, 9th ed, Figure 28–2. Copyright 2008 McGraw-Hill.)

# Initial Management and Prognostic Evaluation

## Management

### *Consultations*

- Medical and Radiation Oncology: assess potential role of radiation and chemotherapy
- Speech and Swallow Therapy: may be considered postoperatively to assess swallowing and speech and provide therapy
- Dental: evaluate dentition and possibility of teeth extraction (before radiation therapy)
- Plastic/Reconstructive/Microvascular Surgery: to evaluate complex reconstructive issues including free-flap transfer, if needed
- Neurosurgery: assist in certain skull base and cranial procedures
- Ophthalmology: assist in surgical management of the eye
- Prosthodontics: if oral/maxillary, orbital, and other head and neck prostheses needed
- Dermatology: consideration of Mohs micrographic surgery for dermal lesions
- Vascular Surgery: for possible carotid resection or bypass
- Thoracic Surgery: for mediastinal extension or pulmonary involvement

- <u>Medicine</u>: preoperative evaluation/clearance, management of coexisting medical conditions
- <u>Gastroenterology</u>: placement of gastrostomy tube, eg, where oral intake is poor or not possible
- <u>Interventional Radiology</u>: also for placement of gastrostomy tube; preoperative angiogram/embolization of certain vascular tumors, embolization of bleeding vessels, CT or US-guided biopsies
- <u>Nutrition/Dietitian</u>: for malnourished patients to assess nutrition status and recommend methods to obtain a positive nitrogen balance
- <u>Palliative Care</u>: if incurable disease and/or limited life expectancy should have end-of-life discussions in order to maintain an optimal quality of life
- <u>Multidisciplinary Tumor Board</u>: discussion of complex head and neck cancer patients with various teams to form a comprehensive treatment plan that is optimal for each patient

### *Treatment Concepts*

- <u>Single Modality Therapy</u>: treatment of early staged disease with surgery or radiation therapy alone
- <u>Multimodality Therapy</u>: combined therapeutic approaches (surgery, radiation, chemotherapy) for advanced disease
- <u>Surgical Therapy</u>: advantages include quicker extirpation of the tumor and provision of specimen for margin analysis; disadvantages include risk of anesthesia, functional disability, and recovery time
- <u>Tumor Extension Regions Considered Unresectable</u>: base of skull, nasopharynx, prevertebral fascia, floor of neck, mediastinum, subdermal lymphatics; carotid artery encasement (>270° circumferentially is generally regarded as unresectable)
- <u>Radiation Therapy</u>: (*see following*) generally indicated as primary therapy for early glottic, hypopharyngeal, and nasopharyngeal cancers and as adjuvant therapy for advanced head and neck cancer; <u>Advantages:</u> easier access for poorly exposed tumors, generally less functional disability; <u>Disadvantages</u>: lengthy treatment course, local radiation side effects, less responsive with larger or deeper tumors, inability for second course radiation therapy if recurrence within previously irradiated fields, difficult to detect recurrent cancer, salvage surgery for radiation failure is associated with higher morbidity (conservation surgery may not be possible for recurrence)
- <u>Intensity-Modulated Radiation Therapy (IMRT)</u>: allows the field of radiation to be more precisely modeled to preserve normal structures, dependent on the expertise of the planning therapist (*see* p. 272)
- <u>Chemotherapy</u>: (*see following*) generally indicated for palliation in disseminated disease, recurrent or unresectable cancer, laryngeal

preservation, esophageal and nasopharyngeal cancers, and clinical protocols; concomitant chemotherapy and radiation have a higher response rate and a higher rate of control for advanced disease than either single modality

- <u>Clinical Trial Designs</u>: **phase 0** trials evaluate pharmacodynamics and pharmacokinetics including oral bioavailability and half-life; **phase I** trials define the dose range and safety as well as side effects; **phase II** trials test the efficacy of the treatment regimen as well as toxicity; **phase III** trials are randomized, prospective trials that evaluate the new treatment effect compared to the standard treatment; **phase IV** trials are performed postapproval and postmarketing to gather additional information such as the treatment's risk, benefits, and optimal use

### *Posttreatment Followup Recommendations (NCCN Guidelines, 2012)*

- based on risk of relapse, second primaries, treatment sequelae and toxicities
- interval history and exam every 1–3 months for year 1 post-therapy, every 2–6 months for year 2, every 4–8 months for years 3–4, every 12 months for year 5
- posttreatment baseline imaging of primary and neck (if treated) recommended within 6 months of treatment, further reimaging as indicated based on signs/symptoms; scans are not routinely indicated for asymptomatic patients
- chest imaging as clinically indicated
- thyroid function tests every 6–12 months if radiation to the neck
- speech/swallow and hearing evaluation and rehab as indicated
- encourage continued smoking and alcohol cessation
- dental evaluation
- consider EBV monitoring for nasopharyngeal carcinoma

## Prognostic Evaluation

- overall 5 year survival for head and neck cancer is **~57%** (SEER database, 1998–2001; varies by subsite); 50–60% of mortality is from failed locoregional control, 20–30% from metastatic disease, and 10–20% from second primaries; premorbid conditions account for the mortality of 30–35% early-staged head and neck cancer patients and 10–15% of late-staged head and neck cancer patients
- <u>Tumor Staging (Presence of Regional and Distant Metastasis)</u>: poorer prognosis associated with invasiveness and metastasis within each site; presence of regional nodal disease is the strongest predictor of

prognosis for most head and neck cancer (may decrease survival as much as 50%)

- <u>Tumor Volume and Thickness</u>: as determined by CT/MRI scan, poorer prognosis associated with increased tumor thickness (especially if >4 mm in depth) and tumor volume
- <u>Tumor Location</u>: presence of abundant lymphatic drainage at the primary site increases risk of regional disease
- <u>Character of Nodal Disease</u>: decreased survival associated with presence of nodal extracapsular spread, metastasis to lower nodal levels (level IV and V), skipped nodes (eg, nodal involvement of level II and IV without involvement of level III), and increased number of positive nodes; lymphocytic predominant immunomorphology of the lymph node has a better prognosis (denotes a host immunologic response) than lymphocyte-depleted patterns
- <u>3 P's of Poor Prognosis with Nodal Disease</u>: **P**oorly differentiated, extraca**P**sular spread, **P**olynodal involvement
- <u>Vascular and Perineural Invasion</u>: histologic predictors of cancer spreading beyond the margins of resection, indicate aggressive cancer behavior suggesting decreased survival
- <u>Cytomorphometric Parameters</u>: (*controversial*) number of chromosome sets (ploidy) may predict prognosis, aneuploidy (abnormal number of chromosomes) associated with worse prognosis than diploidy (euploidy)
- <u>Grade of Differentiation</u>: not an important determinant in prognosis for most head and neck cancers
- <u>Oropharyngeal HPV Status</u>: oropharyngeal carcinomas that are HPV+ have better overall survival and progression-free survival compared to those that are HPV– (*N Engl J Med.* 2010;363:24–35)

# CHEMOTHERAPY AND RADIATION THERAPY

## Chemotherapy

### Indications for Chemotherapy

- **Nasopharyngeal Cancer**: Phase III Intergroup Study 0099 showed increased survival benefit with **chemoradiotherapy** (cisplatin/5-FU) over radiotherapy alone for **stage III–IV** nasopharyngeal cancer (76% versus 46% 3-year survival, *p* <0.001) (*J Clin Oncol.* 1998;16:1310–1317); a more recent phase III trial confirmed these results showing an improved 5 year progression-free and overall survival in stage III–IV nonkeratinizing nasopharyngeal carcinoma (*J Clin Oncol.* 2005;23:6730–6738); this was also shown in **stage II**

patients with a phase III trial showing improved 5 year overall survival and distant metastasis survival when concurrent chemotherapy
(cisplatin) was added to radiotherapy versus radiotherapy alone
(*J Natl Cancer Inst.* 2011;103:1761–1779)

- **Unresectable Head and Neck Cancer**: Phase III Multicenter Study
  showed increased survival benefit with concomitant chemotherapy
  (cisplatin/5-FU) and radiotherapy over radiotherapy alone for
  advanced unresectable head and neck cancer (48% versus 24%
  3-year survival, *p* <0.0003) (*J Clin Oncol.* 1998;16:1318–1324);
  as compared with the standard cisplatin/5-FU regimen, a phase III
  multicenter trial showed that induction chemotherapy with the addition of docetaxel improved progression-free and overall survival in
  patients with unresectable squamous cell carcinoma of the head and
  neck (*N Engl J Med.* 2007;357:1695–1704)

- **Laryngeal Organ Preservation**: VA Laryngeal Study Group showed
  that induction chemotherapy (cisplatin/5-FU) followed by radiotherapy resulted in a 64% chance of preserving a larynx without compromising survival (68% 2-year survival for both groups, *p* = 0.98) (*N
  Engl J Med.* 1991;324:1685–1690); RTOG 91-11 demonstrated that
  at 2 years, radiotherapy with concurrent chemotherapy resulted in
  increased laryngeal preservation compared to induction chemotherapy followed by radiotherapy or radiotherapy alone (*N Engl J Med.*
  2003;349:2091–2098); the 10-year follow-up to this study showed
  that concurrent chemoradiotherapy (cisplatin) had improved locoregional control and larynx preservation compared with the induction
  group (cisplatin/5-FU) and radiotherapy group alone, in addition
  the laryngectomy-free survival was improved in both the induction
  as well as the concurrent group and both were superior to the radiotherapy alone group (*J Clin Oncol.* 2013;31:845–852); several other
  trials have confirmed these 2 landmark studies that support the use
  of chemoradiotherapy with or without induction chemotherapy for
  advanced laryngeal carcinoma with similar survival results and improved larynx preservation

- **Piriform Sinus Cancer Organ Preservation**: 10 year results of the
  EORTC trial 24891 comparing larynx preservation approach (induction chemotherapy with cisplatin/5-FU followed by radiotherapy or
  surgery or both depending on response) versus immediate surgery
  followed by radiotherapy in hypopharynx and lateral epilarynx squamous cell carcinoma showed similar disease control and overall survival and allowed for more than half of responders in the larynx preservation arm to retain their larynx (*Ann Oncol.* 2012;23:2708–2714)

- **Unknown Primary**: the role of chemotherapy is still unclear; one
  study suggested that chemotherapy with cisplatin/5-FU improved
  response rate and median survival when compared to radiation

alone (*Cancer*. 1989;64:510–515); in addition, chemoradiation
should be used for patients with an N2–N3 unknown primary; one
study showed promising 87% 5 year progression-free survival and
75% 5 year overall survival rate by using chemoradiation with follow-
up surgery in patients with N2–N3 disease (*Ann Oncol*. 2003;14:
1306–1311)

- **Recurrent and Distant Metastatic Disease**: original traditional role
  in head and neck cancer, essentially provides palliation for recurrent
  unresectable disease or incurable cancer with distant metastases
- **Investigative Protocols**: numerous multi-institutional studies are
  currently investigating the role of chemotherapy in head and neck
  cancer

## Chemotherapy Strategies

### *Neoadjuvant (Induction)*

- <u>Definition</u>: sequential chemotherapy before local treatment modality
  (surgery, radiation alone, or chemoradiotherapy)
- <u>Advantages</u>: initial chemotherapy may allow better drug penetration
  before vascularity becomes impaired from radiation effects or surgery,
  initial chemotherapy may also reduce tumor bulk or "cure" patient
  of disease (organ preservation); Head and Neck Contracts Program
  (HNCP) and other phase III trials have shown a tendency for
  decreased rate of distant metastasis
- <u>Disadvantages</u>: postchemotherapy patients are often more debilitated,
  which may increase complications of surgical intervention or
  radiotherapy, margins difficult to assess
- randomized phase III trial by the Groupe d'Etude des Tumeurs de la
  Tete Et du Cou (GETTEC) showed that induction chemotherapy
  (cisplatin/5-FU) followed by appropriate locoregional treatment
  had significantly better overall survival versus those who did not get
  induction chemotherapy in patients with treatable oropharyngeal
  carcinoma (*Br J Cancer*. 2000;83;1594–1598)
- a 10-year follow-up of a randomized phase III trial showed that
  patients with unresectable head and neck cancer showed improved
  overall survival at 5 and 10 years with the addition of neoadjuvant
  chemotherapy (cisplatin/5-FU) compared to those who did not;
  there was no improvement in operable head and neck patients
  (*J Natl Cancer Inst*. 2004;96:1714–1717)
- randomized phase III trial by the Groupe Oncologie Radiotherapie
  Tete et Cou (GORTEC) 2000–01 showed that larynx preservation
  was higher when docetaxel was added to cipslatin/5-FU in the
  neoadjuvant setting in patients with laryngeal or hypopharyngeal

cancer requiring total laryngectomy (*J Natl Cancer Inst.* 2009;101:498–506)
- randomized phase III trial (TAX 324) showed improved estimated 3 year overall survival and sustained long-term 5 year overall survival with induction docetaxel plus cisplatin and fluorouracil (TPF) versus cisplatin and fluorouracil (PF) followed by chemoradiotherapy in patients with stage III-IV head and neck cancer (*N Engl J Med.* 2007;357:1705–1715; *Lancet Oncol.* 2011;12:153–159)

### *Concomitant (Radiation Therapy and Chemotherapy)*

- <u>Definition</u>: concurrent chemotherapy and radiation (chemotherapy may be given continuously or interrupted [split course])
- <u>Advantages</u>: simultaneous therapies may synergistically maximize therapeutic effect (chemotherapy sensitizes cells to radiation and simultaneously kills micrometastatic disease, *see following*)
- <u>Disadvantages</u>: increased side effects from concurrent therapies (mucositis, infection, malnutrition, stricture/stenosis)
- concomitant chemoradiation has become the standard of care for the treatment of locally advanced cancers of the larynx, oropharynx, and hypopharynx; several randomized clinical studies have shown improved survival and locoregional control with concomitant chemoradiation compared with radiation alone (*N Engl J Med.* 1998;338:1798–1804, *J Natl Cancer Inst.* 1999;91:2081–2086, *Int J Radiat Oncol Biol Phys.* 2001;50:1161–1171, *J Clin Oncol.* 2005;23:1125–1135, *Int J Radiat Oncol Biol Phys.* 2006;64:983–994)

#### Mechanisms for Increased Effectiveness of Concomitant Radiation and Chemotherapy

- chemotherapy inhibits the repair of cells that may otherwise recover from radiation
- concomitant radiation and chemotherapy result in synchronization of cell cycles, increasing the effectiveness of both therapies
- resistant cells of one mode of therapy may be susceptible to the other mode of therapy
- shrinking the tumor with radiation improves drug delivery for increased effectiveness of chemotherapy
- combined therapy may push cells from the $G_0$ (quiescent) phase of the cell cycle to active (DNA synthesizing or dividing) phases of the cell cycle, rendering the cells more susceptible to therapy
- concomitant modalities damage cells in different ways, increasing chances of cell death

### Adjuvant

- <u>Definition</u>: chemotherapy after primary treatment modality to control microscopic disease
- <u>Indications</u>: locally advanced disease, multiple positive regional neck nodes, nodal extracapsular spread, positive margins, recurrence
- <u>Advantages</u>: may improve survival
- <u>Disadvantages</u>: exposes patient to side effects of chemotherapeutic agents
- the Intergroup Study 0034 showed no significant increased survival advantage with adjuvant chemotherapy (cisplatin/5-FU) followed by postoperative radiation therapy versus postoperative radiation therapy alone for advanced resectable head and neck cancer (*Int J Rad Oncol Biol Phys.* 1992;23:705–713)
- HNCP failed to demonstrate improved survival in advanced resectable head and neck cancer with induction chemotherapy, standard treatment, followed by maintenance therapy (*Cancer.* 1987;60:301–311)
- postoperative concurrent administration of high-dose cisplatin with radiotherapy is more efficacious than radiotherapy alone in patients with locally advanced head and neck cancer (*N Engl J Med.* 2004;350:1945–1952)
- RTOG 9501: adding postoperative chemotherapy to radiation therapy in patients with advanced high-risk head and neck squamous cell carcinoma (HNSCC) improved locoregional and disease-free survival in patients who on postoperative analysis had any of the following poor prognostic factors: extracapsular spread, positive disease in more than 1 lymph node, and/or positive margins (*N Engl J Med.* 2004;350(19):1937–1944);
- the followup study to the 9501 group failed to show any significant differences in outcome after 9 years; however, subgroup analysis in patients with microscopic positive margins and/or extracapsular spread showed that concurrent chemoradiation improved locoregional control and disease-free survival; interestingly, those with 2 or more lymph nodes did not see any benefit from the addition of chemotherapy to radiation (*Int J Rad Oncol Biol Phys.* 2012;84:1198–1205)

### Chemoprevention

- several clinical trials using retinoids have failed to show a consistent benefit in the treatment of oral precancerous lesions and/or prevention of recurrent or second primary tumors in the head and neck

# Standard Chemotherapy Agents

- generally affect rapidly dividing cells

## *Cisplatin*

- <u>Mechanism of Action</u>: heavy metal that acts as an alkylating agent that covalently binds DNA and RNA
- <u>Common Side Effects</u>: nausea, **nephrotoxicity, peripheral neuropathy, ototoxicity** (dose limiting, affects high frequencies, bilateral effects, cumulative toxicity), electrolyte disturbances, anorexia
- <u>Indications</u>: best single agent against squamous cell carcinoma of the head and neck in recurrent disease; common combination agent for neoadjuvant, adjuvant, and concomitant chemotherapy; radiation sensitizer

## *Carboplatin*

- <u>Mechanism of Action</u>: similar to cisplatin (less reactive)
- <u>Common Side Effects</u>: better tolerated than cisplatin (less nephrotoxicity, nausea, neurotoxicity, and ototoxicity), but has an increased myelosuppression risk
- <u>Indications</u>: not fully investigated in head and neck cancer, often used in combination with paclitaxel

## *Taxanes (Paclitaxel and Docetaxel)*

- <u>Mechanism of Action</u>: prevent normal microtubular reorganization
- <u>Common Side Effects</u>: neutropenia, alopecia, mucositis
- <u>Indications</u>: docetaxel has mainly been used in conjunction with cisplatin and 5-FU (TPF) in the neoadjuvant setting for advanced head and neck cancer

## *5-Fluorouracil (5-FU)*

- <u>Mechanism of Action</u>: antimetabolite that binds to thymidylate synthetase blocking the conversion of uridine to thymidine preventing DNA synthesis in S-phase
- <u>Common Side Effects</u>: anorexia and nausea, mucositis, diarrhea, alopecia, **myelosuppression, cardiac toxicity**
- <u>Indications</u>: similar to cisplatin (cisplatin and 5-FU is the most studied combination chemotherapy regimen in head and neck cancer)

### Methotrexate

- <u>Mechanism of Action</u>: antimetabolite that binds to dihydrofolate reductase preventing DNA synthesis in S-phase
- <u>Common Side Effects</u>: **bone marrow suppression**, gastrointestinal disturbances, mucositis, alopecia, dermatitis, nephrotoxicity (renally excreted, thus better if liver disease), teratogenicity, interstitial pneumonitis
- <u>Indications</u>: "standard" palliative therapy for recurrent or metastatic disease
- **Leucovorin (Tetrahydrofolic Acid)**: utilized as a "rescue" agent for methotrexate toxicity, competitively overcomes increases in intracellular pools of dUMP (also used with 5-FU)

### Other Agents

- **Bleomycin and Doxorubicin (Adriamycin)**: bind DNA causing single- or double-stranded breaks, key side effect of bleomycin is pulmonary fibrosis
- **Vincristine**: damages intracellular microtubules (similar to taxanes)
- **Cyclophosphamide**: cross-links DNA, key side effect is hemorrhagic cystitis

## Targeted Chemotherapy Agents

- newer drugs that act on specific molecular targets of particular cancers
- **Monoclonal Antibodies**: **-mab** suffix (-omab mouse origin, -ximab chimeric, -zumab humanized, -umab human); drug is an antibody that targets a specific protein (eg, receptors on surface of tumor cells), various mechanisms may result in tumor cell death (eg, immune system attacks the cell/protein)
- **Tyrosine Kinase Inhibitors**: **-nib** suffix; block activity of specific tyrosine kinases (enzymes that function as a "switch" for cellular functions) involved in signaling that allows cellular division and growth

### Cetuximab

- <u>Mechanism of Action</u>: monoclonal antibody, binds to and inhibits epidermal growth factor receptors (EGFR), which stops the cell from growing and dividing
- <u>Side Effects</u>: acneiform rash, diarrhea, hypomagnesemia
- <u>Indications</u>: locally advanced HNSCC, given with concurrent radiotherapy; phase III randomized control trial showed improved

overall survival at 3 and 5 years when using cetuximab with concurrent radiotherapy in locally advanced HNSCC compared to radiotherapy alone (*N Engl J Med.* 2006;354:567–578, *Lancet Oncol.* 2010;11:21–28); recurrent or metastatic HNSCC when given as first-line therapy; randomized control trial showing improved overall survival in patients treated with cetuximab and platinum-based chemotherapy plus 5-FU compared to those treated with platinum-based chemotherapy plus 5-FU alone (*N Engl J Med.* 2008;359:1116–1127)

## *Ipilimumab*

- <u>Mechanism of Action</u>: monoclonal antibody, binds to cytotoxic T-lymphocyte-associated antigen 4 (CTLA-4), blocks this inhibitory signal to allow the cytotoxic T-cell to destroy cancer cells
- <u>Side Effects</u>: pruritus, rash, fatigue, diarrhea, colitis
- <u>Indications</u>: phase III randomized trial showed improved overall survival in patients with previously treated, unresectable stage III or IV melanoma (*N Engl J Med.* 2010;363:711–723)

## *Vemurafenib*

- <u>Mechanism of Action</u>: tyrosine kinase inhibitor, inhibits MAP kinase pathway in tumors containing V600 mutation in BRAF
- <u>Side Effects</u>: pruritus, rash, fatigue, diarrhea, colitis
- <u>Indications</u>: unresectable or metastatic melanoma

## *Nivolumab*

- <u>Mechanism of Action</u>: monoclonal antibody, blocks ligand activation of the programmed cell death 1 receptor (PD-1) on activated T-cells, promotes antitumor activity
- <u>Indications</u>: several clinical trials underway evaluating its efficacy in advanced and metastatic melanoma as well as other cancers outside of the head and neck; complete or partial responses seen in non-small cell lung cancer, melanoma, and renal cell cancer in a clinical trial with 296 patients (*N Engl J Med.* 2012;366:2443–2454)

## *Cabozantinib*

- <u>Mechanism of Action</u>: tyrosine kinase inhibitor, binds to and blocks RET, MET, VEGF receptors, and other receptor tyrosine kinases
- <u>Side Effects</u>: diarrhea, stomatitis, palmar–plantar erythrodysesthesia (PPE), rare colon perforation/fistula
- <u>Indications</u>: phase III randomized control trial showed improved progression-free survival in progressive, metastatic medullary thyroid carcinoma (*J Clin Oncol.* 2012;30)

### Vandetanib

- Mechanism of Action: similar to cabozantinib
- Indications: medullary thyroid carcinoma

### Gefitinib

- Mechanism of Action: tyrosine kinase inhibitor, blocks EGFR
- Indications: phase III randomized clinical trial did not show improved survival in metastatic or recurrent HNSCC using gefitinib alone versus methotrexate (*J Clin Oncol.* 2009;27:1864); another phase III randomized clinical trial is currently evaluating the use of gefitinib in conjunction with docetaxel in metastatic or locally recurrent HNSCC

### Vismodegib

- Mechanism of Action: **hedgehog inhibitor** (sonic hedgehog [SHH] signaling pathway transmits information to embryonic cells required for proper development, pathway also implicated in the development of some cancers); cyclopamine competitive antagonist of the smoothened receptor (SMO), which is part of the hedgehog signaling pathway
- Side Effects: muscle spasms, alopecia, dysgeusia, fatigue, weight loss
- Indications: metastatic or locally advanced **basal cell carcinoma** that has recurred following surgery, noncandidates for surgery or radiation (*N Engl J Med.* 2012;366:2171–2179)

# Radiation Therapy

## Mechanism of Injury

- **Rad (Radiation Absorbed Dose)**: amount of energy deposited by ionizing radiation per gram of tissue (1 Gy = 100 rads; 1 cGy = 1 rad)
- radiation cell "kill" is expressed as a logarithmic cell survival curve (radiation does not kill a certain number of cells but rather a percentage of cells)
- cells are considered "killed" when they lose clonogenic survival
- **Direct Mechanism of Radiation Injury**: direct damage of radiation to critical elements in a cell (eg, DNA, cell membranes)
- **Indirect Mechanism of Radiation Injury**: secondary damage from direct radiation effects on other cell components, primary mechanism of cell death (eg, DNA injury from production of free radicals)

## Determinants of Sensitivity to Radiation Therapy

- larger tumors have a more hypoxic center, therefore are less sensitive to radiation because fewer free radicals are generated (1 cm tumor = $10^9$ cells; 3 cm tumor = $10^{10}$)
- oxygenated cells are more susceptible to radiation than hypoxic cells (exophytic tumors are typically well vascularized and therefore more susceptible to radiation injury, ulcerative and infiltrative tumors are less vascularized and therefore more resistant to radiation)
- cell death occurs with proliferation (usually 4–5 times before lysis), therefore rapidly growing tumors are more susceptible to injury
- cells tend to be more radiosensitive in mitosis and late $G_1$ and early S-phases of the cell cycle

## Fractionation and the "4 Rs" of Radiation Biology

- **Conventional Fractionation**: radiotherapy given in smaller interval (dosing 5 days a week for 5 weeks) rather than given all at once
- <u>Reassortment</u>: fractionation allows cells to proceed in their cycle to more radiosensitive stages in their cell cycle
- <u>Reoxygenation</u>: fractionation allows for reoxygenation of previously more hypoxic cells (more susceptible)
- <u>Repopulation</u>: prolonged waiting between fractions results in regrowth of tumor cells from sublethal damage
- <u>Repair</u>: normal tissue tends to have better repair than tumor cells, therefore it recovers more quickly from sublethal damage
- fractionation results in less total biological injury due to the greater opportunity for repair, therefore it requires a higher total dose than single or hypofractionated dosing
- fractionation in general is less toxic
- hypofractionation (fewer fractions) are used for tumors with good ability to repair from sublethal injury (malignant melanoma)

## Methods of Fractionation

- **Conventional Fractionation**: typically uses 1 treatment per day (generally 1.8–2.2 Gy) for 5 days a week
- **Pure Hyperfractionation**: increases rate of treatments (eg, twice a day dosing), smaller dose per fraction, same overall duration of therapy, higher total dose than conventional fractionation; decreases late side effects
- **Accelerated (Standard) Fractionation**: decreases overall duration of therapy, increases rate, higher dose per fraction, with same total dose as conventional fractionation; increases acute side effects, decreases

late side effects, increases tumor cell kill (prevents tumor cell proliferation)
- **Accelerated Hyperfractionation**: increases rate of treatments, decreases duration of therapy, increases total dose
- **Concomitant Boost Accelerated Fractionation**: changes rate to twice a day dosing in the last 2 weeks of therapy
- **Hypofractionation:** decreases rate of treatments (less frequently than once per day), higher dose per fraction
- phase III EORTC 22851 trial showed that accelerated fractionation improved locoregional control in comparison to conventional fractionation (59% versus 46% 5-year locoregional control, $p = 0.02$), but no survival benefit (*Radiother Oncol.* 1997;44:111–121)
- phase III trials are currently investigating the effectiveness of hyperfractionation and accelerated fractionation in survival of head and neck cancer

## Radiation Strategies

- **Shrinking Fields**: selective radiation dosing to varying region depending on primary size and shape (eg, 7,000 cGy to primary site as primary therapy, 5,000–5,500 cGy to N0 neck or adjuvant treatment)
- **Brachytherapy**: delivery of radiation to malignant tissue by placement of permanent radioisotopes intraoperatively via a temporarily placed radioactive source within tumor bulk
- **High Dose Rate (HDR) Therapy**: also known as "temporary brachytherapy," provides a very localized single high dose of radiation (eg, iridium-192), delivered and removed via a temporary brachytherapy catheter, performed as an outpatient with no contact exposure risk immediately after therapy
- **Intensity-Modulated Radiation Therapy (IMRT)**: computer 3D-modeled therapy based on the size and location of the primary tumor, delivers higher doses of therapy to the tumor bed and spares uninvolved structures by using combination of several intensity-modulated fields from different beam directions; effectiveness and reduction of complications dependent on skill of planners
- **Three-Dimensional Multiple Treatment Beam Therapy**: uses CT and MRI imaging, multiple treatment fields arranged to maximize radiation dose to target area yet achieves maximum normal tissue sparing
- **Concomitant Radiation Therapy and Chemotherapy**: (*see above*)
- **Hyperfractionation**: (*see above*)
- **Neutron Beam Therapy**: "heavy" neutron particle that results in greater direct mechanisms of injury, less dependence on cell cycle

and proliferation; however, less repair of sublethal damage by normal tissue; often used in treating adenoid cystic carcinoma; currently only available at 3 sites in the United States (University of Washington, Wayne State, and Fermilab/Northern Illinois University)

### Preoperative Radiation Therapy

- <u>Advantages</u>: may reduce tumor bulk, which may cause inoperable lesions to become operable, reduce surgical excision area, or cure (organ preservation); requires smaller portals than postoperative radiation therapy; microscopic tumor is more sensitive than postoperative residual tumor (where microscopic disease may be in scar tissue, therefore more hypoxic)
- <u>Disadvantages</u>: increased difficulty in operating in irradiated tissue, increased postoperative complications (wound infections, carotid blowout)

### Postoperative Radiation Therapy

- <u>Advantages</u>: allows for adequate postoperative healing prior to beginning adjuvant therapy, accurate assessment of pathologic staging and factors for recurrence
- <u>Disadvantages</u>: requires higher dose of radiation due to hypoxia in operated tissue, microscopic disease may be within scar tissue resulting in decreased radiosensitivity, requires larger fields than preoperative radiation therapy
- phase III Radiation Therapy Oncology Group (RTOG) trial did not demonstrate a significant overall survival difference between preoperative and postoperative radiation therapy for advanced head and neck carcinoma, although locoregional control was significantly better with postoperative radiation therapy (*Int J Rad Oncol Biol Phys.* 1991;20:21–28)

## Side Effects

- **Cutaneous Reactions**: may result in dryness, erythema, hyperpigmentation, desquamation, telangiectasis, or subcutaneous fibrosis; <u>Rx</u>: skin moisturizers, mild skin cleaning, oral diphenhydramine (pruritus), corticosteroid creams
- **Mucositis**: tender, erythematous, and swollen mucous membranes; increased risk of coexisting infections with *Candida*, HSV, and bacteria; may result in sepsis for severe cases; <u>Rx</u>: aggressive oral hygiene (oral irrigations), adjust dental appliances, smoking and alcohol cessation, cool food, nutritional supplements, oral and

topical anesthetics (viscous lidocaine, diphenhydramine, aluminum hydroxide-magnesium hydroxide-simethicone mixture)

- <u>WHO Grading System for Oral Mucositis</u>: Grade 1: erythema and unpleasant sensation; Grade 2: erythema and pain but can still eat solids; Grade 3: ulcers, very painful, and can only tolerate liquids; Grade 4: ulcers, severe and intolerable pain, parenteral or enteral feedings as feeding by mouth is impossible

- **Alopecia**: temporary hair loss may occur in radiation field, may be permanent at higher doses

- **Xerostomia/Dental Caries**: salivary acinar cells are extremely sensitive to radiation therapy causing irreversible xerostomia (dry mouth), increased risk of dental caries, change in taste, and tenacious oral secretions; <u>Rx</u>: fluids with meals, artificial saliva, pilocarpine, fluoride treatment, aggressive oral hygiene (prevent with preoperative dental evaluation)

- **Osteoradionecrosis of the Mandible/Chondroradionecrosis of the Larynx**: hypocellularity, hypovascularity, and ischemia of tissue (not infectious); osteoradionecrosis of the mandible increased with doses above 50 Gy, dental extractions performed after radiation, combined chemotherapy; radionecrosis of the larynx may clinically mimic recurrent laryngeal carcinoma; <u>Rx</u>: initially treat conservatively with antibiotics, analgesics, meticulous oral hygiene, and soft diet; debridement may be required; may also consider hyperbaric oxygen; free tissue transfer necessary in recalcitrant painful mandibular disease, orocutaneous fistula, and/or pathologic fracture

- **Radiation-Induced Cancer**: increased risk of thyroid, salivary gland cancer, leukemia, sarcoma (may have lag period of 20 years), temporal bone cancer

- **Otologic Sequelae**: increased incidence of otitis externa, serous otitis media, and auricular chondritis

- **Cataracts**: the lens is the most sensitive part of the body to radiation with as little as 6 Gy needed to cause cataracts

- **Hypothyroidism**: radiation to the neck or larynx can result in decreased thyroid hormone synthesis, TSH should be checked every 6–12 months; 20–25% of patients will be hypothyroid after neck radiation

- **Bleeding**: carotid artery and its main branches are at risk for bleeding after radical neck dissection and radiation therapy, which can lead to a blowout injury (*see* p. 282)

- **Dysphagia/Stricture/Stenosis:** chemoradiation can lead to dysphagia due to fibrosis of the pharynx/cricopharyngeus/esophagus, may require feeding tube; occurs in ≤26% of patients 1 year posttherapy

- **Nonfunctional Larynx:** chemoradiation can cause loss of sensation and movement of the glottis leading to chronic aspiration and inability to phonate, may require tracheostomy; occurs in ≤12% patients at 1 year (*Arch Otolaryngol Head and Neck Surg.* 2009;135:1209–1217, *J Clin Oncol.* 2008;26:3582–3589)

# CANCER OF THE NECK
## Introduction
### Overview

- most malignancies in the neck are from metastasis (~85%), primary neck cancers are less common (~15%), usually from salivary tumors, thyroid cancers, or lymphoma
- bilateral regional metastasis is common with primaries of the base of tongue, supraglottis, ventral tongue, soft palate, and tumors that approach the midline
- <u>Mechanisms of Regional Metastasis</u>: malignant tumors extend to surrounding tissue, tumor cells invade blood vessels and/or lymphatics (via hydrolytic enzymes), microemboli of tumor cells become trapped in the lymph node resulting in seeding for further proliferation (most cells that enter the blood vessels are rapidly destroyed)

## Evaluation and Management of the Neck Mass
### Initial Evaluation

- <u>H&P</u>: complete H&N H&P (*as previous*), attention to nasopharynx, oral cavity, base of tongue, tonsillar fossa, nasal cavity, external ear canal, scalp, thyroid, and salivary glands (also consider breast, rectal, and pelvic exams)
- <u>Primary Cancer Identified</u>: biopsy primary site, treatment based on site of primary
- <u>FNA</u>: indicated for any suspicious nodes without a known primary
- <u>FNA Reveals Benign Lymph Tissue or Is Indeterminate</u>: consider neck CT to re-evaluate criteria for malignancy in the neck mass, may repeat FNA (consider US or CT guided), or may observe if low suspicion
- <u>FNA Reveals Lymphoid Cells</u>: open excisional biopsy (fresh specimen), if frozen section suggests lymphoma proceed per protocol

for lymphomas (*see following*), if frozen section is nonlymphoma then consider complete neck dissection if appropriate
- <u>FNA Suggests Adenocarcinoma</u>: for high-level nodal disease consider neck dissection with submandibulectomy and possible parotidectomy (depending on preoperative imaging), for low-level nodal disease consider excisional biopsy (may also consider thyroid scan)
- <u>FNA Suggests Other Primary Cancer</u>: includes sarcoma, thyroid cancer, salivary gland malignancy; treatment based on type of cancer

## Staging

### Nodal Levels (*see* Figure 7–2)

| | |
|---|---|
| I | **IA**: submental and **IB**: submandibular triangles |
| II | upper jugular (between **hyoid or carotid bifurcation** and **base of skull**); **IIA**: anterior and **IIB**: posterior to CN XI |
| III | middle jugular (between **cricoid or omohyoid** to the **hyoid or carotid bifurcation**) |
| IV | lower jugular (between **clavicle** and **cricoid or omohyoid**) |
| V | posterior triangle (**VA**: superior and **VB**: inferior to omohyoid) |
| VI | anterior neck/central compartment (between carotid sheaths), includes Delphian (precricoid/prelaryngeal) LNs |
| VII | superior mediastinum (suprasternal notch to anterior mediastinum) |

### Nodal Staging (*AJCC Staging Handbook, 7th ed, 2010*)

- *NOTE:* includes most HNSCC including oral, oropharyngeal, hypopharyngeal, laryngeal

| | |
|---|---|
| NX | lymph nodes (LNs) cannot be assessed |
| N0 | no regional LN metastasis |
| N1 | single ipsilateral LN ≤3 cm |
| N2a | single ipsilateral LN >3 cm and ≤6 cm |
| N2b | multiple ipsilateral LNs ≤6 cm |
| N2c | bilateral or contralateral LNs ≤6 cm |
| N3 | any LN >6 cm |

## Management of the Neck in Head and Neck Cancer

### Primary Cancers

- *NOTE:* management for lymphoma, thyroid malignancy, salivary gland tumors is discussed in other sections

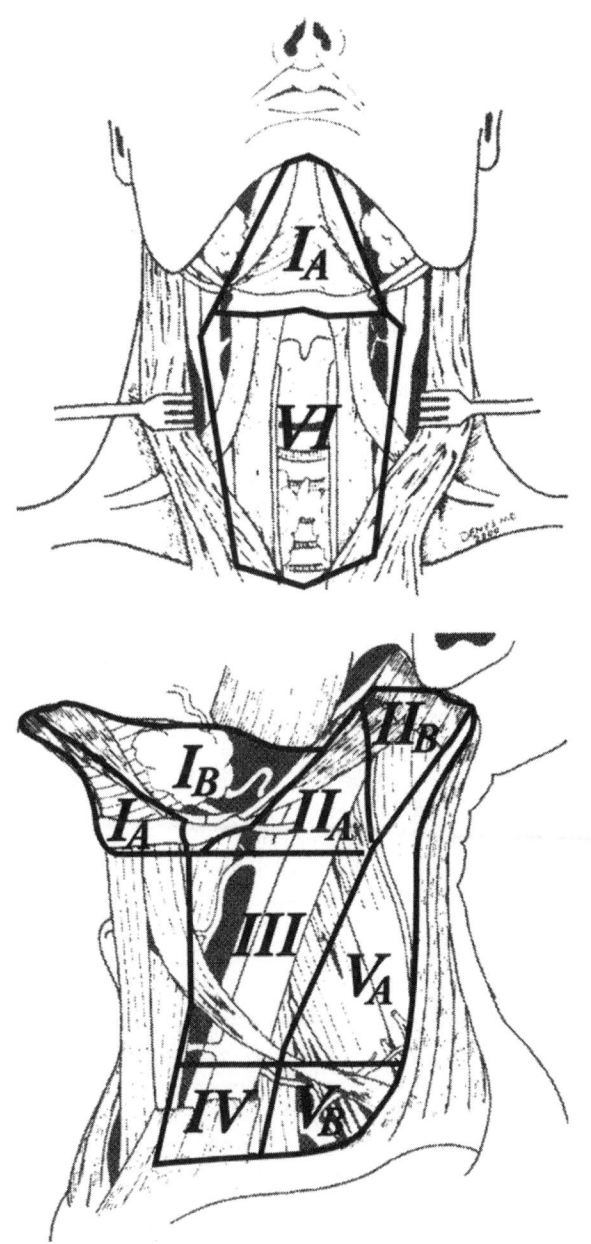

**FIGURE 7–2. A–B.** Lymph node levels of the neck. (From Deschler DG, Day T. *TNM Staging of Head and Neck Cancer and Neck Dissection Classification.* 2008.)

- sarcomas and branchial cleft cyst carcinomas are quite rare and typically require wide resection with neck dissection

### Regional Nodal Metastasis

- <u>Early-Staged Neck Disease (N1)</u>: resection of the primary site with a neck dissection (preferably en bloc if possible) with consideration of adjuvant radiation therapy (to the primary site and neck) for extracapsular spread or advanced primary disease versus primary radiation therapy of **6,500 cGy** (especially if the primary site is being irradiated) with planned or salvage neck dissection
- <u>Late-Staged Neck Disease (N2–N3)</u>: multimodality therapy with a neck dissection and postoperative radiation therapy; alternatively may perform concomitant chemoradiation followed by selective neck dissection for control of residual disease

### Clinically Negative Neck (N0)

- controversial management between observation, elective treatment with neck dissection, or radiation therapy
- <u>Observation</u>: consider if risk of occult metastasis is **<15–25%**
- <u>Elective Neck Dissection</u>: generally indicated if risk of regional metastasis >**15–25%** (eg, supraglottis, base of tongue, tonsil, oral tongue, and advanced staged cancer), typically a selective neck dissection provides the least morbidity with adequate excision, specimen provides histology to evaluate for positive nodes and extracapsular spread (adjuvant therapy)
- <u>Radiation Therapy</u>: may also be considered to eradicate occult neck disease if risk of regional metastasis is >**15–25%**, indicated especially if primary site is being irradiated

### The Fixed Neck (Unresectable)

- fixed nodes suggest adherence to the vertebrae, brachial plexus, major vessels, mastoid process, or other structures that are nonmobile
- unresectability is typically considered for brachial plexus, floor of neck, vertebral involvement, carotid artery encasement (>270° of tumor surrounding the carotid) or invasion (carotid artery can be resected en bloc with the tumor if patient passes a preop balloon occlusion test and understands the risk of stroke)
- multimodality therapy may be offered in form of initial radiation and chemotherapy in hopes of "freeing up" the tumor to allow for later resection

### Bilateral Positive Nodes (N2c)

- therapy typically consists of excision of primary site with bilateral neck dissections and adjuvant radiation therapy
- a modified neck dissection (preserving the internal jugular vein and CN IX) should be attempted first on the least involved side prior to operating on the more involved side; if unable to preserve the internal jugular vein consider staging (temporally spacing) the neck dissections 3–4 weeks apart to allow for dilation of the intracranial venous vasculature to avoid increased intracranial pressure

### Unknown Primary

- <u>Early-Staged Neck Disease (N1)</u>: may manage with a neck dissection and adjuvant radiation therapy to the neck, Waldeyer's ring, nasopharynx versus radiation therapy alone
- <u>Late-Staged Neck Disease (N2–N3)</u>: multimodality therapy with neck dissection and adjuvant radiation therapy to the neck, Waldeyer's ring, and nasopharynx; alternatively may perform concomitant chemoradiation for advanced neck disease
- *see also* pp. 324–326

# Neck Dissection

## Classifications of Neck Dissections

### Radical Neck Dissection

- comprehensive (removes all level nodes) including removal of the sternocleidomastoid muscle, internal jugular vein, and spinal accessory nerve
- rarely performed today because of significant morbidity
- <u>Indications</u>: clinically positive nodes with extracapsular extension and involvement of sternocleidomastoid muscle, internal jugular vein, or spinal accessory nerve
- <u>Technique</u>: removes submandibular gland, tail of parotid, sternocleidomastoid muscle, internal jugular vein, spinal accessory nerve, and cervical nodes
- <u>Advantages</u>: technically easier, lower risk of residual disease
- <u>Disadvantages</u>: neck deformity (removal of sternocleidomastoid muscle), shoulder drop (removal of spinal accessory nerve), risk of facial edema (removal of internal jugular vein), hypesthesia of the neck and periauricular region; higher incidence of carotid blowouts due to lack of tissue (ie, sternocleidomastoid) covering carotid artery

### Modified Radical Neck Dissection

- comprehensive (removes all level nodes)
- **Type I**: spares spinal accessory nerve; **Type II**: spares internal jugular vein and spinal accessory nerve; **Type III (Functional, Bocca)**: spares sternocleidomastoid muscle, internal jugular vein, and spinal accessory nerve
- <u>Indications</u>: clinically positive nodes with primary cancer with a lower risk of occult nodes or the N0 neck; no involvement of sternocleidomastoid muscle, internal jugular vein, or spinal accessory nerve
- <u>Advantages</u>: lower morbidity from preservation of sternocleidomastoid muscle, spinal accessory nerve, and/or internal jugular vein
- <u>Disadvantages</u>: technically more difficult

### Selective Neck Dissection

- does not remove all nodal levels, removes only those at high risk
- **Supraomohyoid (Anterolateral) Neck Dissection**: removes nodal levels **I–III** (expanded supraomohyoid removes level IV); indicated for larger oral cancers with a N0 or select N1 (mobile) neck
- **Lateral Neck Dissection**: removes nodal levels **II–IV**; indicated for select supraglottic, oropharyngeal, hypopharyngeal cancers; typically bilateral
- **Posterior Lateral Neck Dissection**: removes nodal levels **II–V** (also retroauricular and suboccipital nodes); indicated for select posterior scalp cancers

## Complications

- **Wound Infections and Wound Breakdown**: incidence higher in radiated tissue; soilage of wound by saliva, tracheal or gastric secretions; tight wound closure; immunocompromised and malnourished states; and presence of a foreign body, hematoma, or seroma; <u>Rx</u>: aggressive antibiotic regimen, monitor for fistula, control diabetes, optimize nutrition, meticulous wound care (debridement, wet to dry dressings), evaluate potential for carotid blowout (*see following*)
- **Flap Necrosis**: poorly planned incision that compromises vascular supply may result in tissue loss, wound infection, fistula, or vessel exposure; <u>Rx</u>: avoid with properly designed neck incisions (eg, curvilinear, MacFee, modified Schobinger incision; trifurcation should begin at right angles from the main incision), manage wound infection and breakdown as above
- **Shoulder Syndrome**: injury or sacrifice of spinal accessory nerve results in loss of trapezius support, shoulder drop, winged scapula,

and resulting pain (pain is primary source of morbidity); <u>Rx</u>: physical therapy, may also consider early cable grafting or orthopedic reconstruction

- **Injury to the Vagus Nerve**: varying presentation depending on level and branch of injury; superior laryngeal nerve injury may present with only subtle voice changes, recurrent laryngeal nerve injury may result in hoarseness, aspiration, or airway compromise; <u>Rx</u>: may require tracheotomy for airway management (especially for bilateral vocal fold paralysis), management of aspiration and vocal fold immobility (*see* pp. 121–124)

- **Injury to the Marginal Mandibular Branch of the Facial Nerve**: at risk during elevation of the superior cervical/subplatysmal flap, should be identified and protected, most commonly located within the fascia superficial to the submandibular gland and facial vein, bilateral injury may result in oral incompetence; <u>Rx</u>: if discovered intraoperatively immediate neurorrhaphy should be performed, consider facial reanimation procedures (*see* pp. 431–433)

- **Hematoma/Seroma**: prevented with meticulous hemostasis and placement of suction drains (hematoma occurs earlier, seroma occurs later); <u>Rx</u>: consider reopening for major hematomas with removal of clot and controlling bleeding, for minor hematomas may wait 7–10 days to allow for liquification then aspirate, may also consider pressure dressings and prophylactic antibiotics, seromas may also be aspirated

- **Chylous Fistula**: typically left-sided (chy**L**ous = **L**eft sided; 95–97%) from injury to thoracic duct, milky drainage, appears within first few days, incidence from 1–2%; <u>Rx</u>: initial conservative management (pressure drainage, head elevation, restrict fats, place on medium-chain triglyceride diet, manage electrolyte abnormalities), consider tetracycline sclerosing therapy versus surgical re-exploration versus thoracic surgery consult for proximal ligation if failed conservative therapy or if output >600 mL/day

- **Cerebral and Facial Edema**: higher risk with internal jugular vein ligation (especially if bilateral ligation), may present with syndrome of inappropriate antidiuretic hormone (SIADH) or mental status changes; <u>Rx</u>: cerebral edema must be addressed urgently; neurosurgery consultation; consider corticosteroids, lumbar drain, hyperventilation, hyperosmolar agents (mannitol), and diuretics

- **Blindness**: caused by optic nerve infarction (uncertain etiology, may be from hypotension and increased intracranial pressure), rare

- **Postoperative Dyspnea**: possible etiologies include pneumothorax, phrenic nerve injury, intrinsic lung disease (atelactasis), and congestive heart failure

- **Carotid Blowout**: typically from infected wound site and wound breakdown, associated with radiation therapy and radical neck dissection (removal of sternocleidomastoid), high mortality rate (~10%) and risk of stroke; <u>Rx</u>: airway management, digital compression, large-bore catheters with fluid replacement, immediate blood replacement, intraoperative ligation, consider vascular surgery consultation, consider interventional radiology for possible balloon occlusion test and embolization

# ORAL CANCER

## Introduction

### Overview

- **most common head and neck cancer site** (30% of all head and neck cancer)
- oral cavity has the highest rate of second primaries (10–40%)
- >90% of occult metastatic disease in oral cancer involves nodal groups I–III (the supraomohyoid dissection is oncologically sound especially in the N0 neck)
- <u>SSx</u>: nonhealing ulcers, denture difficulties, dysphagia, odynophagia, trismus, halitosis, numbness in the lower teeth (suggests mandible and inferior alveolar nerve involvement)
- <u>Risk Factors</u>: smoking, alcohol, and chewing tobacco; radiation and ultraviolet radiation exposure (lip cancer), Plummer-Vinson syndrome (*see* p. 200), HPV, poor oral hygiene, oral leukoplakia (5–20% malignant potential), and erythroplakia (~25% malignant potential, *see* pp. 205–207)

### Anatomy

- **Oral Cavity**: extends from lips to junction of hard and soft palate and circumvallate papillae
- other than the mandibular periosteum there is no discreet fascial plane to inhibit tumor extension in the oral cavity

### *Subsites and Regional Lymph Node Potential*

- **Lips**: **most common location of oral cancer**, **90%** on lower lip, **90%** 5-year survival if <2 cm, **90%** squamous cell carcinoma (**rules of 90s**), basal cell carcinoma is more common on upper lip; 2–15% regional metastasis (for all stages); lower lip has **bilateral**

**and ipsilateral** lymphatic drainage into level I–III nodal groups and upper lip has **ipsilateral** lymphatic drainage into level I–III nodal groups (no contralateral drainage due to embryologic fusion plates); overall 5-year survival for all stages for squamous cell carcinoma is 70–90% for the lower lip and 40–60% for the upper lip; poorer prognosis is associated with upper lip and commissure involvement

- **Oral Tongue**: second most common location of oral cancer, movable portion, anterior to circumvallate papillae; 25–66% regional metastasis (for all stages); 60–80% 5-year survival for early disease (T1–T2)
- **Buccal Mucosa**: common site near mandibular third molar (site of chewing tobacco), most common site for verrucous carcinoma, more common in India (betel nut); 50% regional metastasis (for all stages), occult neck metastasis in ~10%
- **Alveolar Ridge**: more common in edentulous and molar areas of the mandible, must differentiate from invasive maxillary cancer, high rate of bony involvement; 50–65% 5-year survival
- **Retromolar Trigone**: triangle-shaped region with the base at the last mandibular molar and the apex at the maxillary tuberosity; typically presents in an advanced stage, bony invasion common, 50% regional metastasis (for all stages); ~ 25–55% 5-year survival for all stages (due to advance initial staging and poor salvage potential)
- **Hard Palate**: incisive foramen allows tumor extension into anterior nose, palatine foramen allows tumor extension to pterygopalatine fossa; less aggressive (10–25% occult regional metastasis), minor salivary gland tumors are common
- **Floor of Mouth**: dependent site for alcohol and chewing tobacco, 30% present with regional metastasis, overall 5-year survival is 30–65%

## Staging and Pathologic Classification

**Staging** *(Based on AJCC Staging, 2010)*

*T*

- **T1**: primary tumor ≤2 cm
- **T2**: primary tumor >2 and ≤4 cm
- **T3**: primary tumor >4 cm
- **T4**: primary tumor invades adjacent structures; **T4a**: moderately advanced local disease* (invasion through cortical bone [mandible or maxilla] into deep [extrinsic] muscle of tongue [genioglossus, hyoglossus, palatoglossus, and styloglossus], maxillary sinus, skin of face); **T4b**: very advanced local disease (invasion through masticator

space, pterygoid plates, skull base and/or encases internal carotid artery)

*superficial erosion alone of bone/tooth socket by gingival primary is not sufficient to classify a tumor as T4

***N*** (*see* p. 276)

***M*** (*see* p. 258)

## Pathology

- **Squamous Cell Carcinoma** (SCC): >90% of oral cancers
- **Verrucous Carcinoma**: variant of SCC, broad-based, warty growth, most common site is the **buccal mucosa**, lateral growth, rare metastasis and deep invasion, better prognosis
- **Basal Cell Carcinoma**: more common on the upper lip
- Other Types: lymphoma, Kaposi's sarcoma, salivary gland malignancies, melanoma
- *NOTE: **necrotizing sialometaplasia** and **granular cell tumor** may be mistaken for oral squamous cell carcinoma due to similar histology (pseudoepitheliomatous hyperplasia)*

# Management

## Early Oral Cancer (T1–T2)

- preferred treatment is surgical excision of primary tumor with primary reconstruction (*see following*); may consider primary radiation in the form of brachytherapy, radiation is less ideal due to complications from radiating the mandible
- N0 Neck: elective ipsilateral or bilateral (midline oral tongue cancer) selective neck dissection (supraomohyoid/levels I–III) versus radiation (early-stage hard palate or lower lip do not require elective neck dissections because of lower rate of occult metastasis)
- N1–3 Neck: selective neck dissection (supraomohyoid/levels I–III) or modified radical neck dissection as indicated for clinical nodes, parotid nodes require a superficial parotidectomy
- Adjuvant Therapy
  1. no adverse features → no adjuvant therapy
  2. one positive node without adverse features → radiation therapy optional
  3. adverse features such as positive margins or extracapsular spread (ECS) → chemoradiation (preferred), re-resection, or radiation

4. other risk features → adjuvant radiaton or consider chemoradiation
5. residual tumor postradiation → salvage surgery

## Advanced Oral Cancer (T3–T4a)

- mainstay of treatment is surgical excision of primary tumor with primary reconstruction (*see following*)
- <u>N0 Neck</u>: elective ipsilateral or bilateral (midline tongue cancer) selective neck dissection (supraomohyoid)
- <u>N1–N3 Neck</u>: selective neck dissection including levels I, II, and III or modified radical neck dissection as indicated for clinical nodes, parotid nodes require a superficial parotidectomy
- <u>Adjuvant Therapy</u>
  1. no adverse features → radiation therapy optional
  2. adverse features such as positive margins or extracapsular spread (ECS) → chemoradiation (preferred), re-resection, or radiation
  3. other risk features → adjuvant radiation or consider chemoradiation

## Lip Cancer (T1–T2)

- preferred treatment is surgery with excision of primary tumor (may consider Mohs micrographic excision) with primary reconstruction, may consider primary radiation therapy (5,000–7,000 cGy) to primary site
- <u>N0 Neck</u>: elective ipsilateral or bilateral (midline primary) selective neck dissection (supraomohyoid)
- <u>N1–N3 Neck</u>: ipsilateral or bilateral selective neck dissection (supraomohyoid) or modified radical neck dissection as indicated for clinical nodes, parotid nodes require a superficial parotidectomy
- <u>Adjuvant Therapy</u>
  1. no adverse features → no adjuvant therapy
  2. one positive node without adverse features → radiation therapy optional
  3. adverse features such as positive margins or ECS → chemoradiation (preferred), or re-resection, or radiation
  4. other risk features → can also be managed by adjuvant radiation or consider chemoradiation
  5. residual or recurrent tumor postradiaton → salvage surgery

## Lip Cancer (T3–T4a)

- preferred treatment is surgical excision of primary tumor (may consider Mohs micrographic excision) with primary reconstruction;

may consider primary radiation therapy (5,000–7,000 cGy) or chemoradiation
- <u>N0 Neck</u>: elective neck dissection not recommended
- <u>N1–N3 Neck</u>: selective neck dissection (supraomohyoid) or modified radical neck dissection as indicated for clinical nodes, parotid nodes require a superficial parotidectomy
- <u>Adjuvant Therapy</u>
  1. no adverse features → no adjuvant therapy
  2. adverse features such as positive margins, perineural/vascular/lymphatic invasion → re-resection or radiation
  3. residual or recurrent tumor postradiation → salvage surgery

## Surgical Management of Oral Cancer

- <u>Approach</u>: anterior and small tumors (<2 cm) may be approached intraorally, larger and more posterior tumors require a transmandibular, transcervical, or transoral robotic approach (*see following*)
- <u>Mandible</u>: invasion of the mandible (as diagnosed by CT) requires a **segmental** mandibulectomy, direct abutment of tumor against periosteum requires a mandible-sparing procedure (**marginal** or **rim** mandibulectomy); the term **composite resection** refers to removing multiple types of tissue typically including bone; **COMMANDO** procedure is a historic term (<u>COM</u>bined <u>MA</u>ndibulectomy and <u>N</u>eck <u>D</u>issection <u>O</u>peration)
- <u>Maxilla</u>: invasion of the maxilla requires alveolectomy, palatectomy, or inferior/infrastructure maxillectomy
- <u>Reconstruction</u>: healing by secondary intention, primary closure, or split-thickness skin grafts provide the best speech and swallowing outcomes; large defects require regional or free flaps

# OROPHARYNGEAL CANCER
## Introduction

### Overview

- <u>SSx</u>: sore throat, odynophagia, dysphagia, voice quality changes, neck mass, referred otalgia, globus sensation, trismus, dysarthria, decreased tongue mobility, base of tongue mass (on palpation)
- <u>Risk Factors</u>: smoking, alcohol, and tobacco abuse; Epstein-Barr virus (lymphoepithelioma), HPV

## Anatomy

- **Oropharynx**: anterior boundary at junction of hard and soft palate (*see previous*) and circumvallate papillae (*see following*), superior boundary at level of hard palate, inferior boundary at the superior surface of the hyoid

### Subsites and Regional Lymph Node Potential

- **Tonsil/Lateral Pharyngeal Wall**: **most common site of oropharygeal cancer**, may present as an exophytic mass or an ulcerative lesion, aggressive, usually presents with regional neck disease (65–75%), higher instance of lymphoma and lymphoepitheloma (*see following*)
- **Posterior Pharyngeal Wall**: less common, aggressive although less metastatic potential than base of tongue
- **Soft Palate**: rare; since more visible than other sites, typically found at early stages; 20–45% regional metastasis, 70% 5-year survival
- **Base of Tongue**: more aggressive tumor than oral tongue, high rate of cervical metastasis (>60%, 20% bilateral metastasis), poorer prognosis (approximately 65% 5-year survival for all stages)
- **Vallecula**

## Human Papilloma Virus (HPV) Association

- HPV-associated squamous cell carcinoma can be found in any area of the upper aerodigestive tract, however most common in the oropharynx, particularly the **base of tongue and tonsils**
- incidence increasing
- patients younger by 10 years, associated with multiple sex partners
- better prognosis including decreased local–regional failure, improved progression-free and overall survival (*N Engl J Med.* 2010; 363:24–35)
- many high-risk HPV types exist, **type 16** is most common seen in carcinoma
- <u>Etiology</u>: HPV is a double-stranded DNA virus that infects stratified squamous epithelial cells, oncogenes **E6** and **E7** are responsible for malignancies in both the anogenital and head and neck areas, E6 binds and inactivates the **p53** tumor suppressor gene, E7 binds and inactivates the **Rb** (retinoblastoma) protein leading to release of E2F transcription factor causing cell cycle progression
- <u>Dx</u>: DNA in situ hybridization, PCR, or immunostaining for **p16** (however, p16 is not completely specific for HPV and can be positive in 10–20% of oropharyngeal squamous cell carcinoma in absence

of HPV); testing should be performed for all oropharyngeal cancers (NCCN guidelines)

- <u>Rx</u>: given better prognosis several clinical trials are evaluating the role of deescalated therapy (*see following*), prevention with HPV vaccine (*see* Appendix C)

# Classification and Management

## Staging *(Based on AJCC Staging, 2010)*

### *T*

- **T1**: primary tumor ≤2 cm
- **T2**: primary tumor >2 and ≤4 cm
- **T3**: primary tumor >4 cm or extension to lingual surface of epiglottis
- **T4**: primary tumor invades adjacent structures; **T4a**: moderately advanced local disease (invasion through larynx, extrinsic muscle of tongue, medial pterygoid, hard palate, or mandible*); **T4b**: very advanced local disease (invasion through lateral pterygoid, pterygoid plates, lateral nasopharynx, skull base or encases carotid artery) *mucosal extension to lingual surface of epiglottis from primary tumors of the base of the tongue and vallecula does not constitute invasion of larynx

*N* (*see* p. 276)

*M* (*see* p. 258)

## Pathology

- **Squamous Cell Carcinoma (SCC)**: >95% of oropharyngeal cancer, lymph node metastases may be cystic
- **Lymphoepithelioma**: subgroup of poorly differentiated carcinoma, may present in the tonsil, exophytic, radiosensitive
- **Lymphoma**: (*see* pp. 327–330) 10–15% of base of tongue and tonsillar cancers
- <u>Other Types</u>: sarcoma, salivary gland malignancies, metastatic disease

## Management

### *Early Oropharyngeal Cancer (T1–T2)*

- <u>Primary</u>: options include excision of primary tumor with primary reconstruction (*see following*) versus primary radiation versus chemoradiation for select T2N1 patients

- <u>N0 Neck</u>: elective ipsilateral or bilateral selective neck dissection (levels II–IV) versus radiation
- <u>N1 Neck</u>: selective neck dissection (levels II–IV) or modified radical neck dissection as indicated for clinical nodes or radiation
- <u>N2–3 Neck</u>: concurrent chemoradiation (preferred), induction chemotherapy followed by radiation or chemoradiation, surgery for primary and neck, or multimodality clinical trials
- <u>Adjuvant Therapy</u>
  1. no adverse features → no adjuvant therapy
  2. one positive node without adverse features → radiation therapy optional
  3. adverse features such as positive margins or ECS → chemoradiation (preferred), or re-resection, or radiation
  4. other risk features → can also be managed by adjuvant radiation or consider chemoradiation
  5. residual tumor postradiation → salvage surgery

### *Advanced Oropharyngeal Cancer (T3–T4a)*

- <u>Primary</u>: options include concurrent chemoradiation (preferred) versus excision of primary tumor with primary reconstruction (*see following*) versus induction chemotherapy followed by radiation or chemoradiation versus multimodality clinical trials
- <u>Neck</u>: *see previous*
- <u>Adjuvant Therapy</u>
  1. no adverse features → radiation therapy
  2. adverse features such as positive margins or ECS → chemoradiation
  3. other risk features → can also be managed by adjuvant radiation or consider chemoradiation
  4. residual tumor postradiation → salvage surgery

### *De-escalation of Therapy in HPV-Associated Oropharyngeal Carcinoma*

- due to improved prognosis with HPV association, several clinical trials are investigating de-escalating (de-intensifying) chemoradiation to decrease side effects and morbidity (including ECOG 1013, RTOG 1016)

## Surgical Management of Oropharyngeal Cancer

### *Approaches*

- **Transoral Robotic Surgery (TORS):** *see* p. 333

- **Transoral Laser Microsurgery (TLM):** an ideal treatment for early to intermediate glottic and supraglottic lesions as well as certain oropharyngeal and hypopharyngeal tumors; <u>Advantages</u>: similar to TORS (functional and cosmetic outcomes), added benefit of faster operative time, reduced cost, and presence of tactile (haptic) feedback; <u>Disadvantages</u>: requires line of sight, long instrumentation with limited degrees of motion, presence of tremor and exaggerated movements
- **Transcervical/Visor Flap**: consider for large tumors of the base of tongue or tonsil, access oropharynx from a transoral incision of the floor of the mouth, preserves mandibular integrity, poor exposure, chin numbness
- **Mandibulectomy**: indicated for larger lesions, mandible extension, or multiple sites (composite resection); may be approached laterally or medially with a lip-splitting incision (**mandibular swing**); provides excellent exposure, easier soft tissue closure, risk of malocclusion and plate extrusion (*see* also p. 286)
- **Mandibulotomy**: spares mandible, may be approached laterally or midline with a lip-splitting incision, osteotomy is performed in a stepwise fashion to create a favorable repair followed by rigid fixation, provides excellent exposure, less risk of malocclusion
- **Lateral Pharyngotomy**: consider for small base of tongue or posterior pharyngeal wall tumors; enters pharynx between hypoglossal and superior laryngeal nerves; limited exposure, spares mandible, avoids lip-splitting incision
- **Transhyoid Pharyngotomy**: consider for small base of tongue or posterior pharyngeal wall tumors without significant superior or tonsillar extension; enters pharynx above or through hyoid bone; spares mandible, avoids lip-splitting incision, vallecula must be free of tumor, poor exposure superiorly

## *Reconstruction*

- **Healing by Secondary Intention**: useful in small partial glossectomies, simplest and best functional outcome (speech, swallowing), associated with slightly increased pain; often utilized after TORS resection
- **Primary Closure**: very good functional outcome (speech and swallowing), ideal method of reconstruction if a tension-free closure can be obtained without resulting in significant stenosis
- **Split-Thickness Skin Graft**: allows resurfacing with good functional outcomes, does not provide tissue bulk

- **Pedicled Regional Flap**: provides soft tissue bulk with compromise of speech and swallowing function (*see* pp. 449–452)
- **Free Tissue Transfer**: provides soft tissue bulk with compromise of speech and swallowing function, **radial forearm** flap for large partial glossectomies as well as pharyngeal wall defects and anterolateral thigh or rectus flap for total glossectomies; **fibula**, or **iliac crest** method of choice for mandibular reconstruction of >5 cm of bone loss (*see* pp. 454–456) other options include osteocutaneous radial forearm and scapular flaps for smaller mandibular defects

# HYPOPHARYNGEAL CANCER
## Introduction

### Overview

- usually advanced when diagnosed (poor prognosis)
- <u>SSx</u>: airway obstruction, progressive dysphagia, odynophagia, neck mass, referred otalgia, globus sensation, sore throat, hoarseness, weight loss, laryngeal lesions (ulcerated, exophytic), vocal fold immobility
- <u>Risk Factors</u>: smoking, alcohol, tobacco use, laryngopharyngeal reflux, Barrett's esophagus, Plummer-Vinson syndrome (*see* p. 200)

### Anatomy

- **Hypopharynx**: level of hyoid bone to cricopharyngeus (upper esophageal sphincter), lies behind and around the larynx

#### *Subsites and Regional Lymph Node Potential*

- **Piriform Sinus**: **most common site for hypopharyngeal cancer** (65–75%); may extend into the subglottis, cricoarytenoid joint or muscle (vocal fold fixation), thyroid cartilage, or postcricoid region; 75% regional metastasis; apical primaries are associated with a worse prognosis
- **Posterior Pharyngeal Wall**: 20–25% of hypopharyngeal tumors; may extend into the oropharynx, postcricoid region, or prevertebral fascia (late in disease); 60% regional metastasis
- **Postcricoid Region**: rare (<5%); associated with **Plummer-Vinson syndrome**; may extend into the cricoid cartilage, cricoarytenoid muscle, or cervical esophagus; 40% regional metastasis

# Classification and Management

## Staging *(Based on AJCC Staging, 2010)*

*T*

- **T1**: primary tumor limited to one subsite ≤2 cm
- **T2**: primary tumor invades more than one subsite/adjacent site or >2 cm and ≤4 cm and without fixation of hemilarynx
- **T3**: primary tumor >4 cm or vocal fold fixation or extension into esophagus
- **T4**: primary tumor invades adjacent structures; **T4a**: moderately advanced local disease (invasion of thyroid/cricoid cartilage, hyoid bone, thyroid gland, or central compartment soft tissue*); **T4b**: very advanced local disease (invasion of prevertebral fascia, encases carotid artery, or involves mediastinal structures)
  *central compartment soft tissue includes prelaryngeal strap muscles and subcutaneous fat

*N* (*see* p. 276)

*M* (*see* p. 258)

## Pathology

- **Squamous Cell Carcinoma (SCC)**: poorly differentiated (most common)
- <u>Other Types</u>: adenoma, salivary gland malignancies, metastatic disease

## Management

- tumors of the hypopharynx may extend submucosally resulting in "skip lesions"
- most present in advanced state with clinical cervical nodes (40–75%)

### Early Hypopharyngeal Cancer

- includes most T1–T2 not requiring total laryngectomy
- <u>Primary:</u> definitive radiation with surgical salvage or surgical excision, which entails a partial laryngopharyngectomy (open or endoscopic)
- <u>Neck</u>: elective bilateral radiation, or elective ipsilateral or bilateral (for tumors that cross midline) neck dissection (levels II–IV)
- <u>Adjuvant Therapy</u>
  1. no adverse features → no adjuvant therapy
  2. adverse features such as ECS → chemoradiation, positive margins only should undergo re-resection or consider chemoradiation

3. other risk features → can also be managed by adjuvant radiation or consider chemoradiation
4. residual tumor postradiation → salvage surgery

### *Advanced Hypopharyngeal Cancer*

- includes any tumor requiring total laryngectomy or laryngopharyngectomy
- <u>Primary</u>: options including induction chemotherapy or laryngopharyngectomy with neck dissections including level VI (preferred for T4a tumors) or concurrent chemoradiation or multimodality clinical trials
- <u>Neck</u>: elective radiation therapy to bilateral necks or elective ipsilateral or bilateral (for tumors that cross midline) neck dissection (levels II–IV, VI) or modified radical neck dissection as indicated for clinical nodes
- <u>Adjuvant therapy:</u>
  1. no adverse features → no adjuvant therapy
  2. adverse features such as ECS or positive margins → chemoradiation
  3. other risk features → can also be managed by adjuvant radiation or consider chemoradiation
  4. residual tumor postradiation → salvage surgery

### *Surgical Management*

- <u>Larynx Preservation</u>: indicated for T1–T2 tumors from the medial piriform sinus; contraindications include involvement of thyroid cartilage, apex of piriform sinus, postcricoid region, interarytenoid, cervical esophagus, and vocal fold fixation
- **Transoral Laser Microsurgery (TLM)**: *see* p. 290
- **Transhyoid Pharyngotomy**
- **Mandibulotomy and Median Glossotomy**: (Trotter procedure) mainly historic
- **Partial Laryngopharyngectomy**: laryngeal conservation procedure that may be considered for early T1–T2 piriform sinus cancer if tumor involves primarily the medial wall and >1.5 cm clear from the apex
- **Combined Suprahyoid and Lateral Pharyngectomy**: consider for early T1–T2 posterior cricopharyngeal wall cancer, includes removal of lateral third of the thyroid cartilage
- **Total Laryngectomy with Partial Pharyngectomy**: typically required for most postcricoid primaries, advanced hypopharyngeal disease, recurrence, and radiation failures

- **Total Laryngopharyngectomy with Esophagectomy**: if cervical esophageal involvement
- **Wookey Procedure**: turned-in cervical skin flaps
- Reconstruction: primary closure or skin grafts are rarely appropriate for tension-free closure, typically require regional pedicled flap (pectoralis major or trapezius myocutaneous flap, gastric pull-up) or microvascular free flap

### *Complications of Gastric Pull-Up Reconstruction*

- **Anastomosis Breakdown and Leak**: salivary leak results in wound infection, fistula formation, sepsis, mediastinitis, and death; 10–37% incidence of anastomotic disruption; Rx: prevented with tension-free closure, avoidance of infection, maintenance of vascular supply; may require external diversion or re-exploration and repair (increased risk of mortality)
- **Abdominal Complications**: not common, various potential complications include perforation of the pyloroplasty, peritonitis, wound dehiscence, and splenic injury
- **Cardiopulmonary Complications**: may result from fluid shifts, hemorrhage, pulmonary atelectasis, respiratory failure, pneumothorax
- **Hypocalcemia**: secondary to decreased calcium absorption from decreased gastric acidity and decreased intestinal transit time from the truncal vagotomy and from disruption of the vascular supply to the parathyroid glands; Rx: calcium supplementation
- **Tracheobronchial Injury**: most commonly from injury to the posterior membranous tracheal wall during dissection; Rx: requires primary closure of defect or tissue coverage of defect (eg, adjacent muscle or pedicled flap)

# LARYNGEAL CANCER

## Introduction

### Overview

- 1–5% of all malignancies
- second most common site for head and neck malignancy
- SSx: hoarseness, aspiration, dysphagia, odynophagia, sore throat, hemoptysis, airway obstruction (stridor), referred otalgia, weight loss, globus sensation
- Risk Factors: smoking and alcohol use; radiation exposure; history of recurrent respiratory papillomatosis (HPV), Plummer-Vinson syndrome; exposure to metal, plastics, paint, wood dust, and asbestos

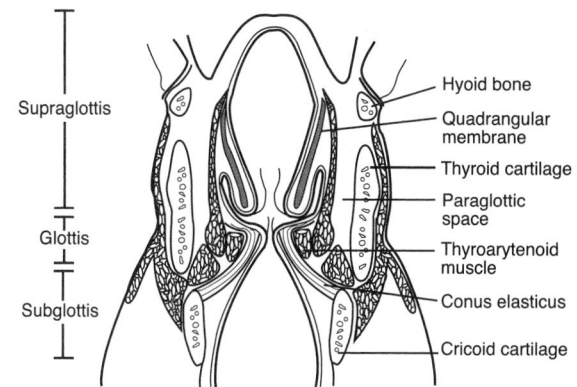

**FIGURE 7–3.** Coronal section of the larynx demonstrating the barriers and divisions of the larynx.

## Barriers and Spaces of the Larynx (*see* Figure 7–3)

- **Quadrangular Membrane**: fibroelastic membrane, supports supraglottis, extends from epiglottis to arytenoid and corniculate cartilage
- **Conus Elasticus**: fibroelastic membrane, supports vocal fold, extends from cricoid cartilage to merge with vocal ligament (resists spread of glottic and subglottic cancers)
- **Pre-epiglottic Space**: midline fibrofatty-filled space bounded by the hyoid bone, thyrohyoid membrane, hyoepiglottic ligament, thyroepiglottic ligament, and epiglottis; tumor may enter from anterior commissure or supraglottic extension; continuous with paraglottic space
- **Paraglottic Space**: fibrofatty-filled space outside of conus elasticus and quadrangular membrane, allows transglottic extension (<u>Borders</u>: superomedial: quadrangular membrane; mid-medial: ventricle; inferomedial: conus elasticus; posterior: piriform sinus mucosa; inferior: space between thyroid and cricoid cartilage; lateral: thyroid cartilage and cricothryoid membrane)
- **Reinke's Space**: superficial lamina propria of true vocal fold, lack of lymphatics and blood vessels permits rapid tumor extension
- **Broyles' Tendon**: insertion of vocalis tendon to thyroid cartilage; *controversial theories:* classically thought to allow tumor spread into thyroid cartilage (no perichondrium found at insertion site), negated by Kirchner's histopathology studies showing it as a barrier to spread, used today as the basis for transoral laser surgery of laryngeal carcinoma

# Supraglottic Site

## Overview

- <u>Anatomic Boundaries</u>: from the epiglottis to the junction of the ventricle and true vocal cord
- ~30–40% of laryngeal cancer
- <u>SSx</u>: **sore throat**, **hemoptysis**, aspiration, dysphagia, odynophagia, airway obstruction (stridor), referred otalgia, weight loss, globus sensation
- <u>Histology</u>: ciliated pseudostratified columnar epithelium
- <u>Subsites</u>: suprahyoid epiglottis, infrahyoid epiglottis (most common supraglottic site for cancer), aryepiglottic folds, arytenoids, false cords
- supraglottis is derived from the third and fourth branchial arches (glottis and subglottis develop from the sixth branchial arch), an embryologic fusion plate forms between supraglottis and glottis that functions as a tumor barrier and creates separate vascular supplies
- tumor invasion typically occurs superiorly toward base of tongue or pre-epiglottic space
- overall 25–75% risk of regional metastasis, primarily to nodal levels II–IV, especially bilateral neck disease (therefore, always treat both necks)
- **Marginal Tumor**: a tumor found at the aryepiglottic fold, usually a basaloid squamous cell carcinoma, aggressive, similar to a hypopharyngeal piriform sinus tumor

## Staging *(Based on AJCC Staging, 2010)*

### T

- **T1**: primary tumor limited to 1 subsite of supraglottis with normal vocal cord mobility
- **T2**: primary tumor invades mucosa of more than 1 adjacent subsite of supraglottis or glottis or region outside the supraglottis (eg, mucosa of base of tongue, vallecula, medial wall of piriform sinus) without vocal cord fixation
- **T3**: vocal fold fixation or primary tumor invades postcricoid area, pre-epiglottic space, paraglottic space, or inner cortex of thyroid cartilage
- **T4**: further invasion; **T4a**: moderately advanced local disease (invasion through thyroid cartilage or tissues beyond the larynx); **T4b**: very advanced local disease (invades prevertebral space, encases carotid artery, or invades mediastinal structures)

***N*** (*see* p. 276)

***M*** (*see* p. 258)

# Glottic Site

## Overview

- <u>Anatomic Boundaries</u>: from the superior surface of the true vocal fold to 1 cm below the true vocal folds
- **most common site of laryngeal cancer**, ~50–75%
- <u>SSx</u>: hoarseness, aspiration, dysphagia, odynophagia, airway obstruction, weight loss, sore throat
- <u>Histology</u>: stratified squamous epithelium
- typically diagnosed at early stages due to early symptomatology (hoarseness) and the barriers of tumor spread (vocal ligament, thyroglottic ligament, and conus elasticus)
- anterior commissure, which does not have an inner perichondrium, allows for thyroid cartilage invasion
- limited regional metastasis, primary drainage to nodal levels II–IV
- vocal fold fixation suggests involvement of thyroarytenoid, lateral or posterior cricoarytenoid, and interarytenoid muscles; extension into cricoarytenoid joint; or perineural invasion

## Staging *(Based on AJCC Staging, 2010)*

*T*

- **T1**: primary tumor limited to vocal folds (may involve anterior or posterior commissure) with normal mobility; **T1a**: one vocal fold involvement, **T1b**: bilateral vocal fold involvement (5% regional metastasis)
- **T2**: primary tumor extends to subglottis or supraglottis, or impaired vocal fold mobility (5–10% regional metastasis)
- **T3**: vocal fold fixation or invasion of paraglottic space or invasion of inner cortex of thyroid cartilage (10–20% regional metastasis)
- **T4**: further invasion; **T4a**: moderately advanced local disease (invades through outer cortex of thyroid cartilage or invades tissues beyond the larynx); **T4b**: very advanced local disease (invades prevertebral space, encases carotid artery, or invades mediastinal structures) (25–40% regional metastasis)

***N*** (*see* p. 276)

***M*** (*see* p. 258)

# Subglottic Site

## Overview

- <u>Anatomic Boundaries</u>: from 1 cm below the true vocal folds to the inferior cricoid cartilage
- **rare** primary site
- <u>SSx</u>: airway obstruction (biphasic stridor), hoarseness, dysphagia, odynophagia, hemoptysis, weight loss, sore throat
- <u>Histology</u>: ciliated pseudostratified columnar epithelium
- often silent, poorly differentiated, usually extends into cricoid cartilage
- poor prognosis
- <20% regional metastasis

## Staging *(Based on AJCC Staging, 2010)*

*T*

- **T1**: primary tumor limited to subglottis
- **T2**: primary tumor involves vocal folds with normal or impaired mobility
- **T3**: primary tumor limited to larynx with fixed vocal folds
- **T4**: further invasion; **T4a**: moderately advanced local disease (invades cricoid or thyroid cartilage, or tissues beyond the larynx); **T4b**: very advanced local disease (invades prevertebral space, encases carotid artery, or invades mediastinal structures)

*N* (*see* p. 276)

*M* (*see* p. 258)

# Pathology

## Squamous Cell Carcinoma

- >95% of laryngeal cancer
- **Basaloid Squamous Cell Carcinoma**: more aggressive high-grade variant

## Verrucous Carcinoma (Ackerman's Tumor)

- slow-growing, locally destructive (rare metastasis)
- excellent prognosis
- glottis most common site in the larynx
- <u>Gross Lesion</u>: rough, exophytic (warty), fungating, gray-white color

- <u>Histopathology</u>: benign-appearing (nonmitotic, no infiltration), well-differentiated squamous epithelium with papillary projections
- extensive hyperkeratosis, basement membrane intact, "**pushing**" margins
- <u>Rx</u>: single-modality radiation versus surgery (controversy surrounds possible malignant transformation of verrucous carcinoma with radiation therapy)

## Adenocarcinoma

- 1% of laryngeal cancer
- primarily supraglottic and subglottic regions (follows distribution of the laryngeal mucous glands)
- more aggressive than squamous cell carcinoma
- presents submucosal and nonulcerative

## Others

- **Adenoid Cystic Carcinoma**: perineural spread, indolent course, may present with distant metastasis years after primary therapy
- **Spindle Cell Carcinoma**: poorly differentiated variant of squamous cell carcinoma with malignant spindle cell stromal component
- **Neuroendocrine Tumors**: paragangliomas, carcinoid tumors, small (oat) cell carcinoma
- **Mucoepidermoid Carcinoma**: low, intermediate, and high grade
- **Sarcomas**: fibrosarcoma, chondrosarcoma, malignant fibrous histiocytoma, rhabdosarcoma
- **Metastatic**: rare; primary sites from kidney, prostate, breast, stomach, and lung

# Premalignant Glottic Lesions

## Introduction

### Histologic Classification

- **Hyperplasia and Hyperkeratosis**: an increase in the number of cells and keratin production, not a significant risk factor for malignant degeneration
- **Mild Dysplasia**: abnormal dyskaryotic squamous cells with mild atypical cytologic alteration involving cell size, shape, color, and organization; not a significant risk factor for malignant degeneration
- **Moderate Dysplasia**: atypical cytologic alteration involving cell size, shape, color, and organization; risk factor for malignant degeneration

- **Severe Dysplasia (Carcinoma in Situ)**: cells demonstrate cytologic features of malignancy without invasion beyond the basement membrane (risk of developing invasive carcinoma varies from 15–25%)
- **Microinvasive Carcinoma**: malignant cells involving entire thickness of mucosa with discrete foci that invade beyond the basement membrane
- **Invasive Carcinoma**: malignant cells that frankly invade through the basement membrane

### *Biopsy Techniques*

- **Incisional Biopsy**: more random, risk of "missing" tumor, less morbidity
- **Excisional Biopsy**: may be therapeutic for early glottic carcinoma
- **Microflap Excision**: excisional biopsy technique that dissects superficial lamina propria, spares vocal ligament, better preservation of the mucosal wave, indicated for superficial and midmembranous lesions
- **Vocal Fold Stripping**: excisional biopsy technique that removes the vocal fold cover, risk of normal tissue stripping, imprecise, impairs mucosal wave

## Management of Severe Dysplasia (Carcinoma in Situ) and Microinvasive Carcinoma

- smoking and alcohol cessation
- may treat initially with radiation therapy versus surgical excision (microflap excision or vocal fold stripping, *see previous*)
- may consider radiation for recurrence after initial excision
- close follow-up every 2–3 months for 5 years with low threshold to repeat biopsy
- may consider excisional biopsy every 3 months until 2 consecutive negative results for microinvasive carcinoma
- consider $CO_2$ laser

# Management of Laryngeal Carcinoma

## Early Supraglottic Carcinoma (T1–T2)

- <u>Single-Modality Therapy</u>: primary radiation to primary site (surgical salvage for failure) versus supraglottic laryngectomy
- <u>N0 Neck</u>: elective bilateral selective neck dissection versus elective radiation therapy to neck regardless of presence of clinically evident

nodes; if the surgical specimen is positive for tumors consider observation, completion of a comprehensive neck dissection, or radiation therapy to neck

- <u>N1–N3 Neck</u>: modified radical neck dissection for clinical nodes
- <u>Adjuvant Therapy</u>: postoperative radiation therapy may be considered for positive or close margins; multiple positive neck nodes or extracapsular extension; perineural or intravascular invasion; bone, cartilage, or soft tissue invasion; or if an emergent tracheotomy is required (increased risk of tumor seeding)

## Advanced Supraglottic Cancer (T3–T4)

- <u>Multimodality Therapy</u>: total laryngectomy (extended supraglottic laryngectomy for select T3 and T4) and postoperative radiation therapy versus chemotherapy and radiation therapy for organ preservation or for nonoperative candidates
- <u>N0 Neck</u>: elective ipsilateral selective neck dissection (lateral) regardless of presence of clinically evident nodes
- <u>N1–N3 Neck</u>: modified radical neck dissection for clinical nodes

## Early Glottic Carcinoma (T1–T2)

- <u>Single-Modality Therapy</u>: limited-field primary radiation therapy or surgical management (cordectomy, endoscopic procedures, or partial laryngectomies) for failed radiation therapy or a patient requesting quick definitive therapy (away from radiation centers)
- <u>Neck</u>: elective neck dissections are **not** indicated for early glottic cancer; however, for rare clinical nodes it may be addressed with radiation or modified neck dissection

## Advanced Glottic Cancer (T3–T4)

- <u>Multimodality Therapy</u>: total laryngectomy (may consider conservation laryngectomy) with postoperative radiation versus organ preservation trial (chemoradiation; or induction chemotherapy then chemoradiation) with salvage total laryngectomy for poor responders (VA Laryngeal Study Group and Intergroup R91–11, *see* p. 263) or primary radiation therapy with surgical salvage
- <u>Neck</u>: elective ipsilateral modified radical neck dissection (may consider selective neck dissection) regardless of presence of clinical nodes
- <u>Laryngeal Organ Preservation</u>: *see* p. 263

## Subglottic Cancer

- no large investigative series exist due to the rarity of subglottic cancer as a primary site
- <u>Single or Multimodality Therapy</u>: extended total laryngectomy with postoperative radiation and/or chemotherapy (for advanced disease) versus primary radiation or chemotherapy and radiation therapy to primary and neck for nonoperative candidates (organ preservation)
- <u>Neck</u>: ipsilateral modified radical neck dissection for clinical nodal disease

# Surgical Techniques

## General Contraindications for Partial Laryngectomy

- now often performed endoscopically with laser (*see* pp. 290, 303 for more on **transoral laser microsurgery [TLM]**) versus open; robot (TORS) is under investigation (*see* p. 333)
- fixed vocal folds (except supracricoid laryngectomies)
- cartilage invasion
- subglottic extension
- significant oropharyngeal extension
- interarytenoid involvement
- tumor spread into neck

## Cordectomy (via Transoral Approach or Laryngofissure)

- <u>Indications</u>: T1 glottic cancer limited to middle third of the vocal fold; no extension of tumor to vocal process or anterior commissure; no invasion into subglottis, ventricle, or false cord
- <u>Technique</u>: transoral approaches may utilize laser (ie, transoral laser microsurgery [TLM], *see* pp. 290, 303), external approach divides laryngeal cartilage at midline (**laryngofissure**), enters glottis at anterior commissure to remove involved vocal fold up to the vocal process of the arytenoid
- <u>Advantages</u>: transoral approach avoids external scar and tracheotomy, external approach provides better access
- <u>Disadvantages</u>: external approach requires initial tracheotomy, morbidity associated with external approach
- <u>European Classification</u>
   I: subepithelial (only epithelium)
   II: subligamental (epithelium, Reinke's space, ligament)

III: transmuscular (above plus vocalis muscle)

IV: total cordectomy (above plus entire muscle to inner pericondrium)

V: extended (Va: anterior resection to contralateral cord; Vb: posterior resection to arytenoid; Vc: superior resection to ventricle, Vd: extended, inferior resection to subglottis up to 1 cm)

## Supraglottic Laryngectomy (Horizontal Hemilaryngectomy)

- <u>Rationale for Procedure</u>: embryologic boundary between false and true vocal folds results in independent lymphatic drainage, supraglottic cancer tends to have pushing borders rather than infiltrating borders
- <u>Indications</u>: T1 or T2 (limited T3) supraglottic tumors; tumor does not involve vocal fold, ventricle, thyroid cartilage, arytenoid, interarytenoid region, piriform, or base of tongue; good pulmonary function tests (forced expiratory volume [FEV1]/forced vital capacity [FVC] >50–60%); patient must also give consent for possible total laryngectomy
- <u>Technique</u>: removes epiglottis, aryepiglottic folds, false vocal folds, pre-epiglottic space, portion of the hyoid bone, and thyroid cartilage (spares true vocal folds and arytenoids)
- <u>Advantages</u>: good voice quality, potential for decannulation, adequate swallow
- <u>Disadvantages</u>: requires initial tracheotomy, extensive postoperative rehabilitation for swallowing (especially after postoperative radiation), increased aspiration risk as superior laryngeal nerve is removed
- **Extended Supraglottic Laryngectomy**: may extend to include excision of base of tongue, hypopharynx, or 1 arytenoid
- **Radiation Salvage**: surgery possible for select small original primaries in which the recurrent cancer correlates with the original primary lesion
- **Endoscopic Laser Supraglottic Laryngectomy (TLM)**: consider for T1–T2 (limited T3) supraglottic tumors that may be accessed endoscopically (eg, suprahyoid epiglottis, aryepiglottic folds, vestibular folds, pharyngoepiglottic folds), tracheotomies are not routinely required, typically provides improved postoperative swallowing function when compared with the transcervical technique (preserves superior laryngeal nerve, tongue base, hyoid bone, and suprahyoid muscles)

## Vertical Partial Laryngectomy (Hemilaryngectomy)

- Indications: select T1–T2 glottic carcinomas; tumor does not extend beyond 1/3 of opposite cord; <10 mm of anterior subglottic extension; or <5 mm of posterior subglottic extension; no posterior commissure, cricoarytenoid joint, aryepiglottic fold, posterior surface of the arytenoid, or paraglottic space involvement, good pulmonary function tests (forced expiratory volume [FEV1]/forced vital capacity [FVC] >50–60%), patient must also give consent for possible total laryngectomy
- Technique: removes one 1 vocal fold from anterior commissure to vocal process (1/2 of the opposite vocal fold may be removed), ipsilateral false cord, ventricle, paraglottic space, and overlying thyroid cartilage (3-mm posterior strip of cartilage preserved)
- Advantages: allows decannulation, functional glottic voice
- Disadvantages: risk of aspiration, requires initial tracheotomy
- **Radiation Salvage**: surgery possible for select small original primaries in which the recurrent cancer correlates with the original primary lesion
- **Extended Hemilaryngectomy**: select T3 lesions or arytenoid involvement; removes 1 vocal fold, arytenoid, and overlying thyroid cartilage (3-mm posterior strip of cartilage preserved)

## Supracricoid Laryngectomy

- Rationale for Procedure: goal is to achieve decannulation, good swallowing, and voice function with comparable local control and survival rates versus a total laryngectomy
- Indications: select T3–T4 glottic and supraglottic cancers that may involve the pre-epiglottic space, paraglottic space, ventricle, limited thyroid cartilage, or epiglottis; good pulmonary function tests (forced expiratory volume [FEV1]/forced vital capacity [FVC] >50–60%); patient must also give consent for possible total laryngectomy
- Contraindications: **arytenoid fixation**; infraglottic extent of tumor reaching upper border of cricoid cartilage; major pre-epiglottic involvement; invasion of the cricoid cartilage, perichondrium of thyroid cartilage, hyoid bone, posterior arytenoid mucosa; extralaryngeal involvement; or poor pulmonary function
- Technique: remove entire thyroid cartilage, bilateral true and false vocal folds, one arytenoid (may spare both arytenoids if not involved), and paraglottic space; spares cricoid cartilage, hyoid bone, and at least 1 arytenoid cartilage (for speech and swallowing); may reconstruct with **cricohyoidopexy (CHP) or cricohyoidoepiglottopexy (CHEP)** if epiglottis is spared

- <u>Advantages</u>: allows decannulation, functional glottic voice
- <u>Disadvantages</u>: risk of aspiration, requires initial tracheotomy, dysphonia
- **Radiation Salvage**: surgery possible for select small original primaries in which the recurrent cancer correlates with the original primary lesion

## Total Laryngectomy

- <u>Indications</u>: standard therapy for any laryngeal cancer that precludes conservative management (advanced disease, recurrence, radiation failure, patients with poor pulmonary function)
- <u>Technique</u>: removes entire larynx (true and false vocal folds, cricoid and thyroid cartilage, both arytenoids, epiglottis, pre-epiglottic and paraglottic spaces, and hyoid bone), creates complete separation between pharynx and trachea
- <u>Advantages</u>: no risk of aspiration
- <u>Disadvantages</u>: requires a permanent stoma, fair voice quality (with tracheoesophageal speech)
- **Near-Total Laryngectomy (3/4 Laryngectomy)**: creates a communication between trachea and pharynx for phonation, must keep 1 arytenoid to prevent aspiration through shunt

## Postoperative Complications

- **Fistula**: increased incidence with radiation therapy; <u>Rx</u>: hold oral feeding (must, however, maximize nutritional status by parenteral or tube feeding for wound healing), medialize fistula if there is possible involvement of carotid artery (to prevent carotid blowout), antibiotic regimen (culture and sensitivity of wound drainage), daily loose wet to dry packing of fistula site to stimulate granulation tissue, local debridement of necrotic tissue, consider flap closure for recalcitrant drainage
- **Tracheotomy Complications**: pneumothorax, hemorrhage, subcutaneous emphysema (*see also* p. 106)
- **Speech Alteration**: variety of postoperative causes including granulation tissue, scar formation, glottic incompetence, vocal fold paralysis; <u>Rx</u>: postoperatively all patients should follow up with speech therapist for videostroboscopy and voice analysis to address phonatory defects
- **Persistent Aspiration, Bronchopneumonia, and Deglutition Problems**: increased incidence with the elderly (poor pulmonary function), conservation laryngectomies, excision of arytenoid or base of tongue, and vagal nerve injury; <u>Rx</u>: postoperatively patients must

follow up with a swallowing therapist to evaluate for aspiration and swallowing disorders; therapy varies depending on etiology from swallowing rehabilitation to laryngeal reconstruction surgery (*see also* pp. 187–192)

- **Delayed Decannulation**: typically secondary to laryngeal edema and laryngeal stenosis (*see following*); <u>Rx</u>: must examine endoscopically for recurrence or persistent disease; may then consider steroid injections, endoscopic excision ($CO_2$ laser) or open thyrotomy with mucosal flap and resurfacing
- **Esophageal or Pharyngeal Stenosis**: typically secondary to scarring; <u>Rx</u>: must examine endoscopically to examine for recurrence; may then consider serial dilation, endoscopic excision ($CO_2$ laser), or pharyngoesophageal reconstruction with regional or free-flap transfer
- **Perichondritis and Chondritis**: increased risk with inadequate coverage of bare cartilage; <u>Rx</u>: antibiotic regimen; may consider local debridement, resection of infected cartilage with reconstruction, or hyperbaric oxygen therapy
- **Stomal Stenosis**: prevented with Bivona prosthesis (laryngectomy tube that acts as a stent) and by making beveled incisions in the distal trachea during laryngectomy, may consider releasing sternal attachments of the sternocleidomastoid; <u>Rx</u>: must evaluate for stomal recurrence, may require surgical dilation
- *see also* complications of neck dissections, pp. 280–282

# Postoperative Voice Management

- postlaryngectomy patients may always select writing as their form of communication rather than voicing

## Artificial Larynx (Electrolarynx)

- <u>Mechanism</u>: buzzing sound introduced into neck tissue from a handheld device and emanated from the mouth, oral type features a straw-like extension (oral tube) that directs sound directly to the oral cavity
- <u>Advantages</u>: easy to learn, inexpensive, loud
- <u>Disadvantages</u>: requires batteries, produces a mechanical voice, requires hands, oral tubes may be required

## Esophageal Speech

- <u>Mechanism</u>: produced by vibration of pharyngoesophageal mucosa; requires trapping air in mouth, injecting air into the esophagus, and expulsion of air ("burping") to create voice

- <u>Advantages</u>: more natural voice, hands free, no appliance required
- <u>Disadvantages</u>: difficult learning (30% success rate), quiet speech

## Tracheoesophageal Puncture

- <u>Mechanism</u>: one-way valve allows air to enter esophagus to allow esophageal speech, which is produced by vibration of the pharyngoesophageal mucosa
- <u>Advantages</u>: more natural voice quality, less conspicuous
- <u>Disadvantages</u>: may not work (most common failure from pharyngeal constrictor spasm, can decrease the risk by performing a generous ~5 cm cricopharyngeal myotomy), requires hands (can improve access by releasing the medial third of the sternocleidomastoid muscles bilaterally), risk of aspiration and esophageal prolapse, may require second procedure to place, requires periodic cleaning and replacement

# NASOPHARYNGEAL CANCER
## Introduction

### Overview

- <u>SSx</u>: **neck mass** (most common initial symptom, 70%, often painless), serous otitis media from eustachian tube obstruction (second most common presentation, 50%), nasal obstruction, cranial nerve palsies (abducens nerve most common), recurrent epistaxis, trismus, headache
- <u>Risk Factors</u>: regional distribution (Southern China, Northern Africa, Southeast Asia, Alaska, Greenland), Epstein-Barr virus (EBV), genetic predisposition

### Epstein-Barr Virus Association

- **Early Intracellular Antigen (EA)**: early antigen
- **Viral Capsule Antigen (VCA)**: late antigen, most specific immunologic finding in nasopharyngeal cancer
- low titers of the IgA EA and IgA VCA and antibody-dependent cell-mediated cytotoxicity (ADCC) for other EBV antigens predict poorer prognosis, higher titers predict better prognosis
- elevated IgA VCA and EA may be used to screen for nasopharyngeal carcinoma in high-risk regions

## Anatomy

- **Nasopharynx**: anteriorly bordered by the choanae, superiorly bordered by the base of skull (body of the sphenoid), inferiorly bordered by the plane of the soft palate, laterally bordered by eustachian tube orifices, posteriorly bordered by the superior constrictor muscles
- **Fossa of Rosenmüller**: slitlike region medial to the medial crura of the eustachian tube orifice, most common site of tumor in the nasopharynx
- **Passavant's Ridge**: interdigitating superior constrictor muscles that form a band at the posterior pharyngeal wall during swallowing that abuts the soft palate
- <u>Subsites</u>: posterior nasopharyngeal wall, lateral nasopharyngeal wall, soft palate
- <u>Histology</u>: lymphoid tissue and epithelium (pseudostratified ciliated columnar cells and stratified squamous cells)

# Classification and Management

**Staging** *(Based on AJCC Staging, 2010)*

*T*

- **T1**: primary tumor confined to nasopharynx, or extends to oropharynx or nasal cavity (without parapharyngeal extension)
- **T2**: primary tumor with parapharyngeal extension
- **T3**: primary tumor invades bony structures of the skull base or paranasal sinuses
- **T4**: primary tumor invasion intracranially or of cranial nerves, hypopharynx, orbit, or with extension to the infratemporal fossa/masticator space

*N*

- *NOTE:* different from most other head and neck cancer N staging
- **NX**: lymph nodes cannot be assessed
- **N0**: no regional lymph node metastasis
- **N1**: unilateral metastasis in cervical lymph node(s), ≤6 cm in greatest dimension, above the supraclavicular fossa, and/or unilateral or bilateral, retropharyngeal lymph nodes, ≤6 cm in greatest dimension (midline nodes are considered ipsilateral)
- **N2**: bilateral metastasis in cervical lymph node(s), ≤6 cm in greatest dimension, above the supraclavicular fossa (midline nodes are considered ipsilateral nodes)

- **N3a**: >6 cm in dimension
- **N3b**: extension to the supraclavicular fossa

*M* (*see* p. 258)

## World Health Organization (WHO) Classification

- based on histopathology
- **WHO Type I: Keratinizing Squamous Cell Carcinoma**, second most common subtype, squamous differentiation, **not** associated with EBV, **sporadic**, worse prognosis, less sensitive to radiation
- **WHO Type II: Nonkeratinizing Squamous Cell Carcinoma**, does not demonstrate definite squamous differentiation, associated with **EBV**, **endemic**, better prognosis, sensitive to radiation
- **WHO Type III: Undifferentiated Carcinoma** (includes lymphoepithelioma, anaplastic, and clear cell variants), **most common** subtype, indistinct cell margins, may have lymphocytic stroma (**lymphoepithelioma**), associated with **EBV**, **endemic** (seen most commonly in southern China), better prognosis, sensitive to radiation
- Other Types: lymphoma, adenocarcinoma, plasma cell myelomas, cylindromas, adenoid cystic carcinoma, melanoma, carcinosarcoma, unclassified spindling malignant neoplasm

## Management

- Stage I–II: not a surgical disease, radiotherapy to primary site and bilateral necks (regardless of nodal status)
- Stage III–IV: concurrent chemoradiotherapy (cisplatin/5-FU) followed by adjuvant chemotherapy (Phase III Intergroup Study 0099, *see* p. 262)
- limited surgical role (neck dissections may be considered for postradiation salvage surgery, tracheotomy if airway issues)

# NASAL AND PARANASAL CANCER
# Introduction

## Overview

- Risk Factors: toxin exposure (nickel, chromium, mustard gas, hydrocarbons, and radium), woodworkers (soft wood type: increased risk for squamous cell carcinoma; hard and soft wood type: increased risk for adenocarcinoma), chronic infection, previous radiation

- <u>SSx</u>: unilateral persistent sinusitis, nasal obstruction, or epistaxis; nasal lesions (exophytic, ulcerative, septal perforation); orbital symptoms (proptosis, diplopia, vision loss); anosmia and taste disturbances; palatal fistula; cranial nerve palsies, headache, facial paresthesia, and pain
- <u>Prognosis</u>: maxillary tumors in general have 5-year survival rates of 20–50%, tumors posterior or superior to **Ohngren's line** (plane from medial canthus to angle of jaw) suggest poorer prognosis due to higher instances of skull base invasion and perineural spread
- maxillary sinus is the most common site for nasal and paranasal cancer (nasal cavity second most common)
- overall low (<10%) risk for occult neck metastases

## Subsites

- **Paranasal Sinuses**: maxillary sinus most common site involved (ethmoid sinus is the second most common sinus), typically presents in an advanced stage (90% invade more than 1 wall), sphenoid sinus has a higher instance of neurologic sequelae (cranial nerve palsies, orbital symptoms, headache), frontal sinus rare site of primary cancer
- **Nasal Cavity**: <10% regional metastatic potential; 60% 5-year survival; worse prognosis for larger tumors, extension outside the nasal cavity, bony involvement, and regional metastasis
- **Anterior Cranial Fossa**: bordered posteriorly by the lesser wing of the sphenoid and optic chiasm, extends to the frontal bone; the floor contains the orbital plates of the frontal bone, fovea ethmoidalis, and cribriform plate
- **Pterygopalatine Fossa**: pyramidal-shaped space below the apex of the orbit and between the posterior wall of the maxillary sinus and the pterygoid plates; contains the foramen rotundum (CN $V_2$), vidian nerve, sphenopalatine nerve, lesser and greater palatine nerves, pterygopalatine (sphenopalatine) ganglion, and maxillary artery; invasion of this space carries a poor prognosis
- **Infratemporal Fossa**: bounded anteriorly by the maxilla, posteriorly by the glenoid fossa and mandible, and medially by the lateral pterygoid plates; roof contains the foramen ovale (CN $V_3$) and foramen spinosum (middle meningeal artery and vein), also contains the pterygoid muscles
- **Orbital Cavity**: invasion into bony orbit or orbital apex requires orbit exenteration

# Pathology

## Epithelial Malignancy

- **Squamous Cell Carcinoma**: most common malignancy in sinonasal tissue, sinonasal lesions are more aggressive and have a higher rate of metastasis, majority are moderately differentiated keratinizing type
- **Adenocarcinoma**: increased instances with wood and leather workers, presents more commonly in the ethmoid sinuses
- **Adenoid Cystic Carcinoma**: salivary gland tumor (more common in the minor salivary glands), insidious growth (distant metastasis may present years later), perineural extension may present with pain
- **Mucoepidermoid Carcinoma**: rare, salivary gland tumor
- **Melanoma (Mucosal Melanoma)**: more common in nasal cavity (anterior nasal septum), high risk of local recurrence, poor prognosis, *see* pp. 326–327
- **Esthesioneuroblastoma (Olfactory Neuroblastoma)**: rare, arises from olfactory epithelium, bimodal frequency (presents in teenagers and the elderly), presents as a pink or brown friable nasal mass, excellent prognosis if confined to nasal cavity; <u>Staging</u>: clinical (Kadish) staging, improved based on radiology (CT/MRI) using the Dulguerov-Calcaterra system (T1: nasal cavity + sinus except sphenoid and superior ethmoids; T2: + sphenoid and cribriform; T3: + orbit and/or extradural anterior cranial fossa; T4: brain involvement) <u>Rx</u>: surgical excision (classically craniofacial resection; however, transnasal endoscopic and more limited transfacial approaches now common) with postoperative radiation (consider neo- or adjuvant chemotherapy)
- **Sinonasal Neuroendocrine Carcinoma (SNEC)**: arises near olfactory groove
- **Sinonasal Undifferentiated Carcinoma (SNUC)**: arises near olfactory groove, extensive tissue destruction, rapidly progressive, extremely poor prognosis
- **Small Cell Carcinoma**: extremely poor prognosis; <u>Rx</u>: nonsurgical, chemotherapy, and radiation
- *NOTE*: differentiation may require immunohistochemical analysis (*see* p. 258)

## Nonepithelial Malignancy

- **Rhabdomyosarcoma**: more aggressive than other head and neck sites; embryologic, alveolar, and pleomorphic (more common in adults) subtypes; management in children is typically radiation and

chemotherapy, adults typically require initial wide surgical excision
with postoperative radiation

- **Hemangiopericytoma (Solitary Fibrous Tumor)**: rare, highly
  vascular, arises from pericytes of Zimmermann (located outside of
  endothelial cells, capable of changing the caliber of the capillaries),
  presents as a lobulated mass and epistaxis, may require preoperative
  embolization prior to excision
- **Neurogenic Sarcoma**: rare, aggressive, associated with
  neurofibromatosis
- **Leiomyosarcoma**: smooth muscle tumor, poor prognosis
- **Fibrosarcoma**: tumors of fibroblasts, associated with trauma and
  radiation
- **Angiosarcoma**: slow growing but locally aggressive with indistinct
  margins
- **Osteogenic Sarcoma and Chondrosarcoma**: aggressive, poor
  prognosis (10–20% 5-year survival), arise from the facial skeleton,
  more common in the mandible than in the maxilla
- **Lymphoma**: typically non-Hodgkin's (*see* pp. 327–330)
- **Metastatic Tumors**: renal cell carcinoma most common
- **Chordoma**: malignant, slow growing, from notochord remnant,
  arises from clivus/skull base, key pathologic finding is physaliferous
  cells

# Management

## Treatment Concepts

- <u>Early Stages</u>: single-modality primarily with surgical resection
  for early maxillary or nasal cavity tumors except for small cell
  carcinoma, lymphoma, and rhabdomyosarcoma (except for
  debulking, postoperative radiation therapy may be considered for
  close or positive margins or bony invasion) versus primary radiation
  therapy (radiation therapy is limited by orbital and intracranial
  complications, eg, blindness, keratitis, brain necrosis)
- <u>Advanced Stages</u>: multimodality therapy with either primary
  radiation therapy with surgical salvage or primary surgical excision
  with postoperative radiation therapy, inoperable patients for whom
  resection would result in severe cosmetic and functional morbidity
  (eg, sphenoid tumors) should undergo primary radiation therapy
  with surgical salvage
- <u>Unresectable/Nonoperative Candidates</u>: consider primary radiation,
  chemotherapy, or combination radiochemotherapy
- <u>N0 Neck</u>: elective neck dissection generally not indicated (may
  be considered if tumor involves the nasopharynx or soft palate)

otherwise treat neck for clinical nodal disease only (<10% occult metastasis)
- <u>N1–N3 Neck</u>: neck dissection, parotid nodes require a superficial parotidectomy
- some nonsquamous tumors (eg, rhabdomyosarcoma, small cell carcinoma) may benefit from chemotherapy

## Surgical Management

- surgery may be considered for cranial base extension (infratemporal fossa), contraindications for surgical resection include involvement of significant brain parenchyma, cavernous sinus, bilateral orbits, optic chiasm, or carotid artery
- orbit exenteration is indicated when there is periorbital bony erosion or tumor is within the orbital apex (via direct bony erosion, perineural or perivascular spread, or infraorbital fissure or nasolacrimal duct extension)
- craniotomy (craniofacial resection) is indicated if tumor is involved superior to cribriform plate or roof of the ethmoid sinuses

### Endoscopic Approaches

- low morbidity, no external scar
- previously limited to small benign lesions, now increasingly common for more aggressive tumors
- approaches include transnasal and others (eg, transorbital)
- may be performed for definitive resection, debulking followed by adjuvant treatment, or for palliation

### Transfacial Open Approaches

- **Lateral Rhinotomy**: incision begins at medial aspect of the eyebrow, follows along the nasal lateral wall, and around alar crease to the philtrum and a sublabial incision; may extend incision to include (split) the lip for exposure of hard palate; standard approach for medial maxillectomy, provides excellent visualization of maxillary wall, ethmoid sinus, sphenoid sinus, medial orbital wall, and nasal cavity
- **Midfacial Degloving**: requires transfixation, bilateral intercartilaginous and gingivobuccal incisions; limited to lesions of inferior and medial maxillary walls (limited superior and anterior visualization); avoids external incisions and allows bilateral exposure
- **Facial Translocation**: indicated for wide exposure of the middle cranial base, infratemporal fossa, pterygopalatine fossa, and nasopharynx, requires extensive facial flaps, more limited degree

of facial nerve transection (requires only transection of the frontal branch)
- **Transpalatal Approach**: indicated for tumors involving the floor of nose or inferior portion of the maxilla, may be used in conjunction with a lateral rhinotomy
- **Weber-Fergusson Approach**: consists of a lateral rhinotomy including a lip-splitting incision that connects with a sublabial incision as well as a subciliary or transconjunctival incision, allows additional exposure of maxilla for a total maxillectomy
- **Infratemporal Fossa Approach**: access obtained via a preauricular or postauricular incision with extension in a hemicoronal and cervical fashion, may gain additional exposure by retracting the temporomandibular joint
- **Combined Craniofacial Approach**: combines the above facial incisions with a bicoronal incision to allow exposure for a craniotomy

### Cranial Approaches

- **Wide Frontal Craniotomy**: standard approach
- **Narrow Frontal Craniotomy**: limited approach
- **Subfrontal Craniotomy**: remove frontal bar complex, allows option to avoid a transfacial approach

### Surgical Resection Types

- **Medial Maxillectomy**: removes lateral nasal wall and medial maxilla, may also include a complete sphenoethmoidectomy, standard resection for inverted papilloma, may be performed endoscopically or open
- **Inferior Maxillectomy**: resects the inferior portion of the maxillary sinus inferior to the infraorbital nerve, indicated for tumors involving the maxillary alveolar process or limited hard palate lesions
- **Total Maxillectomy**: en bloc removal of entire maxilla, indicated for tumors involving the maxillary antrum; bony cuts include zygomaticomaxillary suture line, orbital floor, and medial orbital wall, nasomaxillary suture line, hard palate, and pterygoid plates
- **Radical Maxillectomy**: total maxillectomy with orbital exenteration
- **Craniofacial Resection**: en bloc removal of the anterior cranial base including the cribriform plate and ethmoid sinuses, may require dural excision

### Reconstruction

- **Fascial, Temporalis Muscle, or Pericranial/Galeal Flaps**: provide additional support for watertight closure of skull base and dural defects allowing for adequate cranionasal separation

- **Regional or Microvascular Free Flaps**: provide soft tissue bulk (_see_ pp. 449–458)
- **Prosthetic Obturator**: indicated for inferior maxillary or palatal defects, provides oronasal separation, a surgical obturator (or a patient's denture) is placed initially to allow better speech and swallowing function and is later replaced with a permanent device

### Surgical Complications

- **Intracranial Infections (Meningitis, Cerebritis)**: most significant complication, may occur with a CSF leak, life-threatening; R̲x̲: _see_ pp. 54–55
- **CSF Leak**: prevented by avoiding dissection above cribriform plate, watertight closure of the dura, consider lumbar drainage for high-risk procedures, avoid postoperative straining; R̲x̲: _see_ p. 61
- **Cerebrovascular**: may be secondary to excessive brain retraction
- **Orbital Complications**: extraocular muscle entrapment, optic nerve compression, blindness; R̲x̲: _see_ p. 60
- **Frontal Lobe Syndrome**: frontal lobe dysfunction results in changes in patient's affect, may be permanent
- **Osteitis**: may be secondary to a wound infection or skin flap necrosis
- **Epiphora**: typically from lacrimal duct injury; R̲x̲: consider dacryocystorhinostomy if no resolution
- **Hemorrhage**: increased risk with vascular tumors, may consider preoperative embolization of select tumors; R̲x̲: electrocautery, nasal or surgical cavity packing
- **Tension Pneumocephalus**: occurs from trapped air that enters into the cranial cavity from the sinonasal tract, high risk of brain herniation, may be caused by excessive lumbar CSF drainage; R̲x̲: emergent aspiration, re-exploration to define leak
- **Cranial Nerve Injuries**: combined injuries to CN III, IV, V1, $V_2$, and VI occur in **cavernous sinus syndrome** (versus CN **II**, III, IV, $V_1$, and VI for orbital apex syndrome), which causes total ophthalmoplegia of the affected globe; _see also_ pp. 121–124 for management of vagal nerve injuries; _see also_ pp. 431–433 for facial nerve injuries; other cranial nerve injuries at risk are CN II and V

# CUTANEOUS MALIGNANCIES
## Basal Cell Carcinoma
### Introduction

- most common cancer in humans, ~80% of skin cancer, head and neck is most common location

- indolent course, extends peripherally without vertical invasion
- rare metastasis
- cutaneous lesions located in the embryonic fusion plates ("H" zone) of the face (nasolabial folds, floor of nose, columella, preauricular regions, inner and outer canthus of the eye) are more aggressive and have a higher risk of recurrence, therefore require close follow-up
- 90% cure rate in the head and neck
- <u>Risks</u>: ultraviolet light exposure (UV-B), fair skin, blue-green eyes, sunburns as a child, regions of previous burns (**Marjolin's ulcer**, although less common than with squamous cell carcinoma) and scars, radiodermatitis, arsenic exposure (eg, found in Fowler's solution used for psoriasis), immunosuppression, xeroderma pigmentosum (autosomal recessive disorder caused by a defect in DNA repair), previous basal cell carcinoma
- <u>Dx</u>: excisional biopsy of suspicious lesions

## Histopathology

- principal cells resemble basal cells (small, dark-blue cells with minimal cytoplasm) of the epidermis
- **Undifferentiated (Solid Type)**: proliferation of basaloid cells that extend into the papillary dermis, peripheral columnar cells arranged in palisades
- **Keratotic**: differentiated to hair-like structures
- **Cystic**: differentiated to sebaceous gland-like structures
- **Adenoid**: differentiated to tubular structures, lace-like histologic pattern

## Types

- **Nodular (Noduloulcerative): most common**, pearly, telangiectatic papule, central ulceration, "rolled" appearance at the base
- **Superficial**: typically found in the trunk and extremities (rare in the head and neck), scaly, waxy, indurated, irregular shapes (similar to eczema)
- **Morphea (Sclerosing or Fibrosing)**: common on the face; flat or depressed, indurated, yellow, indistinct borders (similar appearance to a scar); resembles the cutaneous form of scleroderma; **aggressive**, higher rate of recurrence, worst prognosis
- **Pigmented**: similar to nodular type; however, more pigmented, resembles a melanoma or benign nevus
- **Fibroepithelioma**: raised, firm, pedunculated or sessile, red with smooth skin surface

- **Basosquamous Carcinoma**: more aggressive form with features of squamous cell carcinoma

## Management

- avoid excess sun exposure (sunblock)
- careful follow-up for recurrence and second primaries every 4–6 months
- **Excisional Curettage with Electrodesiccation**: most common treatment modality, ideal for small (<2 cm) solid-type, contraindicated for morphea lesions
- **Cryosurgery**: intense cold causes tissue necrosis, requires freeze, thaw, freeze technique for deeper destruction of tissue, requires a 5-mm margin, may be considered for small (<1 cm) lesions
- **Scalpel Excision**: should have 4 mm margin with primary reconstruction (consider intraoperative frozen sections)
- **Radiation Therapy**: consider where cosmetic outcome is important (eyelid, nose, lip) or nonoperative candidates, very radiosensitive, use electron beam radiation because lesions are superficial (as opposed to traditional photon treatment for deeper lesions), advanced stages may be followed by surgical salvage
- **Targeted Chemotherapy**: vismodegib (hedgehog inhibitor) for metastatic or locally advanced basal cell carcinoma that cannot be treated with surgery or radiation (*see* pp. 268–270)

### Mohs Micrographic Surgery (Chemosurgery)

- utilizing intraoperative microscopic examination of all resection margins for complete excision (~96% success)
- Indications: recurrence, morphea type, high risk of recurrence regions ("H-zone"), cosmetic regions in which reconstruction is difficult (eyelids, lips, nose, ears, nasolabial fold)
- Technique: excise lesion while maintaining proper orientation to create a tumor map of the specimen, section specimen and fix to slides, examine microscopically for adequate margins, re-excise regions involved with tumor, repeat until histologic sections are free of tumor

## Nevoid Basal Cell Carcinoma Syndrome (Gorlin's Syndrome, Basal Cell Nevus Syndrome)

- Pathophysiology: autosomal dominant disorder

- <u>SSx</u>: multiple basal cell carcinomas appear at early age, **keratocystic odontogenic tumor** (*see* pp. 219–220), rib abnormalities (bifid ribs), scoliosis, mental retardation, frontal bossing
- <u>Rx</u>: excise malignant lesions, close follow-up every 3–6 months

# Squamous Cell Carcinoma

## Introduction

- second most common skin cancer (approximately 30%)
- 1–4% metastatic potential
- tendency for vertical growth
- more aggressive lesions and higher recurrence rates arise from lesions from previous scars and wounds (**Marjolin's ulcer**), lesions located on embryonic fusion plates (nasolabial folds, floor of nose, columella, preauricular regions, inner and outer canthus of the eye), lesions arising de novo (non-sun-exposed skin), and lesions deep (>6 mm) and large in size (>2 cm)
- <u>Risks</u>: similar to basal cell carcinoma; additional risk factors include **actinic keratosis** (warty, sandpaper-like, scaly lesions on sun-exposed skin), previous squamous cell carcinoma lesions, and infection by HPV (especially types 16, 18)
- <u>SSx</u>: erythematous, hyperkeratotic, opaque nodule, ulcerative, granular base, bleeds easily

## Histopathology Variants

- **Solar Keratosis**: atypical squamous cells extend past the dermal-epidermal junction into the papillary dermis, may not exhibit keratin pearls
- **Spindle Cell**: occurs more commonly at site of a scar, trauma, or burn; elongated nuclei arranged in a swirling pattern, more aggressive
- **Adenoid**: pseudoglandular arrangement, acantholytic dyskeratotic cells, commonly located periauricularly in the elderly, more aggressive
- **Verrucous**: warty appearance, less aggressive (low-grade malignancy)
- **Bowen's Disease**: erythematous patch or plaque, may have scales, noninvasive (**carcinoma in situ**)

## Management

- avoid excess sun exposure (sunblock)
- careful follow-up for recurrence and second primaries initially every 1 month for 6 months then every 4–6 months

- **Surgical Excision**: should have 4–6 mm margins for early disease and 1–2 cm margins for advanced disease
- **Radiation Therapy**: may be considered where cosmetic outcome is important (eyelid, nose, lip) or nonoperative candidates, advanced stages may be followed by surgical salvage
- **Mohs Micrographic Surgery (Chemosurgery)**: similar indications as basal cell carcinoma
- **Neck Dissection and Superficial Parotidectomy**: indicated for clinically positive nodes only
- **Postoperative Radiation Therapy**: may be considered for close or positive margins; multiple positive neck nodes or extracapsular extension, perineural or intravascular invasion, recurrent lesions, or bone or cartilage invasion

# Melanoma

## Introduction

- **10–25%** of melanomas present in head and neck (most common head and neck sites are the skin of the cheek and the occipital scalp)
- <u>Risks</u>: ultraviolet light exposure (UV-B), sunburns in childhood, fair skin (blue–green eyes), immunosuppression, large congenital nevi (>20 cm), sporadic or inherited dysplastic nevi (**familial dysplastic nevus syndrome**, autosomal dominant), genetic disposition, previous melanomas
- <u>ABCDs of Melanoma</u>: **A**symmetry (irregular shaped), **B**order irregularity, **C**olor variation (color changes within the lesion), **D**iameter (>1 cm, increasing size), **E** is sometimes added for evolving (changing lesion), also bleeding and ulceration
- <u>Dx</u>: excisional biopsy of suspicious lesions (shave biopsy, curettage, and laser excision are contraindicated if melanoma is suspected); **HMB-45 tumor marker** fairly specific for melanoma, more recent markers are MART-1 and melan A (*see* p. 258)
- *see* pp. 332–333 for differential diagnosis of neuroendocrine malignancies

## Types and Histopathology

- **Superficial Spreading Melanoma: most common**, 70% from preexisting junctional nevi, radial phase predominates (lateral growth), ulceration suggests vertical phase growth, neoplastic melanocytes form aggregates and invade all levels of the dermis
- **Nodular Melanoma**: very aggressive (rapid vertical phase), may present on non-sun-exposed areas (de novo), worst prognosis, atypical melanocytes invade the reticular dermis

- **Lentigo Maligna**: irregularly hyperpigmented macule, **sun-exposed skin**, more common in the **elderly**, common on the head and neck, confined to epidermis, spreads laterally (extended radial phase), best prognosis, atypical melanocytes tend to remain at the dermal-epidermal junction (*NOTE*: lentigo maligna is carcinoma in situ whereas lentigo maligna melanoma is invasive carcinoma)
- **Acral Lentiginous Melanoma**: presents on **soles of feet and hands**, more common among **blacks**, histologically presents with acanthosis and lentiginous proliferation with lateral growth
- <u>Other Types</u>: **mucosal melanoma** (<10% of head and neck melanoma, poor prognosis; *see* pp. 326–327), **amelanotic melanoma** (nonpigmented, poor prognosis), **desmoplastic**

## Level/Depth Systems

### *Clark's Level*

- **I**: primary tumor involves epidermis only
- **II**: primary tumor invades through basal cell layer
- **III**: primary tumor fills papillary dermis
- **IV**: primary tumor involves reticular dermis
- **V**: primary tumor involves subcutaneous tissue

### *Breslow Thickness*

- measures depth of invasion in mm
- an old staging system stratified with different cutoffs than the current AJCC T system

## Staging *(Based on AJCC Staging, 2010)*

*T* (based on mm measurement of depth, ie, thickness)

- **Tis**: melanoma in situ
- **T1**: ≤1.0 mm thick without ulceration
- **T2**: 1.01–2.0 mm thick
- **T3**: 2.01–4.0 mm thick
- **T4**: > 4.0 mm thick
- <u>T1 Suffix</u>: **a**: without ulceration and mitosis <1/mm$^2$, **b**: with ulceration or mitosis ≥1/mm$^2$; <u>T2–T4 Suffix</u>: **a**: without ulceration, **b**: with ulceration

## *N*

- **N0**: no regional lymph node metastasis detected
- **N1**: 1 metastatic lymph node

- **N2**: 2–3 metastatic lymph nodes
- **N3**: 4 or more metastatic lymph nodes, or matted nodes, or in-transit met(s)/satellite(s) *with* metastatic nodes
- <u>Suffix</u>: **a**: micrometastasis (applied to N1 or N2), **b**: macrometastasis (applied to N1 or N2), **c**: in-transit met(s)/satellite lesion(s) *without* metastatic nodes (applied to N2)

## *M*

- **M0:** no distant metastases detected
- **M1a**: metastases to distant skin, subcutaneous, or distant lymph nodes
- **M1b**: metastases to lung
- **M1c**: metastases to all other visceral sites or distant metastases to any site combined with an elevated LDH

## Management

- prevent by avoiding excess sun exposure (sunblock)
- careful follow-up for recurrence and second primaries every 4–6 months

### *Margins Needed for Surgical Resection*

- **Tis:** 2–5 mm clear margins
- **T1**: 1 cm margins
- **T2**: 1–2 cm margins
- **T3–T4**: 2 cm margins (no difference in survival if larger margins taken)

### *<1 mm Depth (T1)*

- <u>Single-Modality Therapy</u>: excision with 1 cm margin down to fascia
- <u>N0 Neck</u>: elective neck dissection not indicated for superficial lesions

### *1–4-mm Depth (T2–T3)*

- <u>Single-Modality Therapy</u>: excision with up to 2 cm margin down to fascia
- <u>Adjuvant Therapy</u>: may consider interferon α-2b (*see following*)
- <u>N0 Neck</u>: may consider sentinel lymph node biopsy (*see following*), if positive should complete a neck dissection (posterior lateral neck dissections may be considered for scalp lesions); Intergroup Melanoma Surgical Program revealed an overall 5-year survival benefit with elective neck dissections for patients <60 years old with

1 mm to 2 mm melanomas, especially for tumors without ulcerations (*Ann Surg.* 1996;224:255–266)

- N1–N3 Neck: neck dissection (may require a superficial parotidectomy), may consider chemotherapy

### 4 mm Depth (T4)

- Single-Modality Therapy: excision with 2 cm margin down to fascia
- Adjuvant Therapy: consider interferon α-2b (*see following*)
- N0 Neck: elective neck dissections not indicated
- N1–N3 Neck: neck dissection (may require a superficial parotidectomy), may consider chemotherapy

### Metastatic Disease

- dismal prognosis
- Bone Metastasis: single dose of radiation therapy (8 Gy)
- Brain Metastasis: if resectable, surgery; if not resectable, whole-brain radiation therapy
- Chemotherapy: **dacarbazine** or new targeted agents, eg, ipilimumab and vemurafenib (*see* pp. 268–270)

### Interferon α-2b (IFN α-2b)

- Eastern Cooperative Oncology Group (ECOG) Trials 1684, 1690, 1694, and others have demonstrated an improvement in recurrence-free survival of 20–30% with high-dose IFN α-2b and a less clear impact on overall survival, estimated at 3–10% (*J Clin Oncol.* 1996;14:7–17, *J Clin Oncol.* 2002;20:1818–1825, *Clin Cancer Res.* 2004;1670–1677, *Cancer Treat Rev.* 2003;29:241–252, *J Natl Compr Canc Netw.* 2004;2:61–68), FDA approved for stage IIB–III melanoma
- typical duration of therapy is 1 year, durable responses seen in a small number of patients
- Side Effects: cardiac and hepatic toxicity (increased AST), constitutional symptoms (fever, flulike symptoms), myelosuppression, spastic diplegia
- pegylated interferon (PEG-IFN α-2b) FDA approved for stage III melanoma, allows less frequent administration (EORTC 18991)

### Lymphatic Mapping/Sentinel Lymph Node Biopsy

- **Sentinel Node**: first echelon node that drains primary tumor
- **Lymphoscintigraphy and Lymphatic Mapping**: localizes the sentinel node and lymphatic drainage pattern
- **Sentinel Lymph Node Biopsy**: may be recommended for primary tumor that is T2 or greater and/or Clark level IV; in a phase III

trial (MSTL-I) comparing observation versus sentinel node biopsy for intermediate depth melanoma, no difference in overall survival was noted; however, a significant benefit in disease-free survival was observed (*N Engl J Med*. 2006;.355:1307–1317); a phase III trial (MSTL-II) is evaluating the utility of sentinel lymph node biopsy alone versus sentinel lymph node biopsy and completion lymph node dissection in cutaneous melanoma patients with evidence of metastasis in the sentinel node (estimated completion date 2025); recommendation of sentinel node biopsy is thus controversial and a frank discussion with patients is warranted

- elective lymph node dissection is not used for primary disease with no clinical neck nodes
- Technique: preoperatively undergo a lymphoscintigraphy to identify region of the draining basin and sentinel node, intraoperatively inject isosulfan blue dye intradermally to visualize sentinel node during dissection, confirm sentinel node by utilizing a radioactive probe, excise sentinel node and send for frozen section (4–8% false-positive rate)
- if node is **positive** for melanoma should undergo a neck dissection and consideration for interferon therapy
- if node is **negative** for melanoma no neck dissection required, may undergo neck dissection and consideration for interferon therapy if clinical nodes develop
- frozen section positive for tumor 15–20% of time (controversial and institution dependent), however frozen section analysis using MART-1 staining is being tested with promising results for Mohs micrographic surgery

## Prognosis and Metastasis Potential

- overall 5–20% recurrence rate
- *see* Table 7–1
- poorer prognosis also associated with the presence of ulceration, scalp lesions, microscopic satellites, and nodal disease
- distant metastasis has a grave prognosis

**TABLE 7–1.** Melanoma 5-Year Survival and Metastasis Potential Based on Pathologic Staging

| Stage | 5-Year Survival | Nodal Metastasis | Distant Metastasis |
|-------|-----------------|------------------|--------------------|
| pT1   | >95%            | 2–3%             |                    |
| pT2   | 80–94%          | 20–25%           | 8%                 |
| pT3   | 40–84%          | 57%              | 15%                |
| pT4   | 10–30%          | 62%              | 72%                |

## Other Cutaneous Malignancies

### Merkel Cell Carcinoma

- rare, aggressive, head and neck most common site
- third most common cause of skin cancer-related death (after melanoma and squamous cell carcinoma)
- median age 76 years old
- associated with Merkel cell polyomavirus, UV exposure, immunosuppression
- <u>Rx</u>: wide local excision, adjuvant radiation, consider neck dissection or radiation, consider adjuvant chemotherapy

# OTHER HEAD AND NECK NEOPLASMS
## Unknown Primary

### Overview

- defined as a biopsy/FNA-proven cervical metastasis with no demonstrable primary tumor
- incidence decreasing and constitutes <5% of patients
- may originate from an undetected primary tumor that is detected later; alternatively, the primary tumor may undergo immune-mediated spontaneous regression while the metastatic tumor escapes immune surveillance

### Evaluation and Management

- chest imaging (CXR, as part of PET/CT)
- CT with contrast or MRI with gadolinium (skull base through thoracic inlet)
- PET/CT if needed (must do prior to panendoscopy with biopsies)
- HPV, EBV testing suggested for squamous cell or undifferentiated pathology
- panendoscopy (direct laryngoscopy, bronchoscopy, esophagoscopy) with biopsy of suspicious lesions; may consider blind biopsies of nasopharynx, base of tongue, tonsils, and piriform sinuses; also consider bilateral tonsillectomy
- thyroglobulin and calcitonin staining for adenocarcinoma and anaplastic undifferentiated tumors
- consider bone scan, CT of abdomen/pelvis (if level IV–V), mammography, GI imaging (barium swallow), and thyroid scans
- <u>Primary Tumor Identified</u> (≤90%): treatment based on site of primary

- <u>Primary Tumor Unknown</u> (<10%): treatment of neck disease as described in the following, close monthly follow-up with low threshold for biopsy

## Drainage Pathways

- understanding drainage patterns paramount in elucidating possible primary

### *Oral Cavity*

- <u>Anterior Floor of Mouth</u>: IA (early) and IB (late)
- <u>Posterior Floor of Mouth</u>: IIA, IIB
- <u>Buccal Mucosa</u>: IA, IB, IIA
- <u>Lateral Oral Tongue</u>: IIA, III
- <u>Hard Palate</u>: IIA, III, IVA, IVB

### *Oropharynx*

- <u>Soft Palate</u>: IA, IB, IIA, IIB (bilateral)
- <u>Base of Tongue</u>: IIA, IIB, III, IV (bilateral)
- <u>Tonsils</u>: IIB, III (sometimes retropharyngeal nodes)

### *Nasopharynx*

- <u>Nasal Septum and Nasopharynx</u>: retropharyngeal nodes, IIA, IIB, V (bilateral)

### *Larynx and Hypopharynx*

- <u>Supraglottic Larynx</u>: IIA, IIB, III, pretracheal nodes (bilateral)
- <u>Glottic Larynx</u>: (rare unless advanced disease) IIA, III, IVA, IVB, paratracheal nodes
- <u>Hypopharynx</u>: IIA, III, IVA, IVB, paratracheal nodes (bilateral)

## Staging

### *T*

- TX: evaluation ongoing
- T0: primary site not found after full evaluation

*N* (*see* p. 276)

*M* (*see* p. 258)

## Pathology

- **Squamous Cell Carcinoma:** most common
- **Adenocarcinoma:** neck mass is usually supraclavicular, associated with primaries in the abdomen and chest; routine workup should entail PSA in men, mammogram in women, and CT abdomen
- **Lymphoma:** often with multiple/bilateral neck node enlargement
- **Thyroid:** can be found in lateral neck, especially medullary thyroid carcinoma
- **Melanoma:** 4% of melanoma will present as an unknown primary
- **Anaplastic Tumors**

## Management

### Early Neck Disease (N1)

- <u>Primary</u>: site unknown by definition, radiate Waldeyer's ring (bilateral nasopharynx, oropharynx, hypopharynx, supraglottic larynx)
- <u>Neck</u>: single modality therapy with either radiation or surgery of the neck; advantages of surgery include obtaining pathological staging that may be important for directing therapy, especially when ECS cannot be easily determined on imaging; if neck dissection performed and ECS present then follow with chemoradiation; if radiation performed and incomplete response then follow with salvage neck dissection

### Advanced Neck Disease (N2a–N3)

- failures can be as high as 35%–65% with radiation alone or 30%–75% with surgery alone
- <u>Primary</u>: same as early neck disease
- <u>Neck:</u> trimodality approach (role of chemotherapy is not clear but some would advocate the use of concomitant chemoradiation with a planned neck dissection regardless of response), neck dissection (if ECS present then follow with chemoradiation), chemoradiation (if complete response then observe or follow with planned neck dissection, if incomplete response then follow with salvage neck dissection)

## Mucosal Melanoma

- rare (<10% of head and neck melanoma), but more aggressive than cutaneous melanoma
- >50% arise from nasal cavity

- more likely to metastasize to regional and distant locations, high rate of recurrence
- pigmented lesions in nasal or oral cavity should raise suspicion and be biopsied promptly
- depth of invasion has little or no prognostic value (unlike cutaneous form)
- <u>Rx</u>: wide local excision, adjuvant radiation can be considered but benefits have not been proven
- poor prognosis with 5 year survival ~10–15%, slightly better when confined to nasal cavity only

## Staging *(Based on AJCC Staging, 2010)*

*T*

- **T3**: mucosal disease
- **T4a**: moderately advanced disease; tumor involving deep soft tissue, cartilage, bone, or overlying skin
- **T4b**: very advanced disease; tumor involving brain, dura, skull base, lower CNs (IX, X, XI, XII), masticator space, carotid artery, prevertebral space, or mediastinal structures

*N*

- **NX**: regional lymph nodes cannot be assessed
- **N0**: no regional lymph node metastasis detected
- **N1**: regional lymph node metastases present

*M*

- **M0:** no distant metastases detected
- **M1:** distant metastasis

# Lymphoma

## Introduction

- <u>Pathophysiology</u>: lymphoproliferative disorder
- <u>Risks</u>: irradiation, Epstein-Barr virus (Burkitt's lymphoma), HIV, immunosuppression, organic toxins (phenols, benzenes), human T-cell lymphotropic virus (HTLV-1, T-cell malignancies), immunologic diseases (rheumatoid arthritis, celiac disease)
- <u>SSx</u>: nodal masses (may be painful), non-Hodgkin's lymphoma (NHL) may present with extranodal masses as initial presentation (gastrointestinal tract most common extranodal site, also tonsils, paranasal cavity, base of tongue, salivary glands, thyroid, and orbit),

fever, night sweats, weight loss, symptoms from mass effect from extranodal site (throat pain, nasal obstruction, exophthalmos, hoarseness)

### Evaluation

- <u>Complete H&P</u>: including palpation of other nodal sites (supraclavicular, axillary, epitrochlear, inguinal, femoral) and spleen; inquire about fever, weight loss, and night sweats (B symptoms)
- **Fine-Needle Aspirate (FNA)**: may determine immunohistochemical subtype (B-cell or T-cell), DNA character (ploidy, phase), and RNA content (cannot differentiate follicular versus diffuse)
- **Open Biopsy**: usually required for definitive diagnosis prior to treatment, fresh sample required for immunochemistry and flow cytometry
- <u>Labs</u>: CBC, BUN, LDH, $\beta_2$-microglobulin, liver transaminases
- <u>Staging</u>: bone scan (gallium); CT/MRI of neck, chest, abdomen, and pelvis; bone marrow biopsy
- <u>Staging Laparotomy</u>: may be considered for aggressive Hodgkin's lymphoma (not NHL); includes inspection of abdominal cavity, liver biopsy, nodal biopsy, and oophoropexy
- may also consider serum protein electrophoresis, upper gastrointestinal series

## Hodgkin's Lymphoma

- bimodal incidence curve (teenagers and middle-age adults)
- spreads via **contiguous** lymph nodes
- **Reed-Sternberg Cells (R-S cells)**: binucleated, malignant giant cells, eosinophilic inclusions
- <u>Rx</u>: early stages (stage I, II) may consider single-modality radiation therapy; advanced disease (stage III, IV) requires multimodality therapy with radiation and chemotherapy, **MOP(P)** (mechlorethamine, Oncovin [vincristine], prednisone, procarbazine)/ **ABVD** (adriamycin, belomycin, vinblastine, DTIC); no surgical intervention except to obtain biopsy specimen
- <u>Prognosis</u>: dependent on staging (versus NHL, which is dependent on grade), overall >75% 5-year survival; better prognosis for lymphocytic predominance types; worse prognosis with presence of Reed-Sternberg cells, class B symptoms, and higher staging

### Ann Arbor Staging

- **I**: involvement of a single lymph node region or single extralymphatic site

- **II**: involvement of 2 or more lymph node regions on the same side of the diaphragm
- **III**: involvement of lymph node regions on both sides of the diaphragm
- **IV**: involvement of more than 1 extralymphatic organ
- <u>Symptom Classes</u>: **A** (asymptomatic), **B** (weight loss, fever, night sweats)

### Rye Modification of the Lukes and Butler Classification

- **Lymphocytic Predominance**: predominantly lymphocytic cells with few Reed-Sternberg cells, typically presents at an early stage, better prognosis
- **Nodular Sclerosis**: more common in women, typically presents at an early stage
- **Mixed Cellularity**: most common type
- **Lymphocytic Depleted**: rare, few lymphocytes with many Reed-Sternberg cells, usually advanced, poor prognosis

## Non-Hodgkin's Lymphoma (NHL)

- most are **B-cells** or **null cells** (except lymphoblastic lymphomas)
- <u>Rx</u>: typically treated with **CHOP** (cyclophosphamide, doxorubicin, vincristine, prednisone) chemotherapy followed by radiation to involved sites, low-grade B-cell lymphomas and MALT syndrome may be observed
- <u>Prognosis</u>: grading important; better prognosis associated with smaller and nodular types; poor prognosis associated with larger or diffuse types, higher grading, and CNS or bone marrow involvement
- **Mucosa-Associated Lymphoid Tissue (MALT)**: low-grade, B-cell tumors that may occur in the gastrointestinal tract, conjunctiva, lungs, and thyroid, associated with *Helicobacter pylori*, may respond to antibiotics and antiulcer medications

### Rappaport Classification and Working Formulation

- **Low Grade**: typically B-cell lymphomas, better survival (patients can live with disease for a long time); <u>Types</u>:
  1. **Small Lymphocytic**: may be found in the orbit, elderly, consistent with chronic lymphocytic leukemia
  2. **Follicular (Small Cleaved Cells)**: common, indolent course
  3. **Follicular (Mixed Cells)**: small and large cell components
- **Intermediate Grade: most common** type in the head and neck, potentially curable with chemotherapy; <u>Types</u>:
  1. **Follicular (Large Cell)**

2. **Diffuse (Small Cleaved Cell)**
3. **Diffuse (Mixed Cells)**: small and large cell components
4. **Diffuse (Large)**: may involve sanctuary sites (CNS, testes), rapidly fatal, most common NHL type in the head and neck
- **High Grade**: usually presents in the head and neck as part of a more extensive disease, extremely aggressive, requires immediate chemotherapy, chance for cure if treated early; <u>Types</u>:
  1. **Large Cell**
  2. **Lymphoblastic**: usually of T-cell origin
  3. **Burkitt's (Small Noncleaved Cell)**: maxilla or mandible involvement (**EBV** associated, common in Africa), abdominal organ involvement (HIV associated)

# Parapharyngeal Space Tumors

## Introduction

- 80% of parapharyngeal space tumors are benign
- <u>SSx</u>: displaced medial wall of the oropharynx or tonsil (if >3 cm), mass at angle of the mandible, otologic symptoms (mass effect on eustachian tube), cranial nerve palsies (CN IX–XII), dysphagia, obstructive sleep apnea, Horner's syndrome (mass effect on sympathetic chain), trismus, pain

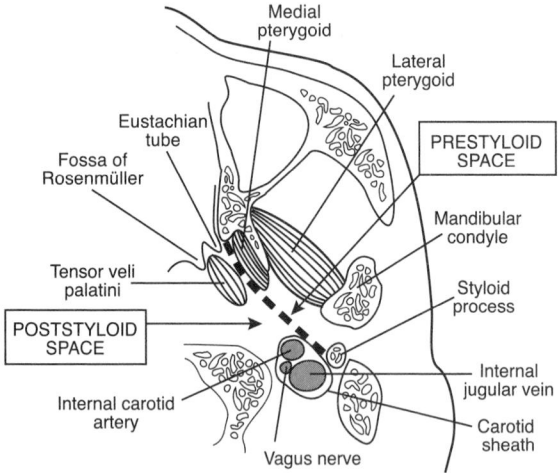

**FIGURE 7–4.** Cross-section at the level of the nasopharynx demonstrating the anatomy of the parapharyngeal space.

- <u>Dx</u>: CT/MRI with contrast, carotid angiography, fine needle aspiration, may consider open biopsy (intraoral route is contraindicated to avoid contamination)

## Anatomy of the Parapharyngeal Space (*see* Figure 7–4)

- potential space shaped like an inverted pyramid that extends from the skull base to the hyoid bone and lies between the angle of the mandible and the tonsil
- attaches to sphenoid bone, foramen lacerum, petrous bone
- <u>Superior Boundary</u>: skull base (sphenoid bone)
- <u>Inferior Boundary</u>: junction of the posterior belly of the digastric muscle and the greater cornu of the hyoid bone
- <u>Medial Boundary</u>: tensor veli palatini, levator veli palatini, and superior constrictor muscles and tonsillar fossa
- <u>Lateral Boundary</u>: ramus of the mandible, lateral and medial pterygoid muscles
- <u>Posterior Boundary</u>: prevertebral fascia
- <u>Anterior Boundary</u>: pterygomandibular raphe and medial pterygoid fascia

### Compartments

- divided by fascia between the styloid process and tensor veli palatini
- **Prestyloid**: maxillary artery, inferior alveolar and lingual nerve (CN $V_3$), deep lobe of the parotid, fat; majority of tumors are **salivary gland tumors**
- **Poststyloid**: carotid sheath (internal carotid artery, jugular vein), cranial nerves IX–XII, sympathetic chain, lymph nodes; majority of tumors are neurogenic and vascular

## Tumors Types

- **Salivary Gland Tumors**: most common primary tumor of the prestyloid parapharyngeal space, pleomorphic adenoma (most common salivary gland tumor in poststyloid parapharyngeal space, dumbbell-shaped)
- **Neurogenic Tumors**: second most common primary tumor of the parapharyngeal space; includes schwannoma (most common neurogenic tumor in the parapharyngeal space, may arise from any myelinated nerve including CN $V_3$, IX, X, XI, XII, sympathetic chain, and upper cervical trunks), paraganglioma (*see* pp. 392–393), neurofibroma, neuroma
- <u>Other Primary Tumors</u>: liposarcoma, chondrosarcoma, lymphoma, meningioma, lipoma

- Secondary Lesions: extension of oropharyngeal, parotid, submandibular, intercranial, or base of skull tumors; metastatic disease from nasopharynx, tongue base, oropharynx, and salivary glands
- Other Masses: lymphadenopathy, branchial cleft cyst, lymphatic malformations, lipomas

## Surgical Approaches

- **Transoral**: poor access, seldom used
- **Transcervical**: access via transverse incision at the level of the hyoid bone, allows direct access to the poststyloid compartment, excellent postsurgical cosmesis, mandibular osteotomy may be used to improve exposure
- **Transcervical Submandibular**: transcervical approach with dissection of the submandibular triangle to gain access to the prestyloid compartment, mandibular osteotomy may be used to improve exposure
- **Parotidectomy–Submandibular**: tumor is excised from the parotidectomy and exposure from the submandibular space, indicated for deep-lobe parotid tumors
- **Lip-Splitting with or without Mandibulotomy**: for pharyngeal malignancies that extend into the parapharyngeal space as part of a composite resection (can also consider a mandibulotomy with a degloving to avoid a lip-splitting incision)
- **Infratemporal Fossa or Craniofacial Approaches:** for tumors involving skull base
- Complications: **first bite syndrome** (parotid pain after first bite of a meal, may be due to loss of sympathetic innervation and denervation hypersensitivity of parotid myopithelial cells), Frey's syndrome (*see* pp. 90–91), facial nerve injury, salivary fistula, infection, hematoma, recurrence

# Miscellaneous

## Differential Diagnosis of Neuroendocrine Malignancies

- Mnemonic for Small Blue Round Cell Tumors ("**MR-SLEEP**"): **M:** melanoma, Merkel cell carcinoma; **R:** rhabdomyosarcoma; **S:** SNUC (sinonasal undifferentiated cancer), small cell cancer, sarcoma; **L:** lymphoma; **E:** Ewing's sarcoma; **E:** esthesioneuroblastoma; **P:** PNET (primitive neuroectodermal tumor)
- Pigmented: melanoma

- <u>Nonpigmented Small Cell</u>: lymphoma, small cell carcinoma, melanoma, neuroendocrine carcinoma, esthesioneuroblastoma
- <u>Nonpigmented Large Cell</u>: lymphoma, melanoma, neuroendocrine carcinoma
- <u>Nonpigmented Mixed Cell</u>: lymphoma, undifferentiated carcinoma, sarcoma, melanoma
- <u>Nonpigmented Spindle Cell</u>: sarcoma, undifferentiated carcinoma, melanoma

# ROBOTIC SURGERY

## Overview

### Introduction

- a minimally invasive approach using the da Vinci surgical system (Intuitive Surgical), the only currently available surgical robotic system in the United States
- role still emerging, interest in procedures with limited visualization/access that require precision
- currently the main clinical application is the oropharynx and the main approach is transoral (**transoral robotic surgery**, **TORS**)
- also employed for benign lesions of the oral cavity, larynx, and pharynx, T1–T2 malignancies; investigation ongoing in skull base, laryngeal, facial plastic, pediatrics, thyroid, reconstructive, neck surgery, and for surgery for obstructive sleep apnea

### Advantages

- 3D endoscopic visualization (depth perception, does not require direct line of site, magnifies ≤10×)
- multiple degrees of motion (flexion, extension, supination, pronation)
- scaling converts large hand movements into small movements of the robotic instruments, tremor may also be reduced
- potentially shorter operative time
- minimally invasive surgery reduces blood loss, infection, and other complications
- less morbidity, pain, and shortened hospital stay
- smaller incision improves cosmetic and functional outcome

### Disadvantages

- no tactile feedback (haptics)

- requires assistant at patient's head
- cost (system, maintenance, limited instrument reusability)
- set up and overall surgical time (improves with experience)
- training can be time-consuming and costly

# Outcomes

## Oncologic Outcomes

- for oropharyngeal carcinoma, 2 year recurrence-free survival was 86% for the entire study; however, a 2 year survival rate of 89% was achieved in patients undergoing primary TORS and recurrences were associated with a previous recurrence and stage III or IV disease (*Arch Otolaryngol Head and Neck*. 2010;136:1248–1252)
- at 2 years after TORS for advanced oropharyngeal carcinoma, disease-specific survival was 90% and overall survival was 82% (*Arch Otolaryngol Head Neck Surg*. 2010;136:1079–1085)

## Functional Outcomes

- postoperative swallowing ability dependent upon location of tumor, preoperative swallowing ability, T stage, and age of the patient
- most patients tolerate an oral diet within 1–2 days after surgery, some may be discharged home with a short-term nasal feeding tube or long-term gastric feeding tube
- TORS for T1–T2 oropharyngeal cancer resulted in a decrease in immediate mean postoperative MD Anderson Dysphagia Inventory (MDADI) scores compared with preoperative baseline scores; however, ongoing improvement in all domains was observed over time (*Arch Otolaryngol Head Neck Surg*. 2011 Nov;137(11):1112–1116)
- TORS for T1–T3 oropharyngeal cancer did not cause aspiration or velopharyngeal insufficiency on endoscopy; there was progressive improvement in diet, swallowing, and oral function from 2 weeks to 2 years (*Arch Otolaryngol Head Neck Surg*. 2011;137(2):151–156)
- combination TORS and adjuvant therapy caused a temporary decrease in Short Form (SF)-8 and Performance Status Scale (PSS) at 6 months, returning to baseline (including swallowing function) in all patients (*Head and Neck*. 2012 Feb;34(2):146–154)

***Acknowledgments:*** *We wish to acknowledge and thank Robert Park and John R. Jacobs for their contributions to this chapter.*

# CHAPTER

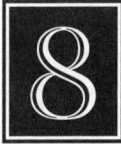

# Otology and Neurotology

Syed F. Ahsan, Dennis I. Bojrab, Douglas R. Sidell, Neil Tanna, Don L. Burgio,
Raza Pasha, and Justin S. Golub

# ANATOMY, EMBRYOLOGY, AND PHYSIOLOGY OF HEARING AND BALANCE

## External Ear and Temporal Bone Anatomy and Embryology

### Auricle

- <u>Embryology</u>: around the sixth week of gestation, the external ear arises from the proliferation of mesenchymal cells from the first and second branchial clefts
    1. **First Branchial (Pharyngeal) Arch (Mandibular Arch/Meckel's Cartilage)**: derives **Hillock of His 1–3** (1. tragus; 2. helical crus; 3. helix)
    2. **Second Branchial (Pharyngeal) Arch (Hyoid Arch/Reichert's Cartilage)**: derives **Hillock of His 4–6** (4. antihelix crus; 5. antihelix; 6. lobule and antitragus)
- auricle is 85% of adult size at 3 years, full adult size at 5 years
- auricle is constructed from a framework of elastic cartilage and perichondrium with tightly adherent skin anteriorly and more loosely adherent skin posteriorly
- attachment of the auricle to the skull is by ligaments (anterior, posterior, and superior ligaments), muscles (anterior, posterior, and superior auricular muscles), skin, and the cartilage of the EAC
- **Darwin's Tubercle**: small protuberance that may arise from the posterosuperior helix around 6 months of gestation

## External Auditory Canal (EAC)

- Embryology: **first branchial groove (cleft)** forms the EAC; in the embryo the EAC fills with epithelial cells that recannulize by apoptosis in a medial to lateral direction around the seventh month (failure of recannulization results in aural atresia, arrest of canalization may result in a normal bony EAC but an atretic membranous EAC with canal cholesteatoma due to trapped squamous debris)
- **Cartilaginous EAC**: lateral 1/3, fibrocartilage, contains pilosebaceous units (cerumen glands, hair follicles, sebaceous glands; thus furuncles and sebaceous cysts may develop)
- **Osseous EAC**: medial 2/3, periosteum, is tightly adherent to the skin, contains no subcutaneous tissue
- Boundaries: infratemporal fossa, bony wall of the mastoid cavity, parotid and temporomandibular joint (TMJ), tympanic membrane (TM), epitympanum
- Sensory Contributions to the Auricle and EAC: **CN $V_3$** (EAC, TM, middle ear), **CN VII** (posterior concha, EAC), **CN IX** (Jacobson's nerve, with Arnold's nerve forms tympanic plexus on the promontory), **CN X** (Arnold's nerve, concha, and antihelix), **great auricular nerve** (cervical plexus), and **lesser occipital nerve**
- **Fissures of Santorini**: lymphatic channels that connect the **lateral** cartilaginous EAC to the parotid and glenoid fossa region, allow for extension of infection and malignant tumors
- **Foramen of Huschke**: embryologic remnant that forms a defect that connects the **medial** EAC to the parotid and glenoid fossa region, allows for extension of infection and malignant tumors outside the temporal bone

## Tympanic Membrane (TM, Figure 8–1)

- Embryology and the Formation of the Three Layers
  1. **First Branchial Groove (Cleft) (Ectoderm)**: forms the **outer epidermal squamous** layer of the TM and the EAC
  2. **Mesoderm**: forms the **middle fibrous** layer of the TM (subdivided further into a radial outer and circular inner layer)
  3. **First Branchial Pouch (Endoderm)**: forms the **inner mucosal** layer of the TM, eustachian tube, and middle ear space
- **Pars Flaccida (Shrapnell's Membrane)**: superior portion of the TM, located in the notch of Rivinus, less stiff, sparse disorganized middle fibrous layer
- **Pars Tensa**: larger, stiff, vibrating surface of the TM, organized middle fibrous layer

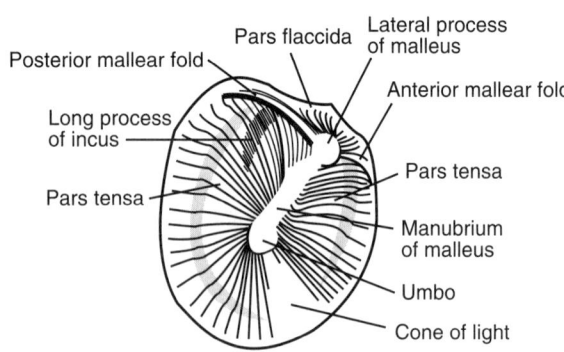

**FIGURE 8–1.** Anatomy of the tympanic membrane.

- **Malleolar Folds (Tympanic Striae)**: run from the lateral (short) process of the malleus to the tympanic spine, composed of anterior and posterior components, divides the pars flaccida from the pars tensa
- **Fibrous Annulus**: thickened circumference of the pars tensa forming a fibrous outer ring for attachment to the temporal bone, lies within tympanic sulcus except where superiorly deficient at the notch of Rivinus
- **Notch of Rivinus**: notch of the squamous portion of the temporal bone located superiorly, within which the pars flaccida attaches directly to the squamous temporal bone

## Mastoid Cavity

- <u>Development</u>: antrum present at birth, increases in size during first year; pneumatization continues into childhood; mastoid fully developed by 3 years
- **Tegmen Mastoidium**: thin plate of bone that serves as the roof of the mastoid cavity, separating it from the middle fossa dura
- **Sinodural (Citelli's) Angle**: region between the sigmoid sinus and the tegmen mastoidium
- **Koerner's (Petrosquamous) Septum**: bony plate that separates the squamous and petrous air cells
- **Mastoid Antrum**: first air cell that allows communication between the middle ear and the mastoid air cells
- **Facial Recess**: triangular space bounded by the short process of the **incus** (fossa incudis) superiorly, **facial nerve** medially, and **chorda tympani** laterally (from its branching off of the facial nerve); potential route to the mesotympanum

- **Donaldson's Line**: imaginary line from the lateral semicircular canal bisecting perpendicularly the posterior semicircular canal, marks the superior limit of where the endolymphatic sac is found
- **Trautmann's Triangle**: bordered by the bony labyrinth, sigmoid sinus, and tegmen mastoideum

## Surface Anatomy of the Temporal Bone

- Four Major Parts of the Temporal Bone
  1. **Petrous**: houses inner ear, medially ends in an apex
  2. **Mastoid**: houses air cells
  3. **Squamous (Squama)**: large superolateral plate, includes posterior zygomatic arch
  4. **Tympanic**: includes majority of bony EAC

### *Lateral Surface*

- **Temporal Line**: bony ridge for the attachment of the temporalis muscle fascia, important landmark in mastoid surgery as it identifies the superior limit of the mastoid dissection and suggests the level of the tegmen
- **Spine of Henle**: eminence located near the posterosuperior wall of the EAC to which the soft tissue of the EAC attaches, important anterior landmark in mastoid surgery as it identifies the beginning of the bony EAC
- **Tympanomastoid Suture Line (Fissure)**: located posteriorly in the EAC, divides the tympanic and mastoid portions of the temporal bone, reliable landmark used in finding CN VII exit the skull during parotidectomy
- **Tympanosquamous Suture Line (Fissure)**: embryonic fusion plane oriented anterosuperiorly in the EAC, divides tympanic and squamous portions of the temporal bone
- **Macewen's (Suprameatal) Triangle (Fossa Mastoidea)**: bordered by the temporal line, spine of Henle, and a line connecting the two; aids in identifying the antrum, which lies deep beneath

### *Superior Surface (Floor of Middle Cranial Fossa)*

- **Arcuate Eminence**: bulging landmark of the superior semicircular canal
- **Foramen Lacerum**: contains the internal carotid artery
- **Facial Hiatus**: contains the greater (superficial) petrosal nerve
- **Tympanic Canaliculus**: superior part contains the lesser (superficial) petrosal nerve, inferior part contains Jacobson's nerve

### Posterior Surface

- **Vestibular Aqueduct**: contains endolymphatic duct; ridge of bone at opening that overlies endolymphatic sac is the **operculum** (*see also* p. 342)
- **Subarcuate Canal**: contains the vestibular, facial, and acoustic (cochlear) nerves
- **Sigmoid Sulcus**: located in medial aspect of the mastoid process
- **Cochlear Aqueduct**: contains periotic duct (*see also* p. 342)
- **Internal Auditory Meatus (Porus Acousticus)**: opening of the **medial** IAC that contains CN VII, CN VIII, nervus intermedius, and labyrinthine (internal auditory) artery and vein (the **fundus** is the **lateral** opening of the IAC)
- **Bill's Bar**: vertical crest of bone in the IAC that helps distinguish CN VII from the superior vestibular nerve
- **Mike's Dot**: marks passage of superior vestibular nerve toward vestibular organs, extreme lateral aspect of the IAC

## Middle Ear Anatomy and Embryology

### Ossicles

- Embryology
    1. **First Branchial Arch**: derives the malleus head and neck, anterior malleal ligament, incus body and lateral (short) process
    2. **Second Branchial Arch**: derives the malleus manubrium, incus long and lenticular processes, stapes (except otic part of footplate)
    3. **Otic Capsule**: otic portion of stapes footplate, annular ligament
- ossicles reach their adult size at birth
- **Malleus**: manubrium (or handle; tip is the umbo), lateral (short) process, anterior process, neck, head; **tensor tympani muscle** (CN V$_3$) attaches to the malleus neck and manubrium by tendon from the **cochleariform process**
- **Incus**: body, short process, long process, lenticular process; articulates with the malleus and the stapes via diarthrodial joints
- **Stapes**: head (capitulum), anterior and posterior crus, footplate (base); **stapedius muscle** (CN VII) attaches to the posterior neck from the **pyramidal eminence**
- **Stapes Footplate**: attaches to the bony margins of the oval window by the **annular ligament** forming a joint (**syndesmosis**)

### Eustachian Tube (Pharyngotympanic Tube)

- Embryology: derived from the **ventral first branchial pouch**
- consists of a posterior osseous portion (1/3, remains open to the middle ear) and an anterior membranous–cartilaginous portion (2/3,

mobile portion); begins in the middle ear, ends in the nasopharynx (**torus tubarius**), 35 mm long
- in adults the eustachian tube is 45° from horizontal; in infants it is shorter (50% adult length) and is 10° from horizontal (more susceptible to regurgitation with feeding)
- <u>Associated Muscles</u>: **tensor veli palatini** (CN V$_3$, predominant dilator, the medial bundle of the tensor veli palatini forms the **dilator tubae**), **levator veli palatini** (pharyngeal plexus), **salpingopharyngeus** (pharyngeal plexus, helps keep closed), **tensor tympani** (CN V$_3$)
- <u>Functions</u>: ventilation (equalization of pressure between nasopharynx and middle ear), clearance (drainage), and protection (from sound and secretions)

## Other Important Landmarks

- middle ear space (**tympanum** or **cleft**) behind the TM divided into **epitympanum** (superior to superior annulus), **mesotympanum**, **hypotympanum** (inferior to inferior annulus)
- **Tegmen Tympani**: thin plate of bone that separates the middle fossa dura from the tympanic cavity (ie, epitympanic space)
- **Scutum**: lateral bony wall of the epitympanic recess
- **Prussak's Space**: superior recess of the tympanic membrane; bounded by lateral malleal fold (roof), short process of the malleus (floor), neck of the malleus (medial), and pars flaccida (lateral)
- **Promontory**: basal turn of the cochlea, floor of the middle ear
- **Jacobson's Nerve**: tympanic branch of **CN IX** located on the promontory
- **Arnold's Nerve**: auricular branch of **CN X**, traverses the tympanomastoid fissure to innervate the posterior aspect of the EAC, causes cough during otoscopy
- **Ponticulus**: ridge of bone posterior to the oval window
- **Subiculum**: ridge of bone between the round window niche and the pyramidal eminence
- **Sinus Tympani**: located in the mesotympanum between the ponticulus superiorly, subiculum inferiorly, and facial nerve laterally

# Inner Ear Anatomy and Embryology

## Embryologic Malformations

- inborn genetic error or teratogen exposure (*in utero* infection, radiation, aminoglycosides, thalidomide) during first trimester results in inner ear malformation

- the earlier the developmental arrest, the more severe the deformity and the worse the hearing will be (3rd week: Michel aplasia; 4th week: common cavity; 5th week: cochlear aplasia; 6th week: cochlear hypoplasia; 7th week: Mondini aplasia; 8th week: normal development)

## Bony Labyrinth

- <u>Embryology</u>: mesenchyme (mesoderm), which encapsulates the otocyst, forms the cartilaginous **otic capsule**; ossification of the otic capsule occurs around the 16th week
- <u>Components</u>: vestibule, semicircular canals, and cochlea
- derived from the labyrinthine capsule from periosteal and endochondral ossification (susceptible to bony diseases such as Paget's disease, osteodystrophies, or otosclerosis)
- **Cochlear Aqueduct**: contains the **periotic duct**, continuous with the subarachnoid space (ends in posterior cranial fossa), inner ear opening is at the base of the scala tympani
- **Vestibular Aqueduct**: contains the **endolymphatic duct** and the veins of the vestibular aqueduct, runs from the vestibule to the posterior surface of the petrous pyramid in the posterior cranial fossa (opening includes the **operculum**, which overlies the endolymphatic sac)

## Membranous Labyrinth

- <u>Embryology</u>: around embryonic day 22–23, ectodermal thickening of the side of the head forms the **otic placode**, which deepens to form the **otic pit**, which later forms the **otocyst**; the otocyst forms the membranous labyrinth
- **Membranous Labyrinth**: enclosed within the bony labyrinth
- **Ductus Reuniens**: narrowest segment connecting cochlea and saccule
- **Periotic Duct**: within the **cochlear aqueduct**, connects the scala tympani to the posterior cranial fossa
- **Endolymphatic Duct**: within the **vestibular aqueduct**, connects the endolymphatic compartment to the **endolymphatic sac**, the endolymphatic sac is the first to appear and the last to stop growth

## Labyrinthine Fluids

- **Perilymph**: fluid within the bony labyrinth, similar in composition to **extracellular fluid** and **CSF** ($[Na^+] > [K^+]$), formed from the filtrate of blood and diffusion of CSF
- **Endolymph**: fluid within the membranous labyrinth, similar in composition to **intracellular fluid** ($[K^+] > [Na^+]$), formed from the filtrate of perilymph

# Semicircular Canals (SCCs)

- sense rotational (angular) acceleration
- **Horizontal (Lateral) SCC**: 30° from horizontal; ampullopetal (toward vestibule) flow of endolymph increases vestibular neuron firing rate
- **Superior (Anterior) SCC and Posterior SCC**: the two vertical canals, share a nonampullated common crus, ampullofugal (away from vestibule) flow of endolymph increases vestibular neuron firing rate
- on each side the 3 SCCs are orthogonal (90° to each other)
- **Ampulla**: pear-shaped expansion located at one end of each SCC near the vestibular opening
- **Cupula**: gelatinous layer located within each ampulla, extends to the roof of the ampulla sealing the SCC
- **Crista Ampullaris**: sensory element of the SCCs; contains hair cells, which extend into the cupula

## *Basic Physiology*

- **rotational** acceleration causes inertial deflection of the cupula, which deflects the hair cells in the crista ampullaris causing depolarization
- **type I** (flask-shaped) and **type II** (cylindrical-shaped) hair cells contain 1 **kinocilium** and ~ 60 stereocilia, deflection of the stereocilia toward the kinocilium results in increased vestibular neuronal firing rate
- in the **horizontal** SCC, the kinocilia are located on the utricular side, therefore displacement of the stereocilia toward the vestibule (**ampullopetal**) causes increased vestibular neuronal firing rate and displacement away from the vestibule (**ampullofugal**) causes decreased vestibular neuronal firing rate
- in the **vertical** SCCs (posterior and superior), the kinocilia are located on the semicircular canal side, therefore the reverse occurs: displacement of the stereocilia away from the vestibule (**ampullo-fugal**) causes increased vestibular neuronal firing rate and displace-ment toward the vestibule (**ampullopetal**) causes decreased vestibular neuronal firing rate
- each canal exhibits a resting basal discharge rate

# Otolith Organs

- composed of the utricle and saccule, located within the vestibule
- **Utricle**: detects horizontal linear acceleration
- **Saccule**: detects vertical linear acceleration and changes in gravity

- **Macula**: sensory element of otolith organs, consists of **supporting cells** and **hair cells** whose stereocilia/kinocilia are within an overlying gelatinous mass on the surface of which lies the **otolithic membrane** and **otoliths (otoconia)** (calcium carbonate)
- **Striola**: line of orientation in the utricle and saccule around which the polarity of the hair cells changes 180°

### Basic Physiology

- **linear** acceleration causes inertial displacement of the otoliths, which displace the stereocilia/kinocilium resulting in hair cell stimulation
- gravity accelerates the otoliths resulting in a sensation of up or down
- the hair cells in the otolith organs act similarly to the SCC in regard to the kinocilia and the stereocilia; however, the utricle and saccule's hair cells are arranged in a specific pattern (striola, *see previous*)

## Vestibular Organ Innervation

- **Scarpa's Ganglion**: contains cell bodies of the vestibular nerve
- **Superior Vestibular Nerve**: superior SCC, horizontal SCC, utricle
- **Inferior Vestibular Nerve**: posterior SCC, saccule

## Cochlea (Figure 8–2)

- **Cochlea**: spiral-shaped acoustic end organ centered on the central **modiolus**, 2½ turns
- **Scala Vestibuli**: contains perilymph, begins in vestibule
- **Scala Media (Cochlear Duct)**: contains endolymph and organ of Corti (*see following*)
- **Scala Tympani**: contains perilymph, begins at the round window
- **Helicotrema**: opening between the scala tympani and the scala vestibuli at the cochlear apex
- **Reissner's Membrane (Vestibular Membrane)**: two-cell-layer membrane between the scala media and scala vestibuli
- **Basilar Membrane**: between the scala media and scala tympani, stiffer and thinner at base, supports the organ of Corti
- **Stria Vascularis**: forms lateral wall of the scala media, Na-K ATPase keeps membrane potential at −80 mV, contains highly metabolically active cells (dense mitochondria, Golgi apparatus, endoplasmic reticulum), supports cochlear function
- **Spiral Ganglion**: contains cell bodies of the cochlear nerve, located within the central modiolus in lateral end of cochlear nerve
- **Osseous Spiral Lamina**: bony plate forms the cochlear framework

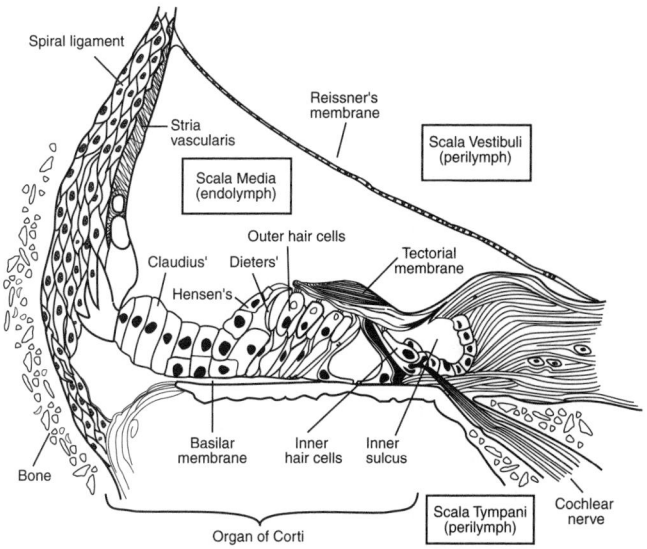

**FIGURE 8–2.** Cross-sectional anatomy of the cochlea. Reprinted with permission from Bailey BJ. *Head and Neck Surgery-Otolaryngology* [Illustration by Tony Pazos]. Copyright 1993, Lippincott, Williams and Wilkins.

## Organ of Corti

- supporting cells (Deiter's, Hensen's, Claudius's) provide nutrients and support
- **Tectorial Membrane:** fibrogelatinous structure arises from the bony spiral lamina, the tips of the stereocilia of the outer hair cells are partially embedded in the tectorial membrane, vibration of the basilar membrane causes shearing forces at the tectorial membrane, which results in stimulation of the hair cells

### Inner Hair Cells

- may act as the principal transducer of motion from the basilar membrane to a nerve impulse
- **single** row, fewer in number than outer hair cells
- **rounded**, flask-like shape with nucleus in the center, low intracellular glycogen
- few stereocilia in a curvilinear shape
- loose connection to tectorial membrane
- completely surrounded by supporting cells
- <u>Afferent Innervation</u>: **type I (radial, bipolar, myelinated)**, form **95%** of fibers of the cochlear nerve, each inner hair

cell is innervated by 10–20 neurons (low hair cell to ganglion ratio) → cochlear nucleus
• <u>Efferent Innervation</u>: sparse

**Outer Hair Cells**

• may act as a motor to amplify motion from the basilar membrane (**cochlear amplifier**)
• source of otoacoustic emissions
• **3 rows**, more numerous than inner hair cells
• **cylindrical** shaped with nucleus at base and organelles aligning the cell membrane, high intracellular glycogen
• many stereocilia in a "W" or "V" shape
• tight connection to tectorial membrane
• supported only at base
• <u>Afferent Innervation</u>: **type II (spiral, pseudomonopolar, unmyelinated)**, form **5%** of fibers of the cochlear nerve, 10 outer hair cells are innervated by one neuron (high hair cell to ganglion ratio) → cochlear nucleus
• <u>Efferent Innervation</u>: from the auditory cortex down to the cochlear nuclei, additional contributions from the superior olive join and terminate predominantly on the outer hair cells

# Physiology of Hearing

## Conductive Pathway

• sound energy from the air is conducted to the inner ear via the auricle (shape funnels sound to the EAC), the TM, and the ossicles; TM and ossicles provide hydraulic (area) advantage and a lever effect
• **Area Advantage**: area of the vibrating portion of TM is 55 mm$^2$, the area of the stapes footplate is 3.2 mm$^2$, advantage (hydraulic) ratio = **17:1**
• **Lever Effect**: lever action of the ossicles affords an advantage ratio of **1.3:1**
• **Transformer Ratio**: area advantage + lever advantage = **22:1** or approximately **25–30 dB gain**
• TM protects the round window by allowing a **phase difference** between sound conducting to the oval window and sound directly reaching the round window; if sound waves would strike the oval and round windows simultaneously the resultant forces would suppress the cochlear fluid wave
• **Tonotopic Organization of the Cochlea**: pressure at the oval window produces a "traveling wave" along the basilar membrane

from the base of the cochlea to the apex, maximal amplitude of **higher** frequencies is at the **base** and **lower** frequencies is at the apex, thus creating a tonotopic arrangement

### Resonance Frequencies

- natural frequencies that vibrate a mass with the least amount of force
- **Concha**: 4000–6000 Hz
- **EAC**: 2000–3000 Hz (primary frequencies of speech)
- **TM**: 800–1600 Hz
- **Ossicles**: 500–2000 Hz
- **Middle Ear**: 800 Hz

## Auditory Nerve Pathway

- Mnemonic: **E COLI** outlines the neural pathway (**E**ighth nerve, **C**ochlear nucleus, superior **O**livary nuclei, **L**ateral lemniscus, **I**nferior colliculus)
- Pathway
  1. stimulation of hair cells from vibration of the basilar membrane stimulates the bipolar neurons of the spiral ganglion that form the cochlear division of CN VIII
  2. the cochlear nerve unites with the vestibular nerve as it courses through the IAC, the cochlear neurons then synapse in the cochlear nuclei (anterior ventral, posterior ventral, dorsal)
  3. **bilateral** innervation from the cochlear nucleus (via the acoustic striae) synapse on the superior olivary nuclei
  4. superior olivary nuclei → lateral lemniscus → inferior colliculus → thalamus (medial geniculate body) → primary auditory cortex at sylvian fissure (lateral sulcus) of temporal lobe (Brodmann area 41, Heschl's or transverse temporal gyri) → secondary auditory cortex (Brodmann area 42, surrounds primary auditory cortex)

## Sound Localization

- **Head Shadow Effect**: head attenuates sound waves with wavelengths shorter than the width of the head (>2 kHz) by 5–15 dB
- **Interaural Time Difference**: ≤0.6 ms time difference for sound hitting one ear to reach the other ear

# Physiology of Balance

## Receptors of Balance

- 5 vestibular receptors per side respond to acceleration (linear and angular changes in velocity), not velocity itself
- **Otolith Organs (2 Per Side)**: linear accelerometers, oriented vertically and horizontally in the erect position; unlike the cristae of the SCCs the maculae of the otolith organs have an extremely complex array of stereocilia; *see also* pp. 343–344
- **Semicircular Canals (3 Per Side)**: rotational accelerometers (sense changes in turning motion), the cristae of the SCCs are arranged orthogonally (at 90° to each other) to create functional pairs, increased output from one canal results in decreased output from its paired contralateral canal thus creating a "push–pull" mechanism that enhances system sensitivity; *see also* p. 343
- SCC Functional Pairs
  1. right horizontal SCC + left horizontal SCC
  2. left anterior (superior) SCC + right posterior SCC ("LARP")
  3. right anterior (superior) SCC + left posterior SCC ("RALP")

## Nystagmus and Reflexes

- **Vestibulo-Ocular Reflex (VOR)**: head rotation in a plane results in an equal but opposite eye rotation to allow the eye (retina) to maintain fixation on an object (ie, head motion 10° to the left produces eye movement 10° to the right)
- **Vestibulospinal Reflex**: the otolith organs modulate the antigravitational muscles in a similar way as the vestibulo-ocular reflex modulates the eye to allow for postural control (ie, simultaneous contraction of the extensor muscles with contralateral flexor muscles to maintain posture), position and motion of muscles and joints may also modify the vestibulospinal reflex via receptors found in intervertebral joint receptors (upper cervical)
- **Nystagmus**: rapid involuntary back-forth movement of the eyes; the **direction** of nystagmus is named after the corrective **fast** phase; the **slow** phase arises from the ear
- use **COWS** ("cold opposite, warm same") to remember direction of nystagmus originating from horizontal canal dysfunction; a **cold** (hypoactive) lesion causes nystagmus (ie, fast phase) **away** from the diseased ear, a **hot** (hyperactive/irritative) lesion causes nystagmus **toward** the diseased ear (*see also* p. 410)
- classically a **right** peripheral disorder results in **left**-beating nystagmus, vertical nystagmus is usually central in origin

- **Alexander's Law**: a pathologic peripheral nystagmus will increase when gaze is in the direction of the fast phase and slow when in the direction of the slow phase
- **Ewald's Law**: (1) peripheral nystagmus is in the plane of the semicircular canal being stimulated and its direction (ie, fast phase) is opposite to the direction of endolymphatic flow; (2) stimulating/excitatory responses are greater than inhibitory responses

## Vestibular Central Nervous System Processing and Compensation

- unlike in the auditory system, the vestibular neural pathways have a balance of bilateral continuous neural output including at rest, unilateral interruption of any vestibular end organ results in vertigo
- imperfect correlation of receptors (vestibular, visual, or somatosensory) produces a "sensory conflict" resulting in vertigo
- habituation (ie, decrease in vertiginous symptoms) occurs with repeated or sustained receptor mismatch resulting in a decreased vestibular response via processing in the brainstem and cerebellum (central compensation)

# AUDIOLOGY AND HEARING DEVICES
## Audiograms

### Units of Measurement

- **Frequency**: **cycles/sec (Hz)**, unit of measurement of pitch
- **Intensity**: **decibels (dB)**, unit of measurement of sound pressure or intensity (ie, "loudness") based on a logarithmic ratio, it is nonlinear and is a relative measure
- Derivation of the Decibel
  1. **Bell** (B) = $\log (I_{output}/I_{reference})$; I = unit of intensity level
  2. dB = $10 \log (I_{output}/I_{reference})$
  3. I = $P^2$; P = unit of sound pressure level
  4. **dB** = $10 \log (P_{output}^2/P_{reference}^2)$ = **$20 \log (P_{output}/P_{reference})$**

### *Reference Levels of the Decibel*

- **Sound Pressure Level (SPL)**: absolute pressure reference level for the dB, 0 dB SPL = pressure force of 20 µPa or 0.0002 dynes/cm$^2$
- **Hearing Level (HL)**: threshold dB based on normative hearing data as a reference (ie, 0 dB HL is the least intensity for the average

normal ear to perceive a specific frequency 50% of the time), is the reference used in most audiometers
- **Sensation Level (SL)**: level in dB above an individual's threshold (ie, if a patient's threshold is 20 dB HL then 50 dB SL = 70 dB HL)

## Basic Audiogram

- **Pure-Tone Audiometry**: utilizes pure tones (single frequency sound) at 250, 500, 1000, 2000, 4000, and 8000 Hz at selected intensities; complete series consists of air and bone conduction thresholds (bone conduction thresholds are not measured at 8000 Hz)
- **Air Conduction (AC) Threshold**: lowest level dB HL (hearing threshold) at which the subject perceives 50% of pure tones introduced via earphones or speakers (soundfield), represents conduction from the auricle to the cochlea
- **Bone Conduction (BC) Threshold**: lowest level dB HL (hearing threshold) at which the subject perceives 50% of pure tones introduced via a bone oscillator apparatus, represents conduction from the bones of the skull to the inner ear (bypassing the TM and ossicles), should always be lower (better) than air conduction
- **Pure-Tone Average (PTA)**: average thresholds for the speech frequencies (500, 1000, 2000 Hz; sometimes also 3000 Hz), typically should be within 10 dB of the speech reception threshold
- **Air–Bone Gap (ABG)**: dB difference between bone and air conduction thresholds
- **Speech Audiometry**: utilizes spoken voice as a sound stimulus at selected intensities
- **Speech (Spondee) Reception Threshold (SRT)**: lowest *dB HL* patient can repeat a **spondee** (2-syllable words with balanced accents) 50% of the time
- **Word Recognition Score (Speech Discrimination Score)**: *percentage* of phonetically balanced monosyllabic words **(phonemes)** repeated correctly after being presented at 20–40 dB above the SRT, **PB max** is the best score obtained after testing at increasing intensities

### *Adult Hearing Loss Levels (Varies by Source/Organization)*

- ≤25 dB: normal
- 26–40 dB: mild
- 41–55 dB: moderate
- 56–70 dB: moderately severe
- 71–90 dB: severe
- ≥91 dB: profound
- *NOTE*: for pediatric levels, *see* p. 570

## *Masking and Crossover*

- **Crossover**: nontest ear detects sound presented to test ear
- **Interaural Attenuation**: the amount of sound intensity needed before crossover occurs (depends on sound insulation provided by the head), difference in sound intensity between what is presented to the test ear and the bone conduction threshold of the nontest ear must not exceed **70 dB** for insert earphones or **40 dB** for over-the-ear earphones (or **0 dB** for bone conduction testing)
- **Masking**: noise introduced with air conduction into the nontest ear to prevent crossover, may be narrowband for pure-tone audiometry or wideband for speech testing
- **Shadow Curve**: in testing a "dead ear," sound will cross over to the contralateral ear; masking can reduce
- bilateral ABG of 50–70 dB cannot be masked (**masking dilemma**)

## *Common Audiogram Patterns*

- **Conductive Hearing Loss (CHL)**: normal bone conduction thresholds with abnormal air conduction thresholds (presence of an ABG), maximal CHL is 60 dB (ossicular chain discontinuity with an intact TM)
- **Sensorineural Hearing Loss (SNHL)**: abnormal bone conduction thresholds, no ABG
- **Mixed Hearing Loss**: hearing loss from conductive and sensorineural components, presence of an ABG with abnormal bone conduction thresholds
- **Low-Frequency SNHL**: endolymphatic hydrops
- **Bilateral High-Frequency (Down-sloping) SNHL**: presbycusis, most ototoxins
- **Carhart Notch**: falsely depressed bone conduction at **2000 Hz** in otosclerosis, secondary to a reduction of the inertial component of bone conduction
- **4 KHz Notch**: high-frequency SNHL at 4000–5000 Hz from noise-induced hearing loss
- **Cookie Bite (U-Shape)**: some forms of hereditary hearing loss
- **Loudness Recruitment**: increasing sound intensity (dB) produces an out-of-proportion perception of loudness, suggests **cochlear hearing loss**, recruitment causes discomfort within a smaller range of the SRT (normally 95 dB above SRT causes discomfort)
- **Rollover**: a paradoxic decrease in word recognition score with increasing sound intensity (dB), suggestive of a **retrocochlear disorder** (eg, vestibular schwannoma, posterior fossa lesions)
- **Tone Decay and Fatigue**: a decrease in auditory perception with a sustained signal stimulus, suggestive of **retrocochlear pathology**

## Acoustic Immittance Testing

- **acoustic immittance** refers to either **acoustic impedance** (opposition to the transfer of acoustic energy) or **acoustic admittance** (ease of sound flow through an acoustic system)
- battery of tests providing information about the middle ear (via tympanometry) and inner ear, acoustic nerve, and brainstem function (via acoustic reflex testing)

### Tympanometry

- indirect tests of middle ear function by the transmission/reflection of sound energy
- **Tympanogram**: plots compliance changes of the TM versus air pressure in the EAC
- **Peak**: point on the tympanogram that represents the point of maximum compliance, in which pressure of the external ear canal equals the pressure of the middle ear space
- Types
- **A**: normal peak between −150 and +50 daPa
- **A$_S$**: "<u>s</u>hallow" peak (reduced compliance), TM <u>s</u>tiff; suggests oto<u>s</u>clerosis or tympano<u>s</u>clerosis
- **A$_D$**: "<u>d</u>eep" peak (hypercompliant), TM flaccid; suggests ossicular <u>d</u>iscontinuity or a "monomeric" TM
- **B**: flat, no peak, nonmobile TM; suggests effusion, perforation, or an open PE (pressure equalization) tube
- **C**: peak shifted to a more negative pressure (<−150), retracted TM; suggests eustachian tube dysfunction or TM atelectasis
- also measures EAC volume (normal for children is <1 mL, adults is <2 mL)

### Acoustic (Stapedial) Reflex Testing

- **Acoustic Reflex**: reflexive contraction of the stapedius muscle in response to high-intensity sound
- measured by introducing acoustic signals at varying frequencies (usually at 500, 1000, and 2000 Hz) in one ear and measuring the TM motility/compliance (stapedial response) via probe in the ipsilateral or contralateral ear
- **Acoustic Reflex Threshold**: lowest sound intensity level (dB) at which middle ear immitance change can be detected (typically elicited at 70–100 dB SL); broadband noise has 20 dB lower threshold compared to pure tones, this difference lessens as hearing worsens
- Reflex Arc: delivered sound → cochlea → action potential via CN VIII → ipsilateral cochlear nucleus → trapezoid body → **bilateral**

superior olives → facial nuclei → CN VII → stapedius contraction
(ipsilateral contraction stronger than contralateral contraction)
- <u>CHL</u>: may not be able to **stimulate** response initially if >40 dB CHL
  in sound delivering ear or may not be able to **receive** signal because
  ossicles cannot transmit stapes signal to TM in probe ear
- <u>SNHL</u>: may not be able to **stimulate** response initially if >60 dB
  SNHL
- **Acoustic Reflex Decay Test**: measures maintenance of the stapedial
  reflex for a sustained signal at 10 dB SL (ie, 10 dB above patient's
  hearing threshold level) for 10 seconds, inability to maintain reflex
  suggests retrocochlear lesion
- <u>Absent Reflexes</u>: minimal CHL (5–10 dB), SNHL (>60 dB), mild
  CN VIII impairment (0–40 dB), brainstem lesion, or CN VII
  dysfunction proximal to the stapedial branch

## Otoacoustic Emissions (OAE)

- **Otoacoustic Emissions**: objective low intensity sounds in the EAC
  emitted from **outer hair cells** spontaneously (spontaneous OAE),
  or more commonly, following acoustic stimulation (evoked OAE);
  presence of OAE suggests a normal cochlea (organ of Corti), middle,
  and external ear
- cochlear disorders >30 dB HL and middle ear disease may not have
  OAE
- retrocochlear lesions (including central auditory disorders) typically
  have normal OAE (as long as audiometric thresholds are within 30
  dB HL)
- <u>Common Reasons for Abnormal OAEs</u>: normal variant, poor
  probe/seal placement, middle and external ear pathology (cerumen
  impaction, otitis media, cholesteatoma, otosclerosis), uncooperative
  patient, cochlear disorders (ototoxicity)

### *Types*

- **Spontaneous OAE**: does not require external stimulus, present in
  ~50% of normal ears (typically not used for screening)
- **Transiently Evoked OAE (TEOAE, Cochlear Echo)**: evoked by
  broadband tones (clicks or tone bursts), indicated for **neonatal
  hearing screening**, present in most normal ears, presence of TEOAE
  suggests hearing threshold at least 20–40 db HL
- **Distortion Product OAE (DPOAE)**: evoked by simultaneous
  application of 2 pure-tone frequencies ($f_1$ and $f_2$); the resulting OAE
  is called the "distortion product" (most prominently $2f_1$–$f_2$); able
  to record at higher and more specific frequencies than TEOAE;

indicated for hearing screening, **ototoxicity, and noise-induced hearing disorders**, present in most normal ears and ears with a mild or moderate SNHL

- **Stimulus Frequency OAE**: evoked with a particular frequency (low tone), present in most normal ears
- **Sustained Frequency OAE**: evoked by a continuous tone, typically not used for clinical screening

### Clinical Application of OAE

- screening of neonates for hearing disorders
- detection of auditory processing disorders and auditory neuropathy (normal OAE, abnormal ABR)
- noise-induced hearing loss (OAE can be used to assess initial signs of cochlear injury)
- monitoring of ototoxic medication (aminoglycosides, cisplatin)
- cross-check behavioral testing
- differentiate sensory and neural hearing loss

## Pseudohypacusis

- subjective hearing loss with absence of organic pathology (**nonorganic hearing loss**); includes **malingering** and **functional hearing loss**
- may be suspected when patient hesitates, shifts pure-tone thresholds (test–retest reliability should be ≤5 dB), expresses confusion, or when the history is inconsistent with the hearing loss recorded on testing
- normally pure-tone average should be within 10 dB of SRT
- normally acoustic reflexes should be absent if tests suggest significant hearing loss
- suspicious if lack of crossover to the good side in purported unilateral hearing loss (crossover should normally occur at 0 dB for bone testing, 40 dB for air testing)
- **Stenger's Test**: the principle is that 2 tones of the same frequency presented to each ear cannot be heard simultaneously if one is louder; subject is given 2 simultaneous tones with matched frequency but the alleged poorer ear receives the tone at a greater intensity; a genuinely hearing-impaired subject or normal subject should hear the tone in the better hearing ear; pseudohypacusis is suggested if the subject reports hearing nothing
- **Lombard Test**: background noise is gradually introduced below the subject's recorded response threshold as the subject is asked to read aloud, pseudohypacusis is suspected if the volume of the reader's voice increases as the masking noise is increased

- **Delayed Auditory Feedback (Lee's Speech Delay Test):** patient's speech is played back at a delay, pseudohypacusis is suspected if patient stutters, hesitates, etc, confirming that he/she can hear his/her delayed speech, less frequently used
- **Doerfler-Stewart Test:** involves repeating spondees in masking noise, time-consuming, rarely used

# Electrical Response Audiometry

## Electrocochleography (ECoG)

- recording of evoked neuroelectrical events from the auditory nerve and cochlea in response to auditory clicks via air conduction
- <u>Technique:</u> probe is placed on the promontory via transtympanic needle electrode (most accurate) or on the TM near the umbo, a reference electrode is placed on the vertex or pinna, wide-band **clicks** or frequency-specific tone **pips** are introduced and electrical potentials are recorded
- <u>Indications:</u> direct measurement of cochlear and auditory nerve function, marked negative summation potential (SP) and an elevated SP amplitude/CAP (compound action potential) amplitude ratio present in certain diseases (eg, SP/CAP **≥0.45** in 66% of **Ménière's disease** as well as in syphilis); intraoperative monitoring with certain diseases (eg, Ménière's disease, perilymphatic fistula, *see also* p. 414)

### Cochlear Potentials

- **Endolymphatic Potential (EP):** determined by the stria vascularis maintaining an electrochemical gradient, produces a direct current potential (280 to 2100 mV)
- **Cochlear Microphonic Potential (CM):** alternating current generated predominantly from outer hair cells, normal CM suggests normal inner ear function
- **Summation Potential (SP):** direct current generated predominantly from the stria vascularis or hair cells, cochlea response to sound reflects changes in endolymphatic pressures
- **Whole-Nerve (Compound) Action Potential (CAP):** represents the summation of many individual nerve fibers, "all or none response," N1 (the first component of the CAP) is identical to the ABR wave I

## Auditory Brainstem Response (ABR, BAER, BAEP)

- also known as brainstem auditory evoked response (**BAER**) or brainstem auditory evoked potential (**BAEP**)

- recording of the activity of CN VIII and CNS's response to an auditory signal, occurs during the first 10–20 milliseconds after the stimulus
- <u>Technique</u>: active and reference electrodes are placed on the vertex, high forehead, mastoid, or earlobe; clicks, filtered clicks, or tone bursts are introduced to the ear between 5 and 50 times per second; surface electrodes utilize **signal averaging** to record specific ABR waves
- <u>Mnemonic for Indications</u>: "**TV DIN**," **T**hreshold testing in patients for whom behavioral testing is difficult to perform (eg, infants, suspected malingering), **V**estibular schwannoma/retrocochlear pathology concern (eg, asymmetric hearing loss, unilateral vestibular weakness, unilateral tinnitus), **D**iagnosis of brainstem lesion/pathology, **I**ntraoperative cochlear nerve monitoring, **N**eonatal/infant hearing screening (eg, high-risk children, failed OAE)
- ABR technique and interpretation vary by indication
- unaffected by sedation; affected by phenytoin, lidocaine, diazepam, and halothane
- waveform ABR may not be measurable with SNHL of >60 dB

## ABR Peaks

- each peak correlates to an anatomic location in the mnemonic **E COLI**
- only waves I, III, and V are observed at birth; I–V is prolonged at birth
- Peaks

| | |
|---|---|
| I–II: | **E**ighth nerve (distal and proximal segments) |
| III: | **C**ochlear nuclei |
| IV: | **O**live (superior) |
| V: | **L**ateral lemniscus (largest wave) |
| VI–VII: | **I**nferior colliculus |

## Retrocochlear Pathology and Vestibular Schwannoma Diagnosis

- abnormal **interaural wave V latency difference** (normal difference
- <0.2 ms), may be relative to size of tumor (reliable)
- abnormal **interaural wave I–V and III–V latency difference** (most reliable in the presence of a CHL)
- prolonged **interwave** latency between I–V or I–III
- increased **absolute** latency measurements (eg, 5.7 ms for wave V), may not be as accurate since latency may be affected by CHL

### *Intraoperative Monitoring of CN VIII*

- guides surgeon in hearing preservation lateral skull base surgery
- **Intraoperative ABR:** wave III typically lost first followed by V then I, long lag time
- **Direct Cochlear Nerve Monitoring:** electrode placed on CN VIII, measures action potentials, provides quicker feedback than ABR

## Auditory Steady-State Response (ASSR)

- newer test with good correlation to behavioral thresholds
- may be used to estimate hearing sensitivity at specific frequencies for patients with >80 dB HL (stimuli for ABR can not exceed 80 dB)
- employs continuous pure-tone signals (steady-state signals) rather than the short broadband clicks and tone bursts used in ABR, continuous pure tones are altered by rapidly modulating the frequency or amplitude

# Sound Amplification Devices

## Introduction

- <u>Components</u>: receiver, filter, amplifier, microphone, battery, volume control
- **Gain**: ratio of the output to the input (amplification)
- **Saturation Sound Pressure Level (SSPL)**: input level that produces the maximum output level
- **Frequency Response**: gain across a range of frequencies
- **Dynamic Range:** listener-specific signal range (of intensity ["loudness"] in this context), the range is from threshold level to loudness discomfort level (LDL)
- **Compression**: allows the dynamic range of the output to be less than the dynamic range of the input in a nonlinear fashion
- **Venting**: a hole within a hearing aid placed in the EAC that reduces low-frequency amplification by increasing resonant frequency, reduces the occlusion effect
- **Head Shadow**: attenuation of signal intensity on the side of the head contralateral to the stimulus
- **Assistive Listening Device:** hearing device designed for specific listening environments (eg, classroom, movie theater); includes soundfield, infrared, FM, and telecoil systems
- in general, binaural aids are preferred for binaural hearing loss to provide better discrimination, loudness, and sound localization

## Conventional Nonimplanted Hearing Aids

- **Analog Hearing Aids**: generally replaced by digital technology
- **Digital Hearing Aids**: provide differential amplification of frequencies to adjust for specific frequency losses, less background and circuit noise, allow **compression** (nonlinear relationship between input and output level, for patients who have limited dynamic range or recruitment) and **programmability** (different optimal programs for different listening situations)

### Body Hearing Aids

- microphone placed on torso
- <u>Advantage</u>: high level output with low feedback, easy to manage
- <u>Disadvantage</u>: conspicuous, clothes and body may rub against microphone, poor sound localization

### Behind-the-Ear (BTE)

- microphone and amplifier placed behind the ear, typically coupled to an earmold
- <u>Advantage</u>: allows adequate gain for mild to profound hearing loss, allows for open ear molds (large vents), less feedback
- <u>Disadvantage</u>: conspicuous

### Over-the-Ear (OTE) (Mini BTE)

- similar to BTE, except advances in miniaturization allow for a far less conspicuous design
- typically coupled to a very slim, clear tube ending in a small dome with a large vent (termed **open-fit**) that fits in ear canal

### In-the-Ear (ITE)

- placed in concha
- <u>Advantage</u>: less conspicuous, allows gain for moderate to severe hearing loss
- <u>Disadvantage</u>: feedback with increased gain, difficult to adjust settings, limited venting, cerumen, moisture damage

### In-the-Canal (ITC)

- placed inside ear canal, lateral aspect protrudes
- <u>Advantage</u>: inconspicuous
- <u>Disadvantage</u>: limited gain because of feedback (restricted to mild to moderately severe hearing loss), difficult to adjust settings, limited venting, cerumen, moisture damage

### Completely-In-Canal (CIC)

- placed deep into ear canal, no visible protrusion
- <u>Advantage</u>: most inconspicuous, for mild to severe hearing loss (does not require as much gain since placed close to TM), less feedback (since requires less gain), reduced noise, less distortion; variations allow extended wearing for months but must be inserted by a health care professional
- <u>Disadvantage</u>: difficult to adjust settings, difficult to insert and remove, limited venting, cerumen and moisture damage

## Middle Ear Implanted Hearing Aids

- surgically placed in middle ear, converts sound into mechanical energy
- an actuator attaches to the ossicles (which ossicle depends on device) and directly drives the ossicular chain
- may be partially implanted (external microphone and speech processor) or totally implanted (periodically charged through transcutaneous induction)
- <u>Advantage</u>: indicated for moderate to severe SNHL, no occlusion effect or feedback, improves word recognition with phone use, possibly improved cosmesis
- <u>Disadvantage</u>: expensive, requires surgery, risk of facial nerve or chorda tympani injury possibly greater than cochlear implant or mastoidectomy, device reliability, some require repeated surgeries for battery change

## Specialized Nonimplanted Hearing Aids for Single-Sided Deafness and Conductive Hearing Loss

- **Contralateral Routing of Signal (CROS)**: for unilateral profound hearing loss (single-sided deafness), microphone placed on poorer hearing ear and sound presented to better ear
- **Bi-CROS**: like CROS, but also amplifies sound on better hearing side
- **Bone Conduction Hearing Aid**: for severe CHL when air conduction aids cannot be used or single-sided deafness, nonsurgical alternative to bone anchored hearing aid (BAHA)
- **Soundbite**: for single-sided deafness, consists of a BTE microphone and processor wirelessly coupled to a custom fit **in-the-mouth** (**ITM**) bone conduction device, transmits sound through the teeth and upper alveolus; <u>Advantage</u>: nonsurgical and removable, superior sound quality and improved speech intelligibility in noisy environment; <u>Disadvantage</u>: expensive, may require removal during eating

## Bone-Anchored Hearing Aid (BAHA)

- also known as bone-anchored hearing implant (BAHI) and osseointegrated auditory implant; BAHA is generic term, Baha is trademarked
- consists of a vibrating sound processor, which couples to a titanium fixture/abutment implanted into the skull behind the ear (abutment-free variation allows coupling through magnets)
- sound conducted via direct bone contact
- <u>Advantage</u>: for congenital ear malformation (atresia, stenosis), chronic inflammation or infection due to presence of conventional hearing aid (can be used in patients with radical mastoid cavity), single-sided deafness (sound conducted to the normal cochlea via bone); superior sound quality and improved speech understanding in noisy environment
- <u>Disadvantage</u>: expensive (although insurance patterns may make more affordable than conventional hearing aids), requires surgery (risk of flap necrosis, skin infection), no sound localization

## Cochlear Implants

### Overview

- converts sound into an electric signal to stimulate the cochlear nerve directly
- <u>External Device</u>: microphone (placed above ear), processor (placed behind the ear or worn), transmitter (directly overlies internal component via magnetics)
- <u>Implanted Device</u>: receiver–stimulator, electrode array (placed in the **scala tympani** via a cochleostomy or the round window)
- <u>Contraindications</u>: acute or chronic infection, retrocochlear disease, Michel's deformity (complete otic capsule aplasia; Mondini and other cochlear deformities are not contraindications), inability to participate in an extensive rehabilitation program (noncompliance), temporal bone fracture involving otic capsule, NF-2 with CN VIII section, absent CN VIII, inappropriate expectations
- <u>Complications</u>: wound issues (most common; infection, skin flap breakdown), device migration or extrusion, meningitis, facial nerve injury, perilymphatic gusher (increased with Mondini's deformity), CSF leak, aberrant facial nerve stimulation (increased with malformations), "hard" (device hardware) failure (eg, electrode malfunction; detected by integrity testing), "soft" failure (normal integrity testing with unexplained performance decline or persistent symptoms when device on such as facial twitching, tinnitus, dizziness, headache)

## Indications

- <u>Adults</u>: **prelingual** if the patient has some sound awareness; **postlingual**, bilateral, severe to profound cochlear hearing loss with minimal benefit from hearing aids; **Hearing-in-Noise Test** (HINT, tests speech recognition in the context of sentences, for candidacy evaluation not performed in noise; similar tests such as **AZ Bio** may also be used) <50% in the ear to be implanted with the best-aided conditions and <60% in the better hearing ear, <50% word recognition score bilaterally, ability to participate in rehabilitation
- <u>Children</u>: ≥1 year old (many centers implant earlier), bilateral, profound (severe to profound if >18–24 months) cochlear hearing loss with minimal benefit from hearing aids (worse than 90 db HL, <20% word recognition score with hearing aids if >5 years old), ability to participate in rehabilitation, may be **pre- or postlingual**; children may be implanted <1 year old if deafness is due to meningitis
- <u>Ear Selection</u>: implant more recently deafened ear if no benefit from amplification bilaterally; in those patients with some benefit from amplification, implant the ear with poorer speech perception; with long-term auditory deprivation, implant the better ear
- implantation for disabling tinnitus and single-sided deafness under investigation

## Types

- **Single Channel**: historically mentioned, provided temporal and intensity information
- **Multichannel**: provides improved sense of pitch by delivering signals to different locations in the cochlea (tonotopic organization), results in better speech recognition; arrays of up to 22 electrodes available; however, only 8–10 electrodes are functionally utilized at any one time
- **Hybrid (Electroacoustic)**: in clinical trials in the United States as of this writing (in use in Europe/Asia), shorter/narrower electrode that preserves native acoustic function of apical cochlea, may incorporate hearing aid into external component, indicated for severe-profound high-frequency hearing loss with relatively good low-frequency hearing
- **Split (Double) Electrode**: for cochlear anomalies such as labyrinthitis ossificans

## Results

- better results associated with shorter duration of deafness, higher word recognition score, postlingual deafness, earlier age of implantation (in kids), and increased implant usage

- shown to reduce tinnitus, improve warble tone thresholds in children, and improve overall communication ability (including speech recognition)
- HINT test improves from average of 5% to 50%, 80% of patients are able to use the telephone
- implantees typically have a reduced dynamic range (difference between hearing threshold and discomfort level)
- labyrinthitis ossificans (ossified cochlea, due to multiple etiologies) may result in suboptimal outcomes and require special surgical techniques and electrode array

# APPROACH TO HEARING LOSS AND TINNITUS

## Evaluation of Hearing Loss

### History

- <u>Character of Hearing Loss</u>: onset and duration, constant versus fluctuating, progression, unilateral versus bilateral, high or low tone loss, decreased speech intelligibility
- <u>Contributing Factors</u>: recent infection (fevers, URI); loud noise exposure; recent trauma (barotrauma, straining, weightlifting, head injury); exacerbating factors of tinnitus (sleep, exercise, caffeine, alcohol, stress); previous otologic history (surgery, infections); toxin exposure and medications (*see* Table 8–1); history of autoimmune disease, hypertension, diabetes, vascular disorders, TMJ disease, neurologic disease (stroke), and depression; family history of deafness
- <u>Associated Symptoms</u>: aural fullness, fevers, vertigo, tinnitus (*see following*), otalgia, otorrhea, weight loss, other neurologic complaints
- think "KITTENS" for differential diagnosis (*see* Table 8–2)

### Physical Exam and Hearing Tests

- <u>Otoscopy/Microscopy</u>: inspection of EAC (cerumen impaction, stenosis, lesions, masses) and TM (color, thickness, presence of fluid, myringosclerosis, perforations, retractions, lesions), Valsalva test (test patency of eustachian tube by having subject perform Valsalva maneuver and inspect TM for mobility)
- <u>Pneumatic Otoscopy</u>: test mobility of TM with positive and negative pressure, **fistula test** (Hennebert's sign: positive pressure causes nystagmus, which reverses with negative pressure, may be seen in perilymph fistula, syphilitic labyrinthitis, superior semicircular canal dehiscense)

- <u>Inspection and Palpation</u>: inspect outer ear for lesions, malformations, auricular pits, scars, edema, swelling, mastoid tenderness, tragal tenderness
- <u>Complete H&N Exam</u>: cervical lymphadenopathy, neurologic and vestibular exam, bruits

## Tuning Fork Tests

- typically use a 512 Hz ($C^1$) or 1024 Hz tuning fork
- **Rinne Test**: compares air conduction (AC) and bone conduction (BC); strike fork then briefly place within 1 cm of the entrance to the ear canal (AC) and then immediately place on the mastoid (BC); when the tuning fork is better heard by AC, the test is referred to as **positive** (normal ear or most SNHL); if BC is louder than AC, the test is referred to as **negative** (CHL >15–30 dB HL or severe to profound SNHL with crossover)
- **Weber Test**: strike fork and place in center of forehead, vertex, or maxillary teeth; perceived sound should normally be heard centrally (or in "both ears"); unilateral **SNHL** should **lateralize to better** hearing ear, unilateral **CHL** should **lateralize to diseased** ear

## Audiometric Tests

- essential to identify auditory function, CHL versus SNHL, cochlear versus neural dysfunction, central auditory dysfunction, and pseudohypacusis (*see* pp. 349–357)

**TABLE 8–1.** Common Ototoxic Medications

| Category | Representative Examples and Comments |
|---|---|
| Antibiotics | aminoglycosides exert their ototoxic effects by damaging vestibular and cochlear hair cells, streptomyocin and gentamicin affect vestibular function more than auditory function (hearing loss occurs initially with supra-audiologic thresholds, >8 kHz), vancomyocin causes synergistic ototoxic effects with aminoglycosides |
| Chemotherapy Agents | cisplatin is toxic to outer hair cells, stria vascularis, spiral ganglion cells, and the vestibular system |
| Diuretics | furosemide and ethacrynic acid are the most common ototoxic diuretic agents, often potentiate other ototoxic medications |
| NSAIDs and Salicylates | aspirin is the most common medication to cause tinnitus (reversible with discontinued use) |

**TABLE 8-2.** Common Differential Diagnosis of Hearing Loss: KITTENS Method

| (K) Congenital | Infectious and Idiopathic | Toxins and Trauma | Tumor (Neoplasms) | Endocrine | Neurologic | Systemic/pSychological |
|---|---|---|---|---|---|---|
| Hereditary progressive | Labyrinthitis | Ototoxic medication | Temporal bone neoplasms | Hypothyroidism | Multiple sclerosis | Ménière's disease |
| Congenital auricular malformations | Otitis media | Noise-induced hearing loss | Cholesteatoma | Dyslipidemia | Meningitis | Paget's disease |
| Congenital hearing loss | Syphilis (leutic) | Head trauma | | | Stroke | Otosclerosis |
| | Presbycusis | Lead and mercury toxicity | | | Central auditory processing disorder | Presbycusis |
| | | Barotrauma | | | | Cerumen impaction |
| | | | | | | Pseudohypacusis |
| | | | | | | Autoimmune disorders |

## Ancillary Tests

### Imaging

- **CT Temporal Bone**: to evaluate complications of suppurative ear disease, tumors, cholesteatoma, mastoiditis, temporal bone fracture, petrous apex lesions, or congenital disorder
- **MRI of Brain and Brainstem with Gadolinium**: if suspect cerebellopontine angle tumor (vestibular schwannoma, meningioma), demyelinating lesions (multiple sclerosis), or petrous apex lesions (cholesterol granuloma)
- **Radiographs**: special views of temporal bone (Schuller's, Stenver's, Towne's views) largely replaced by CT and MRI

### Ancillary Laboratory Studies

- considered for specific circumstances
- **CBC**: may suggest active inflammation or leukemic process
- **Treponemal Studies**: Lyme titers and VDRL/FTA-ABS
- **Lipid Profile**: high risk of atherosclerotic disease (associated with hearing loss)
- **Immunologic/Autoimmune Profiles**: *see following*
- **Glucose**: screen for diabetes (associated with hearing loss)
- **Coagulation Profile**: coagulopathies associated with hearing disorders

# Evaluation and Management of Tinnitus

## Introduction

- **Subjective Tinnitus**: perception of sound in the absence of any acoustic, electrical, or external stimulation; more common than objective tinnitus; typically associated with a high-frequency hearing loss (pitch of tinnitus may correlate with the frequency of hearing loss, most common is 3000–5000 Hz)
- **Objective Tinnitus**: perception of sound caused by an internal body sound or vibration, may be exacerbated with a CHL
- Pathophysiology: pathophysiology of subjective tinnitus is largely unknown; however, current models center around subcortical auditory pathways rather than cochlear dysfunction; objective tinnitus is typically caused by an underlying vascular or mechanical disorder
- affects ~1/3 of those >50 years old; of these, 50% experience daily

## Workup for Tinnitus

- similar workup as hearing loss (*see* pp. 362–365) with special attention to retrotympanic masses, audible bruits, history of trauma, medications (**especially aspirin-containing products**), TMJ, and psychologic factors
- consider appropriate evaluation for retrocochlear lesions if suspected (vestibular schwannomas may present with tinnitus)
- may use Toynbee stethoscope to auscultate for objective tinnitus
- <u>Character of Tinnitus</u>: unilateral or bilateral, high-pitched (ringing, hissing) or low-pitched (roaring, buzzing), pulsatile (pulse synchronous versus non-pulse synchronous) or nonpulsatile, clicking, progression and frequency, loudness, pure or multiple tones, level of discomfort (eg, difficulty sleeping)
- <u>Labs</u>: thyroid function tests, lipid panel, VDRL/FTA-ABS

## Causes and Management of Objective Tinnitus

### Vascular Causes

- usually **pulse synchronous** (pulsatile in synch with heartbeat)
- **Benign Intracranial Hypertension (Pseudotumor Cerebri)**: most common cause of pulsatile tinnitus (especially in overweight females, 20–30 years old), increased intracranial pressure without focal neurologic signs, caused by systolic pulsations of CSF transmitted to dural venous sinuses, diagnosis is by lumbar puncture to measure CSF pressure, may be associated with mild SNHL; <u>Rx</u>: weight loss and diuretics such as acetazolamide (subarachnoid-peritoneal shunts in select cases)
- **Arteriovenous Malformation (AVM)**: pulse synchronous, may be secondary to trauma; <u>Rx</u>: surgical excision or embolization
- **Arterial Bruits and Venous Hums**: "whooshing" pulse synchronous sound, may be caused by turbulent blood flow in nearby vessels (stenosis, eg, from atherosclerosis) or by aberrant vessels (dehiscent or high riding jugular bulb or carotid, persistent stapedial artery)
- **Hypertension**: may present with pulsatile tinnitus
- **Vascular Tumor**: most common are glomus tympanicum (pulsatile tinnitus is most common presentation) and glomus jugulare (*see* pp. 392–393)

### Mechanical Causes

- may be pulsatile but **non–pulse synchronous**
- **Patulous Eustachian Tube**: eustachian tube abnormally open causing an abnormal flow of air between the nasopharynx and middle ear; presents with autophony (hyperacusis to one's

own speech and bodily sounds), hyponasal speech; may have a hypermobile TM that moves with respiration; causes include postradiation, significant weight loss (postpartum, cancer), stroke, injury to CN V, or iatrogenic (injury to the tensor veli palatini from cleft palate surgery); also associated with gum chewing, dental malocclusion, TMJ subluxation; <u>Rx</u>: address underlying cause, in children typically self-limiting, consider placing a catheter into the protympanic portion of the eustachian tube (often requires a PE tube, which is often of limited benefit), consider estrogen nasal drops to attempt to create swelling of vasoactive tissue of the torus tubarius

- **Palatal Myoclonus**: rapid clicking sound (~0.7–3.3 Hz) caused by contraction of the palatal muscles and eustachian tube; <u>Dx</u>: may be evaluated by nasopharyngoscopy in an awake patient, EMG; <u>Rx</u>: consider muscle relaxants

- **Tensor Tympani/Stapedius Syndrome**: spasm or myoclonus of the tensor tympani or stapedius muscles resulting in a fluttering, low-frequency tinnitus, accentuated by external sound; <u>Dx</u>: tinnitus synchronous with TM movement; <u>Rx</u>: avoidance of stimulants, reassurance, rarely requires section of the tensor tympani or stapedius

### Miscellaneous

- **Spontaneous Otoacoustic Emissions**: rare cause of objective tinnitus

## Causes and Management of Subjective Tinnitus

### Causes (*see* Table 8–3)

### Conservative Management

- evaluate medications for possible causes or contributing factors (eg, aspirin, NSAIDs, and alcohol may exacerbate subjective tinnitus)
- broadband masking at night (eg, placing the radio between stations)
- smoking and caffeine cessation
- relaxation techniques (biofeedback) and improvement of sleep hygiene
- regular exercise
- consider referral for habituation/retraining therapy and support groups

### Hearing Aids

- indicated for tinnitus associated with hearing loss
- reduces tinnitus by amplifying ambient sound to mask the tinnitus
- simplest method of "direct masking"

**TABLE 8–3.** Differential Diagnosis of Subjective Tinnitus

Hearing Loss and Otologic Disorders
- Hearing loss (presbycusis, autoimmune hearing loss)
- Retrocochlear lesions (vestibular schwannoma)
- Ménière's disease

Medications: (*see* Table 8–1)
- Aspirin/NSAIDs
- Antihypertensive agents
- Aminoglycosides
- Numerous medications have been reported to have the potential to cause tinnitus

Trauma
- Head injuries (whiplash)
- Loud noise exposure
- Barotrauma

Systemic Diseases
- Hypertension
- Depression and anxiety
- Neurologic disease (multiple sclerosis, brainstem stroke, meningitis)

Metabolic
- Hyperthyroidism and hypothydroidism
- Hyperlipidemia
- Vitamin deficiency (A, B, zinc)

## *Maskers*

- masking devices utilize a band of white noise centered around the tinnitus frequency (pitch matched)
- may be combined with hearing aid
- indicated for intractable tinnitus in patients with normal or near-normal hearing
- **Pitch and Loudness Matches**: determine frequency and intensity of tinnitus, difficult to obtain and often inaccurate
- **Minimal Masking Level**: intensity of sound (pure tone, narrowband, or broadband of noise) required to cover the tinnitus (requirements of >10–15 dB are associated with a poor success rate)
- **Residual Inhibition**: length of time of decreased or absent tinnitus after exposure to 1 minute of masking, typically lasts seconds to minutes

### Medical Management

- treating concurrent anxiety/depression reduces impact of tinnitus
- consider benzodiazepines, tricyclic antidepressants, carbamazepine, gabapentin, lipoflavinoids; poor evidence to support use of supplements
- may result in a >50% improvement of tinnitus (substantial placebo effect)

### Surgical Management

- cochlear implant for bothersome tinnitus associated with single-sided deafness under investigation

## Hyperacusis

- painful sensitivity to sounds
- 25–40% association with tinnitus
- may develop overprotection (overzealous earplug use) and phonophobia
- <u>Rx</u>: auditory desensitization

# INFECTIONS OF THE EAR AND TEMPORAL BONE

## Infections of the External Ear

### Acute Otitis Externa (Swimmer's Ear)

- **Acute Otitis Externa**: infection involving the skin of the EAC, usually bacterial (*see* Otomycosis, *following, for fungal otitis externa*)
- <u>Pathophysiology</u>
  1. aggressive washing of cerumen or retention of water ("swimmer's ear") results in a more alkalotic EAC and decreased production of antibacterial agents (eg, lysozyme), which are permissive for bacterial overgrowth and penetration into the pilosebaceous unit
  2. microtrauma (eg, cotton swabs, fingernails, or hairpins) directly injures EAC soft tissue
  3. moist, dark, warm environment of EAC is ideal for pathogen growth
- <u>Pathogens</u>: *Pseudomonas aeruginosa* (most common, opportunistic infection), *Staphylococcus*, and other gram-negative bacilli
- <u>Risks</u>: immunocompromised (diabetics, HIV), swimmers
- <u>SSx</u>: pain with posterosuperior manipulation of auricle, tragal tenderness, otalgia, and pruritus; edematous and erythematous EAC,

exudative or purulent discharge (may be difficult to distinguish from a coexisting otitis media); may have a CHL
- <u>Dx</u>: H&P (perforation of the TM may suggest underlying chronic otitis media)

### Management

- thorough and frequent ear canal debridement with fine suction
- aggressively manage diabetes
- evaluate for signs and symptoms of necrotizing otitis externa (granulation tissue in the canal, cranial nerve involvement)
- **Otic Drops**: acidification (eg, acetic acid), drying, antibiotic (eg, quinolone, aminoglycoside [neomycin], polymyxin B), or antibiotic/corticosteroid combination drops for 7–10 days (consider placing an otowick to aid drops in reaching medial EAC if canal is too edematous to visualize TM); avoid aminoglycoside drops in patients with PE tubes or TM perforations, especially if healthy middle ear mucosa (ototoxicity risk)
- **Oral Pain Medication**: may require opioids
- **Oral Antibiotics**: typically not required unless cellulitis, concurrent otitis media, persistent or severe symptoms, or systemic illness
- for refractory cases or noncompliance, may apply gentian violet in clinic
- consider culturing the EAC for recalcitrant infection
- educate patient to not instrument ear (no cotton swabs or fingers) and to maintain dry ear precautions (waterproof earplugs when showering, swimming; especially if recurrent)

## Otomycosis

- <u>Common Pathogens</u>: *Aspergillus* (most common) and *Candida* (10% of otitis externa)
- <u>Risks</u>: immunocompromised (diabetics, HIV), poor hygiene, increased ear moisture, long-term topical antibiotics
- often occurs as a superinfection with bacterial otitis externa
- <u>SSx</u>: moist, "tissue-paper" sheets of keratin within the EAC; dotted white, black, or gray membrane (removal of membrane reveals an erythematous canal); musty exudate; pruritic; *Aspergillus* produces distinct small black conidiophores on top of fluffy white filamentous hyphae
- <u>Dx</u>: H&P, may see fungal hyphae under microscope, culture
- <u>Rx</u>: similar to bacterial acute otitis externa (*see previous*); debridement; acidifying (eg, acetic acid), drying, or fungicidal otic drops; for refractory cases consider gentian violet or methyl-cresyl acetate

# Chronic Otitis Externa and Eczematous Otitis Externa

- **Chronic Otitis Externa**: thickening of the EAC from a persistent low-grade infection or inflammation
- **Eczematous Otitis Externa**: broad term that describes the dermatologic conditions affecting the EAC (eg, atopic dermatitis, contact dermatitis, psoriasis, lupus)
- **risk of secondary infection** by bacteria or fungal agents
- <u>SSx</u>: dry and flaky erythematous EAC, pruritus, mild pain
- <u>Dx</u>: H&P
- <u>Rx</u>: clean/debride EAC, corticosteroid cream/lotion or a combination of steroid lotion with nystatin can be applied TID, consider dermatology consult for eczematous otitis externa, surgical intervention (canalplasty with STSG) considered for recalcitrant disease

# Necrotizing Otitis Externa (Malignant Otitis Externa)

- <u>Pathophysiology</u>: extension of infection from the EAC into the temporal bone or skull base resulting in severe, **progressive osteomyelitis** ("malignant" otitis externa is a misnomer)
- <u>Pathogens</u>: *Pseudomonas aeruginosa* (most common)
- <u>Risks</u>: debilitated and immunocompromised patients (diabetics, HIV), radiation exposure
- <u>SSx</u>: **granulation tissue** in EAC typically at the bony-cartilaginous junction, persistent otalgia and otorrhea, cranial nerve involvement (CN VII > X > XI)
- <u>Dx</u>: H&P, CT temporal bone, technetium-99 bone scan (evaluates osteoblastic activity, excellent for localization of acute or chronic process, stays positive for prolonged period), gallium-67 bone scan (evaluates inflammation, used to follow course, will fade if disease resolves), indium-111 bone scan (newer), consider biopsy and culture of EAC, elevated ESR
- <u>Complications</u>: cranial neuropathy, sinus thrombosis, sepsis, meningitis, intracranial infections, high mortality (particularly in immunocompromised)

## *Management*

- prolonged parenteral anti-*Pseudomonas* antibiotics
- acidic, antibiotic, or antibiotic/corticosteroid combination otic drops
- aggressive diabetic control
- meticulous cleaning and debridement
- follow course with periodic gallium bone scans

- hyperbaric oxygen may be considered for recalcitrant cases
- rarely surgical debridement of involved tissue if failed medical management

## Perichondritis

- <u>Pathophysiology</u>: infection of the auricular cartilage possibly from extension from inadequately treated auricular cellulitis, exposed cartilage, trauma, otitis externa, or infected endaural incision
- <u>Pathogens</u>: *Pseudomonas aeruginosa* (most common), *S. aureus, Streptococcus*
- risk of cauliflower ear from cartilage erosion if not treated aggressively
- <u>SSx</u>: tender, erythematous, warm, edematous auricle; occasional systemic symptoms (fever, cervical adenopathy)
- <u>Dx</u>: H&P (also consider relapsing perichrondritis, *see* p. 372)
- <u>Rx</u>: aggressive systemic antibiotic regimen (anti-*Pseudomonal*)

## Bullous Myringitis

- <u>Pathophysiology</u>: inflammation of TM with formation of serous/hemorrhagic bullae on epithelial surface
- <u>Pathogens</u>: associated with virus or *Mycoplasma* after URI
- <u>SSx</u>: otalgia, serosanguinous otorrhea, hearing loss
- <u>Rx</u>: decompression of painful vesicles, analgesia, antibiotics; prednisone if SNHL

# Infections of the Middle Ear

## Acute Otitis Media (Acute Suppurative Otitis Media)

- acute infection (<3 weeks) causing inflammation of the middle ear space
- second most common disease in children (URI is the most common)
- most common <2 years old
- <u>Pathophysiology</u>: eustachian tube dysfunction results in negative middle ear pressure leading to transudative fluid collection in the middle ear space and subsequent infection
- <u>Common Pathogens</u>: **S. pneumoniae** (most common), *H. influenzae, Moraxella catarrhalis*; gram-negative bacilli, and Group B streptococcus may be found in infants; viral infection may often predispose/precede bacterial infection
- <u>Risks</u>: factors that contribute to eustachian tube dysfunction (craniofacial or skull base abnormalities, recurrent URI, allergic rhinitis), attendance at a child care facility, bottle feeding or supine baby feeds

(reflux into ear), smoking or secondhand smoke, immunologic disorders (especially IgA and IgG subclass 2 and 3 deficiencies) or ciliary dysfunction (Kartagener syndrome), GERD, prolonged nasotracheal intubation or nasogastric tube, adenoid hypertrophy, cholesteatoma, mass in nasopharynx at eustachian orifice

- <u>SSx</u>: otalgia (irritability and tugging of ears in children), aural fullness, hearing loss, tinnitus, fever, hyperemic or thickened TM, fluid in middle ear space (nonmobile or bulging TM, air-fluid levels or bubbles, yellow hue)
- <u>Dx</u>: H&P, audiogram (CHL <30 dB), tympanometry

### Medical Management of Acute Otitis Media

- 60% of cases will spontaneously resolve in 24 hours, 80% within 2–3 days
- <u>Topical Antimicrobial Therapy</u>: ototopical drops indicated if TM is perforated
- <u>Oral Antimicrobial Therapy</u>: first-line antimicrobials should include gram-positive and gram-negative coverage, may consider β-lactamase-resistant agents due to increasing β-lactamase activity in certain regions; treat for at least 7–10 days (typically resolves within 72 hours); if no resolution may consider broader spectrum coverage or β-lactamase-resistant agents
- <u>Adjunctive Therapy</u>: antipyretics, analgesics, oral or nasal decongestants (relieve associated nasal congestion, no proven benefit in the treatment of acute otitis media), myringotomy may be considered for severe otalgia or toxic patients
- <u>Antibiotic Prophylaxis</u>: indicated for recurrent acute otitis media, full course of antibiotics for 10 days followed by reduced bedtime dose for 5–6 weeks (eg, amoxicillin 250 mg tid for 3–10 days then 250 mg every night for 3–6 weeks)

### Surgical Management of Acute Otitis Media (*see pp. 376–377*)

## Serous Otitis Media (Otitis Media with Effusion)

- persistence of fluid in the middle ear space without evidence of infection
- **most common cause of pediatric hearing loss**, associated with language delay and behavioral issues
- <u>Pathophysiology</u>: may be from persistent fluid from suppurative acute otitis media (50% of acute otitis media patients have persistent fluid at 1 month, **10%** have fluid at 3 months) or secondary to eustachian tube dysfunction

- <u>SSx</u>: serous fluid (amber, dull, or gray) in middle ear space with air-fluid levels or bubbles, nonmobile (or retracted) TM, aural fullness, hearing loss, tinnitus
- <u>Dx</u>: H&P, audiogram (CHL <30 dB) and tympanometry (type B [flat] or type C [negative pressure])
- <u>Rx</u>: observation for 3 months in non "at risk" patients, frequent autoinflation, management of nasal congestion if present (eg, nasal corticosteroids for allergic rhinitis, routine decongestants not effective), consider myringotomy with PE tube, and/or adenoidectomy (if adenoids enlarged/obstructing) after failed conservative measures, antimicrobials (similar to acute otitis media) reduce the risk of secondary infection
- *NOTE*: any adult with unilateral, persistent middle ear effusion should undergo inspection of the nasopharynx (ie, nasopharyngoscopy) for nasopharyngeal tumor with biopsy of suspicious lesions

## Eustachian Tube Dysfunction

- <u>Pathophysiology</u>: obstruction of eustachian tube due to increased inflammation/infection of the sinonasal passage (URI or allergies) prevents ciliary motion and leads to decreased fluid clearance in the middle ear, chronic ETD results in underaeration of the middle ear leading to negative middle ear pressure, hypoxia and hypercapnia increase mucosal disease by an increase in number of goblet cells, negative pressure can cause retraction pockets and cholesteatoma
- <u>SSx</u>: constant or intermittent aural fullness, possible CHL, recurrent or chronic otitis media with effusion, inability to equalize middle ear pressure with swallowing or Valsalva maneuver, otalgia with pressure changes (descending in an airplane or scuba diving)
- <u>Dx</u>: H&P (diagnosis of exclusion), consider sudden SNHL and endolymphatic hydrops, audiogram and tympanogram (Type C)
- <u>Rx</u>: if associated with an acute infection (URI) usually resolves with resolution of infection; for chronic ETD consider corticosteroid nasal sprays, allergy management, oral and topical decongestants; address nasopharyngeal obstruction (adenoids and tumors); consider PE tubes for refractory cases; simple mastoidectomy may be considered for multiple PE tubes, retracted TM, and poorly pneumatized mastoids

## Chronic Otitis Media (with Otorrhea)

- **Chronic Otitis Media**: persistent (>6 weeks) or recurrent drainage from infection of the middle ear and/or mastoid in the presence of a TM perforation (or ventilation tube)

- <u>Pathophysiology</u>: chronically inflamed or infected middle ear space or mastoid secondary to poor aeration (chronic eustachian tube dysfunction), chronic perforation, or the presence of a cholesteatoma
- <u>Pathogens</u>: mixed infections; gram-negative bacilli (*Pseudomonas, Klebsiella, Proteus, E. coli*), *Staphylococcus (rates of MRSA increasing)*, and anaerobes
- <u>Risks</u>: abnormal eustachian tube function (cleft palate, Down syndrome), cholesteatoma, immune deficiency, ciliary dysfunction (Kartagener syndrome), gastroesophageal reflux
- <u>SSx</u>: otorrhea (mucopurulent, odorous), TM perforation, inflamed middle ear mucosa, CHL
- **Tuberculous Otitis Media**: uncommon; presents as insidious, painless, odorless, scant otorrhea, lymphadenopathy, multiple minute TM perforations with pale granulation tissue; usually from pulmonary source via hematological spread; nontubercular mycobacteria may also cause chronic otitis media
- **Granulomatosis with Polyangiitis (Wegener's)**: uncommon; may present with middle ear mass (granuloma) and serous otitis media, otorrhea or a SNHL secondary to cochlear vasculitis
- <u>Dx</u>: H&P, audiogram (CHL); CT is controversial, however, it should be obtained if suspect labyrinthine fistula, presence of facial weakness, or possible intracranial complications; relative indications for CT include previous surgery (revisions), only hearing ear, and inability to visualize TM
- <u>Complications</u>: *see* pp. 379–383

## *Medical Management of Chronic Otitis Media*

- <u>Aural Hygiene</u>: cleaning of discharge and debris from EAC (vinegar irrigations, periodic office cleaning), water protection (waterproof ear plugs during swimming and bathing)
- <u>Otic Drops</u>: antimicrobial or antimicrobial/corticosteroid combination drops
- <u>Systemic Antimicrobial Therapy</u>: consider 3–4 weeks of oral antimicrobials (broad spectrum including antipseuodomonal coverage), may consider parenteral antibiotics for persistent drainage; culture any drainage if not responsive to routine treatment
- <u>Address Eustachian Tube Dysfunction/Sinonasal Disease</u>: topical nasal corticosteroids, decongestants (results unimpressive)

## *Surgical Management of Chronic Otitis Media* (*see* following)

# Surgical Management of Otitis Media

## Myringotomy with Pressure Equalization (PE, Tympanostomy) Tubes

- <u>Indications</u>: recurrent otitis media (>3 episodes of acute otitis media over 6 months or >4 episodes over 1 year) with middle ear effusion at time of evaluation, persistent effusion (>3 months), poor response to antibiotic regimen, immunocompromised patient, cleft palate, impending complication (hearing loss), severe retraction pocket, barotitis media, autophony from eustachian tube dysfunction
- <u>Complications</u>: persistent otorrhea (10%), early extrusion, persistent perforation, tympanosclerosis, granuloma formation, cholesteatoma, hearing loss (similar complications may occur with nonsurgically treated recurrent otitis media)

## Adenoidectomy

- adenoids may harbor infection or obstruct eustachian tube especially in children
- <u>Indications</u>: consider in children >1–4 years old (age criteria controversial) with recurrent infections or hyperplastic adenoids; consider when patients require repeat PE tube placement

## Mastoidectomy

- <u>Indications</u>: persistent chronic otitis media despite appropriate medical therapy, coalescent mastoiditis, subperiosteal abscess, cholesteatoma; also used for various surgical approaches (eg, cochlear implantation, facial nerve decompression)
- <u>Goals</u>: create a "safe" ear by eradicating infection and removing cholesteatoma (first priority), preservation of hearing and vestibular function (second priority)
- **Canal Wall-Up Mastoidectomy**: includes simple/cortical and total mastoidectomy, preserves the posterior and superior wall of the EAC, procedure of choice to avoid mastoid bowl and provide a water-safe ear, indicated for limited disease and a reliable patient for follow-up (to check for recurrent disease), faster healing rate, increased risk of undetected recurrence or residual cholesteatoma (may require a "second look" procedure)
- **Modified Radical Mastoidectomy (Canal Wall Down)**: posterior EAC is removed creating a "mastoid cavity" or "bowl"; indicated for advanced disease (eroded canal wall, erosion of lateral SCC, large cholesteatoma), noncompliant patients, only hearing ear; provides good exposure and easier recognition of recurrent disease; disadvantages

include required cleaning of mastoid cavity, difficulty with hearing aid fitting, and increased risk of infection with water exposure
- **Radical Mastoidectomy**: totally exteriorizes the middle ear, attic, and mastoid cavity and obliterates eustachian tube; no attempt to reconstruct the middle ear; rarely indicated today
- **Tympanomastoidectomy**: tympanoplasty performed at the same time as mastoidectomy
- Complications: facial nerve injury; chorda tympani injury; worsening of CHL, SNHL, vertigo, infection

## Tympanoplasty

- **Myringoplasty**: isolated repair of the TM, surgery confined to the surface of the tympanic membrane
- **Tympanoplasty**: reconstruction of the TM and/or the securing of a sound-conducting mechanism to the inner ear fluid; can involve exploration, eradication of disease, and/or reconstruction of the middle ear with techniques such as ossicular chain reconstruction (this term is sometimes also used to refer to isolated myringoplasty)
- **Simple Closure (Paper Patch) Technique**: may be considered for small perforations, involves "rimming" the perforation (freshening the edges) to stimulate regrowth and subsequent placement of a scaffold material to encourage cellular migration (eg, cotton disk, onionskin paper, cigarette paper, Silastic film, collagen film)
- **Graft Technique**: repair of TM utilizing a tissue graft such as temporalis fascia (most common), perichondrium, cartilage, fat, areolar tissue, periosteum, vein, dura; may also employ bioengineered or synthetic materials
- Graft Technique Types
  1. **Medial (Underlay) Technique**: graft placed under (medial to) the annulus and remnant TM, and either lateral or medial to the malleus, adequate for most TM perforations (especially smaller posterior perforations), technically easier, shorter operating time, fewer complications
  2. **Lateral (Overlay) Technique**: graft placed lateral to the annulus, indicated for larger perforations (especially anterior perforations) and problem perforations, longer operating time, risk of lateralizing and anterior blunting of the graft, longer healing process, risk of entering the glenoid fossa, greater postoperative CHL
- Zollner-Wullstein Tympanoplasty Classification
  **Type I**:   repair of TM only
  **Type II**:  for malleus erosion, TM placed onto incus or malleus remnant

**Type III**:    for malleus and incus erosion; TM (or **PORP**) placed
              onto intact mobile stapes superstructure

**Type IV**:    for malleus, incus, and stapes superstructure erosion; TM
              (or **TORP**) placed onto mobile stapes footplate

**Type V**:    for fixed stapes fooplate; **Va** is horizontal canal
              fenestration (historic); **Vb** is stapedectomy

# Ossicular Chain Reconstruction (OCR, Ossiculoplasty)

- re-establishes the sound conduction mechanism from the TM to the cochlear fluids
- most common disruption is erosion of the lenticular process of the incus to the capitulum of the stapes (most susceptible site of avascular necrosis)
- in addition to discontinuity of the ossicles, ossicular fixation must also be assessed
- *see previous* for classic Zollner-Wullstein classification
- Incudostapedial Joint Reconstruction
    1. **Incudostapedial Joint Prosthesis**: composed of titanium or hydroxyapatite, can be used to bridge the gap when incus is partially eroded
    2. **Hydroxyapatite Cement (eg, OtoMimix)**: bone cement can be molded around incus and stapes
- Incus Replacement
    1. **Transposed or Sculptured Incus (Autograft)**: incus is removed, sculpted, and interposed between the malleus and the stapes superstructure
    2. **Allograft (Homograft)**: well-tolerated, provides excellent sound conduction, may be presculpted, requires storage, risk of disease transfer (fallen out of favor in United States)
    3. **Synthetic Incus Strut**: constructed from a variety of materials (eg, titanium, hydroxyapatite, porous polyethylene) to recreate the connection from the malleus to the stapes superstructure
    4. **Partial Ossicular Replacement Prosthesis (PORP)**: replaces malleus and incus, connects the TM to the stapes capitulum, constructed from a variety of material (eg, titanium, hydroxyapatite, predesigned gold, or porous polyethylene with a cartilaginous cap)
- Incus-Stapes Replacement
    1. **Transposed or Sculptured Incus Autograft**: incus is removed, sculpted, and interposed between the malleus and the stapes footplate
    2. **Allograft (Homograft)**: similar to allograft for incus replacement

3. **Synthetic Incus-Stapes Strut**: similar to synthetic incus strut for incus replacement, recreates connection from malleus or the TM to the stapes footplate

4. **Total Ossicular Replacement Prosthesis (TORP)**: replaces malleus, incus, and stapes superstructure, connects the TM to the stapes footplate, material similar to PORP

# Complications of Otitis Media

## Introduction

- High-Risk Pathogens: **type III pneumococcus** (intracranial predilection), **H. influenzae type B** (higher risk of meningitis), and presence of coexisting anaerobes
- Routes of Intracranial Spread: direct extension from bone erosion, lymphatic or hematogenous spread, invasion through normal anatomic structures (labyrinth), spread through iatrogenic or traumatic defects, extension through **Hyrtle's fissure** (**tympanomeningeal hiatus**; embryologic remnant that connects hypotympanum to the subarachnoid space)
- Dx: CT head with contrast or MRI brain with gadolinium, lumbar puncture (LP) may be required if meningitis is suspected (LP contraindicated with increased intracranial pressure to avoid herniation)
- *see also* pp. 387–388 for tympanosclerosis and TM perforation

## Extracranial Complications

### *Mastoiditis*

- Pathophysiology: suppurative infection of the middle ear spreads to the mastoid resulting in an osteitis of the mastoid air cells, continued infection within the mastoid may become purulent and result in breakdown of bony septae and coalescence of air cells (**acute coalescent mastoiditis**)
- may be acute coalescent, acute noncoalescent, or chronic; the term mastoiditis alone may refer to any, thus must specify
- SSx: in acute mastoiditis may have tenderness over the mastoid, associated suppurative otitis media, edema over the mastoid (indicates involvement of the cortex), fever, adenopathy
- Dx: CT temporal bone (look for coalescence or lack of septations of the mastoid with the presence of fluid or soft tissue)
- Rx: for acute mastoiditis, parenteral antibiotics, possible wide myringotomy or PE tube; for chronic or acute coalescent mastoiditis, consider mastoidectomy

### Subperiosteal Abscess

- <u>Pathophysiology</u>: acute mastoiditis results in spread of infection to involve the outer mastoid cortex elevating the periosteum
- <u>SSx</u>: edema, erythema, and tenderness over site of abscess, associated suppurative otitis media, fever
- **Postauricular Abscess**: most common site, spread through emissary veins or through bone, may present with a pinna protruding outward from mass effect
- **Bezold's Abscess**: spread through a perforation in the mastoid cortex, tracks into sternocleidomastoid muscle, presents as a mass in the posterior triangle of the neck
- <u>Dx</u>: CT temporal bone
- <u>Rx</u>: parenteral antibiotics, mastoidectomy with drainage of the abscess

### Petrous Apicitis (Petrositis)

- <u>Pathophysiology</u>: extension of infection into the air cell tracts around the labyrinthine capsule
- <u>SSx</u>: **Gradenigo's triad** (otorrhea, retroorbital pain, diplopia [abducens palsy occurs from involvement of **Dorello's canal**]), fever
- <u>Dx</u>: CT temporal bone
- <u>Rx</u>: parenteral antibiotics, consider mastoidectomy and petrous apicectomy

### Labyrinthine Fistula

- <u>Pathophysiology</u>: chronic suppurative otitis media from a cholesteatoma erodes the bone of the labyrinth (most commonly at the horizontal canal)
- <u>SSx</u>: may be asymptomatic, vertigo, SNHL
- <u>Dx</u>: CT may reveal bony erosion of the labyrinth, **fistula test** (nystagmus induced with pneumatic otoscopy, low sensitivity)
- <u>Rx</u>: surgical exploration via mastoidectomy with exteriorization of the cholesteatoma (matrix [shell] should be left intact over the horizontal canal), graft site if fistula is exposed (eg, with fascia), parenteral antibiotics if infected

### Facial Nerve Paralysis

- <u>Pathophysiology</u>: infection from suppurative otitis media adjacent to a dehiscent facial nerve in the middle ear space or elsewhere in the fallopian canal, injury may occur due to swelling of nerve

(inflammatory edema), direct pressure from suppuration, or bacterial toxic effects
- Rx: consider urgent surgical exploration/decompression or wide myringotomy, antibiotics for acute otitis media
- *see also* p. 429

## Intracranial Complications

### Meningitis

- most common intracranial complication of otitis media (especially in children <5 years old)
- increased risk with Mondini deformity
- Pathogens: **H. influenzae type B**, pneumococcus, hemolytic *Streptococcus*
- SSx: headache, lethargy, nuchal rigidity, irritability, fever, **Kernig's sign** (with hip in flexion, pain is elicited with leg extension), **Brudzinski's sign** (flexion at neck causes a reflexive flexion of legs), seizures, photophobia
- Dx: lumbar puncture (after verifying no increased intracranial pressure with CT or assessing for papilledema) for cells and culture (elevated pressure, decreased glucose, presence of inflammatory cells and bacteria, increased protein content), may consider MRI
- Rx: high-dose parenteral antibiotics, wide myringotomy, with culture of middle ear fluid, possible mastoidectomy, and surgical exploration (may cause ossification of the labyrinth or cochlea), audiogram when stable (10–20% risk of postmeningitic partial or total, unilateral or bilateral SNHL)

### Epidural (Extradural) Abscess

- purulent collection between skull and dura
- most commonly from direct extension via bone erosion
- associated with lateral sinus thrombosis
- SSx: may be asymptomatic, headaches, low-grade fevers, malaise
- Dx: CT/MRI reveals **biconvex disk-shaped enhancement**
- Rx: high-dose parenteral antibiotics and surgical drainage (debride diseased bone until normal dura is exposed, approach usually through mastoidectomy)

### Subdural Abscess

- purulent collection between dura and arachnoid membrane
- SSx: rapid neurologic deterioration (may develop quickly to seizures, delirium, hemiplegia, aphasia, or coma), nausea/vomiting

- <u>Dx</u>: CT/MRI reveals **crescent-shaped enhancement**
- <u>Rx</u>: high-dose parenteral antibiotics and neurosurgical consultation for drainage, surgical exploration with mastoidectomy and exploration of middle ear once patient is stable

### Brain Abscess

- most common sites are temporal lobe and cerebellum
- <u>SSx and Stages</u>
  1. **Encephalitis:** (initial invasion) fevers, headache, nuchal rigidity
  2. **Latency:** (organization of abscess, liquefaction necrosis) minimal symptoms, may last weeks
  3. **Expanding Abscess:** intracranial hypertension, seizures, localizing signs (nominal aphasia, quadrantic homonymous hemianopia, and motor paralysis for a temporal lobe abscess; nystagmus and gait disturbances for cerebellar lesions)
  4. **Termination:** rupture of abscess, death
- <u>Rx</u>: high-dose parenteral antibiotics, neurosurgical consultation for drainage, surgical exploration with mastoidectomy and exploration of middle ear once patient is stable

### Lateral Sinus Thrombophlebitis

- inflammation with subsequent thrombus formation of the sigmoid and/or transverse sinus
- <u>Pathophysiology</u>: mural thrombus forms in vessel wall (thrombophlebitis) → propagates distally and begins to seed
- <u>SSx</u>: "picket fence" spiking fevers, headache, papilledema, **Griesinger's sign** (edema and pain over mastoid from occlusion of the mastoid emissary vein), torticollis
- <u>Dx</u>: typically with imaging (CT may reveal enhancement within the sinus, MRI reveals increased signal intensity in both T1- and T2-weighted images, MRA/MRV may reveal total/partial occlusion), **Tobey-Ayer or Queckenstedt's test** (normally external compression of jugular vein results in a rapid increase in CSF pressure of 60–100 mm Hg, compression on the side of lateral sinus thrombosis results in a slow rise or no rise in CSF pressure secondary to obstruction), consider blood cultures or LP for cells and culture
- <u>Rx</u>: parenteral antibiotics, possible surgical exploration via mastoidectomy with removal of thrombus, may require ligation of internal jugular vein for recalcitrant disease, anticoagulants (*controversial*)

### *Otitic Hydrocephalus*

- raised intracranial pressure associated with otitis media
- *Misnomer*: does not cause hydrocephalus (dilation of the ventricles) but mimics its symptoms
- <u>Pathophysiology</u>: lateral sinus mural thrombus formation prevents CSF absorption, which results in intracranial hypertension (*theoretical*)
- <u>SSx</u>: chronic course (weeks), papilledema, diplopia, nausea, headache, lethargy, abducens palsy
- <u>Rx</u>: address thrombophlebitis (*as previous*), lower intracranial pressure (corticosteroids, mannitol, acetazolamide, serial LPs), consider surgical exploration with debridement once patient is stable
- <u>Complications</u>: risk of blindness secondary to compressive optic neuropathy

# Infections of the Inner Ear

## Labyrinthitis

- **auditory and vestibular dysfunction** (versus vestibular neuritis, which is only vestibular)

### *Viral Labyrinthitis*

- <u>Pathophysiology</u>: viral mediated, can occur in the absence of systemic viral illness, may complicate course of measles, mumps, varicella, or influenza
- <u>Histopathology</u>: atrophy of organ of Corti, stria vascularis, tectorial membrane
- <u>SSx</u>: severe vertigo, hearing loss, tinnitus, irritative nystagmus toward the affected ear, may develop lingering disequilibrium
- <u>Dx</u>: H&P, audiogram (SNHL)
- <u>Rx</u>: limited course of vestibular suppression, parenteral hydration if needed, early restart of activities (3–5 days), management of underlying infectious process (if possible), oral or transtympanic steroids if SNHL
- **Luetic Labyrinthitis**: *Treponema pallidum* infection that may present in primary, secondary, or tertiary syphilis; may present with **Tullio's sign** (vertigo and nystagmus elicited with loud noise)

### *Serous (Toxic) Labyrinthitis*

- toxin containing serous inflammation of the labyrinth resulting in hearing loss and vertigo

- <u>Pathophysiology</u>: presumed diffusion of toxic inflammatory products into the labyrinth, typically from the middle ear, can be a result of acute or chronic otitis media, trauma, or surgery
- <u>SSx</u>: vertigo, hearing loss, tinnitus, irritative nystagmus toward the affected ear
- <u>Dx</u>: H&P, audiogram (SNHL)
- <u>Rx</u>: same as viral labyrinthitis

### Suppurative Labyrinthitis

- bacterial invasion into labyrinth, associated with permanent hearing loss and vestibular dysfunction, can cause meningitis
- <u>Pathophysiology</u>: bacterial invasion from the middle ear space through the round window membrane or oval window niche or bone erosion with spread though the otic capsule (may occur secondarily from meningitis from invasion through the cochlear aqueduct)
- <u>SSx</u>: sudden vertigo and permanent hearing loss, typically in the presence of a middle ear infection, tinnitus, nystagmus away from the affected ear
- <u>Dx</u>: H&P, audiogram (SNHL)
- <u>Rx</u>: high-dose parenteral antibiotics, limited course of vestibular suppressants, surgical management of middle ear infection (if indicated); consider oral or transtympanic steroid administration after the initial infection is resolved and there is no improvement in hearing

## Vestibular Neuronitis (Neuritis)

- **vestibular dysfunction only** (versus labyrinthitis, which also includes hearing loss)
- <u>Pathophysiology</u>: presumed viral infection of the vestibular nerve
- <u>SSx</u>: vertigo lasting several hours to **days**, no hearing loss, may be associated with a prodromal URI, full recovery may require weeks or months, chronic imbalance possible, may later develop benign paroxysmal positional vertigo (BPPV)
- <u>Dx</u>: H&P, unilateral vestibular weakness (decreased caloric response) on ENG, no associated hearing loss on audiogram
- <u>Rx</u>: hospitalization with parenteral hydration if severe, high-dose corticosteroids, vestibular suppressants and antiemetics (long-term antivertiginous medications decrease central compensation, limit to ≤72 hours), vestibular rehabilitation

# NONINFECTIOUS DISORDERS OF THE EAR AND TEMPORAL BONE

## Noninfectious Diseases of the External Ear

### Cerumen Impaction and Foreign Body

- <u>Cerumen Risk Factors</u>: cotton swabs, hearing aids, earplugs
- <u>SSx</u>: CHL (if >95% of canal is occluded), tinnitus, aural fullness
- <u>Dx</u>: otoscopic inspection
- <u>Rx</u>: manual removal under magnification, consider low-pressure irrigation if no perforation, cerumen-softening agents (eg, mineral oil) for severely impacted cerumen, prevention (eg, discontinue cotton swabs)

### Keratosis Obturans

- <u>Pathophysiology</u>: keratin debris obliterates the EAC due to abnormal epithelial migration and/or hyperplastic epithelium with increased desquamation
- usually **bilateral** and affects **younger** patients with bronchiectasis and chronic sinusitis
- now considered distinct entity from canal cholesteatoma (*see following*)
- <u>SSx</u>: keratin debris in EAC with widening of the medial EAC, otorrhea, otalgia, CHL, often underlying inflammation
- <u>Dx</u>: H&P, CT shows diffuse widening of the EAC
- <u>Rx</u>: regular debridement of EAC, antibiotics/steroid drops if infected, routine use of acetic acid solution or hydrogen peroxide solution may reduce accumulation; surgery for recalcitrant cases involves canalplasty with skin graft

### Canal Cholesteatoma

- <u>Pathophysiology</u>: EAC cholesteatoma caused by blockage of the EAC (typically after trauma) permitting accumulation of epithelial debris, bone remodeling from pressure of the keratin plug may cause bony enlargement; may be acquired (due to surgery, trauma, chronic inflammation) or spontaneous
- usually **unilateral** and affects **older** patients
- <u>SSx</u>: keratin debris in EAC, chronic otalgia, otorrhea, CHL, may become secondarily infected, may erode into middle ear or attic
- <u>Dx</u>: H&P, CT shows focal erosion

- <u>Rx</u>: debridement of EAC, cleansing with ototopical (softening) drops, surgical removal with canalplasty (including replacement of diseased skin with healthy skin graft or cartilage/perichondrial grafts)

## Relapsing Polychondritis (Perichondritis)

- <u>Pathophysiology</u>: autoimmune disease of unknown etiology, inflammation of elastic cartilaginous tissue with high concentration of glycosaminoglycans
- <u>SSx</u> (episodic and progressive)
  1. auricular chondritis, cochlear and vestibular injury (vertigo, hearing loss)
  2. respiratory chondritis (laryngeal collapse)
  3. nasal chondritis (saddle-nose deformity)
  4. polyarthritis (nonerosive, migratory)
  5. cardiac valve insufficiency
- <u>Histopathology</u>: perichondrial inflammation, fibrous tissue replacement
- <u>Dx</u>: H&P, elevated nonspecific immunologic markers (eg, ESR, IgG), elevated antibodies to type II and type IV collagen (must differentiate from rheumatoid arthritis, gout, and other connective tissue diseases)
- <u>Rx</u>: NSAIDs, corticosteroids for severe attacks, dapsone

## Exostoses

- <u>Pathophysiology</u>: unknown etiology (associated with **cold water and cold wind activities**; also called **surfer's ear**) resulting in benign bony outgrowths from bony EAC
- <u>SSx</u>: most commonly asymptomatic; single or **multiple**, unilateral or **bilateral** smooth sessile protrusions of the **medial** bony EAC (often anterior and posterior walls), results in narrowing of the canal with progressive growth
- <u>Dx</u>: H&P
- <u>Rx</u>: excise (canalplasty) if symptomatic (CHL, recurrent external ear infections, chronic wax accumulation)

## Osteoma

- <u>Pathophysiology</u>: true neoplastic benign outgrowth in the bony canal
- <u>SSx</u>: **single, unilateral** protrusion at the **bony-cartilaginous junction**, asymptomatic unless it becomes obstructive
- <u>Dx</u>: H&P
- <u>Rx</u>: excise (canalplasty) if symptomatic

## Aural Polyp

- <u>Pathophysiology</u>: EAC inflammatory tissue associated with PE tubes, middle ear disease, cholesteatoma, foreign bodies, and malignant tumors
- <u>SSx</u>: well-circumscribed, soft, fleshy mass; symptoms related to obstruction or secondary infection, otherwise usually painless
- <u>Dx</u>: H&P, biopsy if unclear etiology (possibly in conjunction with middle ear exploration)
- <u>Rx</u>: debridement, topical steroid/antibiotic drops; nonresolution suggests more concerning underlying process

## Painful Auricular Nodules

- **Chondrodermatitis Nodularis Helices (Winkler's Nodule)**: benign nodular growth on helix of older men (may look like basal cell or squamous cell carcinoma), may be due to pressure or trauma to cartilage; <u>Rx</u>: full thickness excision
- **Gout**: pink nodules filled with chalky substance, due to uric acid deposits; <u>Rx</u>: medical control of gout, analgesia as indicated
- **Ochronosis**: occurs in alkaptonuria (homogentisic acid metabolic disorder), connective tissue black when oxidized, deposits in cartilage

# Noninfectious Disease of the Tympanic Membrane and Middle Ear

## Tympanic Membrane Perforation

- <u>Pathophysiology</u>: **acute/chronic suppurative otitis media** (most common cause), persistent perforation after extrusion of a **PE tube, trauma** (cotton swab/foreign body, hard blow to the ear, barotrauma, diving, water skiing, explosion, forceful irrigation, slag burn), **iatrogenic, cholesteatoma** (associated with peripheral perforations)
- spontaneous closure of a perforated TM results in a dimeric membrane ("monomeric" is a *misnomer* as it contains two layers: outer epidermal and inner mucosal)
- <u>Types</u>
  1. **Central**: perforation does not involve the annulus, typically infectious
  2. **Marginal**: involves the annulus, less likely to resolve spontaneously, higher association with cholesteatoma
  3. **Subtotal**: involving nearly the entire TM
  4. **Total**: involving entire TM
- <u>SSx</u>: CHL, tinnitus, otorrhea

- <u>Dx</u>: otoscopic exam, audiogram
- <u>Rx</u>: keep ear dry, may consider tympanoplasty for a persistent perforation (*see* pp. 377–378)

## Tympanosclerosis

- **Myringosclerosis**: hyalin and calcified deposits within the TM only, seen as visible white plaques on the TM, occurs as sequela of otitis media or TM trauma (eg, prior PE tubes), does not affect hearing; <u>Rx</u>: none
- **Tympanosclerosis**: same process as myringosclerosis except occurs in the middle ear mucosa as well, may fix ossicles and cause CHL; <u>Rx</u>: tympanoplasty ± OCR if warranted

## Cholesteatoma (of Middle Ear/Mastoid)

- *NOTE:* this section concerns cholesteatoma of the middle ear/mastoid (most common), cholesteatoma may also occur in the EAC (*see* pp. 385–386) or the petrous apex/CPA (*see* pp. 396, 397–398; then also called epidermoid cyst)
- *Misnomer:* does not contain fat or cholesterin ("keratoma" or "squamoma" would be more appropriate terms)
- results from squamous epithelium in the middle ear or mastoid, desquamation results in continued accumulation (growth) of keratin debris, and associated bone and soft tissue erosion and recurrent infections
- <u>Types</u>
  1. **Primary Acquired**: forms from invagination of a **retraction pocket**, associated with negative ear pressure (eustachian tube dysfunction); pars flaccida pockets are most common and initially invade the epitympanum via **Prussak's space** (*see* p. 341), pars tensa retraction pockets more directly invade the middle ear
  2. **Secondary Acquired**: forms from ingrowth of keratinizing epithelium into the middle ear space through a pre-existing TM perforation (previous otitis media) or secondary to trapping canal skin from surgery (iatrogenic) or trauma
  3. **Congenital**: forms from embryonic epithelial tissue (rests) within the temporal bone (commonly associated with the tensor tympani muscle), presents as a white mass generally in the anterosuperior middle ear with an intact TM
- <u>Pathophysiology</u>: cholesteatoma forms as described previously; bony resorption can occur through proteolytic enzymes released by the cholesteatoma, pressure necrosis, or secondary infection; presence of cholesteatoma may harbor infection, resulting in a chronically draining ear, may be associated with biofilms

- <u>SSx</u>: white "pearly" mass within the middle ear or mastoid space, nonresolving chronic suppurative otitis media, progressive CHL ("silent cholesteatoma" may occur when a large cholesteatoma acts as a sound conductor)
- <u>Dx</u>: visualization of squamous epithelium by otomicroscopic evaluation, CT temporal bone considered in select cases (abnormal soft tissue mass within middle ear, epitympanum, or mastoid cavity with associated bony erosion, most commonly of the scutum), audiometry (CHL)
- <u>Histopathology</u>: compact sac of keratinizing squamous epithelium with a central core of keratin debris
- <u>Complications</u>: destruction of the ossicular chain, chronic otitis media, labyrinthine fistula, intracranial complications, facial nerve paralysis
- <u>Rx</u>: surgical removal or exteriorization via tympanoplasty or tympanomastoidectomy with primary or secondary ossicular chain reconstruction, address chronic otitis media (*see* pp. 374–379)

## Otosclerosis

- historically also called otospongiosis
- abnormal resorption and deposition of bone in all 3 layers of the otic capsule (endosteal, endochondral, and periosteal) and ossicles
- autosomal dominant with incomplete penetrance, 60% have family history
- <u>Pathophysiology</u>: increased osteoclastic activity results in perivascular bony resorption forming fibrotic spaces (**lytic phase**), osteoblasts within the fibrotic spaces produce immature bone (**bone production phase**), cycling of resorption and bone formation results in otosclerotic bone (**remodeling phase**)
- most common involved site is anterior to oval window (**fissula ante fenestrum**), second most common site is the border of the round window (**round window otosclerosis**)
- disease process may involve the inner ear, causing SNHL (cochlear otosclerosis)
- ~10% of Caucasians have histologic evidence of otosclerosis (<1% develop clinical otosclerosis)
- frequent bilateral involvement (not necessarily associated with hearing loss, ≤85%, varies widely among studies)
- pregnancy may be associated with acceleration of otosclerosis
- **Carhart notch**: depressed bone conduction threshold at **2000 Hz,** which typically improves after stapedectomy causing **overclosure** of the air–bone gap (postoperative AC thresholds are better than preoperative BC thresholds) suggesting that the cause of this audiologic phenomenon is artifactual

- <u>SSx</u>: slowly progressive CHL beginning at 20–40 years old without history of otitis, tinnitus (80%), **Schwartze sign** (red hue behind TM from hyperemia of the promontory mucosa from increased vascularity, represents active phase)
- <u>Dx</u>: H&P including tuning forks, audiogram (CHL, normal word recognition, Carhart notch, SNHL in late disease), absent stapedial (acoustic) reflex, tympanometry (may be type $A_S$); must rule out superior semicircular canal dehiscence syndrome with CT or acoustic reflexes (absent in otosclerosis, normal in superior canal dehiscence); confirmation of otosclerosis through exploratory tympanotomy
- <u>Histopathology</u>: active lesions reveal spongy bone (**otospongiosis**) seen as blue with staining (**blue mantles of Manasse**), hyper-cellularity, active osteocytes and osteoblasts, increased resorption spaces, and increased vascular channels; inactive lesions reveal resorption spaces filled with collagen and osteoid, sclerotic bone, and narrowed vascular spaces
- **Cochlear (Labyrinthine) Otosclerosis**: presents as an SNHL, rarely associated with vertigo

### Differential Diagnosis

- **Superior Semicircular Canal Dehiscence Syndrome**: rarely presents with only CHL
- **Ossicular Fixation**: may be congenital, secondary to infection or trauma, or a result of bony ankylosis or ossification of suspensory ligaments; <u>Rx</u>: surgical reconstruction
- **Paget's Disease (Osteitis Deformans)**: rare, autosomal dominant with variable penetrance, excessive absorption of bone with fibrovascular replacement forming weak haphazard trabecular bone (mosaic bony changes), similar histologically to otosclerosis except begins in periosteal layer, diffuse involvement of the skull (eg, enlarged calvaria; otosclerosis only involves the temporal bone), usually does not involve the stapes footplate, typically causes SNHL (may also have CHL), onset in 50s, increased alkaline phosphatase on labs; <u>Rx</u>: hearing aid, medical management to inhibit bone resorption (*see also* pp. 225–226)
- **Osteogenesis Imperfecta (van der Hoeve Syndrome)**: rare, autosomal dominant (most subtypes), characterized by increased bone resorption and abnormal remodeling, usually presents in childhood, multiple fractures, blue sclera, may result in stapes fixation; <u>Rx</u>: may consider stapedectomy for stapes fixation
- **Osteopetrosis (Albers-Schönberg Disease)**: rare, autosomal dominant or recessive, results in ossicular anomalies (otic capsule is resistant to the disease), thickened bones of the skull base, blindness (optic nerve atrophy), absent paranasal sinuses, choanal atresia, facial paralysis, hepatosplenomegaly, brittle bones; <u>Rx</u>: hearing aid

## Nonsurgical Management

- **Hearing Aid/Observation**: option for those who do not want to undergo elective stapes surgery, only hearing ear, failed surgical management, high-risk patients, and nonoperative candidates
- **Medical Management**: sodium fluoride (may prevent progression of hearing loss), vitamin D, calcium (*controversial*)

## Stapedectomy/Stapedotomy

- Indications: CHL (>20 dB ABG, negative [abnormal] Rinne with 512 Hz tuning fork) secondary to otosclerosis with adequate cochlear reserve and good speech discrimination (initial stapedectomy should be carried out on the poorer hearing ear, the better ear may be addressed 6–12 months later)
- Contraindications: only hearing ear, active infection, suspected active endolymphatic hydrops, TM perforation; advanced age is not a contraindication; however, success may be slightly lower >70 years of age
- **Stapedectomy**: totally or partially removes stapes footplate with placement of a prosthesis from the incus to the vestibule
- **Small-Fenestra Stapedotomy**: creates a fenestration in the footplate for placement of a prosthesis, fenestrations may be completed with a microdrill or laser ($CO_2$ or KTP)
- Complications: SNHL (1–3%, may be profound), facial nerve injury (<1%), chorda tympani nerve injury (taste disturbance), displaced prosthesis, tinnitus, vertigo/disequilibrium
- Hearing Results: 90% closure of ABG <10 dB, 10% unchanged, 1% worse, 1% deaf (revision procedures have 65% success rate, but with 7× increased risk of iatrogenic profound SNHL)

### Intraoperative Considerations in Stapes Surgery

- **Perilymphatic Gusher**: rare, may occur secondary to a defect in the cribrose area of the IAC fundus (actually CSF gusher), risk of permanent SNHL; Rx: seal vestibular opening with a graft, place prosthesis, pack, and close; management for perilymph fistula; may consider lumbar puncture or drain
- **Facial Nerve Dehiscence**: facial nerve may block access to oval window; Rx: if significant may abort procedure, otherwise consider gently retracting nerve superiorly (*controversial*)
- **TM Perforation**: may occur intraoperatively; Rx: repair small perforations with fascia, perichondrium, or fat graft; larger perforations may require deferring stapedectomy
- **Floating Footplate**: fixed footplate suddenly becomes mobile after the stapes superstructure is removed, risk of depressing the

footplate into the vestibule; <u>Rx</u>: if control hole is in place may attempt to remove (creating a control hole may be difficult) or abort and wait for the footplate to refix and reoperate later (laser techniques minimize floating footplate)

- **Biscuit Footplate**: primary focus of otosclerosis causes a very thickened footplate; <u>Rx</u>: use microdrill on thickened bone, then usual technique
- **Persistent Stapedial Artery**: if involves anterior half of footplate procedure can be completed posterior to the vessel, if not enough uninvolved space on the footplate then abort; persistent stapedial artery may be difficult to coagulate with bipolar cautery or laser
- **Lateral Ossicular Chain Fixation**: after separation of incudostapedial joint, it is essential to evaluate for stapes versus lateral chain fixation; if lateral chain fixated, perform ossiculoplasty or mobilize lateral chain instead

# Temporal Bone and Lateral Skull Base Tumors

## Paraganglioma (Glomus Tumor, Chemodectoma)

- slow-growing, benign tumor, although locally destructive (expansive, bone eroding) of the chemoreceptive cells (paraganglion cells, neural crest in origin) distributed along parasympathetic nerves in the base of skull, neck, and chest
- most common benign tumor of the temporal bone of adults (rare in pediatrics)
- **10%** multiple
- **<5%** malignant degeneration
- genetic predisposition (**20% family history**)
- female > male
- **1–3%** associated with a paraneoplastic syndrome (paroxysmal hypertension, headache, and palpitations, eg, in MEN syndrome) from secretion of vasoactive catecholamines and other neuropeptides
- <u>Types</u>
  1. **Carotid Body (Glomus Caroticum)**: arises from carotid body, most common type in the head/neck, typically does not involve the temporal bone
  2. **Glomus Jugulare**: arises from the region of the jugular foramen (the adventitia of the jugular bulb), most common type in the temporal bone, supplied by ascending pharyngeal artery
  3. **Glomus Tympanicum**: arises from the promontory along the course of Jacobson's nerve (tympanic branch of CN IX), confined to the middle ear space, supplied by ascending pharyngeal artery

4. **Glomus Vagale**: arises from paraganglia around the vagus nerve at the base of skull

- <u>SSx</u>: pulsatile tinnitus (most common symptom), aural fullness, hearing loss, cranial nerve palsies (CN IV–XII), Vernet syndrome (CN IX–XI), Collet Sicard syndrome (CN IX–XII), Villaret's syndrome (CN IX–XII and sympathetic chain defects), aural discharge, otalgia, dizziness (invasion of the labyrinth), reddish middle ear mass, **Brown's sign** (blanching of the TM with positive pressure in glomus tympanicum), **Aquino's Sign** (pulsation of paraganglioma decreases with carotid artery compression), rare cases of bloody otorrhea
- <u>Dx</u>: otomicroscopic exam, neurologic exam, CT temporal bone with contrast; MRI/MRA ("salt and pepper" lesion on T2-weighted images, may miss small tumors), bilateral four-vessel angiography (assesses collateral circulation and allows for preoperative embolization), audiometry (baseline hearing), and 24-hour urine catecholamine screen (vanillylmandelic acid, metanephrine, normetanephrine)
- <u>Histopathology</u>: nests of nonchromaffin-staining cells clustered among vascular channels lined by epithelioid cells (Zellballen)
- <u>Staging</u>: *see* Table 8–4
- <u>Rx</u>: surgical resection (endaural versus extended facial recess approach for glomus tympanicum, Fisch type A infratemporal fossa approach for glomus jugulare) with possible preoperative embolization; primary radiation therapy for nonoperative candidates, advanced tumors, or presence of residual disease

## Vestibular Schwannoma (Acoustic Neuroma)

- **Vestibular Schwannoma: most common** CPA tumor (~85%), arises from the Schwann cells of the vestibular portion of CN VIII (hence vestibular schwannoma, **acoustic neuroma is a misnomer** since it typically does not arise from the cochlear nerve and is not a neuroma), indolent growth rate, benign and encapsulated, very rare malignant potential (<1%)
- **Cerebellopontine Angle (CPA)**: space in the posterior fossa bordered anterolaterally by the petrous bone and clivus, posterolaterally by the cerebellum, inferiorly by the cerebellar tonsil, and superiorly by the cerebellar peduncles and pons; includes CN V–XII and the anterior inferior cerebellar artery (AICA)
- CPA tumors account for 10% of all intracranial masses
- 95% sporadic, 5% associated with neurofibromatosis type 2 or familial

**TABLE 8–4.** Classification of Glomus Tumors of the Temporal Bone

**Glasscock-Jackson Classification**

Glomus Tympanicum

  I.  small mass limited to the promontory

 II.  tumor filling the middle ear space

III.  tumor extending into the mastoid

IV.  tumor extending into the mastoid, EAC, and anterior to carotid artery

Glomus Jugulare

  I.  small tumor involving jugular bulb, middle ear, and mastoid

 II.  tumor extending under IAC with or without intracranial extension

III.  tumor extending into petrous apex with or without intracranial extension

IV.  tumor extending into the clivus, infratemporal fossa, may have intracranial extension

**Fisch Classification**

A.  tumor involves middle ear only (glomus tympanicum)

B.  tumor involves middle ear and mastoid

C.  tumor extend in the infralabyrinthine region toward petrous apex

D.  tumors with <2 cm intracranial extension (D1) or >2 cm (D2)

- **Neurofibromatosis Type 2 (NF2)**: autosomal dominant disorder associated with bilateral vestibular schwannomas and other intracranial and spinal cord tumors (*see also* p. 405)
- Vestibular Schwannoma Histologic Types
    1. **Antoni Type A:** histologically parallel nuclei, uniform spindle cells, compact cells
    2. **Antoni Type B:** histologically less uniform, may have fatty or hyaline degeneration, less cellular
- SSx: progressive, high frequency, unilateral SNHL (most common presenting symptom); 10–20% may present with sudden SNHL; tinnitus (typically high frequency); vertigo or imbalance with increased growth; advanced tumors may present with facial nerve (facial paresis, **Hitselberger's sign** [reduced sensation of the EAC and conchal bowl]) or trigeminal nerve (unilateral facial numbness) involvement, papilledema, occipital headache, lower cranial nerve involvement, or ataxia

## *Diagnosis*

- **Audiometry**: initial screening, asymmetric SNHL with a word recognition score poorer than expected from the amount of pure-tone loss, **acoustic (stapedial) reflex decay** (inability to maintain the stapedial reflex for a sustained signal at 10 dB SL for 10 seconds), **rollover** (paradoxic decrease in word recognition ability with increasing signal intensity [dB])
- **Auditory Brainstem Response (ABR)**: most sensitive and specific audiologic test (10–15% false-negative rate), may be used for selective screening of asymmetric hearing loss or vestibular weakness (*see* pp. 355–357), may miss tumors <1 cm in size
- **MRI with Gadolinium of IAC**: gold-standard, sensitive to submillimeter tumors, brightly enhance with gadolinium
- **CT with Contrast**: indicated if MRI is unavailable or contraindicated, may miss tumors <1 cm, suspect with asymmetric widening of the internal auditory canal
- **Vestibular Tests**: normal or asymmetric caloric weakness (an early sign)

## *Management*

- **Surgical Excision**: *see following* for approaches, subtotal or staged excision considered if total resection risks neurologic function or in the elderly
- **Stereotactic Radiation Therapy**: eg, Gamma Knife, linear accelerator (LINAC, eg, CyberKnife); considered for tumors <2.5 cm, nonoperative candidates, elderly; prevents tumor growth (does not remove tumor); risk of facial nerve injury and hearing loss may be less than surgical excision for small tumors <2.5 cm (*controversial*); complications (eg, hearing loss) can occur many year after finishing therapy; no pathologic diagnosis
- **Observation**: consider in select patients (eg, elderly and nonoperative candidates) or for small tumors to assess for growth before treatment, follow with serial MRIs every 9–12 months
- <u>NF2</u>: *see* p. 405

# Other Cerebellopontine Angle Tumors

- **Meningioma**: second most common CPA tumor (3–15%), arises from cap (endothelial) cells from the tips of the arachnoid villi, female predilection (2:1), presentation similar to vestibular schwannoma, imaging typically distinguishes difference (meningiomas are more homogeneous, dense, contain calcifications, and have a flat dural base/tail), histopathology reveals large endothelial cells with uniform nuclei occurring in whorls and psammoma bodies; <u>Rx</u>: surgical excision, stereotactic radiation therapy, external beam radiation

- **Epidermoid Cyst**: congenital cholesteatoma of the CPA; may erode bone; may present with cranial nerve palsies, headache, or hearing loss (*see* pp. 385–386, 388–389, 397–398 for cholesteatoma of other locations)

- **Arachnoid Cyst**: thin-walled sac within the arachnoid, filled with CSF, may be differentiated with diffusion-weighted MRI; <u>Rx</u>: incision and drainage for symptomatic lesions

- **Facial Nerve Schwannoma**: usually involves geniculate, skip lesions, on MRI may see extension to IAC with enlarged fallopian canal; <u>Rx</u>: initial observation, decompression, resection with nerve graft

- **Venous Malformation**: rare, venous vascular malformation (formerly classified as hemangioma) may involve CN VII particularly in the IAC and perigeniculate region (rather than the CPA), may erode into cochlea, causing pulsatile tinnitus, may ossify

- **Metastatic Lesions**: rare, primaries from glial tumors, breast, lung, prostate, and others

- **Malignancies**: present with more rapid growth, earlier cranial nerve involvement, and destructive rather than expansive growth

- <u>Others</u>: lipoma, lymphoma, glioma, dermoid, teratoma, melanoma, paraganglioma, chordoma (typically at the clivus), chondrosarcomas, endolymphatic sac tumor

## Surgical Approaches to the Cerebellopontine Angle

### *Translabyrinthine*

- <u>Indication</u>: approach of choice for nonserviceable hearing
- <u>Advantages</u>: most direct route, excellent exposure, minimal cerebellar retraction, less risk of facial nerve injury than retrosigmoid/suboccipital, retrolabyrinthine, middle cranial fossa approach
- <u>Disadvantages</u>: sacrifices hearing, higher incidence of CSF leak than middle cranial fossa

### *Retrosigmoid/Suboccipital*

- <u>Indication</u>: large tumors, tumors of the medial IAC, hearing preservation
- <u>Advantages</u>: provides wide exposure, brainstem identified early, hearing preservation possible
- <u>Disadvantages</u>: higher incidence of postoperative headaches, limited exposure to lateral IAC, higher incidence of CSF leak, higher risk of facial nerve injury than translabyrinthine approach, requires cerebellar retraction (postoperative imbalance, less retraction required with retrosigmoid than classic suboccipital), air embolism

### Middle Cranial Fossa

- <u>Indication</u>: small intracanalicular (intra-IAC) lesions (<1 cm), serviceable hearing
- <u>Advantages</u>: hearing preservation possible
- <u>Disadvantages</u>: requires retraction of temporal lobe (small risk of aphasia or seizure), more difficult technically, poor exposure to posterior fossa, higher risk of facial nerve injury than translabyrinthine

### Retrolabyrinthine

- <u>Indication</u>: not indicated for vestibular schwannomas (does not allow adequate exposure), indicated for vestibular nerve section
- <u>Advantages</u>: preserves hearing, easier technically (shorter operative time)
- <u>Disadvantages</u>: limited exposure and narrow field of view (cannot access IAC lesions or porus acousticus)

### Comparison (May Vary by Source)

- <u>Facial Nerve Injury</u>: translabyrinthine < middle fossa < retrosigmoid
- <u>CSF Leak</u>: middle fossa < translabyrinthine < retrosigmoid
- <u>Hearing Loss</u>: middle fossa < retrosigmoid <<< translabyrinthine (destroys hearing)

## Petrous Apex Lesions (*see* Table 8–5)

- **Petrous Apex**: pyramid-shaped portion of the temporal bone medial to the otic capsule
- <u>SSx</u>: headache (dural pressure), cranial compression symptoms, vertigo or imbalance, eustachian tube dysfunction and CHL (serous otitis media), Gradenigo's syndrome (otorrhea, lateral rectus palsy, trigeminal/retroorbital pain)
- <u>Dx</u>: CT and MRI of temporal bone, audiometry
- **Cholesterol Granuloma**: cystic lesion of the petrous apex, foreign body response to cholesterol crystals causing a giant cell reaction; contains brown, thick fluid; diagnosed by CT (smooth, round, expansive lesions, smooth remodeled bone, may have cyst wall enhancement) and MRI (bright images on both T1- and T2-weighted sequences, unlike epidermoids [cholesteatomas], which are hyperintense on T2-weighted images only); <u>Rx</u>: surgical decompression and exteriorization
- **Epidermoid Cyst (Cholesteatoma)**: cystic lesion formed from embryologic-entrapped epithelial remnants, slow growth, presents as a young adult; <u>Rx</u>: surgical removal and exteriorization

**TABLE 8–5.** Cystic Lesions of the Petrous Apex

| Lesion | CT | Expansile | MRI T1 | MRI T2 | Enhancing |
|---|---|---|---|---|---|
| Mucocele | Smooth bony remodeling | Yes | Low signal | Bright | No |
| Petrous apicitis | Irregular bony remodeling | No | Low | Bright | Yes |
| Cholesteatoma | Smooth bony remodeling | Yes | Low | Bright | No |
| Cholesteral Granuloma | Smooth bony remodeling | Yes | Bright | Bright | No |

- <u>Others</u>: meningioma, glomus tumor, lymphoma, or metastatic tumors

## Other Benign Lesions of the Temporal Bone

- **Fibrous Dysplasia**: developmental disease, medullary bone replaced with fibro-osseous tissue, usually monostotic, presents as a painless asymmetric swelling of the temporal bone, CHL, EAC narrowing, "ground glass" expansive mass on CT; <u>Rx</u>: excision
- **Langerhans Cell Histiocytosis**: granulomatous disease of unknown etiology, characterized by a proliferation of histiocytes, localized and chronic disseminated forms, presents with chronic otorrhea and granulation tissue; <u>Rx</u>: excision, radiation therapy, chemotherapy, or multimodality therapy (depends on histology type and sites involved)
- <u>Embryonic Tumors</u>: dermoids, teratomas, chordomas

## Malignant Tumors of the Temporal Bone

- numerous pathways of tumor invasion that allow easy spread of tumor (typically presents in an advanced stage)
- <u>SSx</u>: EAC mass or granulation tissue, chronically draining ear, insidious CHL, aural fullness, bloody otorrhea, pain, facial nerve and other cranial nerve palsies, vertigo
- <u>Dx</u>: CT temporal bone, biopsy, full H&N workup (*see* pp. 254–262), audiogram (baseline hearing)

### Types

- **Squamous Cell Carcinoma**: most common, arises from the auricle or EAC; <u>Rx</u>: wide surgical resection with consideration of adjunctive radiation therapy (for advanced disease) versus primary radiation (for unresectable disease or nonoperative candidates)

- **Basal Cell Carcinoma**: second most common, often arises from auricle, may extend into EAC and temporal bone; <u>Rx</u>: local resection (with negative margins)
- **Melanoma**: third most common, arises from auricle or EAC
- **Rhabdomyosarcoma**: most common temporal bone malignancy of childhood, may arise from tensor tympani or stapedius muscles; <u>Rx</u>: chemotherapy and radiotherapy (surgical management rarely indicated)
- **Adenoid Cystic Carcinoma**: uncommon in the temporal bone, may arise from ectopic salivary gland tissue in middle ear, may invade neural tissue causing pain, histologically may have skip areas (high recurrence), unpredictable incidence of late metastasis; <u>Rx</u>: resection with consideration of adjunctive radiation therapy versus primary radiation
- **Metastasis**: breast most common in women, lung and prostate most common in men
- <u>Others</u>: ceruminous adenocarcinoma, adenocarcinoma, carcinoid tumor, verrucous carcinoma, giant cell tumor, chondrosarcoma, osteosarcoma, papillary (endolymphatic sac)

## *Temporal Bone Resection*

- **Sleeve Resection**: indicated for tumors of the concha, periauricular, or cartilaginous canal regions with sparing of the bony EAC, parotid, and TMJ; removes cartilaginous EAC and bony canal wall skin without bone removal
- **Lateral (Partial) Temporal Bone Resection**: indicated for tumors lateral to the TM (may involve outer layer of the TM); removes en bloc the entire osseous and cartilaginous EAC, TM, malleus, and incus
- **Subtotal Temporal Bone Resection**: indicated for malignancies involving the middle ear or mastoid; removes en bloc the entire temporal bone lateral to the petrous carotid artery, spares the petrous apex and portions of the bony labyrinth
- **Total Temporal Bone Resection**: indicated for tumors invading the cochlea, petrous apex, and carotid canal (*controversial*); removes en bloc temporal bone lateral to the IAC; results in anacusis, initial vestibular dysfunction, and facial nerve paralysis

# Trauma to the Ear and Temporal Bone

## Barotrauma

- <u>Pathophysiology</u>: ambient pressure changes (such as from diving or flying) or forceful nose blowing (particularly with mouth closed) results in pressure differentials affecting the air-containing spaces of the temporal bone, which may cause otalgia (pressure differential of 60 mm Hg), eustachian tube dysfunction (pressure differential of 90 mm Hg), or middle ear hemorrhage or TM perforation (pressure differential of 100–500 mm Hg)
- <u>SSx</u>: acute otalgia, acute hearing loss (SNHL or CHL), tinnitus, hemotympanum, bloody otorrhea, vertigo, facial nerve paralysis (usually brief, possibly due to pressure over natural defects in the fallopian canal)
- <u>Dx</u>: H&P, possible audiogram
- <u>Rx</u>: analgesics, anti-inflammatory agents (eg, possible steroid course), antivertigo medications, prophylactic oral and topical decongestants; consider tympanostomy tubes for progressive hearing loss or failure of symptom resolutions after 4–5 days; do not recompress (except for "the bends")

### Types of Barotrauma

- **Middle Ear Squeeze**: on descent the eustachian tube may close, thus failing to relieve pressure in the middle ear; as ambient pressure increases may cause the TM to rupture or middle ear hemorrhage resulting in hemotympanum (*theoretical*)
- **Round Window Rupture**: may occur as the diver attempts a Valsalva maneuver: the TM snaps into a neutral position pulling the stapes and causing negative pressure in the cochlea (implosion of the round window), or as the diver attempts a Valsalva maneuver there is an increase in CSF pressure that is transmitted through the perilymph causing a rupture of the round window (*theoretical*)
- **Inner Ear Decompression Sickness (Caisson Disease, "The Bends")**: with increased pressure (diving), nitrogen becomes more soluble and enters the blood and body fluids; if decompression (ascent) occurs rapidly, small gas emboli may form and enter the cerebral circulation leading to blindness, deafness, paralysis, or death; <u>Dx</u>: no middle ear pathology or CHL (may have SNHL), vertigo more common than with other barotraumas (>50%); <u>Rx</u>: immediate recompression (hyperbaric oxygen)

## Acoustic Trauma (*see* p. 403)

**Temporal Bone Fracture** (*see* pp. 659–662)

# Inner Ear and Central Hearing Disorders

## Presbycusis (Presbyacusis)

- progressive deterioration of hearing associated with aging
- most common cause of adult hearing loss (~50% of people >75 years old have hearing impairment)
- <u>Pathophysiology</u>: loss of sensory hair cells (majority of cases; possibly due to age-related degeneration, cumulative noise-induced trauma or cumulative ototoxin-induced injury over life); also possibly due to vascular disorders causing atrophy of the stria vascularis, loss of ganglion cells, or degeneration of nerve fibers (also associated with hair cell loss), stiffening of the basilar membrane
- <u>SSx</u>: progressive, symmetric SNHL initially of frequencies >2000 Hz (downsloping configuration)
- <u>Dx</u>: history of high-frequency SNHL without other sources of hearing loss
- <u>Rx</u>: sound amplification, cochlear implant if severe–profound

## Sudden Sensorineural Hearing Loss (SSNHL)

- ≥**30** dB SNHL in at least **3** adjacent frequencies that occurs over ≤**3** days, typically unilateral; 1/3 return to normal hearing, 1/3 result in profound hearing loss (rule of 3s)
- worse prognosis if associated with vertigo (diagnosis is then more correctly labyrinthitis), total deafness, delay in treatment initiation, advanced age, downsloping audiogram (high-frequency loss), or associated vascular risk factors
- better prognosis if minimal hearing loss and low-frequency hearing loss, no change in ECoG N1 latency
- <u>Causes</u>: most commonly no etiology found (**idiopathic SSNHL**); may be autoimmune (*see following*), viral, vascular, CPA mass (1–5%), traumatic; may be the first episode of hearing loss in patients who go on to develop Ménière's disease
- <u>Evaluation</u>: similar to hearing loss evaluation (*as previous*); however, must keep a high suspicion of reversible causes of SSNHL (eg, ossicular trauma, perilymphatic fistula); initial investigations should include an immediate audiogram and immittance testing; MRI to rule out a CPA mass (or uncommonly multiple sclerosis) if SSNHL does not reverse; consider ABR and CT for MRI contraindications, routine CT in acute period not recommended
- <u>Rx</u>: in the absence of a known cause, medical treatment is empirical and controversial; high-dose oral corticosteroids is the most

commonly employed therapy; diuretic; consider transtympanic steroid injection for oral corticosteroid contradictions (diabetes, intolerance) or after failed oral course; hyperbaric oxygen optional; antivirals generally ineffective and not recommended; vasodilators and agents to improve cochlear blood flow (anticoagulants, dextran) or reverse vasospasm are controversial and have not been shown to be effective in prospective randomized trials

## Autoimmune Hearing Loss

- may be associated with systemic immune disease (rheumatoid arthritis, lupus, etc), allergy, and vasculitis
- most common between 20–50 years old, females > males
- Pathophysiology: may arise from host's defense from infection causing autoimmunity, cross-reactivity from distant antigens, or circulating immune complexes affecting circulation in the stria vascularis
- SSx: rapidly progressive (weeks to months) or fluctuating SNHL (bilateral), normal otoscopic exam, tinnitus; up to 50% may have vestibular symptoms
- Dx: rapidly progressive SNHL with serologic evidence of immune dysfunction, steroid-responsive
- Serologic Evaluation for Autoimmunity in Hearing Loss: CBC, ESR, CRP, ANA, rheumatoid factor (RF), ANCA, C1q binding test, Raji cell assay (for circulating immune complexes), cryoglobulins, complement profiles, lymphocyte transformation test (exposes patient's lymphocytes to known inner ear antigens to evaluate for reactivity), Western blot (looks for antibodies against a 68-kD inner ear protein antigen), lymphocyte migration inhibition test (targets type II collagen)
- Rx: high-dose oral corticosteroid trial for at least 30 days with audiogram follow-up to assess response; if an immunologic diagnosis is highly suspected (positive serology), immunosuppressive medications (eg, cyclophosphamide, methotrexate) for nonresponsive cases, consider adjunctive plasmapheresis

## Noise-Induced Hearing Loss (NIHL)

- includes **occupational hearing loss**
- according to OSHA regulations, **≥85 dB** average exposure for **8 hours** requires hearing protection programs (action level or **50% allowable** exposure); **≥90 dB** exposure for **8 hours** is **100% allowable** exposure (or 95 dB × 4 hours, 100 dB × 2 hours, 130 dB × 2 minutes)

- **Temporary Threshold Shift (TTS)**: loud noise exposure can cause a temporary SNHL that typically resolves within 24 hours
- **Permanent Threshold Shift (PTS)**: permanent hearing loss from noise exposure that does not improve after the acoustic trauma event
- increased damage with higher intensities (dB), longer durations, and higher frequencies
- rifle gunfire poses a risk to the opposite side ear of the shooting arm, the same side ear is protected by being pressed ("muffled") against the shoulder; pistol gunfire poses a risk to the same side of the shooting arm
- stapedial reflex has a latency of 10 ms, thus it will not protect cochlea from unexpected sounds
- Pathophysiology: outer hair cells are susceptible to damage from chronic loud noise exposure, loss of hair cells may be due to oxygen radical formation with subsequent membrane and cellular damage, *see following* for acoustic trauma
- SSx: SNHL (typically bilateral), high-pitched tinnitus
- Dx: history and audiogram findings (initially see **4-kHz notch**)
- Rx: hearing protection programs (prevention), hearing aids if indicated, yearly audiograms until hearing is stable or no longer in at-risk environment

## Acoustic Trauma

- Pathophysiology: a single intense exposure (>140 dB, eg, explosion or gunfire) may mechanically damage the middle or inner ear directly from acoustic energy; may rupture cochlear membranes, resulting in mixing of perilymph and endolymph, injuring cells
- distinct from noise-induced hearing loss
- >140 dB can result in permanent threshold shift
- >180 dB can rupture TM, fracture ossicles

## Ototoxin-Induced Hearing Loss

- Common Ototoxic Agents: aminoglycoside antibiotics (eg, gentamicin), cisplatin, loop diuretics, antimalarials (eg, quinine, chloroquine), ASA/NSAIDs (causes tinnitus)
- Pathophysiology: causes death of sensory hair cells and degeneration of stria vascularis
- generally affects high-frequency hearing first as damage progresses from base to apex of cochlea
- may prevent by regular screening for hearing loss when administering known ototoxic agents

## Auditory Neuropathy

- SNHL with poor word recognition due to abnormal inner hair cell or CN VIII function, normal outer hair cell function
- Pathophysiology: unclear, may be secondary to cochlear hair cells' discharging dyssynchronously, may also be due to abnormal CN VIII function
- Dx: audiogram (mild to profound SNHL in pure tones with decreased word recognition score out of proportion to level of hearing loss), elevated or absent acoustic reflexes, **absent or abnormal ABR, normal otoacoustic emissions**, normal ECoG
- Rx: trial of amplification, cochlear implant can bypass the abnormally firing hair cells and stimulate the auditory nerve synchronously

## Central Auditory Processing Disorder

- central receptive language disorder of adults and children from difficulty in decoding and storing auditory information
- higher risk among children with learning disabilities, family history, attention deficit disorder, other neurologic disorders (many children have normal hearing and intelligence)
- SSx: perceptual hearing loss (especially with background noise), delayed communication abilities (eg, speech problems, delayed responses, use of gestures instead of speech), echolalia (repeating back words without comprehension), easy distraction, behavior problems
- Dx: normal audiogram, testing by audiologists (series of auditory processing tests) and child psychologists; rule out auditory neuropathy (*see previous*)
- Rx: preferential seating, reduction of background noise (consider FM devices in school), speech therapy, behavior–cognitive therapy

## Neurofibromatosis

### *Neurofibromatosis Type 1 (NF1, von Recklinghausen Disease, Classic Neurofibromatosis)*

- Pathophysiology: mutation in neurofibromin 1 on chromosome 17
- Otologic SSx: 5% risk of unilateral vestibular schwannoma (retrocochlear hearing loss)
- Other SSx: café-au-lait spots (giant melanosomes >1.5 cm); neurofibromas are most commonly cutaneous although may involve the CNS (mental retardation), viscera, orbit (optic gliomas), or peripheral nerves; Lisch nodules (hamartomas of the eye); groin and axillary freckling; associated with pheochromocytoma

- <u>Dx</u>: requires 2 of the following characteristics: ≥6 café-au-lait spots, ≥2 neurofibromas, or ≥1 plexiform neurofibroma, axillary or groin freckling, optic nerve glioma, ≥2 Lisch nodules, distinct bony lesions, first-degree relative with neurofibromatosis 1

### Neurofibromatosis Type 2 (NF2, Central Neurofibromatosis)

- <u>Pathophysiology</u>: mutation in merlin (schwannomin, neurofibromin 2), a tumor suppressor gene on chromosome 22; 50% of cases due to a spontaneous (ie, noninherited) mutation
- <u>Otologic SSx</u>: 95% risk of bilateral vestibular schwannomas, often <21 years old
- <u>Other SSx</u>: fewer NF1 symptoms, other central tumors possible
- <u>Dx</u>: bilateral vestibular schwannomas; or first-degree relative with neurofibromatosis 2 plus either a unilateral vestibular schwannoma at <30 years old or any two of meningioma, glioma, schwannoma, or specific juvenile cataract
- <u>Rx</u>: remove larger vestibular schwannoma first, consider placement of auditory brainstem implant if cochlear nerve sacrificed (if cochlear nerve preserved then consider cochlear implantation), if hearing is preserved consider removal of second tumor, for only hearing ear may follow with serial MRIs every 9–12 months, also consider stereotactic radiation and bevacizumab (Avastin, VEGF anatogonist); screen relatives with MRI of brain/spine and audiometry

## Congenital and Hereditary Hearing Loss
(*see* pp. 573–582)

# VESTIBULAR PATHOLOGY
## Evaluation of the Dizzy Patient

### History

- a specific diagnosis may be made in a majority of dizzy patients by an adequate history and physical exam
- **dizziness** is a term used to describe any of a variety of sensations that produce spatial disorientation
- <u>Describe Dizziness</u>
  1. **Vertiginous**: illusion of rotational, linear, or tilting movement such as "spinning," "whirling," or "turning" of the patient or the surroundings
  2. **Disequilibrium**: sensation of instability of body positions; walking or standing described as "off-balance" or "imbalanced"

3. **Oscillopsia**: blurred vision and inability to focus on objects with motion, such as reading a sign while walking; seen with loss of the vestibulo-ocular reflex in bilateral or central vestibular dysfunction
4. **Lightheadedness**: sense of impending faint, presyncope
5. **Physiologic Dizziness**: motion sickness, height-related vertigo
6. **Multisensory Dizziness**: diabetes, aging resulting in partial loss of multiple sensory systems

- <u>Onset and Duration of Symptoms</u>: seconds to minutes (BPPV, VBI, migraine-associated vertigo, epilepsy, arrhythmia), hours (Ménière's, migraine), days (vestibular neuronitis, labyrinthitis), constant (central causes); frequency and time of the day; initial and last spell
- <u>Character of Dizziness</u>: associated otologic factors (hearing loss, aural fullness, tinnitus), intensity and fatigability, fluctuating versus constant, precipitating factors (head movement or motion, stress, diet), systemic complaints (nausea, vomiting), central symptoms (numbness, weakness, diplopia, blurred vision), *see* Table 8–6
- <u>Contributing Factors</u>: medications (antipsychotics, antihypertensives, ototoxic medications, sedative/hypnotics); medical history (hypertension, cardiac arrhythmia and ischemia, diabetes, thyroid disorder, vascular disease, otologic problems, depression, neurologic disease, migraine, or premenstrual syndrome); recent head trauma, loud noise exposure (Tullio's phenomenon), flying, diving, or heavy lifting; new eyeglasses; family history of hearing loss, neurologic disease, or otologic disease
- <u>Associated Symptoms</u>: falls, confusion, weakness, weight loss, nervousness, headache

**TABLE 8–6.** General Characteristics of Peripheral and Central Causes of Vertigo

| Characteristic | Peripheral | Central |
|---|---|---|
| Intensity | severe | mild |
| Fatigability | fatigues, adaptation | does not fatigue |
| Associated Symptoms | nausea, hearing loss, sweating | weakness, numbness, falls more likely |
| Eye Closure | symptoms worse with eyes closed | symptoms better with eyes closed |
| Nystagmus | horizontal, may be unilateral, rotary | vertical, bilateral |
| Ocular Fixation | suppresses nystagmus (may not suppress during acute phase) | no effect or enhances nystagmus |

---

**TABLE 8–7.** Common Causes of Peripheral, Central, and Systemic Vertigo

<u>Peripheral Vertigo</u>

- benign paroxysmal positional vertigo (BPPV)
- Ménière's disease
- vestibular neuronitis and labyrinthitis
- perilymph fistula
- cerebellopontine angle tumors
- otitis media
- traumatic vestibular dysfunction (labyrinthine concussion)
- autoimmune, hereditary, or ototoxin-induced inner ear disease
- labyrinthine apoplexy

<u>Central and Systemic Vertigo</u>

- multiple sclerosis
- other neurologic disorders (stroke, seizures, middle cerebellar lesions, parkinsonism, pseudobulbar palsy, basilar impression)
- metabolic disorders (hypo/hyperthyroidism, diabetes)
- medications and intoxicants (psychotropic drugs, alcohol, analgesics, anesthetics, antihypertensives, antiarrhythmics, chemotherapeutics)
- vascular causes (vertebrobasilar insufficiency, basilar migraine syndrome, vascular loop compression syndrome)

---

- *see* Table 8–7 for differential diagnosis of peripheral, central, and systemic vertigo

## Physical Exam

- <u>H&N and General Physical Exam</u>: vital signs (including for orthostatic hypotension), general medical exam with particular evaluation for general neurologic, cardiovascular, and peripheral vascular disorders (hypertension, carotid bruits)
- <u>Otoscopy</u>: pneumatoscopy (positive fistula test [Hennebert's sign] if induce nystagmus or dizziness, *see* p. 417), inspection of TM and middle ear (otitis media, presence of fluid, masses)
- <u>Vestibular Testing</u>: eye motility (check pursuit with convergence and divergence) test using **Frenzel lenses** (prevents ocular fixation that may suppress nystagmus), spontaneous and gaze-evoked nystagmus (*see following*), Dix-Hallpike maneuver (*see following*), head shake (head motion in horizontal plane for 20–30 seconds, then suddenly

stop to evaluate for nystagmus), head thrust (>50% reduced response), caloric testing
- <u>Neurologic Exam</u>: cranial palsies, vestibulospinal reflexes (eg, Romberg test, gait, past pointing test, Fukuda test) lateralizing signs (eg, weakness, paresthesias), tuning forks
- <u>Dynamic Visual Acuity</u>: have patient read Snellen eye chart with 2-Hz head oscillation and compare to stationary evaluation, positive if acuity drops 2–3 lines

## Vestibular Testing

- *see also* pp. 348–349 *for overview of nystagmus and reflexes*

### *Electronystagmography (ENG) / Videonystagmography (VNG) Battery*

- **ENG/VNG**: battery of tests (oculomotor evaluation, positional/positioning testing, caloric testing) that record eye movements either with corneoretinal potentials (ENG, *see following*) or video (VNG); provides information regarding localization of lesion (peripheral versus central, side of lesion); dependent on anatomy of the ear canal and temporal bone, only induces a low-frequency response to caloric stimuli; difficult to perform in children, well-tolerated, does not correlate with function
- **Corneoretinal Potential**: an electrical voltage between the cornea and the retina exists with ocular axis changes (does not change with torsional ocular motion), ENG records changes in the corneoretinal potential by placing electrodes around the eyes to record eye movement (in contrast, VNG records actual eye movement with video), may be effective in evaluating blind patients

#### Oculomotor Testing

- **Spontaneous Nystagmus and Fixation Testing**: spontaneous nystagmus may be observed with eyes centered and head upright; patient is first asked to visually fixate on an object that is then followed by loss of fixation (ie, close eyes, turn lights off, or use Frenzel lenses), nystagmus due to peripheral lesions usually decreases with fixation (**fixation suppression**)
- **Gaze-Evoked Nystagmus**: may be induced by having the subject gaze 20–30° to the left and right of center for 30 seconds each (may be done with and without fixation)
- **Rebound Nystagmus**: may occur after prolonged gaze holding after the eye is returned to primary position
- *see also* pp. 348–349 *for nystagmus laws*

- **Saccadic System**: saccades allow rapid shifting of gaze from one object to another, maintaining the target image on the fovea; tested by presenting targets at 10–20° right and left of center gaze, patient asked to rapidly shift gaze to each target; evaluates CNS components of the vestibular system; cerebellar or brainstem injury may cause **ocular dysmetria** (overshooting or undershooting of eye rotation)
- **Pursuit System**: pursuits allow ocular fixation on moving objects, maintaining the target image on the fovea; tested with **sinusoidal-tracking tests** by having the patient follow a spot moving in a sinusoidal pattern, at faster speeds the eyes may not be able to "keep up" causing saccadic eye jerks; saccadic eye jerks at low velocity (rotational frequencies <0.1–0.3 Hz or target velocities <30° per second) suggest CNS pathology
- **Optokinetic System**: the optokinetic system allows fixation on a moving field, maintaining the image on the whole retina rather than specifically on the fovea as in the saccadic and pursuit systems; tested by having the patient stay still while the environment is "moved" (eg, a series of black and white stripes on a moving field that encompasses the whole field of vision); brainstem disease may cause bilateral reduced gain, cerebellar lesions may induce ataxia, peripheral lesions may demonstrate asymmetry

### Positional/Positioning Nystagmus Testing and Dix-Hallpike Maneuver

- **Positional Testing**: tests for nystagmus evoked by a new static head position (positional nystagmus is maintained as long as head remains in the evoked position)
- **Positioning Testing**: tests for nystagmus evoked by the action of motion of the head
- **Dix-Hallpike Maneuver**: positioning vestibular test designed to stimulate the posterior SCC, induction of nystagmus is a hallmark for benign paroxysmal positional vertigo (*see* pp. 412–413)
- <u>Dix-Hallpike Maneuver Technique</u>: to test the right posterior SCC, patient sits upright with head turned 45° to the right, patient then lays flat with the head hanging slightly backward and the right ear down, eyes are observed for nystagmus (rotary to the downward side, delayed 2–15 seconds, transient lasting 10–60 seconds, associated with vertigo) for at least 20 seconds, patient is returned to the upright position, eyes are observed again for nystagmus for at least 20 seconds; test may then be repeated for left posterior SCC

**Caloric Testing**

- only test that evaluates horizontal SCC function in each ear independently; determines right, left, or bilateral vestibular weakness
- <u>Technique</u>: in supine position, head is elevated (chin toward sternum) 30° to bring the horizontal canal into a vertical position, each ear is irrigated with cool and warm water (or air), nystagmus is recorded with eyes open and closed
- <u>Theoretical Normal Response</u>: **cool** water or air (30° C) to **right** ear with patient in upright position causes flow in the ampullofugal direction, which decreases the electrical activity of the ipsilateral vestibular nerve with a corresponding (relative) increase in electrical activity of the opposite vestibular nerve resulting in **left**-beating nystagmus (warm water or air [40° C] produces the opposite response); the mnemonic **COWS**, "**C**ool **O**pposite, **W**arm **S**ame," represents the direction of the (fast beating component of the) nystagmus with warm and cool water
- **Maximum Slow Phase Velocity**: determined by dividing the amplitude by the duration of the slow phase, standard measure of caloric response intensity
- **Directional Preponderance**: denotes that the nystagmus response in a particular direction is weaker than the evoked response in the opposite direction, determined by comparing the duration or velocity of right-beating nystagmus from both ears with left-beating nystagmus from both ears, **>20–25%** difference between sides may suggest a unilateral weakness
- **Unilateral Caloric Weakness**: denotes that the response of one side to a stimulus is reduced in comparison to the other side, determined by comparing the duration or velocity response from left and right ears, approximately **>20–25%** difference between sides suggests a unilateral peripheral weakness
- **Bilateral Caloric Weakness**: suggested when the total caloric maximum slow phase velocity from each ear (all 4 irrigations) is **<12–24°/second**
- **Postcaloric Fixation**: determined by dividing the maximum slow phase velocity with fixation and without fixation, an inability to suppress nystagmus suggests a central lesion

## Rotation Tests (Rotary Chair)

- **Sinusoidal (Slow) Harmonic Acceleration Test**: patient is seated in the chair, eye movements are recorded while patient (chair) is rotated along the horizontal plane; evaluates the vestibulo-ocular reflex

- Vestibulo-ocular Reflex Measurements
  1. **Gain**: ratio of slow phase eye velocity to chair (head) velocity, normal gain is 1
  2. **Phase**: compares maximum responses of the slow component of the eye velocity with the maximum velocity of the chair, determines the timing relationship between stimulus and response, eye velocity normally leads chair velocity (**phase lead**)
  3. **Symmetry**: compares eye movements during rightward chair rotation versus eye movements during leftward chair rotation, normally should be completely symmetric
- Indications: procedure of choice to evaluate bilateral vestibular dysfunction, may detect mild vestibular dysfunction undetected by traditional ENG testing, may follow progress of vestibular compensation
- abnormalities are primarily seen at low frequencies (abnormal phase and gain reduction) and high frequencies (asymmetry)
- normal vestibulo-ocular response results in similar slow eye phase velocity and chair velocity
- acute unilateral peripheral lesions typically reveal low-frequency phase leads and high-frequency asymmetry (the absence of asymmetry suggests vestibular compensation, eg, vestibular schwannoma)
- bilateral vestibular disease typically demonstrates reduced gain at low frequencies but normal gain at high frequencies

## Posturography (Computerized Dynamic Posturography)

- measures postural stability while variably changing the visual field references and support structures
- patient tries to maintain balance on a level platform with eyes open, eyes closed, and with a simulated moving visual environment; test is then repeated on a physically swaying platform
- functional evaluation of spinal/proprioceptive, visual, and vestibular systems
- controversial applications in diagnosis (nonspecific), may be used to quantify functional vestibular impairment, evaluate malingering, and for vestibular rehabilitation

## Vestibular Evoked Myogenic Potential (VEMP)

### Cervical VEMP (cVEMP)

- provide 95 dB auditory click stimulation, gauge EMG response in ipsilateral sternocleidomastoid muscle (measures sacculocolic reflex)

- <u>Pathway</u>: acoustic signal → **saccule** → **inferior** vestibular nerve → vestibular nucleus → vestibulospinal tract → sternocleidomastoid muscle action potential
- useful in evaluation of Ménière's disease, superior semicircular canal dehiscence (20 dB increase in sensitivity, decrease in threshold), inferior vestibular nerve lesion (eg, compressing schwannoma), and saccule function

### Ocular VEMP (oVEMP)

- EMG response of contralateral ocular muscles in response to bone conducted vibration or air conducted sound; air conduction elicits contralateral response, bone conduction elicits bilateral responses (represents vestibulo-ocular pathway)
- <u>Pathway</u>: signal → **utricle** → **superior** vestibular nerve → contralateral inferior oblique (for air conduction) or bilateral response (for bone vibration)
- superior vestibular neuritis causes absent/reduced oVEMP but no effect on cVEMP

## Management Concepts

- <u>Safety</u>: avoid heights, ladders, driving, operating heavy machinery
- <u>Acute Vestibular Suppression</u>: indicated for intolerable symptoms but may delay central compensatory mechanisms in the long-term; common drugs include meclizine, diazepam, promethazine, transdermal scopolamine, corticosteroids, and antiemetics
- <u>Vestibular Rehabilitation</u>: indicated for chronic symptoms, consists of a series of positional tasks, head movements, and oculomotor exercises to facilitate central compensation
- <u>Surgical Management</u>: may be indicated for specific diagnoses

## Peripheral Vestibular Disorders

### Benign Paroxysmal Positional Vertigo (BPPV)

- most common peripheral vestibular disorder
- <u>Causes</u>: spontaneous, posttraumatic, and postviral (labyrinthitis, vestibular neuronitis)
- typically self-limiting, may have recurrent episodes
- <u>SSx</u>: recurrent episodes of brief (seconds to minutes) positional vertigo (turning over in bed, getting up, turning head, bending over, looking up); may be associated with nausea and prolonged light-headedness; induced positional nystagmus is torsional (rotary to

the downward side [geotropic]), typically exhibits a latency of 2–15 seconds with a crescendo and decrescendo of nystagmus associated with vertigo, usually fatigable and transient (seconds); no associated hearing loss; horizontal canal variant is more severe (shorter latency, greater magnitude, less fatigable)
- <u>Dx</u>: H&P (Dix-Hallpike maneuver), may need more sensitive tests for horizontal canal BPPV (eg, supine roll test); audio and VNG not indicated for routine BPPV (obtain when persistent or when other pathology is suspected)

## Pathophysiology

- affects posterior (90%), horizontal (10%), or superior (rare) semicircular canal
- **Canalithiasis Theory**: free-floating debris (dislodged otoconia) in the endolymph of the semicircular canal moves when placed in a dependent position, the inertial drag of the endolymph causes displacement of the cupula resulting in latent vertigo, which resolves when the debris settles
- **Cupulolithiasis Theory**: debris adheres to the cupula of the semicircular canal resulting in an ampulla that is gravity-sensitive (objections to theory include no account for the transient nature of vertigo and the torsional nystagmus exhibited in BPPV)

## Management

- education, reassurance, and observation
- **Canalith Repositioning Procedure (Epley Maneuver)**: series of head positionings typically completed in the office, based on "repositioning" free-floating particle in the posterior canal, requires patient to be upright after repositioning for 48 hours (90% effective), reassess within 1 month
- <u>Other Treatment Maneuvers</u>: Semont, Brandt-Daroff (induces vertigo to stimulate vestibular compensation), more specialized maneuvers for horizontal canal BPPV
- antivertigo medications typically are not useful due to the sporadic and brief nature of the vertigo, consider short-term antiemetics for patients with severe vegetative symptoms
- **Semicircular Canal Occlusion**: occludes ampullated end to prevent movement of endolymph, considered for intractable BPPV (uncommon)
- **Vestibular Nerve Section or Singular Neurectomy**: transection of vestibular nerve (via craniotomy) or branch to the affected semicircular canal (eg, posterior ampullary [singular] neurectomy for posterior canal BPPV), largely replaced by canal occlusion

## Ménière's Disease (Endolymphatic Hydrops)

### Signs and Symptoms

- Symptomatic Triad
    1. **episodic vertigo** lasting minutes to hours
    2. **fluctuating SNHL** (usually unilateral), recovery between episodes may be incomplete, resulting in a progressive SNHL (initially at lower frequencies)
    3. **tinnitus**
    4. ± **aural fullness** sensation
- classic Ménière's disease presents with all of the previously mentioned symptoms; however, Ménière's disease may also present as any combination of those symptoms (*see* Variants *following*)
- *see* Table 8–8 for AAO-HNS criteria for Meniere's disease
- bilateral in 25–30%

### Diagnosis and Other Causes of Endolymphatic Hydrops

- H&P and audiologic findings (initial low-frequency SNHL) with exclusion of other causes of hearing loss and vertigo are adequate for diagnosis and initiating empirical therapy
- vestibular testing may reveal unilateral weakness on affected side
- **Electrocochleography (ECoG):** may exhibit marked negative summation potential from basilar membrane distortion (hydrops) and a larger SP amplitude/AP amplitude ratio (SP/AP ratio > 0.5, normal = 0.2)

**TABLE 8–8.** AAO-HNS Criteria for Meniere's Disease

| | |
|---|---|
| Certain | Definite Meniere's + histopathologic confirmation |
| Definite | ≥2 definitive spontaneous episodes of vertigo ≥20 min + all other criteria in probable Meniere's disease |
| Probable | 1 definite episode of vertigo<br>Audiometric hearing loss on ≥1 occasion<br>Tinnitus or aural fullness in affected ear<br>Other causes excluded |
| Possible | Episodic vertigo of Meniere's type with no documented hearing loss, or<br>SNHL, fluctuating or fixed, with disequilibrium but without definitive episodes<br>Other causes excluded |

*Source*: Committee on Hearing and Equilibrium guidelines for the diagnosis and evaluation of therapy in Meniere's disease. *Otolaryngol Head Neck Surg.* 1995. 113(3):181–185.

- **Vestibular Evoked Myogenic Potential (VEMP)**: may see diminished or absent response (*see* pp. 411–412)
- **Glycerol (Dehydration) Test**: oral glycerol ingestion or mannitol acts as an osmotic diuretic that in the presence of active hydrops may improve symptoms temporarily within 30–60 minutes (~50% sensitive, not commonly utilized)
- <u>Rule Out Other Causes of Endolymphatic Hydrops</u>: allergy, syphilis, mumps, hypothyroidism, Mondini's aplasia, trauma, viral, bacterial infection

### *Pathophysiologic Theories and Histologic Findings (Controversial)*

- classically patients with Ménière's disease have histologic raising of Reissner's membrane and dilation of the endolymphatic spaces (endolymphatic hydrops)
- altered glycoprotein metabolism may result in dysregulation of inner ear fluid causing abnormal osmotic pressure and quantitative volume differences between perilymph and endolymph resulting in endolymphatic hydrops
- fibrosis of endolymphatic duct and sac impairs endolymph absorption and may result in overdistention of membranous labyrinth (endolymphatic hydrops)
- membranous labyrinth distention may cause microtears (rupture), which mixes endolymph and perilymph resulting in some permanent damage to hair cells and instant vertigo; the tear then spontaneously seals, after 2–3 hours the inner ear fluid re-equilibrates with resolution of the vertigo, repeated ruptures may cause progression of the SNHL
- newer theory suggests abnormal regulation of an endolymphatic sac hormone, saccin, may cause excessive production of fluid in sac with retrograde filling

### *Variants*

- **Cochlear Hydrops**: isolated cochlear variant characterized by hearing loss, aural fullness, tinnitus, without vertigo
- **Vestibular Hydrops**: isolated vestibular variant characterized by episodic vertigo without hearing loss or tinnitus
- **Lermoyez Syndrome**: rare, initially presents with increasing tinnitus, hearing loss, and aural fullness with sudden relief after a spell of vertigo
- **Crisis of Tumarkin (Drop Attack)**: sudden loss of extensor function causing a "drop attack" without loss of consciousness and with complete recovery

- **Delayed Endolymphatic Hydrops**: loss of hearing later followed by typical Ménière's symptoms

## Medical Management

- **Dietary Restrictions**: first-line therapy; avoid fluid shifts by restricting salt (<1.5 g/day), alcohol, monosodium glutamate, sugar, and caffeine; evenly space out meals (avoid binge eating or skipping meals) and water consumption
- **Diuretics**: first-line therapy (eg, hydrochlorothiazide); encourages constant renal output (must avoid dehydration, which would exacerbate symptoms)
- **Vestibular Suppressants**: consider for symptomatic treatment of attacks (eg, diazepam)
- **Corticosteroids**: consider for acute exacerbations and for management of hearing loss; transtympanic steroids may increase chance of hearing improvement and reduce vertigo attacks when diuretic and diet are not sufficient
- **Transtympanic Aminoglycoside Injections**: reduces vertigo attack frequency/severity, typically gentamicin or streptomycin, risk of SNHL
- **Allergy Management**: *see* pp. 37–40
- **Stress Reduction**: symptoms are exacerbated by stress

## Surgical Management of Vertigo

- needed in 10–15% of patients
- **Endolymphatic Sac Surgery**: first choice for failed conservative management of episodic vertigo (*controversial*); may consider wide bony decompression of endolymphatic sac or endolymphatic shunt to the mastoid cavity; preserves auditory and vestibular function, low morbidity, less successful than ablative procedures, rate of success 60–80% (however, 70% usually recover spontaneously)
- **Vestibular Nerve Section**: selective section of vestibular nerve (spares cochlear nerve, preserving hearing); higher risk of hearing loss and postoperative dizziness than endolymphatic sac surgery, 90% effective, requires craniotomy
- **Labyrinthectomy**: ablative procedure (contraindicated if other ear has reduced vestibular function) that may be considered for nonserviceable hearing (>50–60 dB HL or <50% word recognition) with failed conservative management, high rate of success (≤90%), must take into account risk of development of Ménière's disease in the contralateral ear

*Vestibular Neuronitis and Labyrinthitis* (*see* pp. 383–384)

# Labyrinthine Concussion

- <u>Pathophysiology</u>: posttraumatic disorder of inner ear function without fracture of the labyrinth
- <u>SSx</u>: self-limited acute vertigo, recoverable SNHL and tinnitus, normal otoscopic and radiologic findings, may result in residual BPPV-like symptoms
- <u>Dx</u>: H&P, audiology
- <u>Rx</u>: reassurance and observation, consider symptomatic medications (transient vestibular suppression)

# Perilymph Fistula

- <u>Pathophysiology</u>: abnormal fistula opening between inner and middle ear (or mastoid cavity) results in progressive hearing loss and vertigo
- <u>Causes</u>: barotrauma (Valsalva maneuver, straining, sneezing, head trauma, birth trauma), iatrogenic (stapedectomy), congenital (associated with Mondini dysplasia and abnormalities of the stapes or round window), spontaneous (*controversial*)
- <u>SSx</u>: sudden SNHL with vertigo subsequent to a traumatic event, positive **fistula test** (Hennebert's sign; nystagmus from pressure pneumatoscopy that causes stimulation of the membranous labyrinth, 10–40% sensitivity)
- <u>Dx</u>: **no definitive preoperative test**, exploration often not definitive, may visualize fluid at or near the oval or round window
- <u>Rx</u>: bed rest with head elevation and avoidance of any straining (sneezing with mouth open, stool softeners) for 5–10 days, for persistent symptoms or progression of hearing loss consider exploration surgery (often nondiagnostic) with grafting site of leak
- *NOTE:* perilymphatic fistula diagnosis and management is controversial, many neurotologists question the existence of spontaneous (nontrauma associated) form

# Cogan Syndrome

- <u>Pathophysiology</u>: unknown, autoimmune etiology, produces hydrops similar to Ménière's disease
- <u>SSx</u>: **interstitial keratitis** (nonreactive VDRL, blurriness, rapidly progresses to blindness), **episodic vertigo, bilateral fluctuating SNHL** (associated with tinnitus), disease progresses over months

- <u>Dx</u>: H&P; elevated ESR, CRP
- <u>Rx</u>: high-dose oral corticosteroids (usually resolves hearing and vestibular dysfunction), may consider cyclophosphamide, azathioprine
- **Vogt-Koyanagi-Harada Syndrome**: similar to Cogan syndrome (hearing loss, vertigo), also associated with granulomatous uveitis, depigmentation of hair and skin, aseptic meningitis, and loss of eyelashes

## Superior Semicircular Canal Dehiscence Syndrome (Minor's Syndrome)

- <u>Pathophysiology</u>: dehiscence of bone covering the superior semicircular canal (congenital predispositon, increased CSF pressure, posttraumatic) results in a third window to inner ear (in addition to round and oval windows); rarely other semicircular canals may be dehiscent
- <u>SSx</u>: vertigo and oscillopsia due to loud sound or pressure (Tullio phenomenon, Hennebert sign), autophony (hearing eyes move in head, heels hitting ground), aural fullness
- <u>Dx</u>: H&P, audiogram (CHL, supranormal bone conduction thresholds), cVEMP (lower threshold and increased amplitude compared to normal side), CT temporal bone formatted in plane of canals (gold standard), stapedial reflexes (should be normal; versus in otosclerosis where reflexes are absent)
- <u>Rx</u>: most patients have minimal symptoms managed with avoidance of loud sounds, if severe consider resurfacing defect or plugging the superior canal through a middle cranial fossa (more common) or transmastoid approach

## Other Peripheral Vestibular Disorders

- **Labyrinthine Apoplexy**: thrombosis of the internal auditory artery resulting in acute vertigo, hearing loss, and tinnitus
- **Autoimmune Inner Ear Disease**: usually presents with SNHL (*see* p. 402)
- **Ototoxin Induced**: aminoglycosides, cisplatin, *see following*
- **Bilateral Vestibular Hypofunction/Areflexia (Anastasis)**: most commonly due to ototoxins, bilateral absence of vestibuloocular reflex (VOR) results in debilitating **oscillopsia** (visual blurring with head motion including with walking); <u>Rx</u>: rehabilitation ineffective, vestibular implantation under investigation

# Central Vestibular Disorders

## Wallenberg Syndrome (Lateral Medullary Syndrome)

- <u>Pathophysiology</u>: embolic event or thrombosis of the ipsilateral vertebral or posterior inferior cerebellar artery (PICA) resulting in an infarction of the lateral medullary region of the brainstem (serving CN V–X, cerebellum, and sympathetic ganglion), **spares cochlear** nucleus
- <u>SSx</u>
  1. ipsilateral loss of **facial sensation** (CN V)
  2. ipsilateral loss of lateral rectus (CN VI) and facial musculature (CN VII)
  3. acute **vertigo**, nystagmus, nausea, vomiting (vestibular portion of CN VIII)
  4. **dysphagia** from weakness of palate and pharynx, **dysphonia** from weakness of larynx (pharyngeal plexus, nucleus ambiguus, CN IX, X)
  5. **ataxia** from incoordination of ipsilateral limbs (fall toward the lesion), dysmetria (cerebellum)
  6. contralateral loss of pain and temperature sensation (spinothalamic tract crossed fibers)
  7. ipsilateral **Horner's syndrome** (ptosis, miosis, anhydrosis; preganglionic sympathetic fibers)
- <u>Dx</u>: angiogram, CT (wedge-shaped infarct)
- <u>Rx</u>: per cerebrovascular accident protocols

## Vertebrobasilar Insufficiency (VBI)

- <u>Pathophysiology</u>: compression of the vertebral artery compromises flow to the posterior and anterior inferior cerebellar arteries
- <u>SSx</u>: transient vertigo with neck hyperextension or excessive rotation; **"4 Ds" (dizziness, diplopia, dysphagia, drop attacks)**; also associated with dysarthria, headaches, hallucinations, ataxia, and hemiparesis (normal neurologic exam between attacks)
- <u>Dx</u>: H&P, radiography (evaluate for cervical spine disease)
- <u>Rx</u>: anticoagulation (antiplatelet medication)

## Other Central Vestibular Disorders

- **Migraine-Associated Vertigo, Basilar Migraine Syndrome**: migraine headache accompanied by symptoms of brainstem lesions including vertigo, vertigo may also present as an aura, may occur without headache; <u>Rx</u>: migraine therapy

- **Vestibular Epilepsy**: disequilibrium that may present as an aura or as an absence seizure, symptoms vary in severity and may present episodically similar to Ménière's disease
- **Multiple Sclerosis (MS)**: demyelinating disorder of the CNS may result in plaques within the central vestibular system causing vertigo, may present initially with vertigo (10–15%)
- **Subclavian Steal Syndrome**: occlusion of the subclavian artery proximal to the vertebral artery results in reverse flow of the vertebral artery in favor of the ipsilateral arm resulting in intermittent vertigo, occipital headaches, blurred vision, upper extremity pain, supraclavicular fossa bruit, blood pressure differential between arms, and a weak radial pulse
- **Hyperinsulinemia/Diabetes**: may contribute to acute vertiginous attacks or Ménière's-like complaints

# Pediatric Vestibular Disorders (see pp. 585–586)

# THE FACIAL NERVE
## Anatomy and Physiology

- the facial nerve is composed of ~10,000 neurons; 7,000 are myelinated and innervate the nerves of facial expression; 3,000 comprise the nervus intermedius and are somatosensory and secretomotor

### Facial Nerve Course
#### Brainstem Nuclei

- **Motor Nucleus (Pons)**
- **Superior Salivatory Nucleus (Pons)**: sends general visceral efferents to lacrimal, nasal, palatine, sublingual, submandibular glands
- **Nucleus Solitarius (Medulla)**: receives afferents from anterior 2/3 tongue and skin

#### Intracranial Segment

- segment from brainstem to internal auditory canal (IAC)
- **Nervus Intermedius (Nerve of Wrisberg)**: parasympathetic and sensory root of the facial nerve (contribute to the superficial petrosal and chorda tympani nerves)
- motor root joins with the nervus intermedius in the CPA/IAC to form the common facial nerve

## Intratemporal Segment

### 1. Meatal: Porus Acousticus → Fundus

- CN VII transverses in the **superior anterior** quadrant of the IAC separated by the **falciform crest** (horizontal crest) inferiorly and **Bill's bar** (vertical crest) posteriorly (other quadrants include the superior vestibular nerve [superior posterior], inferior vestibular nerve [inferior posterior], and the cochlear nerve [inferior anterior]; superior/inferior relationship between CN VII and cochlear nerve can be remembered by "7-Up, Coke [Cochlear nerve] Down")
- the meatal segment is ensheathed within an extension of the meninges
- 8–10 mm length

### 2. Labyrinthine: Fundus → Geniculate

- narrowest segment of the fallopian canal (**0.61–0.68 mm diameter**), 4 mm length
- **Geniculate Ganglion**: located at the **first genu**, houses cell bodies of sensory cells and taste cells from the anterior two-thirds of the tongue and palate
- **Greater (Superficial) Petrosal Nerve (GSPN)**: first branch (branches off the geniculate ganglion and exits fallopian canal via the facial hiatus), carries preganglionic parasympathetic fibers to the lacrimal gland

### 3. Tympanic (Horizontal): Geniculate → Second Genu

- inferior to the horizontal semicircular canal
- courses above the oval window and stapes
- **most common site of dehiscence (40–50%)**
- 11 mm length

### 4. Mastoid (Vertical): Second Genu → Stylomastoid Foramen

- branches to the **stapedius** and the **chorda tympani** (preganglionic parasympathetic to the submandibular and sublingual glands and special sensory taste fibers)
- becomes more lateral as it descends
- 13 mm length

## Extratemporal Segment

- begins at the stylomastoid foramen
- **Posterior Auricular Nerve**: branch to the posterior auricular and occipitofrontalis muscles
- **Nerve to the Stylohyoid**
- **Nerve to the Posterior Digastric**
- **Pes Anserinus:** branching point of the extratemporal segments in the parotid gland, most commonly divides into two divisions, the **temporozygomatic** and **cervicofacial** branches (many variants)

- Branches of Pes Anserinus ("To Zanzibar By Motor Coach")
  1. **Temporal**: innervates the frontalis, corrugator supercillii, procerus, and upper orbicularis oculi
  2. **Zygomatic**: innervates the lower orbicularis oculi, abundant anastomotic supply with buccal branch
  3. **Buccal**: innervates the zygomaticus major and minor, levator anguli oris, buccinator, and upper orbicularis oris (smile); abundant anastomotic supply with the zygomatic branch
  4. **(Marginal) Mandibular**: innervates the lower orbicularis oris, depressor anguli oris, depressor labii inferioris, and mentalis
  5. **Cervical**: innervates the platysma

## Nerve Fiber Components

- **Endoneurium**: surrounds each nerve fiber (axons), tightly adherent to the Schwann cell layer, provides the endoneural tube for regeneration, poorer prognosis for regeneration when disrupted
- **Perineurium**: surrounds endoneural tubules, provides tensile strength, maintains intrafunicular pressure, and protects from infection
- **Epineurium (Nerve Sheath)**: outer layer, contains the vasa nervorum for nutrition

## Facial Nerve Components

### *Branchial Motor (Special Visceral Efferent)*

- **premotor cortex** → **motor cortex** → *corticobulbar tract* → **bilateral facial nuclei** (pons) → muscles of facial expression
- fibers that innervate the forehead receive bilateral innervation from upper motor neurons, fibers that innervate the lower face receive contralateral fibers only from upper motor neurons
- also supplies stapedius (**stapedial reflex**), stylohyoid, posterior digastric, and buccinator

### *Parasympathetic (General Visceral Efferent)*

- **superior salivatory nucleus** (pons) → *nervus intermedius* → **greater (superficial) petrosal nerve** → through facial hiatus → middle cranial fossa → joins the *deep petrosal nerve* (sympathetic fibers from cervical plexus) → through pterygoid canal (now called *nerve of the pterygoid canal* or *vidian nerve*) → pterygopalatine fossa → **spheno/pterygopalatine ganglion** → *postganglionic parasympathetic fibers* →

joins the *zygomaticotemporal nerve (CN V₂)* → **lacrimal gland** (also innervates the seromucinous glands of nasal and oral cavity)
- **superior salivatory nucleus** (pons) → *nervus intermedius* → **chorda tympani** → carried on *lingual nerve* → **submandibular ganglion** → *postganglionic parasympathetic fibers* → **submandibular and sublingual glands**

### Sensory *(General Sensory Afferent)*

- supplies sensation to the auricular concha, postauricular skin, wall of the EAC, and part of the TM
- cell bodies housed in the **geniculate ganglion** (also holds the cell bodies of the taste fibers)

### Taste *(Special Visceral Afferent)*

- bilateral **postcentral gyrus** → **nucleus solitaries** (gustatory nucleus) → *tractus solitarius* → *nervus intermedius* → **geniculate ganglion** (taste fibers and sensory cell bodies) → **chorda tympani** → joins *lingual nerve* → anterior 2/3 of the tongue and hard and soft palate
- **Iter Chordae Posterior**: canal through which the chorda tympani enters the middle ear branching from the facial nerve
- **Iter Chordae Anterior (Canal of Huguier)**: canal through which the chorda tympani exits the middle ear

## Sunderland Nerve Injury Classification

- **Class I (First-Degree) Injury (Neuropraxia)**: **compression** of the nerve causes loss of axoplasmic flow, results only in a conduction block, complete recovery anticipated
- **Class II (Second-Degree) Injury (Axonotmesis)**: **axon** transected, endoneurium preserved, Wallerian degeneration occurs distal to site of injury, complete recovery anticipated (axon regenerates through an intact neural tube at **1 mm/day**)
- **Class III (Third-Degree) Injury (Neurotmesis)**: **neural tube** (axon, myelin sheath, and **endoneurium**) transected, Wallerian degeneration occurs distal to site of injury, unpredictable outcome (loss of endoneural tubules results in high risk for **synkinesis**, the contraction of multiple muscle fibers simultaneously if regrowth occurs)
- **Class IV (Fourth-Degree) Injury**: violates **perineurium**
- **Class V (Fifth-Degree) Injury**: **complete** transection (violates **epineurium**), risk of a neuroma from nerve sprouts outside of nerve sheath

# Evaluation of Facial Nerve Paralysis

## History

- <u>Character of Facial Paralysis</u>: onset (immediate versus delayed), duration, and progression of paralysis (complete versus incomplete)
- <u>Contributing Factors</u>: recent infection or illness, trauma (birth trauma in neonates), surgery (otologic, parotid, or neurologic surgery); recent tick bites or outdoor activity; history of syphilis, HIV, tuberculosis, or herpes infections; toxin exposure (lead); history of otologic, neurologic, diabetic, or vascular disorders; previous history of facial nerve paralysis
- <u>Associated Symptoms</u>: fever, facial pain, hearing loss, aural fullness, otalgia, vertigo, other neurologic deficits, change in taste sensation, vision changes, drooling, cheek biting, epiphora, dysacusis, pain (auricular, postauricular, or facial)
- think "KITTENS" for differential diagnosis (*see* Table 8–9)

## Physical Exam

- <u>Facial Nerve</u>: observe facial symmetry at rest and with movement, paresis versus paralysis, hemifacial spasms, and facial tics at rest; determine unilateral versus bilateral weakness, eye closure, quality of **Bell's phenomenon** (globe turns up and out during attempts to close eyes), tear production, corneal reflex, and visual acuity
- <u>House-Brackmann Grading</u>: (*see* Table 8–10) used to evaluate recovery of paralysis (eg, recovery from Bell's palsy, preoperative versus postoperative results)
- <u>Other H&N Assessment</u>: evaluate for mass or fluid in the middle ear, presence of vesicles in the EAC and concha, **Hitselberger sign** (hypesthesia of the sensory division of the facial nerve at the superior posterior concha), other cranial nerve involvement, other lateralizing signs (hemiparesthesias, hemiparalysis, aphasia), parotid mass

## Ancillary Studies

### Electromyography (EMG)

- electrodes inserted into muscle, measure muscle response to voluntary contraction
- useful to demonstrate the existence of functional motor units
- **fibrillations** from **denervated** nerve appear after 1–2 weeks
- **polysynaptic** signals indicate **reinnervation**
- presence of voluntary action potentials indicates at least partial continuity of nerve

TABLE 8-9. Differential Diagnosis of Facial Nerve Paralysis: KITTENS Method

| (K) Congenital | Infectious and Idiopathic | Toxins and Trauma | Tumor (Neoplasms) | Endocrine | Neurologic | Systemic/ PSychological |
|---|---|---|---|---|---|---|
| Möbius syndrome | Idiopathic facial paralysis (Bell's palsy) | Head trauma | Parotid tumors | Diabetes mellitus | Guillain-Barré | Sarcoidosis |
| Myotonic dystrophy | Melkersson-Rosenthal syndrome | Temporal bone trauma | Facial neuroma | Pregnancy | Multiple sclerosis | Amyloidosis |
| | Ramsay-Hunt syndrome | Iatrogenic injuries | Vestibular schwannoma | Hyperthyroidism | Myasthenia gravis | Hyperostoses (Paget's disease, osteopetrosis) |
| | Otitis media/mastoiditis | Birth trauma | Cholesteatoma | | Stroke | |
| | Necrotizing otitis externa | Barotrauma | Glioma | | | |
| | Meningitis | | Temporal bone tumors | | | |
| | Lyme disease | | Paraganglioma | | | |
| | Tetanus | | | | | |
| | TB, HIV, EBV, syphilis | | | | | |

| Grading | Function |
|---------|----------|
| **TABLE 8–10.** House-Brackmann System of Grading Facial Nerve Paralysis | |
| I | **normal function** |
| II | mild dysfunction: weakness on close inspection, normal symmetry and tone at rest, moderate to good facial function (slight mouth asymmetry, complete eye closure with minimal effort) |
| III | moderate dysfunction: obvious weakness, and/or asymmetry (not disfiguring), contracture, and/or hemifacial spasms, normal symmetry and tone at rest; moderate facial function (weak mouth and forehead function, complete eye closure with effort) |
| IV | moderately severe dysfunction: disfiguring symmetry and/or obvious weakness, normal symmetry and tone at rest, incomplete eye closure, no forehead motion, symmetric mouth motion with maximal effort |
| V | severe dysfunction: barely perceptible motion, asymmetry at rest, incomplete eye closure, no forehead motion, slight mouth motion |
| VI | **total paralysis** |

*Source:* From House JW and Brackmann DE. Facial nerve grading system. *Arch Otolaryngol Head Neck Surg.* 1985; 93:146–147.

## Electroneuronography (ENoG)

- essentially an evoked EMG (muscle response is recorded by electromyogram)
- only obtain for House-Brackmann VI
- records muscle response via electrodes after stimulation of the facial nerve with a transcutaneous impulse at the stylomastoid foramen
- objectively compares muscle compound action potential amplitudes (related to intact motor axons) and latencies from the paralyzed and normal sides
- in an acute setting ENoG is typically not useful until after 24–72 hours when Wallerian degeneration occurs
- can distinguish neuropraxia versus more severe injuries
- valuable in determining prognosis for idiopathic paralysis

## Other Ancillary Studies

- may be considered in select cases
- no electrophysiological test can distinguish axonotmesis (likely full recovery) from more severe injury
- **Nerve Excitability Text (NET)**: nerve stimulator used at stylomastoid foramen, (minimum) thresholds for eliciting facial twitching compared

between the left and right sides of the face, difference ≥3.5 mA suggests significant degeneration, subjective and rarely used
- **Maximal Stimulation Test (MST)**: similar to NET except uses maximum current that does not cause discomfort and measures movement instead of current, subjective and rarely used
- **Audiogram**: indicated for all intratemporal injuries and for preoperative baseline hearing
- **Topognostic Tests**: (Schirmer's test, stapedial reflex, salivary flow test) in general are not useful and have been replaced with electrophysiologic testing
- **CT Temporal Bone**: may detect temporal bone lesions and fractures
- **MRI of Temporal Bone**: most sensitive imaging for examining the intratemporal segment of the facial nerve; gadolinium enhancement may reveal vestibular schwannoma, facial neuroma, or other tumors
- **Treponemal Studies:** Lyme titers and VDRL/FTA-ABS
- **CBC**: may suggest inflammatory process
- **ACE level**: may suggest active sarcoidosis

# Congenital Facial Palsy (see pp. 586–587)

# Infectious and Idiopathic Causes of Facial Palsy

## Idiopathic Facial Paralysis (Bell's Palsy)

- most common cause of facial paralysis (~50%)
- if underlying cause of facial paralysis known, condition is **not** Bell's palsy
- <u>Pathophysiology</u>: unclear, facial paralysis or paresis may be due to impaired axoplasmic flow from edema of the facial nerve within the fallopian canal secondary to a herpes simplex virus type 1 (HSV-1) infection (may be reactivated from dormancy in geniculate ganglion), other possible etiologies include immunologic or vascular (ischemic) pathology
- <u>Risks</u>: diabetes, pregnancy, past history (7–12% recur)
- <u>SSx</u>: acute, unilateral paresis (~1/3) or paralysis (~2/3) of the face, rapid onset (<48 hours); may have a viral-like prodrome 3–4 days prior to paralysis, postauricular pain, dysgeusia (chorda tympani), hyperacusis (stapedius), decreased lacrimation
- approximately 70–85% will have full recovery by 6 months; approximately 15–30% will have incomplete recovery
- favorable prognosis is associated with the presence of any facial movement

- poorer prognosis is associated with complete facial paralysis (ENoG reveals >90% weakness) within 2 weeks of onset
- <u>Dx</u>: diagnosis is based on exclusion of other causes of facial nerve paralysis as well as H&P

### Initial Management

- <u>Medical Management</u>: oral corticosteroid (~10 day course) and antivirals (valacyclovir) for acute phases
- <u>Eye Protection</u>: artificial tears, ocular ointment and eye patch at night
- follow progression with serial exams (may consider ENoG)

### Surgical Decompression

- <u>Indications</u>: (*controversial*) Gantz et al. suggest consideration of surgical decompression if ENoG reveals >90% weakness within 2 weeks after onset and no voluntary movement on EMG (*Laryngoscope.* 1999;109:1177–1188)
- most effective if performed ≤2 weeks of onset
- typically requires a transmastoid and middle cranial fossa approach with decompression of the tympanic segment, geniculate ganglion, labyrinthine segment, and meatal foramen

## Herpes Zoster Oticus (Ramsay Hunt Syndrome)

- herpes zoster induced facial nerve palsy, may also affect other cranial nerves
- <u>Pathophysiology</u>: primary infection or reactivation of latent varicella (herpes) zoster virus in the geniculate ganglion
- 30–50% risk of residual facial weakness after an acute episode (higher risk than Bell's palsy), worse prognosis if complete paralysis
- <u>SSx</u>: acute peripheral facial palsy, painful vesicular lesions in the concha or EAC (often precedes palsy, often misdiagnosed as otitis externa), dysgeusia (chorda tympani), hyperacusis (stapedius), hearing loss, vertigo, may involve other cranial nerves
- <u>Dx</u>: H&P, complement fixation and serum titers confirm diagnosis
- <u>Rx</u>: antivirals (valacyclovir) and corticosteroids for 10 days, analgesics, and eye protection; rare to consider surgical facial nerve decompression (*see previous*)

## Melkersson-Rosenthal Syndrome

- <u>Pathophysiology</u>: unknown etiology
- <u>SSx</u>: chronic or recurrent edema of the face (defining feature), recurrent unilateral or bilateral facial motor dysfunction (50–90%), fissured tongue, cheilitis granulomatosa

- facial swelling and facial paralysis begins in childhood and early adolescence
- <u>Dx</u>: H&P, lip biopsy reveals dilated lymphatics and granulomatous changes with giant cells, may have elevated ACE levels during attacks
- <u>Rx</u>: empiric management with corticosteroids, may consider surgical decompression (*controversial*)

## Lyme Disease

- <u>Pathophysiology</u>: ***Borrelia burgdorferi*** (spirochete) transmitted by *Ixodes* tick
- <u>SSx</u>: 10% of patients with Lyme disease have ipsilateral or bilateral facial nerve involvement after 1–4 weeks incubation period (higher risk with tick bite of the head); initial erythema migrans (bull's-eye rash), flu-like symptoms (stage 1); meningitis, multiple neuropathies (stage 2); cardiac conduction disorders, meningoencephalitis, swollen joints (stage 3)
- facial paralysis resolves in 6–12 months (full recovery anticipated)
- <u>Dx</u>: identification of a tick bite or erythema migrans rash, antibodies in serum or CSF
- <u>Rx</u>: parenteral penicillin, ceftriaxone, or cefotaxime for severe cases; for rash only consider oral therapy (penicillin, erythromycin, or tetracycline); rare to consider surgical facial nerve decompression (*see previous*)

## Otitis Media, Cholesteatoma

- <u>Pathophysiology</u>: in acute otitis media, toxic effects from infectious spread into the nerve sheath results in facial nerve dysfunction; in chronic otitis media, facial nerve paralysis may occur from compressive effects from a cholesteatoma or from granulation tissue
- <u>SSx</u>: progressive unilateral facial palsy with suppurative otitis media
- <u>Dx</u>: H&P (otoscopic exam), CT/MRI may reveal cholesteatoma or soft tissue compression
- <u>Rx</u>: *see* pp. 373, 376–377

## Necrotizing Otitis Externa

- <u>Pathophysiology</u>: facial nerve injury from the effect of temporal bone osteomyelitis
- <u>SSx</u>: progressive unilateral facial palsy with a necrotizing otitis externa
- <u>Dx</u> and <u>Rx</u>: *see* pp. 371–372

# Facial Nerve Trauma

## Penetrating and Blunt Trauma

- <u>Causes</u>: penetrating injury to the extratemporal facial branches or blunt trauma resulting in a temporal bone fracture
- <u>Dx</u>: assess facial nerve integrity (*as previous*) and possible temporal bone fractures (CT)
- <u>Rx</u>: *see* pp. 659–662 *for evaluation and management of temporal bone fractures*; penetrating injury resulting in total facial nerve paralysis should be explored and repaired with an end-to-end anastomosis (*see following*) within 48–72 hours while the distal branches may be stimulated; however, injuries medial to a line perpendicular to the lateral canthus usually recover spontaneously and do not require exploration; if wound is contaminated or there is significant tissue loss consider identifying distal and proximal ends of the facial nerve with plans for a second stage procedure within 3–4 weeks

## Iatrogenic Injury

- tympanic and vertical segments are the most commonly injured segments in otologic surgery (tympanic most common site of facial nerve dehiscence)
- facial nerve injury may also occur with salivary gland surgery, neck dissection, rhytidoplasty, and branchial cleft excision

### Management

- intraoperative injury may be addressed with primary anastomosis or cable grafting
- for immediate postoperative facial palsies wait for local anesthetic to wear off (2–3 hours) then re-evaluate
- for postoperative paralysis (with intraoperative confirmation of facial nerve preservation) consider corticosteroids and follow progression with serial electrodiagnostic testing
- facial weakness or delayed onset of facial paralysis usually results in complete recovery
- may consider re-exploration for complete paralysis in select cases

# Other Causes of Facial Nerve Paralysis

## Tumors

- <u>SSx</u>: tumors may present as an acute ipsilateral facial paralysis or progression of facial paralysis

- **Parotid Tumors**: most common malignancy to cause facial nerve paralysis, mucoepidermoid carcinoma is the most common parotid tumor to cause facial dysfunction, although adenoid cystic carcinoma has a higher rate of neural involvement
- **Nerve Tumors (Facial Nerve Schwannoma, Vestibular Schwannoma)**: uncommon, large tumors may cause facial paralysis
- Other Tumors: cholesteatoma, vascular malformation, glomus jugulare or tympanicum, meningioma, metastatic carcinoma, leukemia, rhabdomyosarcoma

### Neurologic Disease

- **Stroke**: presents with acute, **forehead sparing** facial paralysis associated with other lateralizing neurologic signs
- **Guillain-Barré Syndrome**: common cause of acute **bilateral** facial nerve palsy, associated with generalized weakness, central nervous and autonomic dysfunction
- **Myasthenia Gravis**: autoimmune disease with antibodies against the acetylcholine receptor at the neuromuscular junction, which causes progressive motor weakness with repetitive function; associated with ptosis, difficulty chewing, talking, weakness, and thymic tumors

## Facial Nerve Repair and Reanimation

### Introduction

- Goals of Facial Rehabilitation: protect eye from corneal exposure, provide a balanced smile (cosmesis), resolve drooling, improve mastication, improve articulation
- no irreversible procedure that interrupts the continuity of the facial nerve should be considered if there is a possibility of spontaneous recovery
- if paralysis has occurred <12–18 months (before significant muscle atrophy or loss of motor end plates) consider end-to-end anastomosis (preferred), interpositioning, crossover grafting, and upper eyelid weighted implants (gold weight, platinum chain)
- if paralysis has occurred >12–18 months with significant muscle atrophy or the facial nerve cannot be grafted consider musculofacial transpositions, static procedures, and upper eyelid weight or spring implants
- best result for any nerve repair surgery is House-Brackmann grade III

## End-to-End Anastomosis (Neurorrhaphy)

- <u>Indications</u>: best choice when tension-free closure is possible and motor end plates are intact (recent injury), provides best chance of rehabilitation (facial muscle movement with the least synkinesis)
- <u>Technique</u>: microsurgical anastomosis of the epineurium (nerve sheath) or perineurium (if feasible), avoidance of tension is essential (may require releasing proximally and distally or rerouting at the mastoid segment)
- ideally completed before three days (**distal branches may be stimulated up to 3 days following transection**)

## Interposition (Cable) Grafting

- <u>Indications</u>: method of choice if unable to achieve a tension-free end-to-end anastomosis and motor end plates are intact
- <u>Technique</u>: nerve cable graft interposed between nerve endings, greater auricular or sural nerves are most common nerve grafts
- typically provides resting muscle tone and spontaneous facial expression

## Nerve Crossover (Transposition)

- <u>Indications</u>: proximal stump unavailable (eg, temporal bone tumors), distal segment intact, and functioning motor end plates (<12–18 months of injury, evaluated with EMG or muscle biopsy)
- <u>Technique</u>: connects **hypoglossal** nerve to distal segment of facial nerve via a cable graft or direct end-to-side grafting with a mobilized facial nerve ("12-7")
- restores some voluntary motion and resting tone typically by 6 months
- may result in significant synkinesis, requires patient re-education of motor coordination
- **Crossface Nerve Graft**: connects the branches of the opposite facial nerve to distal segment of facial nerve via a cable graft (*controversial*)

## Static Procedures

- <u>Indications</u>: may be used as an adjunctive procedure to enhance facial symmetry by providing static support
- <u>Types</u>: fascial, allograft, or synthetic (Gore-Tex) slings; browlifts, rhytidoplasty, canthoplasty
- simpler techniques than dynamic procedures

## Dynamic Procedures

- <u>Indications</u>: unavailable facial nerve or atrophic facial muscles
- **Temporalis Muscle Transposition**: reanimates the mouth (superior vector, may also be used for the eye)
- **Masseter Muscle Transposition**: reanimates the mouth (horizontal vector)
- **Free Nerve Muscle Transfer**: two-stage procedure, initial procedure creates a sural nerve anastomosis to the facial branch of the unaffected side with distal graft end left free in preauricular region of the paralyzed side, after 6–12 months a pectoralis minor or gracilis free flap is transposed and anastomosed to the nerve graft

## Ocular Rehabilitation Techniques

- **Tarsorrhaphy**: partial suturing of the eyelids, does not reanimate, results in visual field deficits and cosmetic deformity
- **Upper Eyelid Weight Implant**: enhances closure by utilizing gravity, implants include gold weight and platinum chain, may be used with reversible or irreversible paralysis, risk of implant extrusion or migration, contraindicated with glaucoma (may aggravate ocular hypertension)
- **Lateral Canthoplasty/Lid Shortening Procedures**: indicated to correct senile ectropion from lower lid laxity
- **Botox Injections**: for synkinesis or hypertonia

# CHAPTER

# Reconstructive and Facial Plastic Surgery

Richard A. Zoumalan, Joseph F. Goodman, Neil Tanna, Richard L. Arden,
Justin S. Golub, and Raza Pasha

# FUNDAMENTALS OF WOUND HEALING

## Overview

### Skin and Adjacent Layers

*Skin* (*see* Figure 9–1)

- **Epidermis**: outer layer, predominant cell is the **keratinocyte** (epidermis rarely referred to as cuticle)
- Epidermal Layers
  1. **Stratum Corneum**: most superficial, dead cells (no nucleus), loosens then desquamates
  2. **Stratum Lucidum**: absent in thin skin
  3. **Stratum Granulosum**: 3–5 layers thick, flattened, keratohyalin granules
  4. **Stratum Spinosum**: (prickle layer) initiates keratin synthesis, basophilic cells
  5. **Stratum Basale**: deepest, continuously dividing to renew outer layers, single layer of cuboidal cells at basal lamina
- **Epidermal–Dermal Junction:** "blueprint" for overlying skin, must be re-established in repair
- Epidermal–Dermal Junction Elements
  1. **Rete Pegs**: epidermal projections into dermal layer
  2. **Papillae**: dermal, vascularized projections into epidermal layer

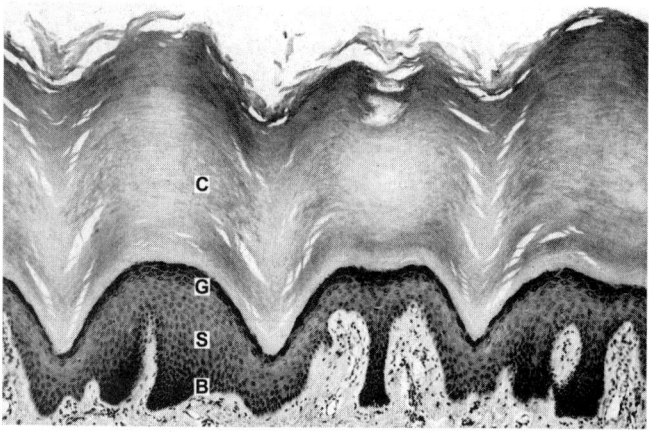

**FIGURE 9–1.** Layers of epidermis (C = stratum corneum, G = stratum granulosum, S = stratum spinosum, B = stratum basale). Image is from the sole of the foot, thus the stratum corneum is much thicker than in the head/neck. Reprinted with permission from B Young, *Wheater's Functional Histology: A Text and Colour Atlas*: 159. Copyright 2000 Elsevier.

- **Dermis**: inner layer, predominant cell is the **fibroblast** (dermis rarely referred to as subcuticle, as in **subcuticular** stitch, which is simply intradermal)
- Dermal Layers
  1. **Papillary**: lies immediately deep to the epidermis, made of loose connective tissue, contains small blood vessels and nerve endings
  2. **Reticular**: made of dense connective tissue; contains blood vessels, hair follicles, sweat glands, lymphatics, nerves, and sebaceous glands

### Subcutaneous Layer (Hypodermis)

- deep to skin
- contains fat and fibrous tissue

## Methods of Wound Closure

- **Primary (First Intention)**: skin edges are approximated within hours, optimal cosmesis, typically for clean wounds
- **Secondary (Second Intention)**: wound is left open, wound bed granulates, contracts → increased scar, typically for contaminated or very small wounds
- **Tertiary (Third Intention, Delayed Primary)**: delayed closure after initial secondary healing (and possible debridement)
- chronic wounds are >4–6 weeks old

# Stages of Cutaneous Wound Healing

## Inflammatory (Substrate) Phase

### Hemostasis

- initial vasoconstriction for 10–15 minutes (thromboxane $A_2$) followed by vasodilation (histamine, serotonin [platelets], and nitric oxide [endothelium])
- endothelial cells contract → expose collagen, fibronectin, and laminin → forms platelet plug with fibrin from coagulation cascade
- the coagulation and complement cascades, along with activated platelets, release a variety of biologically active substances, including prostaglandins, growth factors, and cytokines (chemotactic and proliferative factors), which activate their target cells

### Inflammatory (Cellular)

- **Neutrophils (PMNs)**: appear within 6 hours, maximum cellular influx at 24–48 hours (not critical for wound healing); clean wound

of debris and bacteria by phagocytosis, then they are extruded or phagocytosed in turn
- **Macrophages**: essential for wound healing (regulatory function); predominant cell type by 48–96 hours; attracted by PDGF; transition wound into stage of repair; attract fibroblasts via PDGF; secrete TNF-$\alpha$, TNF-$\beta$, IGF-1, and IL-1
- **Fibroblasts**: appear by 48 hours, maximum cells at 15 days; predominant producer of collagen, elastin, and fibronectin (differentiate into **myofibroblasts,** which are important for wound contraction, disappear by apoptosis once a scar is formed)

## Proliferative Phase

### *Reepithelialization*

- begins in hours with basal epithelial cell differentiation and separation from basement membrane (may be stimulated by epidermal growth factor), collagenase and plasmin begin dissolution of eschar matrix, matrix metalloproteinases also important for degradation and remodeling
- initial cellular detachment from loss of desmosomes, pseudopod formation and migration of fibroblast from dermis into wound bed
- migration in "leap frog" pattern with fibronectin and others at 12–21 µm/hr (moist environment aids in migration)

### *Neovascularization*

- **Granulation Tissue**: begins ~day 4; scaffold for cell migration made of fibrin, fibronectin and hyaluronic acid in matrix
- **Angiogenesis**: migration of epithelial cells into perivascular spaces, forms channels and capillary buds
- increases delivery of neutrophils, macrophages, and fibroblasts
- modulated via vascular endothelial growth factor (VEGF)

### *Collagen Deposition*

- initial deposition of **type III collagen**, later forms **type I collagen**
- maximum deposition at 2–3 weeks
- <u>Collagen Synthesis</u>: polypeptide chains → hydroxylation of proline and lysine (requires vitamin C and iron) → combine into a helix → glycosylation → secreted by fibroblasts as **procollagen** → cleavage to **tropocollagen** → aggregates into fibrils → combines into **collagen fiber**
- collagen fiber cross-linking aids in increasing local tissue strength
- tensile strength begins to increase at 4–5 days

- Collagen Types
    - **I**   most common, bone ("b-one"), tendon, **late scar**, fascia, skin
    - **II**  hyaline cartilage ("car-two-lage")
    - **III** skin, uterus, arteries, **early scar**
    - **IV**  basement membrane

### Wound Contraction

- mediated by myofibroblasts
- maximal at 12–15 days
- contracts at 0.6–0.75 mm/day

## Remodeling (Maturation) Phase

- increase in **type I collagen** and more parallel alignment of collagen fibers results in increased tensile strength with decreased scar dimensions (4:1 ratio of type III to type I ultimately)
- **3 weeks**: **15%** original tensile strength (highest level of collagen)
- **6 weeks**: **60%** original tensile strength
- **6 months**: **70–80%** original tensile strength (maximum achieved)
- fetal skin does not form scars (due to ↓TGF-b and ↑MMP)

# Compromised Wound Healing

## Causes

- Local Factors: infection, irradiated tissue, contamination, hematoma, neoplasm, wound desiccation, hypoxia, ischemia
- Medications: corticosteroids, NSAIDs, chemotherapy, immunosuppressants
- Medical Conditions: diabetes, obesity, severe malnutrition (specifically protein or loss of 20% lean body mass), cofactor deficiency (vitamin A, $B_{12}$, C, zinc, folate, iron, selenium), smoking, peripheral vascular disease, hypothyroidism, connective tissue disorders (Ehlers-Danlos syndrome, osteogenesis imperfecta), immunodeficiency (cancer, HIV, transplant), and fibroproliferative disorders (keloids, hypertrophic scars)
- Technical Factors: traumatic handling of tissues, poor incision design, closure tension, poor hemostasis

## Management

### Assess Medical Condition

- assess nutrition (albumin and prealbumin, total lymphocyte count, transferrin, nitrogen balance)

- dietary modifications with protein and micronutrient supplementation, consider parenteral nutrition
- assess diabetes (fasting glucose) and hypothyroidism (TSH, $T_4$)
- the catabolic state induced by stress (trauma, surgery) leads to excess protein metabolism

### Address Infection

- culture and sensitivities with appropriate antibiotics (oral versus parenteral)
- defined as $10^5$ bacterial colonies per gram of tissue
- topical antibiotics (moist environment aids in reepithelization)
- silver-based dressings prophylactic against superinfection (eg, MRSA)

### Local Wound Care

- debridement and irrigation (healthy tissue bleeds)
- occlusive wound dressing changes (wet-to-dry for debridement)
- consider hydrogen peroxide, sodium hypochlorite (Dakin's solution), or povidone–iodine (Betadine) dressings to aid in local debridement and decrease bacterial load
- **Negative Pressure Dressing** (eg, Wound VAC [vacuum-assisted closure]): promotes angiogenesis, actively debrides, faster healing, use to bolster STSG (eg, burns) or save distal pedicle flap necrosis (eg, scalp), helps promote granulation tissue over exposed bone, may decrease bacterial load, not indicated over exposed dura, may be painful (*Head Neck.* 2006;28:974–981).
- **Skin Substitutes**: for large areas, stimulate wound bed to granulate, prevent fluid loss, contracture; options include cadaver versus bovine (neither for permanent use) or autologous skin grafts consisting of dermal and epidermal components

### Hyperbaric Oxygen (HBO)

- beneficial for poorly healing tissue secondary to hypoxia
- creates a steep oxygenation gradient that aids in oxygen delivery
- reduces edema, activates fibroblasts and macrophages, stimulates collagen synthesis/angiogenesis, bacteriostatic/bacteriocidal
- Complications (Rare): pneumothorax, lung toxicity (ARDS), seizures, middle ear barotrauma (may require myringotomy prior to initiating HBO)
- Absolute Contraindications: untreated pneumothorax, select medications (eg, cisplatin, doxorubicin, disulfiram, mefenamic acid, steroids)

- <u>Relative Contraindications</u>: emphysematous blebs, eustachian tube dysfunction, sinusitis, seizure disorder, history of thoracic surgery, pregnancy

# HEAD AND NECK RECONSTRUCTIVE FLAPS

## Overview

### The Reconstructive Ladder

- each option for wound closure is considered before moving to the next more complicated option, based on the complete clinical picture (*Curr Opin Otolaryngol Head Neck Surg.* 2003;11:251–254)
- concerns for defect analysis include size of defect, available tissue and type needed, type of injury (burn, cancer, trauma), patient comorbidities (chronic disease, infection, previous surgery, trauma, radiation, future treatments), functional status, cosmesis
- <u>Reconstructive Ladder</u> (from least to most complex)
  1. **Second Intention**: small defects, best in concave areas, eg, medial canthus
  2. **Primary Closure (First Intention)**: small–moderate defects
  3. **Skin Grafts**: split thickness (STSG), full thickness (FTSG), dermal grafts
  4. **Local Skin Flaps**: (eg, advancement, rotational)
  5. **Tissue Expansion**: recruits local skin
  6. **Regional Pedicled Flaps**: skin, muscle, bone (eg, pectoralis or latissimus dorsi flap)
  7. **Free Tissue Transfer (Free Flap)**: skin, muscle, bone (eg, radial forearm or fibular free flap)

### Vascular Anatomy of the Skin

- **Angiosome Theory**: 40 distinct regions of body consisting of skin paddle and underlying tissue supplied by a named artery
- **Fasciocutaneous Plexus Theory**: 6 distinctive types of deep fascia perforators (can be considered direct or indirect)
  1. direct cutaneous branch of a muscular artery
  2. septocutaneous perforator (direct)
  3. direct cutaneous perforator
  4. direct septocutaneous artery
  5. musculocutaneous perforator (indirect)
  6. perforating cutaneous branch of a muscular vessel (indirect)

### Musculocutaneous Vessels

- dominant blood supply to skin
- ubiquitous
- small variable size of perfusion area
- run perpendicular to skin
- basis of **random flaps** (most local facial skin flaps)
- based off subdermal plexus, limited 3:1 length-width ratio

### Direct Cutaneous Vessels

- supplementary blood supply to skin
- limited number
- larger size of perfusion area
- run parallel to skin
- associated with a vein
- basis of **axial and island flaps** (eg, paramedian forehead flap)

## Types of Flaps (By Tissue Type)

### Skin Flaps

- <u>Examples</u>: cutaneous, fasciocutaneous, adipofascial, septocutaneous, musculocutaneous

### Muscular Flaps

- **Perforator Flaps**: indirect muscle perforator, indirect septal perforator, direct cutaneous perforator; <u>Advantages</u>: able to incorporate muscle, bone, fat; decreased donor site morbidity; <u>Disadvantages</u>: tedious, variable, fat necrosis
- **Musculocutaneous Flaps**: <u>Advantages</u>: compared to fasciocutaneous flap, better ability to obliterate dead space, reduce infection, and increase collagen deposition
- <u>Musculocutaneous Flap Types</u> (classified based on vascular pedicle; types I, III, and V are most reliable)
  Type I:   1 dominant pedicle (eg, tensor fascia lata flap)
  Type II:  1 dominant + 1 or more minor (eg, gracilis flap)
  Type III: 2 dominant (eg, gluteus maximus flap)
  Type IV:  multiple segmental (eg, sartorius flap)
  Type V:   1 dominant, multiple segmental (eg, latissimus flap)

### Visceral Flaps

- <u>Examples</u>: omentum, colon, jejunum
- used as free tissue transfer for pharyngoesophageal reconstruction

### *Osseous Flaps*

- <u>Examples</u>: fibula, humerus, radius, iliac crest, scapula

### *Innervated Flaps*

- innervation can occur spontaneously, however, innervated flaps produce better results (*Plast Reconstr Surg.* 1999;104(5):1307–1313); almost any flap can be innervated
- **Sural Nerve**: for facial reanimation
- **Radial Forearm**: for oral sensation (lateral antebrachial cutaneous nerve)
- **Lateral Arm**: allows sensation to face and/or movement of face/tongue (lower lateral brachial cutaneous nerve and/or motor to triceps)
- **Anterolateral Thigh**: for partial glossectomy (cutaneous nerve below inguinal ligament to lingual nerve)
- **Rectus Abdominus**: for partial glossectomy (anterior cutaneous branches of the intercostal nerves to lingual nerve)

# Local Skin Flaps

## Introduction

- also referred to as **adjacent tissue transfer**
- factors for consideration include underlying disease (tumor, wound healing problems), smoking status (increases risk of flap necrosis), size, depth, quality of skin, adjacent structures, function (movement, sensation), cosmesis (color match, potential scarring, relaxed skin tension lines, anatomic subunits)
- <u>Basic Technique</u>: undermine, orient to relaxed skin tension lines (RSTLs), 4:1 ratio of length to width for elliptical excision, avoid dog-ears (eg, employ Burow's triangles); develop flap, tack sutures, evaluate for anatomic distortion, reduce tension on closure; consider letting some areas heal by secondary intention
- almost all local flaps in the head and neck have an element of random pattern vascular supply based on the subdermal plexus
- axial flaps are based on a septocutaneous artery with associated venae comitantes (eg, forehead)
- estimated length–width ratio of local flaps is 4:1 in the face and 2:1 in the neck
- local skin flap types are defined by the direction of tissue movement (eg, advancement flap is linear, rotational flap is radial)

## Advancement Flap

- characterized by **linear movement**
- **Single Advancement Flap**: placed over defect, long axis oriented parallel to RSTLs (relaxed skin tension lines), should not be longer than 2–3 times the width (Figure 9–2)
- **Bilateral Advancement Flap**: flaps begin on opposing ends of defect (for larger defects)
- **T-plasty**: converts triangular or circular defect into inverted-T scar (upper lip, forehead)
- typically requires **Burow's triangles** (*see* Figure 9–2) to prevent **dog-ear (standing cone deformity)** formation
- **V–Y Plasty**: versatile advancement technique, which can provide lengthening of some structures, V-shaped flap with underlying tissue advanced into defect (good for lip and columella)
- <u>Advantages</u>: simple, avoids unwanted or secondary movement, avoids deformity of facial structures by favorably orienting incisions (eg, brow, lateral canthus)
- <u>Disadvantages</u>: restricted flexibility
- <u>Common Uses</u>: forehead, chin/mentum

## Rotational Flap (Figure 9–3)

- semicircular flap, raised in subdermal plane, **radial pattern of movement** along a defined arc with a fixed pivot point, shares a common side with the defect
- length-width ratio is ideally 2:1

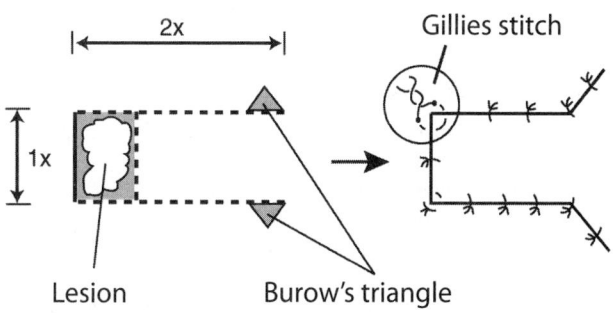

**FIGURE 9–2.** Illustration of the single advancement flap. Burow's triangles are utilized on the ends to prevent dog-ear deformity. Ideally, the length should not be longer than 2–3 times the width. A Gillies stitch, which is constructed similar to a mattress suture, is utilized to reduce tension at the corners.

A.

B.

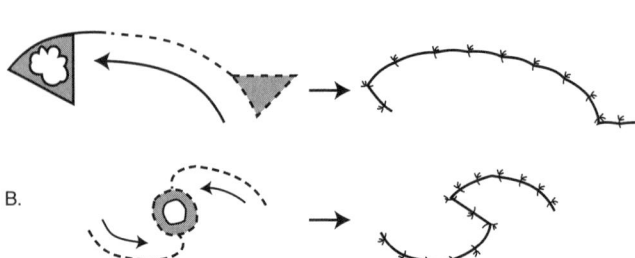

**FIGURE 9–3. A.** Rotational flap to close a triangular defect. Triangular excision at opposite end of defect allows for a flat closure. **B.** Bilateral rotational flaps utilized to close an elliptical defect.

- the effective length decreases with increased angle of rotation
- may use Burow's triangle or a back cut to facilitate
- <u>Advantages</u>: allows closure of large lesions by recruiting lax skin
- <u>Disadvantages</u>: requires a wider base than the advancement flap, requires extensive undermining and long peripheral incision (4–5× diameter of the defect)
- <u>Common Uses</u>: cheek defects using lax neck skin

## Transposition Flap

- raised from a donor site and **rotated over adjacent tissue** to be placed in the defect site
- 3:1 length–width ratio
- most important principles are to minimize tension and develop a wide flap base

### *Classic Rhomboid Flap (Limberg)*

- transposition flap constructed typically from equal length segments around two 120° and two 60° angles (Figure 9–4)
- **Dufourmentel Flap**: defect diamond is created similarly, however, the extending segments are constructed with more acute angles (<120° and <60° angles); allows improved blood supply to flap base and shares closing tensions
- <u>Advantages</u>: better distribution of tension (tension is away from defect, *see* Figure 9–4), reliable, may be designed so the final closure will be parallel to the RSTLs
- <u>Disadvantages</u>: forces a facial defect into an arbitrary design
- <u>Common Uses</u>: cheek, temple

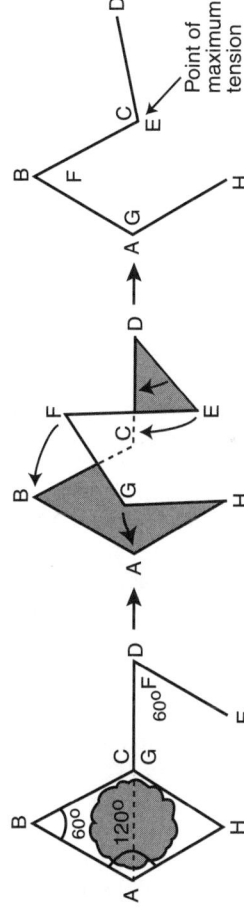

**FIGURE 9–4.** Classic rhomboid flap utilizes 120° and 60° angles to allow the point of maximal tension to be away from the defect. (Adapted with permission from Lore JM. *An Atlas of Head and Neck Surgery.* 3rd ed. Philadelphia, PA: W.B. Saunders; 1988.)

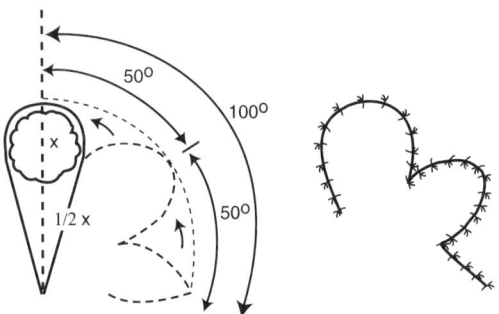

**FIGURE 9–5.** Bilobed flaps are designed with a primary flap and a smaller secondary flap to distribute the tension of wound closure more evenly.

### Bilobed Flap

- transposition flap that recruits lax tissue (secondary flap) from a nearby site that allows primary flap to effect closure of the defect (Figure 9–5)
- primary flap should be slightly smaller than the defect, secondary flap should be 1/2-3/4 the width of the primary flap (except on nasal tip where defect:primary flap = 1:1)
- <u>Advantages</u>: distributes tension evenly
- <u>Disadvantages</u>: risk of pincushioning, lengthy incision that rarely exploits ideal RSTLs
- <u>Common Uses</u>: nasal tip/dorsum (medial lesions generally employ laterally based flaps, lateral lesions generally employ medially based flaps), lateral cheek

### Z-plasty and W-plasty (*see also* pp. 514–516)

- break up scar profiles into smaller, irregular units; useful for scar revision
- **Z-plasty**: versatile method for excising lesion or scar, reorienting and lengthening new incision; relies on health of adjacent skin; may not be optimal for burn contractures (*see* pp. 514–516, Figure 9–13)
- **W-plasty**: preplanned excision with alternating angle which can be interdigitated, does not provide increase in length but can camouflage scar profile (*see* p. 516, Figure 9–14)

## Interpolated Flap

- flap **passed over or under a bridge of skin**, separates donor site from defect (eg, subcutaneous island flap, paramedian forehead flap), useful in ear and nose defects

- random pattern of blood supply
- <u>Advantages</u>: healthy vascular supply, can fill deep defects
- <u>Disadvantages</u>: requires second procedure to divide pedicle, trapdoor effect from excess donor skin
- **Paramedian Forehead Flap:** based on supratrochlear artery; similar to a regional flap; great for extensive nasal defects; pedicle is divided at 3–4 weeks after inset and nasal defect healing; 2 or 3 stages can be used, based on when to thin the underlying frontalis muscle and subcutaneous tissue; forehead defect can close by secondary intention if large flap taken

# Regional Pedicled Flaps

## Introduction

- <u>Advantages</u>: shorter operating times, provides coverage of radiated or traumatized tissue especially when local vasculature is tenuous, microsurgical training is not necessary (important in geographic areas with access challenges)
- <u>Disadvantages</u>: limited range of mobility, bulkiness, and distal necrosis (causing regional pedicled flaps to become less in favor for head and neck reconstruction)

## Pectoralis Major

- most common pedicled flap, very reliable
- <u>Type</u>: myocutaneous (can be raised with skin paddle to recreate mucosa, or muscle alone)
- <u>Advantages</u>: reliable, excellent reach (up to lateral canthus), one-stage procedure, potential for simultaneous harvesting, easy to harvest, good for neck reconstruction, can be taken with fifth rib for bone reconstruction (eg, mandible)
- <u>Disadvantages</u>: bulky (although will atrophy if medial and lateral pectoral nerves cut during harvest), potential for breast deformity in women, potential hair transfer, loss of pectoralis function (may be significant with concurrent ipsilateral injury to CN XI)
- <u>Arterial Supply</u>: **pectoral branch of thoracoacromial artery**
- <u>Common Uses</u>: internal and external defects of the oral cavity, oropharynx, hypopharynx
- incision is made along the inframammary crease in women to camouflage closure line

## Trapezius

- <u>Type</u>: myocutaneous
- <u>Advantages</u>: 3 forms allow for versatility, relatively flat and thin flap, one-stage procedure
- <u>Disadvantages</u>: relatively limited arc of rotation, significant donor site morbidity (weakness of upper extremities, may require skin graft for closure), weaker blood supply, awkward positioning
- <u>Common Uses</u>: oropharyngeal and hypopharyngeal defects, lateral neck, posterior face

### *Flap Designs* (Figure 9–6)

1. **Superiorly Based (Upper) Trapezius Flap**: main vascular supply from the occipital artery and paraspinal perforators; reliable flap; limited arc of rotation; donor site may require a skin graft; based on three angiosomes, including transverse cervical artery supply in middle of flap and a branch of the thoracoacromial artery laterally

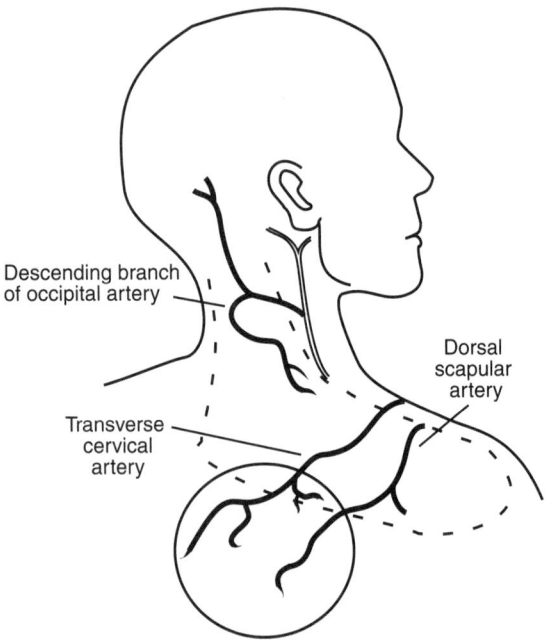

**FIGURE 9–6.** Diagram of the superiorly based (upper) trapezius flap (*dashed line*) based on the occipital artery and the inferior (lower) trapezius island flap (*solid line*) based on the transverse cervical and dorsal scapular arteries.

2. **Lateral Island Trapezius Flap**: vascular supply from the superficial branches of the transverse cervical artery; may cover defects of the oropharynx, posterior oral cavity, and hypopharynx; skin island based anteriorly; requires meticulous dissection of artery and vein from posterior neck
3. **Inferior (Lower) Trapezius Island Flap**: vascular supply from the descending branches of the transverse cervical artery and the dorsal scapular artery, provides the longest pedicle, most commonly used trapezius flap to reach auricle or side of face

## Latissimus Dorsi

- <u>Type</u>: myocutaneous
- <u>Advantages</u>: versatile and dependable, large amount of available skin and soft tissue, long vascular pedicle with extended arc of rotation (to vertex of scalp), less hair transfer, potential for bilobed skin islands, out of irradiated field
- <u>Disadvantages</u>: requires repositioning (lateral decubitus), propensity for seroma formation at donor site, may be bulky in large patients, requires extended tunneling between pectoralis major/minor
- <u>Arterial Supply</u>: thoracodorsal artery (up to 15 cm length, includes vena comitans and nerve)
- <u>Common Uses</u>: similar to pectoralis major flaps (although not as common)
- skin paddle should be based in central portion of muscle if needed

## Sternocleidomastoid

- <u>Type</u>: myocutaneous
- <u>Advantages</u>: donor site located close to defect
- <u>Disadvantages</u>: tenuous blood supply to skin, especially superior portion (platysma limits role of skin perforators), rotation limited by accessory nerve and vascular supply
- <u>Arterial Supply</u>: perforating vessels from the occipital (superior portion) and posterior auricular, superior thyroid, and thyrocervical arteries (middle and inferior portions); preserve at least 2 supplies
- <u>Common Uses</u>: small defects in anterolateral oral cavity and lateral oro- or hypopharynx, parotid defects superiorly, can be raised with periosteum of clavicle to repair laryngeal/tracheal defects

## Platysma

- <u>Type</u>: myocutaneous
- <u>Advantages</u>: donor site located close to defect, thin and pliable skin

- <u>Disadvantages</u>: inconsistent and weak blood supply (not a true axial flap) from facial artery branches
- <u>Arterial Supply</u>: random perforators from external carotid system
- <u>Common Uses</u>: floor of mouth, buccal mucosa, pharyngeal wall (prone to infection)

## Temporoparietal Fascia

- <u>Type</u>: fasciocutaneous
- <u>Advantages</u>: easy access, direct closure
- <u>Disadvantages</u>: temporal branch of facial nerve may be injured
- <u>Arterial Supply</u>: parietal branch or the superficial temporal artery
- <u>Common Uses</u>: coverage of ear cartilage, orbit, oral cavity, anterior skull base, upper/mid third of face

## Deltopectoral

- <u>Type</u>: fasciocutaneous (fascia from pectoralis muscle)
- <u>Advantages</u>: strong blood supply, large amount of donor tissue available, tunnel forms a favorable fistula (inferiorly located), can raise 10×20 cm flap
- <u>Disadvantages</u>: requires second-stage procedure for detachment (6–8 weeks), requires skin graft at donor site
- <u>Arterial Supply</u>: first 4 perforating vessels of internal mammary artery (the second vessel is the largest)
- <u>Common Uses</u>: internal and external defects of the oral cavity, oropharynx, hypopharynx

# Microvascular Free Flaps

## Introduction

- <u>Preoperative Examination</u>: history of arterial lines or peripheral vascular disease, consider duplex studies for radial forearm and fibular free flaps, consider arteriograms for ankle-brachial index (ABI) <1.0 or toe-brachial index (TBI) <0.7
- <u>Advantages</u>: single-stage procedure, excellent perfusion, ability to preselect tissue characteristics of donor tissue for given recipient site defect, potential 2-team approach, possible functional restoration (sensation/motor), improved ability for spatial positioning of donor tissue
- <u>Disadvantages</u>: requires microsurgical expertise and specialized instrumentation, may require longer operating time, possible color and texture mismatch

- **5–15%** failure, most occur in first 24–72 hours; ~**50%** salvage rate on re-exploration
- neovascularization complete after **8 days** (except jejunal flaps, serosa prevents neovascularization)
- vascularized muscle reduces to ~20% of its mass, vascularized fat reduces to 40–60% of its mass (fat required for tissue bulk)
- monitor flap by examining color, turgor, capillary refill, temperature, and quality of dermal–mucosal bleeding (eg, 25G needle prick should produce bright red blood); additional information afforded by monitoring devices (eg, implantable or laser Doppler)
- venous anastomosis failure (purple flap, copious dark blood on needle poke) more common than arterial failure (pale flap, no bright red blood on needle poke)
- revisions should be completed as soon as possible to avoid no-reflow phenomenon, survival time may be extended with free-radical scavengers, or NSAIDs
- <u>Critical Time of Warm Ischemia</u>: jejunal flaps ≈ **2 hours**, skeletal flaps ≈ **6 hours**, cutaneous flaps ≈ **8 hours**

## Microvascular Anastomosis Pearls

- removal of atherosclerotic plaques may lead to thrombosis from intimal damage
- avoid intraoperative and postoperative hypothermia, hypovolemia, and hypotension
- avoid vasospasm by minimizing trauma to vessels (only grasp adventitia); signs of trauma include cobweb sign, measles sign, thrombus sign (low spurt test), and telescope sign
- avoid intraluminal introduction of adventitia (thrombogenic)
- vessels for anastomosis should be similar in size and ideally oriented longitudinally in the neck (avoid kinking)
- arterial anastomoses typically are end-to-end
- venous anastomoses are accomplished either end-to-end or end-to-side
- if a lumen size mismatch beyond 2:1 exists, the surgeon can fish-mouth the smaller vessel and take unequal bites to achieve adequate approximation (the end-to-side anastomosis can also be used for large-vessel mismatch); longitudinal wedge of larger vessel may also allow size match
- avoid stasis and collagen deposition by irrigating with heparin
- may consider aspirin for 10 days postoperatively
- vascular pedicle is susceptible to damage from infection and salivary contamination (prophylactic antibiotics, watertight seal from oral cavity and pharynx)

## Osseous Free Flaps

### Radial Forearm

- <u>Type</u>: fasciocutaneous or osseocutaneous
- <u>Advantages</u>: thin skin, typically hairless, potentially sensate, rapid harvest, long pedicle (20 cm), 10 cm of bone available
- <u>Disadvantages</u>: potential for pathologic fractures (if taking bone), bone does not accept endosseous implants (only take 30–40% circumference of bone), donor defect requires a skin graft, damage to superficial branch of the radial nerve may cause numbness, sacrifices a main artery
- <u>Neurovascular Transfer</u>: **radial artery** and venae comitantes, superficial forearm vein, lateral and medial antebrachial cutaneous nerve (stays in superficial plane), superficial branch of radial nerve (pierces through brachioradialis in mid to distal third)
- <u>Common Uses</u>: most frequently used free flap in head/neck, good for moderately large defects that require a thin flap, may be tubed for pharyngeal reconstruction
- preoperatively must check collateral circulation with **Allen's test** (compress radial and ulnar arteries → patient clenches/unclenches fist several times → hand pallor results from reduced perfusion → release compression on ulnar artery → if sufficient ulnar collateral circulation, hand pallor should fade in ≤10 seconds) or Doppler studies
- protect arm from IV placement immediately preop (wrap arm in gauze with note)

### Lateral Arm

- <u>Type</u>: fasciocutaneous
- <u>Advantages</u>: minimal donor site defect, does not sacrifice major artery, thin skin, quick harvest, typically hairless, may include humerus
- <u>Disadvantages</u>: shorter vascular pedicle than a radial forearm free flap, sensory deficit on extensor surface of forearm, may require skin graft for defects >6 cm, difficult to position for two-team approach
- <u>Neurovascular Transfer</u>: profunda brachii artery and posterior radial collateral artery, venae comitantes, posterior cutaneous nerve (antebrachial)
- <u>Common Uses</u>: moderately large defects that require a thin flap, cheek, may be tubed for pharyngeal reconstruction

## *Scapula*

- <u>Type</u>: osseocutaneous
- <u>Advantages</u>: 8–14 cm of bone available (lateral border), primary closure of donor defect (≤12 cm), color and texture matches facial skin well, typically hairless, can develop two separate skin paddles
- <u>Disadvantages</u>: requires detachment of shoulder girdle muscles resulting in significant weakness, smaller volume bone stock for endosseous implants, requires lateral decubitus positioning restricting ease of two-team approach, skin can be thick in obese patients
- <u>Vascular Transfer</u>: circumflex scapular artery (horizontal cutaneous branch) and vein
- <u>Common Uses</u>: complex through and through bone and soft tissue defects, facial defects, mandible defects (can be harvested together with latissimus or serratus muscle, common vascular pedicle)

## *Fibula*

- <u>Type</u>: osseocutaneous
- <u>Advantages</u>: up to 40 cm of bone available, excellent to reconstruct large bony defects, consistent diameter, good segmental periosteal supply allows for segmental osteotomies, thin fasciocutaneous flap, sensory potential (lateral sural cutaneous nerve), allows for osseointegrated implants (excellent for mandible), limited functional morbidity
- <u>Disadvantages</u>: variable and tenuous blood supply to skin paddle, septocutaneous perforators make for a precarious skin island, skin graft may be required at donor site for osseocutaneous harvest (skin paddle >6 cm)
- obtain preoperative Doppler, consider arteriogram in peripheral vascular disease (peroneal artery is dominant for foot in 10%)
- <u>Neurovascular Transfer</u>: endosteal and periosteal branches of **peroneal (fibular) artery**, peroneal vein, lateral cutaneous branch of peroneal nerve
- <u>Common Uses</u>: mandible reconstruction for bone only or bone with limited soft tissue requirements (can cover entire length of mandible with multiple osteotomies)

## *Iliac Crest*

- <u>Type</u>: osseomyocutaneous or primary bone flap
- <u>Advantages</u>: 3–4 cm of muscle and 14 cm bone available, excellent bone reconstruction, can be transferred as free bone graft material, large cancellous component favors endosseous implants and bone healing, concealed scar placement, allows for primary closure of large flap

- <u>Disadvantages</u>: bulky soft tissue that cannot be thinned because of retention of obligatory muscle cuff and abdominal fat thickness, large amount of dissection required (painful donor site), temporary hip weakness with paresthesia, risk of abdominal hernia
- <u>Vascular Transfer</u>: deep circumflex iliac artery and vein (may need additional anastomosis with superficial circumflex iliac artery in bulky flaps)
- <u>Common Uses</u>: mandible reconstruction with larger soft tissue requirements (floor of mouth, hemitongue)

## Soft Tissue Free Flaps

### *Rectus Abdominus*

- <u>Type</u>: myocutaneous
- <u>Advantages</u>: large soft tissue availability, reliable, flexible flap design, long vascular pedicle, potential motor innervation (25 × 6 cm muscle)
- <u>Disadvantages</u>: risk of ventral hernia (especially below arcuate line; need to reapproximate anterior sheath below arcuate line), poor color match to facial skin
- <u>Neurovascular Transfer</u>: two dominant pedicles → inferior and superior epigastrics (with perforators), lower 6 intercostal nerves
- <u>Common Uses</u>: orbit, maxilla, tongue, skull base; the deep inferior epigastric perforator (DIEP) flap is a variation that spares most of the muscle, separates out only the deep inferior epigastric artery pedicle with cutaneous flap

### *Latissimus Dorsi*

- <u>Type</u>: myocutaneous
- <u>Advantages</u>: massive soft tissue with large surface area, bulky, may be split into 2 islands, reinnervation potential maintains bulk, closed primarily, and possible to transfer as a pedicled flap
- <u>Disadvantages</u>: marginal flap necrosis (pass pedicle carefully between pectoralis major and minor), poor color match, potential shoulder disability when included with radical neck dissection or pectoralis muscle flap, difficult positioning for 2-team approach, may have delayed healing from mobility of donor site, requires 1 week immobilization (eg, arm flexed across chest), higher risk of seroma formation
- <u>Neurovascular Transfer</u>: thoracodorsal artery (primary) and 9–11 intercostals (secondary), thoracodorsal nerve
- <u>Common Uses</u>: massive defects, scalp defects

## Lateral Thigh

- <u>Type</u>: fasciocutaneous
- <u>Advantages</u>: intermediate thickness, may close donor site primarily, potentially sensate
- <u>Disadvantages</u>: more difficult to harvest, occasional hair-bearing, higher risk of seroma formation
- <u>Neurovascular Transfer</u>: third perforator of profunda femoris artery, lateral femoral cutaneous nerve (can create two separate paddles based on separate perforators)
- <u>Common Uses</u>: large sensory skin requirements (up to 16 × 30 cm flaps), tongue, pharynx

## Anterolateral Thigh

- <u>Type</u>: fasciocutaneous
- <u>Advantages</u>: can be thinned, close primarily 60% of time (>9 cm wide), can be sensate
- <u>Disadvantages</u>: more difficult to harvest, occasional hair-bearing, higher risk of seroma formation
- <u>Neurovascular Transfer</u>: descending branch of the lateral circumflex femoral artery and its venae comitantes, anterior branch of the lateral femoral cutaneous nerve (based on musculocutaneous and septocutaneous perforators)
- <u>Common Uses</u>: large sensory skin requirements (up to 12 × 28 cm)

## Jejunum

- <u>Type</u>: visceral
- <u>Advantages</u>: similar diameter to the esophagus, tolerates radiation, operation is extrathoracic, 90% tolerate soft diet afterward
- <u>Disadvantages</u>: laparotomy required, total flap necrosis dangerous (risk of carotid blowout), limited tolerance for warm ischemia (2 hours), inferior speech rehabilitation quality following puncture, requires multiple anastomoses, may inhibit swallowing if redundant tissue folds (flex neck to inset)
- <u>Vascular Transfer</u>: superior mesenteric arcade (5 jejunal branches)
- <u>Common Uses</u>: esophageal and long circumferential pharyngeal defects
- <u>Contraindicated</u>: ascites, carcinoma below thoracic inlet, inflammatory bowel disease, significant abdominal adhesions

## Gracilis

- <u>Type</u>: muscle
- <u>Advantages</u>: thin muscle sheet excellent for facial reanimation

- <u>Neurovascular Transfer</u>: adductor artery (arises from profunda femoris), 2 venae comitantes, anterior branch of obturator nerve
- <u>Common Uses</u>: facial reanimation for facial paralysis

### *Temporoparietal Fascia*

- <u>Type</u>: fascia
- <u>Advantages</u>: thin, easily harvested because it is a distinct layer, lies superficial to temporalis muscle
- <u>Disadvantages</u>: frontal branch of facial nerve easily damaged, alopecia
- <u>Vascular Transfer</u>: superficial temporal artery and vein

# GRAFTS, IMPLANTS, AND EXPANDERS
## Introduction

### Overview

- in plastic surgery, a **graft** is transferred living or synthetic material that does not require preservation or anastomosis of a blood supply (as opposed to a **flap**); eg, the blood supply to a skin graft is entirely disconnected upon harvesting, it initially survives in the recipient site by nutrient diffusion from the underlying wound bed until the blood supply is later re-established
- <u>Ideal Implant</u>: inert, noninflammatory, resist foreign body reaction, noncarcinogenic, resist mechanical stress, sterilizable, easy to sculpt, easily removed, inexpensive, resist extrusion and mobility, radiopaque
- <u>Types</u>
  1. **Autograft** (autogenous graft): patient's own tissue
  2. **Allograft** (allogeneic graft; homograft is older term): same species, often cadaveric
  3. **Xenograft**: different species
  4. **Alloplast**: synthetic material
- when possible autografts are generally preferred to avoid complications such as immediate graft rejection, foreign body reaction (delayed rejection or encapsulation), and graft resorption (incorporation [eg, bone] may be desired)
- allografts and xenografts are processed to not contain living cells to reduce immunogenicity

## Graft Types and Materials

### Bone

- <u>Advantages</u>: does not warp, living tissue, limited resorption, resists infection

- <u>Disadvantages</u>: requires bone-to-bone contact to avoid resorption with fibrosis (except for nasoseptal and turbinate bone for uncertain reasons), soft tissue coverage, and immobility (8–12 weeks)
- **Cortical Bone**: outer layer, provides strength
- **Cancellous Bone**: inner, trabecular layer, contains more osteocytes and osteoblasts
- <u>Phases of Osteogenesis</u>
  1. **Osteoid Formation**: primarily a function of transplanted osteoblastic cells in cancellous bone, occurs for 1 month, forms framework
  2. **Remodeling**: function of osteoblasts, osteoclasts, and fibroblasts (require pluripotent cells), begins at 2 weeks, mediated by bone morphogenic proteins (BMPs) found in cortical bone
- <u>Common Donor Sites</u>: calvarium, iliac crest, rib, fibula, radius
- <u>Common Uses</u>: mandible reconstruction, midfacial defects, craniofacial surgery, rhinoplasty

## Cartilage

- <u>Advantages</u>: easy to shape, maintains structural integrity, easy to harvest and store, does not require direct contact with cartilage or bone, minimal resorption and displacement
- <u>Disadvantages</u>: requires soft-tissue coverage (attached perichondrium prevents resorption)
- <u>Types</u>
  1. **Hyaline**: most common, contains only type II collagen; found in articular joints and the nasal septum
  2. **Elastic**: contains elastic fibers for flexibility; found in the ear, epiglottis, and parts of the larynx
  3. **Fibrocartilage**: sparse ground substance; more dense than hyaline cartilage; found in the pubic symphysis, attachments of tendons and ligaments, and intervertebral disks
- <u>Common Donor Sites</u>: nasal septum, auricular concha, rib
- <u>Common Uses</u>: rhinoplasty, nasal reconstruction, otoplasty, orbital reconstruction

## Dermis, Skin, and Fat

### Split-Thickness Skin Graft (STSG)

- *see pp. 437–438 for skin anatomy*
- contains epidermis and variable amount of dermis (thin STSG [Thiersch graft]: 0.008–0.012 inch; medium STSG: 0.012–0.018 inch; thick STSG: 0.018–0.030 inch)

- primary contraction occurs immediately after harvesting (up to 20%), secondary contraction occurs on the wound during healing (more on burns, large wounds)
- STSG has less primary contraction but more secondary contraction than FTSG
- grafting onto fascia can reduce contraction, grafting onto granulation tissue and/or mobile areas (eg, joints) produces more contracture
- <u>Advantages</u>: better survival (quicker healing, less nutritional needs), easy to mesh, does not require closure of donor site
- <u>Disadvantages</u>: hypertrophic scars more than FTSGs, poor color and texture match, less durable (particularly over bone), donor defect
- <u>Common Uses</u>: defects with chance of recurrent tumor or for temporary coverage prior to definitive reconstruction, coverage of donor site defects

### Full-Thickness Skin Graft (FTSG)

- contains entire epidermis and dermis
- initial attachment to wound bed within 24 hours via fibrin, replaced by granulation tissue, nourished by plasmatic imbibition over 72 hours before new capillary ingrowth starts, within a week lymph and blood flow is restored
- <u>Advantages</u>: better color match, multiple donor site options, less contracture, resists trauma
- <u>Disadvantages</u>: higher graft failure, slower revascularization
- <u>Common Donor Sites</u>: postauricular and preauricular skin (thin, hairless, similar facial skin color), upper eyelid (from excess skin), supraclavicular region, melolabial skin (thick, similar nasal skin color)
- <u>Common Uses</u>: nasal defects (dorsum, sidewall, ala, tip), auricle, eyelids

### Dermal Graft

- contains dermis after removal of epithelium and subcutaneous fat
- <u>Advantages</u>: resistant to infection, may be buried under skin, capable of re-epithelialization, limited resorption
- <u>Disadvantages</u>: loss of thickness at donor site (although more cosmetically acceptable than STSG)
- <u>Common Uses</u>: intraoral, vessel, or dural coverage; subcutaneous implantation for soft tissue bulk

### Fat

- <u>Advantages:</u> does not undergo complete resorption, acts as a permanent filler, natural feeling substance for full face rejuvenation

- <u>Disadvantages</u>: can clump if improperly placed (especially along infraorbital rim, tear trough), granuloma formation (rare), up to 50% resorbs, resorpotion is unpredictable, irregularities/asymmetries difficult to treat
- <u>Common uses</u>: facial augmentation, reconstruction-related augmentation
- <u>Common donor sites</u>: abdominal (periumbilical), thigh, flank

## Common Synthetic Materials

- **Silicone Rubber**: low reactivity and rejection, autoclavable, resists infection, easy to sculpt, becomes encapsulated, high extrusion rate (especially in the nose)
- **Mersilene (Polyester Fiber)**: resists infection, minimal degradation, allows for tissue ingrowth
- **Expanded Polytetrafluoroethylene (ePTFE, Gore-Tex)**: nonresorbable, allows some tissue ingrowth, low infection rate, can extrude or become palpable
- **Acrylics**: (eg, polymethylmethacrylate, PMMA) rigid, able to be molded in situ, does not allow tissue ingrowth
- **Metals**: includes gold (low tissue reactivity, malleable), titanium (anticorrosive, osseointegration, lightweight, low tissue reactivity), stainless steel (strong, anticorrosive, no osseointegration)
- **Medpor (Porous Polyethylene)**: contains pores (100–200 μm) that are interconnected allowing soft tissue ingrowth, resistant to infection, harder than silicone, autoclavable
- **Calcium Hydroxyapatite**: type of ceramic, bioreactive properties (can conduct osteogenic cells), resists infection, minimal inflammation, dense and porous varieties, allows ingrowth, difficult to shape
- **Resorbable Materials:** include **polylactic acid (PLA)**, **polyglocolic acid (PGA)** and mixtures **(PLGA)**, used for rigid craniofacial fixation (lasts 1 year, good for pediatrics); **Gelfilm** (absorbable gelatin film) for small defects (lasts 2–3 months)

# Tissue Expanders

## Introduction

- produce additional tissue adjacent to defect
- <u>Advantages</u>: avoids distant flaps (poor color and texture match, donor site morbidity), allows for hair-bearing skin, can plan scar placement
- <u>Disadvantages</u>: requires multiple procedures, deformity from expansion device, requires serial insertions, delayed reconstruction, possible complications (extrusion, infection)

- <u>Common Uses</u>: face and neck (eg, forehead expansion for nasal flaps), scalp (eg, alopecia), preauricular region (eg, otoplasty), up to 50% skin loss (eg, burns), concurrent procedure with serial excisions

## Biomechanical Properties

- <u>Biomechanical Components</u>: collagen (stores energy), elastin (determines elastic property), glycosaminoglycans (GAGs; bind collagen and elastin fibers), hyaluronate (type of GAG that binds fluid to form a gel)
- long-term remodeling occurs in the epidermis (thickens, increased mitotic activity, normalizes after 6 months), dermis (thins, increased fibroblasts, normalizes after 2 years), muscle (decreases mass but not function), fat (loses up to 50% mass permanently), capsule forms with myofibroblasts and collagen
- **Biological Creep**: property of conventional tissue expanders, permanent changes in microanatomy and collagen production, increases epidermal expansion and subdermal vasculature proliferation, results in a net increase in surface area after long-term stretch
- **Mechanical Creep**: no change in microanatomy, displaces fluid and extracellular substances, realigns collagen fibers by breaking bonds with glycosaminoglycans and elastin fibers (eg, rapid intraoperative expansion), no net increase in surface area but can recruit adjacent tissue
- **Stress Relaxation**: decrease over time in tension on skin when held under constant pressure

## Types of Injection Ports

- **Self-Contained**: risk of implant rupture, less dissection required
- **Remote**: variable-length connector tubing separates expander from injection port, requires more tissue dissection to place, essentially eliminates risk of expander rupture
- **External Valve**: port outside of patient, pain is avoided because there is no percutaneous injection (excellent for children)

## Techniques

- base should be 2.5 times the area of the defect (rectangular expander has the best expander volume-to-skin area [38%] versus round [25%])
- available skin after tissue expansion is calculated by subtracting the width of the base from the circumference of the skin over the

expander; the capsule overlying the implant may be scored to further mobilize although this may compromise underlying blood supply to skin

- shape based on site of expansion (not shape of flap)
- expansion should only form slight blanching, not pain or intractable blanching
- start expansion 2–3 weeks after placement, lasts 6–12 weeks

### Conventional Tissue Expansion Technique

- expand over 4–6 weeks of use, can be done 1–2 times weekly
- relies on **biological creep**

### Rapid Intraoperative Tissue Expansion

- expansion and deflation of prosthesis in operating room over 3-minute intervals (typically 3 cycles)
- no true net gain of skin surface area
- relies on **mechanical creep**

## Complications

- minor complications include pain, transient neuropraxia, vascular compromise from placement over a nerve or vessel, scar widening
- **Infection**: consider antibiotic trial, drainage, and irrigation before removing implant
- **Extrusion and Leakage**: may not necessarily require removal, may provide antibiotics and continue process
- **Bone Resorption**: from placement of expander near bone
- **Hematoma or Skin Necrosis:** treat with local wound care (aspiration, deflation, or debridement)

# FACIAL RECONSTRUCTION TECHNIQUES

## Eyelid Reconstruction

### Structural Support and Anatomy

- eyelid serves critical functional and aesthetic role
- support is key to reconstruction and avoiding malposition, ectropion, contracture
- Horizontal Support (strongest support system)
  1. **Medial Canthal Tendon**: three attachments are the maxillary bone (anterior), lacrimal sac (superior), and posterior lacrimal crest (Horner's muscle, pretarsal orbicularis)

2. **Lateral Canthal Tendon**: dense fibrous insertion from upper and lower tarsal plates, continuous with levator aponeurosis superiorly, inserts 7 mm vertical dimension
- Vertical Support
  1. **Levator Aponeurosis**: upper
  2. **Lower Lid Retractors**: lower
- Lamellae (Layers)
  1. **Anterior**: skin and orbicularis
  2. **Middle**: orbital septum
  3. **Posterior**: eyelid retractors/elevators, tarsal plates, conjunctiva
- Upper Eyelid: margin lies 3–4 mm above center of pupil, covers superior limbus usually (8–12 mm above lower lid), upper eyelid crease 6–12 mm above lash (less or nonexistent in Asians), maintaining mobility most important for upper eyelid reconstruction
- Lower Eyelid: usually lies at inferior limbus, lower eyelid crease 3–5 mm below margin

## Reconstruction Techniques

- defects <25% of width can be closed primarily
- **Lateral or Medial Cantholysis**: provides laxity for closure ≤50%
- **Tenzel Semicircular Advancement Flap**: used for defects ≤75% (with cantholysis)
- **Hughes Tarsoconjunctival Flap**: can be raised from posterior lamella of upper lid, transposed to recreate posterior lamella of lower lid (preserve 4 mm of inferior tarsal border), covered with a local flap to reconstruct anterior lamella, divided 2–6 weeks later

# Auricular Reconstruction

## Reconstruction Principles

- *NOTE: for total auricular reconstruction and microtia repair, see* pp. 611–613
- auricular reconstruction poses one of the most difficult challenges in reconstructive surgery because of multiple concavities and convexities of the cartilage framework, which are enveloped anteriorly by a very thin, tightly adherent skin envelope (posteriorly skin is mobile over a subcutaneous fat layer)
- all reconstructive efforts must preserve size, location, orientation, and anatomic landmarks of the auricle
- large defects may deform ear if left to heal by secondary intention
- primary goal for reconstruction is achieving the general shape of a normal auricle and preservation of the EAC

- <15% height difference between ears not appreciated
- position and height are secondary considerations
- a useful way to approach auricular reconstruction is by classification based on region of the defect

## Reconstruction Techniques Based on Region

### Conchal Bowl

- reconstruction typically can be successful by providing adequate skin coverage alone
- as long as peripheral auricular cartilage framework is intact, an absence of a conchal bowl cartilage is relatively inconsequential (no cosmetic deformity results) and can be left to heal by secondary intention
- FTSG can work well in resurfacing defects in this region as long as perichondrium is intact (resect cartilage and use posterior perichondrium if necessary)
- if more substantial amount of tissue is required for resurfacing and bulk, donor sites from the postauricular and retromastoid regions can be used
- **Postauricular/Retroauricular Skin Flaps**: utilizes a postauricular pedicled flap tunneled through the cartilage with a second-stage division 1 month later
- **Postauricular Myocutaneous Flaps**: single-stage procedure utilizes a postauricular pedicled myocutaneous flap that is transposed to the anterior surface with primary closure of the donor defect

### Helical Root/Rim

- ~50% of auricular skin cancers
- defects in the helical root can be reconstructed with a superiorly based preauricular flap with or without the introduction of cartilage to replace the missing tissue
- if defect >25% of rim, can be reconstructed from composite graft from contralateral ear
- wedge resection for <15% of height (~20 mm), **star-shaped** wedge excision avoids cupping
- **Rotational Flap**: utilizes the adjacent portion of the helix (cartilage and skin) with primary closure of donor defect, may be considered for smaller defects
- **Tubed Flaps**: 3 stage procedure using tubed skin constructed from the adjacent postauricular region; <u>Stage 1</u>: raise flap (0.5 cm longer than defect) and approximate edges creating a tube with superior and inferior pedicles; <u>Stage 2</u>: divide superior pedicle and attach to defect; <u>Stage 3</u>: divide inferior pedicle and attach to defect

## Upper Third of the Ear

- includes region superior to the upper portion of the concha cymba
- often needs cartilage graft (contralateral ear, nasal, or rib origin) for structural support
- simple skin grafts or healing by secondary intention considered for small defects
- postauricular and mastoid skin are convenient and suitable donor sites for reconstruction because they are thin and usually nonhair bearing
- may use temporoparietal fascia (based on superficial temporal vessels, tunneled under skin) to cover cartilage with STSG
- **Helical Chondrocutaneous Advancement Flap**: for small marginal defects, advances a chondrocutaneous flap by excising a wedge of antihelix and scaphoid fossa and advancing mobilized segment
- **Conchal Chondrocutaneous Rotation Flap**: utilizes a composite graft pedicled from the concha for larger defects, skin graft used to repair donor defect

## Middle Third of the Ear

- main consideration is reestablishing the appropriate auricular contour
- postauricular and mastoid tissue advancement flaps are useful
- interpositioned cartilaginous grafts may be required for larger defects
- a full-thickness composite graft with replacement of both skin layers, as well as the intervening cartilage structure, can be used to restore appropriate helical architecture and contour
- **Postauricular Turnover Flap**: utilizes a pedicled flap with the base at the defect border and extended to the posterior surface of the ear and the postauricular skin, flap is redraped over a cartilage graft, skin graft used to repair postauricular donor defect
- **Free Transfer Composite Graft from Opposite Ear**: transfers composite skin and cartilage, half the size of the defect, from the mirrored region of the opposite ear with primary closure

## Lower Third of the Ear and Lobule

- predominant tissue in this area is skin and subcutaneous fatty tissue, can be closed primarily if small but never use STSG alone (contracture)
- local tissue along with or without contralateral auricular cartilage (to prevent contracture) can be used to recreate the normal lobule architecture (auriculomastoid flap, should be 30% larger to account for contracture)

### Preauricular Tissue

- defects can be reconstructed with recruitment and mobilization of cervical facial skin
- when the defect involves the preauricular temporal hair, reconstruction can be performed using a hair-bearing scalp flap recruited from the postauricular region

# Nasal Reconstruction

## Reconstruction Principles

- <u>Aesthetic Subunits</u>: dorsum, sidewall (paired), tip, ala (paired), columella, soft triangle (paired)
- if >50% of subunit involved, consider replacing the entire subunit versus only the defect
- plan reconstruction of three distinct layers (skin, structural support, and inner mucosa)
- immobility of skin in the lower nose limits the use of primary closure (risk of rotating the nasal tip or distorting the alae)
- soft tissue defects in areas of concavity heal well through secondary intention

## Reconstruction Techniques

1. examine condition of skin, general nutrition, general medical condition, smoking history
2. examine location and extent of missing subunits and external skin (ie, thick versus thin, concave versus convex)
3. plan superficial defect donor sites
   - <u>Small Thick-Skinned Regions (<1.5 cm)</u>: bilobed local flap, nasalis myocutaneous flap
   - <u>Large Thick-Skinned Regions (>1.5 cm)</u>: consider local pedicled flaps (*see following*)
   - <u>Thin-Skinned Regions</u>: consider FTSG (eg, preauricular, postauricular, or supraclavicular donor sites)
4. address bone and cartilage replacements
   - <u>Lateral Support</u>: consider septal and conchal cartilage or helical rim free grafts, septal hinge flap (middle 1/3)
   - <u>Midline Support</u>: dorsal onlay grafts using cartilage, cantilever bone graft (attached to nasal radix to tip of nose), chondromucosal (composite) septal flaps, or costal-chondral grafts
5. address nasal lining
   - donor sites from inferior turbinates and nasal septum (lower and middle thirds)

- pericranial flap can be used for nasal mucosa lining (in conjunction with forehead flap)
- septal hinge flaps middle third
- bipedicled flap for lower third
- STSG or FTSG (vascularized recipient site)

### Regional Pedicled Flaps for Nasal Reconstruction

- **Sliding Nasal Dorsal Flap (Modified Reiger)**: single-stage V–Y advancement glabellar flap continuous with nasal dorsal skin, useful for midnasal and nasal tip wounds, nasal scars tend to be more visible (requires back cut)
- **Direct Cheek Advancement and Rotational Flaps**: capable of closing large lateral nasal defects, major disadvantage is violation of principle of segmental facial composition

#### Nasolabial Flap

- based on blood supply from facial artery
- transfer from cheek tissue lateral to melolabial crease (may need anchoring sutures to recreate nasolabial fold)
- <u>Advantages</u>: abundant mobile skin, scar may be hidden within melolabial crease
- <u>Disadvantages</u>: may result in some facial asymmetry (flattening), pincushioning, tip edema
- **Superiorly Based Design**: for defects of the lower 2/3 of the nose (lateral nasal wall, nasal ala), allows for one-stage reconstruction
- **Inferiorly Based Design**: for defects of upper lip, nasal sill, and columella
- **Island Pedicled Flap**: for whole subunit alar surface replacements

#### Paramedian Forehead Flap

- <u>Advantages</u>: reliable, good color and texture match, reliable blood supply, single pedicle allows for rotation
- <u>Disadvantages</u>: long vertical forehead scar, two stages required, length limited by supraorbital rim and anterior hairline, interferes with eyeglasses (for 2–3 weeks)
- <u>Arterial Supply</u>: supratrochlear artery (axial pattern) and subdermal plexus feeds random component
- <u>Common Uses</u>: large full-thickness defects of the lower 2/3 of the nose

# Lip Reconstruction

## Introduction

- <u>Goals</u>: oral competence, prevent microstomia, preserve sensation, speech, cosmesis
- bony and dental defects should be addressed first to allow for favorable projection of the lip
- proper soft tissue contour of the lip is achieved with precise apposition of the dermal scroll (vermilion cutaneous border) and layered closure of skin, muscle, and mucosa

## Anatomy

- <u>Aesthetic Subunits</u>: two upper (lateral, philtral), one lower
- <u>Landmarks</u>: philtral columns, Cupid's bow, tubercle, white roll, red line (dry versus wet vermilion)
- <u>Sphincter</u>: orbicularis oris
- the modiolus is the common attachment of the muscles of facial expression (lateral to oral commissure)
- <u>Upward Movement</u>: levators (anguli oris, labii superioris, LSAN) and zygomaticus major/minor
- <u>Downward Movement</u>: depressors (anguli oris, labii inferioris) and platysma
- <u>Lateral Movement</u>: risorius
- <u>Lip Protrusion</u>: mentalis (lower lip) and orbicularis oris
- <u>Lymphatics</u>: both upper and lower to submental/submandibular nodes; upper does not cross midline, lower does; upper also to preauricular and infraparotid nodes

## Minor (<1/3 Lip) Defect Reconstruction

- analyze the size (percent total), depth (partial versus full thickness), and commissure involvement
- for volume deficit may use dermal-fat graft
- for vermilion defect may use axial or V–Y advancement, or lip-switch procedures
- **Vermilion Flap**: axial pattern orbicularis oris flap based on the labial artery
- **Labial Mucosal Advancement Flap**: indicated after shave excisions (vermilionectomy)
- **Primary Closure**: indicated with full-thickness defects, may consider V or M-plasty excision of lower lip, generally achieved without distortion for upper lip defects ≤1/4 or lower lip defects ≤1/3

## Intermediate (1/2–2/3 Lip) Defect Reconstruction

- for vermilion defects >50%, perform 2-stage tongue flap or buccal mucosa advancement

### Gillies Fan Flap (Figure 9–7)

- orbicularis oris myocutaneous flap based on labial vessels, unilateral advancement
- <u>Advantages</u>: allows for one-stage repair, more tissue than cross-lip flaps, less microstomia
- <u>Disadvantages</u>: delayed muscle function and sensation may occur, may have oral incompetence

### Karapandzik Labioplasty (Figure 9–8)

- modifies the Gillies fan flap, bilateral advancement (melolabial creases are lateral extent), good for lower lip but can also be used for upper lip
- <u>Advantages</u>: excellent oral competence, can recruit cheek tissue
- <u>Disadvantages</u>: unsightly circumoral scar, risk of microstomia, blunting of oral commissure, tedious dissection of neurovascular bundle between orbicularis oris and underlying facial musculature

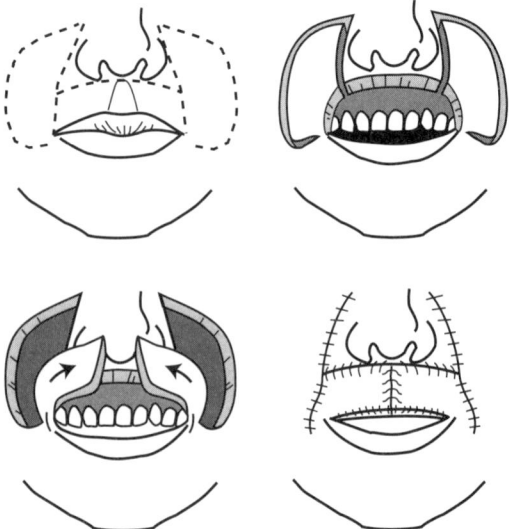

**FIGURE 9–7.** Gillies fan flap is based on an inferior medial pedicle constructed from full-thickness cheek flaps.

### *Abbe-Estlander Flap* (Figure 9–9)

- transfers full-thickness segment of lip to opposing lip
- single (lateral) or two-stage procedure for medial defects (separation of flap pedicle and commissuroplasty completed later for the Abbe flap), requires an intact labial artery.
- height of flap = height of defect, width of flap = 1/2 width of defect
- <u>Advantages:</u> may be used for commissure defects (Estlander), good color match
- <u>Disadvantages</u>: needs second stage, tissue is denervated (delayed return of sensation, may be reinnervated), reduces stomal size, liquid diet required if pedicle used

## Major (>2/3 Lip) Defect Reconstruction

- **Bernard-Burow Flap**: advancement flap from cheek, indicated for midline lower lip defects (Webster modification for upper lip defects)
- **Nasolabial Flaps**: inferiorly designed, indicated for lateral defects, bilateral nasolabial flaps required for defects >80%
- **Johanson Technique**: may be used to close defects from <1 cm to entire lip, bilateral lateral advancement flaps with stepwise

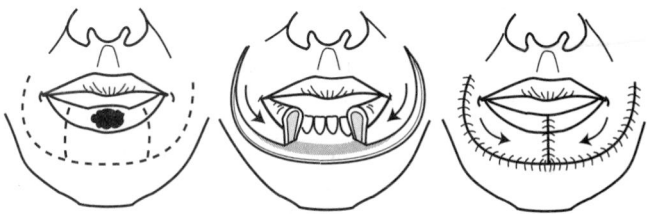

**FIGURE 9–8.** Karapandzik labioplasty requires circumoral incisions for closure of defects involving greater than 1/2 of the lip.

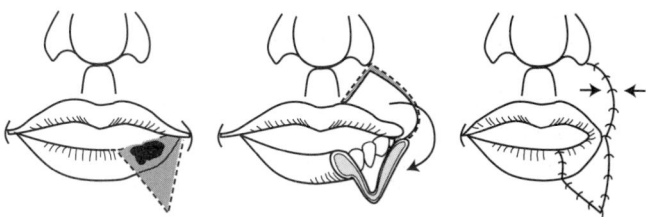

**FIGURE 9–9.** Abbe-Estlander flap allows for repairs of defects involving the commissure of the lip.

inferolateral skin incisions, preserves neuromuscular bundle and oral commissure, however, loses sensation to the lip
- **Total Reconstruction Techniques**: radial forearm free flap, fascial sling with mucosal advancement flap (palmaris longus tendon graft to modiolus), may also consider cutaneous and myocutaneous flaps

# Cheek Reconstruction

## Introduction and Anatomy

- largest subunit of face
- place incisions at boundaries to hide scar if possible (superior at infraorbital rim and zygomatic arch; medial at nasofacial junction, nasolabial fold, and labiomandibular crease; inferior at border of mandible; lateral at preauricular crease)
- retaining ligaments provide support and fix soft tissue to bony skeleton (orbicularis, zygomatic, upper masseteric, and mandibular)
- malar fat pad provides convex contour
- <u>Vascular Supply</u>: from facial artery → angular artery and anastomosis with infraorbital artery; rich subdermal plexus is basis for local flaps

## Reconstruction Techniques

- <u>Primary Closure</u>: can be ideal, undermine, convert defect to elliptical shape (use RSTLs)
- <u>Secondary Intention</u>: reserved for small defects on concave surfaces due to risk of contracture and distortion
- <u>Skin Grafts</u>: useful for small defects (harvest from scalp or supraclavicular area), FTSG better cosmesis, allow 1–2 weeks granulation for STSG for better contour
- <u>Local Flaps</u>: place incisions at borders of subunits, plan flap base to account for tension
  1. medial defect (posterior or inferior base)
  2. lateral defect (inferior or anterior base)
  3. elevate in sub-SMAS plane lateral to zygomaticus major muscle to avoid facial nerve
  4. plan infraorbital incisions to avoid ectropion
  5. V–Y island advancement flap → melolabial/perialar area (superficial to SMAS)
- <u>Regional or Free Flaps</u>: if large volume of composite tissue needed
- <u>Reconstructive Principles Based on Subunits</u>
  1. **Lateral**: adherent to SMAS over parotid, close primarily <1 cm only
  2. **Superior** (Zygomatic): consider M-plasty to avoid tension on lateral canthus

3. **Medial**: can close larger areas primarily, consider V–Y advancement
4. **Inferior (Buccal)**: adjust bites of suture to recreate lateral mound of melolabial fold

# Mandibular Reconstruction

## Introduction

- immediate reconstruction prevents soft tissue contraction (compromising function and cosmesis) and mandibular segment displacement from muscle vector forces
- in general, the more anterior the defect the greater the functional and cosmetic morbidity and the more difficult to reconstruct; defects >5 cm have 10-fold increase in complications
- high, limited, posterior defects may compensate well without reconstruction (less loading requirements); however, may have chin deviation, tongue elevation
- a proximal segment that contains only a coronoid process, condyle, and portion of the ramus may benefit from a coronoidectomy to avoid upward and medial displacement from vector force of the temporalis and pterygoid muscles
- <u>Goals of Mandibular Reconstruction</u>: mandible contour restoration, mastication, speech, sensation of lower lip and oral cavity, restoration of dentition

## Reconstruction Techniques

### Bone Grafting

- <u>Indications</u>: limited defects <6 cm (failure 75% if >6 cm)
- <u>Advantages</u>: tolerates higher level of stress and strain than other nonvascularized neomandibles
- <u>Disadvantages</u>: requires jaw immobilization for weeks or months; high rate of infection, resorption, and exposure; contraindicated with radiation therapy or anterior defects
- <u>Donor Sites</u>: rib, iliac crest

### Osseous Free Flap

- <u>Indications</u>: reliable method for restoration of the mandible
- <u>Advantages</u>: may allow for later placement of osseointegrated dental implants, excellent functional restoration, can reconstruct radiated tissue

- Disadvantages: requires microsurgical expertise and specialized instrumentation (*see* Microvascular Free Flaps for general advantages and disadvantages of each composite free flap transfer)
- Common Types: fibula, iliac crest, radial forearm (does not allow implants), scapula

### *Osseous Regional Pedicled Flap*

- Indications: limited posterior mandibular defects
- Advantages: provides soft tissue bulk for mandibular contour, may resist some muscle force of remaining mandibular segment, quick
- Disadvantages: does not allow osseointegrated implants, poor functional outcome, high rate of bone necrosis, minimal bone volume
- Common Types: pectoralis major (with rib), trapezius (with spine of scapula), latissimus dorsi (with rib), deltopectoral, sternocleidomastoid (with clavicle), temporalis (with calvarial bone), platysma (intraoral coverage)

### *Soft Tissue Regional Pedicled Flap with Reconstruction Plate*

- Indications: limited defects (<5 cm), rapid repairs (comorbidities), elderly (less opportunity for extrusion)
- Advantages: quick, avoids donor defect (eg, in setting of poor wound healing such as cancer)
- Disadvantages: poor oral functioning, high rate of extrusion and fractures (especially with defects >5 cm and anterior defects), failures occur within 18 months (extrusion or plate failure)
- Common Types: pectoralis major, trapezius, latissimus dorsi

# FACIAL AESTHETIC SURGERY
## Facial Analysis

### Facial Anatomic Landmarks

- **Trichion**: midline at hairline
- **Glabella**: prominence in midsagittal plane, superior to root of nose
- **Nasion**: **n**asofrontal suture, superior to sellion
- **Sellion**: **s**oft tissue, deepest point of the nasofrontal angle
- **Radix**: root of the nose (contains the sellion and nasion)
- **Rhinion**: cartilaginous–bony junction (**thinnest skin of nose**)
- **Supratip Break**: just cephalic to tip-defining point
- **Tip-Defining Point**: 2 points representing the highest point of the crural arch (medial cephalic portion of the lateral crura)

- **Infratip Lobule**: portion of lobule inferior to the tip-defining point, superior to nostril
- **Infratip Break**: junction of the columella and lobule
- **Alar Crease**: most posterior portion of nose
- **Stomion**: embouchure of lips
- **Pogonion**: anterior-most border of chin
- **Menton**: inferior-most border of chin
- **Cervical Point**: menton and neck intersection
- **Tragion**: supratragal notch of ear

## General Facial Assessment

- <u>Shape</u>: oval, round, or triangular
- **Facial Thirds**: facial **height** divided into three equally spaced segments demarcated by trichion, glabella, subnasale, menton
- **Lower Facial Thirds**: lower third further divided into 1/3 (subnasale → stomion) and 2/3 (stomion → menton)
- **Facial Fifths**: facial **width** divided into 5 equally spaced segments demarcated by lateral auricle, lateral canthus, medial canthus, medial canthus, lateral canthus, lateral auricle

## Effects of Aging on the Face

- <u>Skin</u>: thinned epidermis, decreased subcutaneous fat, dermis loses elastic fragments (elastosis), decreased melanocytes and Langerhans cells, decrease in type I (mature) collagen and increase in type III (immature) collagen, reduced vascular supply (especially in smokers)
- <u>Skeletal</u>: thinned skull and mandible (especially if edentulous) resulting in excess skin envelope, laryngeal skeleton and hyoid descends
- <u>Forehead Midface</u>: weakened supportive matrix between SMAS (superficial muscular aponeurotic system) (*see* p. 494) and overlying fat pad results in deepened melolabial crease, hypotonic facial muscles result in festooning (undulating) and facial rhytids
- <u>Neck</u>: jowling, chin ptosis, ptotic submandibular glands, platysma banding from loss of tone resulting in loss of cervicomental angle

## Poor Candidates for Cosmetic Facial Plastic Surgery

- unrealistic expectations
- multiple physician visits
- psychiatric instability (eg, depression, anxiety)
- smokers have >12× increased risk of skin sloughing and scarring

## Preoperative Photography

- **Frankfort Horizontal**: horizontal line from superior border of EAC (or superior tragus) to infraorbital rim, reference plane used for photos and analysis
- <u>Recommended Photographic Settings</u>: slower speeds (ISO-equivalent ≤ 100), focal length 90–105 mm, medium blue background most common, two light sources/diffused flashes to reduce shadowing effects
- <u>Rhinoplasty Views</u>: left and right lateral, 3/4 oblique, lateral with smile, frontal, and base
- <u>Blepharoplasty, Rhytidoplasty, and Forehead/Brow Views</u>: full frontal face, lateral, 3/4 oblique, close-up eyelids (straight and upward gaze, eyes closed), and facial animation (smiling, raising eyebrows)

# RHINOPLASTY

## Surgical Nasal Anatomy

### Nasal Thirds

- <u>Upper Third</u>: nasal bones, skin
- <u>Middle Third</u>: upper lateral cartilages, septum, skin (thinnest)
- <u>Lower Third</u>: lower lateral cartilages, septum

### Nasal Tip Support

*Major Tip Support*

- direction, strength, and resiliency of **lower lateral (alar) cartilage**
- **medial crura** attachment to the inferior septal angle
- attachment of the **lower and upper lateral cartilage (scroll)**

*Minor Tip Support*

- interdomal ligament between lower lateral cartilage
- sesamoid complex
- skin/soft-tissue envelope (SSTE; includes overlying skin/muscle and its attachment to the alar cartilage)
- anterior nasal spine
- cartilaginous septal dorsum
- membranous septum

## Anatomic Terms

- **Nasal Length**: distance from nasofrontal angle to tip-defining point of domes, determined mainly from the length, width, and direction of the lateral crura
- **Scroll**: continuous roll of the cephalic margin of the lateral crus that overlies the upper lateral cartilage (may be trimmed to reduced bulbousness of the tip)
- **Keystone Area**: region of overlap of the upper lateral cartilage by nasal bones
- **Angle**: junction of the medial and lateral cartilage (narrowest portion of alar cartilage)
- **Dome**: concavity formed by the inner surface of most superior extent of the lateral crus (lateral to angle)
- **Sill**: continuation of alar margin toward base of columella

# Initial Consultation and Analysis

## Introduction

- <u>History</u>: nasal trauma, cocaine, smoking, granulomatous disease, sinusitis, nasal obstruction, previous surgery, bleeding disorders
- assess motivational factors for surgery
- preoperative photography (*see previous*)
- **Non-Caucasian Nose**: usually address nasal tip projection, nasolabial angle, dorsal hump, and alar base; risk of overprojected look, limited by maximum projection

## Internal Nose

- evaluate functional nasal airway (resistance, nasal valve)
- assess for septal deflection/deformities and turbinate hypertrophy
- *see also* pp. 19–20 for nasal valve and septum evaluation

## External Nose

### Skin

- ideal skin is not too thick or thin, minimal sebaceous glands
- <u>Thicker Skin</u>: more postoperative edema, more subcutaneous scarring (increased risk of a "polly beak" deformity)
- <u>Thinner Skin</u>: reveals minor irregularities

### Profiles

- **Nasofrontal Angle**: angle between external nose and forehead, ~**120°** (approximately at the level of the upper eyelid folds)

- **Columellar–Labial Angle:** male ~90–105°, female ~95–110°
- **Dorsal Hump:** may be straight, slight hump (males), slight scoop (females), suggestion of dorsal prominence at rhinion
- **Dorsal Height:** rule of **facial thirds**, nasion to subnasale = middle 1/3 of facial length (*see previous*)
- **Dorsal Width:** rule of **facial fifths**, nasal width = 1/5 facial width = intercanthal distance (*see previous*)
- **Fronto-Naso-Orbital Line:** frontal view should reveal a smooth line from eyebrows along the lateral edge of the dorsum then diverging slightly at the tip

### Nasal Tip

- **Double Break**: characterizes a refined nasal tip, **supratip break** (separates dorsum from lobule) located 1–3 mm above the tip-defining point and an **infratip break** between the infratip lobule and columella
- **Light Reflex**: two symmetric reflections defined by the tip-defining points (5–6 mm apart)
- **Tip-Defining Point**: should lie 2.8 mm anterior to line connecting nasofrontal angle to the upper lip vermilion–cutaneous junction
- **Tip Rotation**: determined by **columellar–labial angle**
- **Tip Projection**: distance between facial plane and tip of the nose
- **3:4:5 rule = columella:base:dorsum**
- **Tip Recoil**: tip of nose is depressed and degree of resistance is assessed, adequate recoil required for manipulation of lower lateral cartilage
- have patient smile in profile to see effect/significance of depressor septi during smile, when well-developed draws nasal tip downward when smiling widely

### Lobule and Columella

- alar rim should arch 2–3 mm above columella (**columellar show**)
- alar–columellar margin forms a "gull in flight" outline
- basal view should reveal an isosceles triangle
- lobular height should be 1/3 of total height on basal view

## Chin

- chin should align with a vertical line dropped from the vermilion border of the lower lip (in women may be slightly behind this line)
- *see* p. 501

# Surgical Techniques

## Introductory Points

- *NOTE:* for functional septorhinoplasty, *see also* p. 20
- minimize reduction of upper lateral cartilage to maintain an adequate nasal valve
- avoid transection of nasal dome to maintain alar spring
- preserve nasal tip support, especially caudal septal cartilage
- always err on the side of conservation of tissue rather than resection
- tip rhinoplasty generally should be performed first to determine nasal profile (to determine amount of hump to remove)

## Incisions

- **Intercartilaginous**: disrupts attachment of lower and upper lateral cartilage, scarring may result in nasal obstruction since incision involves nasal valve
- **Marginal**: follows caudal margin of the lower lateral cartilage, may be combined with intercartilaginous incisions to form a bipedicle flap (intact strip)
- **Trans/Intracartilaginous**: splits lower lateral cartilage, lessens risk of nasal obstruction
- **Transcolumellar**: used for open rhinoplasty

## Approaches

### Nondelivery Approach

- <u>Types</u>
  1. **Cartilage Splitting (Trans/Intracartilaginous):** for minimal refinement of nasal tip
  2. **Retrograde Approach:** for minimal refinement of nasal tip with thick skin, uses an intercartilaginous incision
- <u>Advantages</u>: no major tip support affected, preserves intact caudal rim, one incision, no external scar, reduced surgical trauma and edema
- <u>Disadvantages</u>: minimal exposure of lower lateral cartilage, limited to conservative tip work, risk of asymmetric incisions

### Delivery Approach

- combines intercartilaginous and marginal incisions
- allows delivery of lower lateral cartilage as a bilateral pedicled chondrocutaneous flap

- <u>Advantages</u>: visualize entire lower lateral cartilage, good access to tip and nasal dome, no external scar
- <u>Disadvantages</u>: compromises major support by removing the attachment of the alar cartilage and the upper lateral cartilage, causes more edema (postoperative distortion), requires 2 incisions

### *Open (External) Rhinoplasty*

- combines marginal and transcolumellar incisions
- <u>Indications</u>: extensive tip work, revisions, non-Caucasians, cleft lip, crooked nose, major reconstructions, academic teaching
- <u>Advantages</u>: affords maximal nondistorted exposure, allows accurate placement and direct suture ability for grafting, does not disrupt major tip support mechanisms
- <u>Disadvantages</u>: compromises one minor support by separating the skin/soft tissue envelope (SSTE) from the lateral cartilage, external scar, more postoperative edema, sensory tip disturbances

## Nasal Tip Projection and Rotation

- **Nasal Tripod Model**: predicts changes in nasal length, tip projection, and tip rotation in relation to changes in the 3 legs (legs of the tripod include the **conjoined medial crura** and the **two lateral crura**)
- should maintain a minimum of 6–8 mm of alar cartilage for support

### *Tip Correction Methods*

#### Complete Strip Technique

- reduces volume of the cephalic margin of the lower lateral cartilage leaving the caudal margin intact from the foot of the medial crus to the piriform aperture
- results in a slight cephalic rotation, accentuates domes, and decreases the convexity of the lower lateral cartilage
- <u>Advantages</u>: better preserves tip projection (intact medial crus), allows for more symmetric healing, resists tip retrodisplacement
- <u>Disadvantages</u>: flaring of nostrils may result from any tip rotation

#### Interrupted Strip Technique

- "interrupts" the lower lateral cartilage
- indicated for tips requiring maximal rotation, overprojected tips from excessively large alar cartilage, wide boxy tips

- contraindicated in thin-skinned patients (subtle irregularities cannot be camouflaged)
- **Rim Strip**: interrupts anterior border of lower lateral cartilage lateral to dome and proximal to piriform (loss of tip support), provides maximal tip rotation
- **Lateral Crural Flap**: similar to rim strip procedure, however, leaves triangular portion of lateral crura at piriform to prevent alar margin retraction and pinching, limits supra-alar definition
- **Dome Division**: complete interruption of lower lateral cartilage near dome, corrects asymmetric tips, allows increased or decreased projection, and narrowing of tip

## Methods to Increase Tip Projection

- suture the medial crura together (transdomal or interdomal sutures)
- may increase cephalic rotation
- permanent septocolumellar suture
- **Supradomal Graft or Shield Graft**: adds 1–2 mm additional projection
- **Columellar Strut**: placed between medial crura (does more to maintain projection than actually increase projection)
- **Plumping Grafts**: placed at base of columella, changes the columellar–labial angle with an illusion of increased projection

## Methods to Decrease Tip Projection (Retrodisplacement Techniques)

- complete transfixion of caudal septum
- full-thickness excision and suture of segments of the lateral and/or medial crura
- release lower lateral cartilage attachments to septum and scroll and reposition cartilages
- free medial and lateral crura, incise and overlap

## Methods to Increase Tip Rotation

- reduce caudal septum edge
- shorten lateral crura (must avoid excessive reduction to prevent valve collapse)
- augment the premaxilla
- removal of dorsal hump, augmenting the columellar–labial angle, and rotating the infratip lobule causes an apparent increase in tip rotation
- augment medial crura (ie, tripod concept)
- *see also* Tip Correction Methods *previous*

### *Methods to Decrease Tip Rotation*

- excise caudal septum near spine and shorten medial crura
- dorsum augmentation causes an apparent decrease in tip rotation
- consider an infratip button graft for a retruse infratip lobule

## Nasal Hump

- most nasal hump deformity is caused from the cartilaginous dorsum
- nasal skin is thinnest at middorsum (rhinion), therefore it must create a slight middorsal hump to avoid saddle-nose deformity
- use a sharp downbiting rasp to reduce hump, take care not to avulse upper lateral cartilage from the nasal bones
- an illusion of increased nasal length is achieved by leaving a small dorsal hump
- Dorsal Augmentation Graft Materials
  1. **Septal Cartilage**: does not resorb, ample supply, low infection rate
  2. **Conchal Cartilage**: more difficult to sculpt
  3. **Split Calvarium**: may be too rigid
  4. **Costal Cartilage**: may warp
  5. **Allografts**

## Medial and Lateral Osteotomies

- osteotomies reduce open roof defects caused by removal of a nasal hump, straighten a crooked nose, and flatten convex nasal bones
- **Medial Osteotomy**: completed first, frees nasal bones from perpendicular plate of ethmoid
- **Lateral Osteotomy**: low, curved (low to high) cut (along nasomaxillary groove), leaves a triangular wedge at piriform ledge superior to level of inferior turbinate to protect airway
- **Intermediate Osteotomies**: may be utilized to correct the deviated nose with one sidewall longer than the other or to straighten an excessively wide or convex nasal bone
- damage to the lacrimal crest is rare
- to avoid nasal obstruction, for short nasal bones or when dorsal hump reduction is >3 mm consider **spreader grafts** (placed between the septum and upper lateral cartilage), osteotomies may considerably narrow the nasal valve

## Postoperative Care

- **Nasal Splints**: remove after 1 week
- **Intranasal Packing**: remove after 1–2 days

- **Septal Splints:** help prevent synechiae, remove after 1 week
- avoid strenuous activity
- cold packs to reduce swelling
- oral antibiotics while nasal packing in place

## Correction of the Crooked Nose

- **Septoplasty:** may necessitate swinging door (releasing caudal septum to other side of maxillary crest) or extracorporeal septoplasty
- <u>Upper Third</u>: osteotomies
- <u>Middle Third</u>: spreader grafts, onlay camouflage grafts
- <u>Lower Third</u>: septoplasty, reshaping of lower lateral cartilages, camouflage grafting

# Revision Rhinoplasty and Complications

## Overview

- **10–15%** of rhinoplasties require revision work
- typically wait 1 year for revision.
- <u>Immediate and Short-Term Postoperative Complications</u>: epistaxis, infection, septal perforation, septal hematoma, skin necrosis, transient epiphora

## Late Postoperative Defects and Complications

### Polly Beak Deformity

- supratip prominence resulting in a convexity of the lower 2/3 of nasal dorsum
- <u>Types</u>: soft tissue versus cartilaginous defects
- <u>Causes</u>
  1. excess resection of nasal dorsum resulting in increased dead space and soft tissue scarring resulting in a paradoxic polly beak deformity
  2. inadequate removal of cartilaginous dorsum
  3. loss of nasal tip support
  4. insufficient lowering of dorsal septal borders
  5. shortened columella
  6. excessive excision of domes of alar cartilage
- <u>Management Techniques</u>
  1. in first 2–3 months, inject steroid with supratip taping, this can help if deformity is due to dead space and soft tissue scarring
  2. after healed and with residual scar, resect prominent tissue or scar for soft-tissue deformities versus resect excess cartilaginous

dorsum; other options include grafting dorsum, augmenting lower lateral cartilage, and columellar struts to maintain desired projection and rotation

### Retracted and Notched Ala

- notched or retracted intranasal tip
- <u>Causes</u>: excess lower lateral cartilage excision, excess vestibular skin removal (soft triangle), improper closure of a marginal incision
- <u>Rx</u>: for minimal retraction/notching, cartilage graft placed as either an alar batten, lateral crural strut graft, or alar rim graft; for significant retraction, composite graft from ear

### Columellar Defects

- **Retracted Columella**: deficient columella show resulting in an acute nasolabial angle (<90°), caused by excessive resection at base of columella or caudal septum; <u>Rx</u>: plumping graft at columella base, premaxillary implant cartilage, composite graft if skin required
- **Hanging Columella**: caused by persistent overly convex medial crura or abnormally elongated caudal septum

### Saddling

- concavity of nasal dorsum from excess removal of nasal dorsum or an open roof deformity
- <u>Rx</u>: lateral osteomies to close open roof for mild deformities, dorsal implant or graft for more severe deformities

### Nasal Obstruction

- transient nasal obstruction should be expected from mucosal edema and crusting for 2–4 weeks
- **Persistent Septal Deformity**: preoperatively may not have been obstructing; <u>Rx</u>: revision septoplasty
- **Intranasal Synechia**: more common with concurrent turbinectomies; <u>Rx</u>: prevented by avoiding mucosal injuries and placement of septal splints, managed with lysis with Z-plasty, intralesional corticosteroids, septal splints, or mucosal flaps
- **Narrowing of the Nasal Vault**: may occur from overresection of caudal end of upper lateral cartilage or lower lateral crura (**nasal tip pinching**), overaggressive infracture of nasal bones, high intercartilaginous incisions; <u>Rx</u>: revision with placement of spreader grafts

### Tip Defects

- **Tip Ptosis**: caused by loss of tip support, unfavorable healing factors, uncorrected depressor septi, or false tip projection from surgical tip edema; <u>Rx</u>: reconstruct tip, address depressor septi
- **Bossae**: knoblike protuberances in the dome area caused by irregular scarring; <u>Rx</u>: add a small alar graft to opposite side or shave excision
- **Pinched Tip**: caused by excessive reduction of dome, failure to maintain intact rim strip, internal adhesions, or excision of vestibular skin

### Midnasal Asymmetry

- <u>Causes</u>: subluxation or asymmetric removal of upper lateral cartilage, deviated septum
- <u>Rx</u>: onlay graft, septoplasty

### Inverted V Deformity

- <u>Causes</u>: collapse of upper lateral cartilage grafts, which leaves demarcated visible edges of nasal bones; seen years after primary rhinoplasty due to lack of adequate bony narrowing, weakening of attachment of upper lateral cartilages to nasal bones, and/or lack of spreader graft placement
- <u>Rx</u>: revision rhinoplasty with placement of spreader grafts, possible osteotomies versus onlay grafts

# OTOPLASTY

## Introduction

### Initial Evaluation

- determine auriculocephalic angle (auricular protrusion from the skull normally **20–30°**) and distance of helical rim to mastoid skin (2–2.5 cm)
- evaluate slope of ear (normally ~20° from vertical or approximately the slope of the nasal dorsum)
- measure vertical height (normally ~6 cm)
- evaluate the auricular components and convolutions (helix, antihelix, scaphoid fossa, fossa triangularis, lobule)
- compare ear to opposite side
- evaluate for other associated defects (eg, branchial arch deformities, cleft palate, urogenital and cardiovascular malformations)
- prior to reconstruction consider CT of temporal bone (for microtia/ anotia) and audiologic evaluation

- preoperative photodocumentation
- <u>Common Syndromes with Auricular Malformations</u>: Treacher Collins, hemifacial microsomia, Goldenhar, Down

## Common Auricular Defects

- **Protruding Ear**: auriculocephalic angle >30°, caused by loss of formation of the antihelical fold or overgrowth or protrusion of the conchal cartilage
- **Cryptotia**: pocket ear deformity
- **Cup Ear Deformity**: constriction of the helix and scapha; <u>Rx</u>: requires unfurling of the helical rim by dividing the helical-scaphoid cartilage to allow for expansion followed by redraping of skin over the excess cartilage
- **Colobomata**: clefts
- **Lobule Deformities**
- **Microtia and Anotia** (*see* pp. 611–612)

## Surgical Techniques

### Correcting the Protruding Ear

- best age for reconstruction is at 5–6 years old when ear is at 85% of adult size and before the age of social stigmatization
- **Suture Techniques (Mustardé)**: mattress sutures placed along the scapha through a posterior incision to create an antihelical fold with resulting reduction of the auriculocephalic angle, does not address conchal bowl, simple technique
- **Cartilage Sculpting Techniques**: reshaping (scoring, thinning) or splitting of auricular cartilage to weaken the cartilage surface to create a convexity for the antihelical fold
- **Farrior Technique**: combination suture and cartilage sculpting techniques, removes wedges of cartilage from posterior surface to allow bending to supplement the mattress sutures (additionally may place a wedge of cartilage anteriorly to help form the antihelical fold)
- **Concha Setback Technique (Conchomastoid Suture Technique of Furnas)**: sutures the conchal bowl to the mastoid periosteum to reduce the auriculocephalic angle

### Complications

- similar to auricular reconstruction (hematomas, infection, *see* p. 613)
- **Telephone Ear Deformity**: "telephone" appearance (upper and lower poles of the auricle protrude on anterior view); may occur from over-

correcting the middle antihelix, improper placement of mattress sutures, inadequate skin or cartilage excision; <u>Rx</u>: revision with possible skin excision and suturing the root of the helix to the temporal fascia

- **Malposition and Reprotrusion**: varied causes including suture splitting, overcorrection, and undercorrection; <u>Rx</u>: revision

# BLEPHAROPLASTY

## Introduction

### Anatomy

- **Orbital Septum**: continuous with periosteum, houses orbital fat, barrier to both neoplastic and inflammatory invasion, upper eyelid septum fuses with **levator aponeurosis**, lower lid septum fuses with capsulopalpebral fascia
- **Medial Canthal Tendon**: constructed from medial heads of the pretarsal and preseptal muscles, attaches to the **lacrimal crest** (*see also* pp. 463–464)
- **Lateral Canthal Tendon**: constructed from lateral heads of the pretarsal and preseptal muscles, attaches inside **orbital tubercle of Whitnall**
- **Superior Palpebral Sulcus**: formed from insertion of **levator aponeurosis** to the lid skin
- **Whitnall's Ligament**: dense fibrous connective tissue that functions as a fulcrum for levator muscle
- **Lockwood's Ligament**: dense fibrous connective tissue that functions as a fulcrum for lower lid
- <u>Superior Tarsal Plate Height</u>: 8–9 mm
- <u>Inferior Tarsal Plate Height</u>: 4–5 mm
- <u>The East Asian Eye</u>: insertion of the levator aponeurosis may attach lower in the lid than in Caucasians resulting in a less developed superior palpebral sulcus (superior tarsal crease), the orbital fat tends to be more fibrous

### *Layers Above Eyelid Crease* (Figure 9–10)

1. skin (devoid of subcutaneous fat)
2. orbicularis oculi muscle (composed of orbital [outer, thicker], preseptal, and pretarsal [inner, thinner] bands)
3. orbital septum
4. orbital fat
5. levator aponeurosis
6. Müller's muscle (sympathetic smooth muscle)
7. tarsal portion

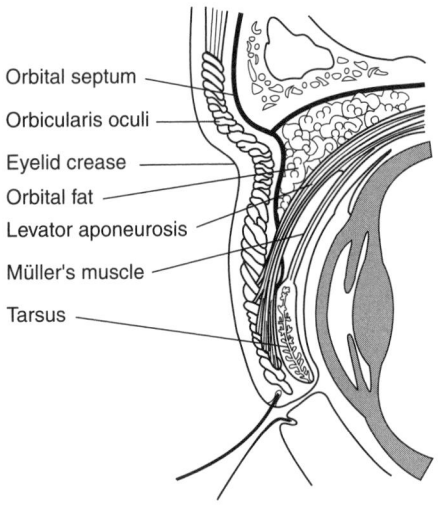

**FIGURE 9–10.** Cross-section of the layers of the upper eyelid.

### *Orbital Fat Compartments (lie beneath orbital septum)*

1. <u>Lower Medial</u>: lighter color, denser, separated by inferior oblique muscle
2. <u>Lower Central</u>: darker than medial compartment
3. <u>Lower Lateral</u>: separated by fascial barrier
4. <u>Upper Medial</u>: separated by superior oblique muscle
5. <u>Upper Central</u>: medial to lacrimal gland (which replaces most of the upper lateral compartment)

## Indications

- **Dermatochalasis**: acquired draping of excess skin over lids, usually from actinic damage, thins eyelid skin, allows for prolapse of orbital fat, progressive ptosis occurs with aging (not to be confused with blepharochalasis)
- **Blepharochalasis**: rare condition of unknown cause, may be familial, characterized by recurrent attacks of lid edema resulting in swelling and edema of the lids, progressive tissue breakdown, prolapse of the orbital fat (and possibly the lacrimal gland), and drooping of the lid
- **Pseudoherniation**: orbital fat protrudes through a lax orbital septum behind orbicularis muscle, baggy lids
- **Orbicularis Hypertrophy**: may be cause of residual bagginess, obvious with squinting
- **Blepharoptosis**: droopy eyelid caused by levator muscle malfunction

### Blepharoplasty Does Not Correct

- crows feet (lateral rhytids) caused by the orbicularis muscle insertion to skin; <u>Rx</u>: temporal lift, collagen injection, botulinum toxin injections, peels
- asymmetric brow or brow ptosis; <u>Rx</u>: requires a brow-lifting procedure
- malar or cheek pads (fluid); <u>Rx</u>: corrected with cheek implants or deep plane facelifts
- fine wrinkles and hyperpigmented lesions; <u>Rx</u>: consider a chemical peel or another resurfacing procedure

### Causes of False Pseudoherniation of Fat

- prominent orbital rim
- allergic edema
- lacrimal gland ptosis
- orbicularis oculi hypertrophy
- malar or cheek bags
- myxedema
- festooning (hammock-like bags in the lower eyelid from folds in the orbicularis oculi, must consider hypothyroidism)

## Evaluation

### History

- family history of baggy eyes, fluid retention, thyroid disorders, allergic dermatitis, ophthalmic history (corrective lenses, dry eyes, tearing), collagen vascular diseases, previous keloids, bleeding disorders
- assess motivational factors for surgery
- preoperative photography (*see* p. 476)

### Ophthalmic Evaluation

- check visual acuity (Snellen chart), visual field tests, motility, ocular tension, measure scleral show, proptosis, fundoscopic exam
- **Normal Bell's Phenomenon**: assesses adequate protection of the globe, evaluated by forcing the lids open and observing the upward rotation of the globe to protect the cornea
- **Schirmer's Test**: Schirmer strip (filter paper) is draped over the lower lid margin (lateral to the cornea), the distance between the leading edge of wetness and the lid is measured after 5 minutes (abnormal is <5 mm with topical anesthesia)

## Evaluate Brow and Upper Lid

- examine for brow ptosis (brow should be at orbital rim in males or just above orbital rim in women) if present patient is at risk of worsening ptosis with upper lid blepharoplasty (consider repositioning brow with brow lift procedures before blepharoplasty)
- the superior orbital sulcus (eyelid crease) should be <10 mm from lid margin and below bony margin of superior orbital rim (should also note symmetry)
- evaluate for fat herniation, skin redundancy, ptotic lacrimal gland, and muscle hypertrophy
- evaluate skin type, thin skin requires conservative resection to avoid a retracted or "hollow" look, thick skin results in an ill-defined superior orbital sulcus and requires considerable amount of fat and muscle excision
- determine presence and degree of ptosis by measuring the margin-reflex distance (MRD), the distance between the corneal light reflex and the upper lid margin (normally between 3–4.5 mm)
- access levator functioning by measuring the upper lid margin excursion in downward and upward gaze (normally >12 mm)
- evaluate for presence of **lagophthalmos** (incomplete closure of eye) and **lateral hooding**

## Evaluate Lower Lid

- the inferior orbital sulcus (eyelid crease) should be <5–6 mm from lid margin (a second crease may be located inferiorly corresponding to an area of tissue thickness)
- evaluate fat herniation (have patient look superiorly), skin redundancy, and muscle hypertrophy
- palpate inferior orbital rim, may imitate fat herniation
- **Lid Distraction Test (Snap Test)**: tests lateral lower lid laxity; outwardly displace the lower lid and observe for a normal snap, if >10 mm displacement or if lid settles slowly patient at risk of ectropion or scleral show, patient requires a lid-tightening procedure at the same time as the blepharoplasty
- **Lid Retraction Test**: tests lateral lower lid laxity; inferiorly displace the lower lid, if the puncta moves >3 mm it indicates a lax canthal tendon and suggests the need of a tendoplication to avoid ectropion or scleral show
- examine for skin crepe (fine wrinkles), festooning, malar bags, and lateral orbital rhytids (crow's feet), which cannot be corrected with blepharoplasty

# Surgical Techniques

## Brow Lift Procedures

- should be completed first
- *see* pp. 498–499

## Addressing the Upper Lid

- completed before addressing the lower lid
- mark estimated skin to be excised by bringing together redundant skin with forceps while patient is in an upright position (pinch technique), correct amount should begin to move the eyelashes upward but not move the lid margin, ideally lid should leave a slight (1–2 mm) lagophthalmos intraoperatively, lower incision begins at the superior lid crease (hooding may be addressed by extending the incision lateral to the orbital rim)
- a strip of orbicularis muscle may be excised in the heavy lid with thick skin, allows for better definition of lid crease
- open the orbital septum and excise the pseudoherniated fat (amount typically determined by excising the fat that extrudes out of the septum when placing gentle digital pressure on the globe)
- ptotic lacrimal gland may be addressed by plicating to the periosteum
- accentuation of the superior eyelid crease may be considered by plicating the skin margin of the inferior skin incision to the levator aponeurosis

## Addressing the Lower Lid

- <u>Approaches</u>: skin–muscle flap (most common, more avascular dissection), skin flap (allows for independent modification of skin and muscle, more skin trauma, increased risk of vertical eyelid retraction), and transconjunctival (indicated for excessive fat herniation with minimal skin redundancy, no external scar, avoids eyelid retraction, may be combined with a chemical peel or laser resurfacing to address rhytids)
- excise redundant skin (marked similarly to the upper lid)
- excise orbicularis oculi if needed
- excise pseudoherniated fat (medial compartment typically requires more aggressive excision)
- **Repositioned Orbital Fat Technique**: releases the orbital fat by opening the orbital septum and allowing the pseudoherniated fat to be repositioned inferiorly with the suborbicularis oculi fat (SOOF), allows for a more subtle change (avoids hollowing of the orbit)

## Postoperative Care

- cold compress
- limit physical activity
- avoid downward gaze (may cause skin flap to slide)
- contact lenses may be used after postoperative day 10

## Complications

- **Milia**: inclusion cysts, most common complication; <u>Rx</u>: pinpoint cautery and marsupialization
- **Hematoma**: more common in lower lid; <u>Rx</u>: consider reopening for major hematomas with removal of clot and controlling bleeding; minor hematomas may evacuate through incisions or wait 7–10 days to allow for liquefaction then aspirate, antibiotics, pressure dressings; in emergency canthotomy/cantholysis may be required
- **Blindness**: can occur ≤5 days postoperatively, usually from retrobulbar hematoma from lower eyelid fat removal (intraocular pressure >80 mm Hg increases risk of blindness), pain typically precedes ocular symptoms; <u>Rx</u>: prevent permanent blindness with urgent decompression via lateral canthotomy and orbital decompression
- **Subconjunctival Ecchymosis**: usually only a temporary cosmetic problem; <u>Rx</u>: self-limiting, typically resolves in 3 weeks
- **Lagophthalmos**: normally present for a short period postoperatively, persistent lagophthalmos is caused by excess upper lid excision or sutured orbital septum with skin closure; <u>Rx</u>: often resolves, ophthalmic drops, night taping of lids, consider FTSG for persistent lagophthalmos
- **Scleral Show**: 1 mm considered a normal variant, caused by excess lid reduction or excess laxity, may resolve with edema in 1–2 weeks; <u>Rx</u>: postoperative squint exercises, upward massage, superotemporal taping
- **Ectropion (Eversion)**: caused by excessive lower lid skin or muscle excision, lid contracture, lateral laxity; <u>Rx</u>: initially treat conservatively with tape closure, cold compress, squinting exercises, and perioperative corticosteroids; if no resolution consider lid lengthening with a FTSG from the upper eyelid (best color match) or a FTSG from postauricular skin; if from lateral lid laxity a horizontal lid-shortening procedure is required
- **Ptosis**: caused by levator aponeurosis dehiscence from edema, hematoma, excess cautery, or infection; <u>Rx</u>: intraoperative aponeurosis injury should be corrected immediately, transient ptosis may be caused by edema (resolves within days), may consider a Müller's muscle resection or other ptosis-correcting procedures

- **Pseudoepicanthal Folds (Webbing)**: caused by extending incision too medially (<1 mm of punctum); <u>Rx</u>: Z-plasty
- **Epiphora**: caused by eversion of punctum, lacrimal pump injury, disregard for eyelid laxity, or removal of too much skin beneath punctum; <u>Rx</u>: transient epiphora from edema typically resolves within the first few days; persistent epiphora may be addressed with a punctoplasty, horizontal eyelid-shortening procedure, or dacryocystorhinostomy
- **Dry Eyes**: avoided by assessing tearing function (eg, Schirmer's test); <u>Rx</u>: topical wetting agents and ophthalmologic ointments at night
- **Ocular Palsy**: may be caused by too much fat excision in the nasal pocket causing superior oblique or inferior rectus injury; <u>Rx</u>: diplopia usually resolves in 6 months, may release scar tissue
- **Conjunctival Lymphedema**: skin and muscle flaps may compromise lymphatics; <u>Rx</u>: usually resolves in 1–2 months
- **Chemosis (Conjunctival Edema)**: affects bulbar conjunctiva; <u>Rx</u>: usually resolves in 6 weeks, consider prednisolone/sulfacetamide ophthalmic drops, severe cases may need tarsorrhaphy
- **Persistent Lower Fat Pocket**: lateral compartment is the most common; <u>Rx</u>: revision

# RHYTIDOPLASTY (RHYTIDECTOMY, FACELIFT)

## Introduction

### Anatomy

#### *Layers of Facial Planes*

- skin
- subcutaneous fat
- SMAS (*see following*)
- mimetic muscles
- deep facial fascia
- deep elements (eg, facial nerve, parotid duct, buccal fat)

#### *Facial Nerve Relationships*

- **Temporal (Frontal) Branch**: courses along line from earlobe to zygomatic arch at point midway between tragus and lateral canthus, over zygomatic arch, then penetrates deep temporal fascia into the undersurface of the superficial temporal fascia
- **Zygomatic Branch**: courses 1 cm below the zygomatic arch in a superior and medial direction from tragus to lateral canthus

- **Marginal Mandibular Branch**: exits the parotid 1 cm below the mandibular angle, deep to the platysma within the submandibular gland fascia (superficial to the facial vein)
- the facial nerve innervates facial muscles deeply except the **buccinator, levator anguli oris, and mentalis**

## Superficial Muscular–Aponeurotic System (SMAS)

- translates facial muscle action to dynamic action in the facial skin
- continuous with platysma, superficial temporal fascia, perioral, nasolabial, and periorbital muscles
- adherent to **parotidomasseteric fascia** (continuation of deep cervical fascia in the neck and deep temporal fascia above zygomatic arch), dermis of the cheek, and zygomatic arch
- located above parotid fascia, facial nerve, and facial artery
- plicated for lift in rhytidoplasty
- **Melolabial Crease (Nasolabial Fold)**: insertion of muscles from the zygoma and the SMAS

## Osseocutaneous Retaining Ligaments

- skin attachments to bone
- **Zygomatic Ligament**: attaches from zygomaticomaxillary suture (McGregor's patch) to overlying malar skin
- **Mandibular Ligament**: attaches from anterior mandible to overlying parasymphyseal skin

## Fascia–Fascia Retaining Ligaments

- skin attachments to fascia
- **Parotid Ligament**: attaches to overlying skin
- **Masseter Ligament**: supports soft tissue of the medial cheek superiorly over the mandibular body (attenuation results in jowls)

## Malar Fat Pad

- triangular-shaped fat pad, superficial to SMAS, adherent to overlying skin
- volume of fat pad does not change with relative changes in body adiposity
- with aging loss of malar support results in inferior migration of the malar fat pad about the melolabial crease resulting in the illusion of a deepened melolabial crease

# Evaluation

## History

- history of sun exposure (most common factor in premature aging from actinic damage from **UVA**)
- smoking history (increases skin slough 12×)
- history of recent weight loss (if patient is losing weight should wait until weight is stable)
- complete medical history including thyroid disorders, allergic dermatitis, collagen vascular diseases, previous keloids, and bleeding disorders

## Diseases of Premature Aging

- **Cutis Laxa**: autosomal recessive, associated with hernias, emphysema, aneurysms; rhytidoplasty **helpful**
- **Progeria**: autosomal recessive, associated with growth retardation, early atherosclerosis; rhytidoplasty **not helpful**
- **Werner Syndrome**: autosomal recessive, high-pitched voice, diabetes, osteoporosis; rhytidoplasty **not helpful**

## General Assessment

- ideal candidates are in their 40s–50s, good bony framework, strong cheekbones and chin, normally placed hyoid bone, thin face, good elasticity, and stable weight
- screen for precancerous lesions
- must have favorable medical and psychological conditions
- preoperative photography (*see* p. 476)

## Middle, Lower, and Neck Assessment

- evaluate for well-demarcated mandibular line and jowling (loss on contour at the angle of the mandible)
- assess for deepened melolabial crease, chin ptosis, increased distance from ciliary margin to malar crescent
- **Turkey Gobbler Deformities**: loss of cervicomental angle (>120°) from laxity in platysma (does not decussate across midline), addressed with liposuction and approximating platysma at midline
- **Ptotic Submandibular Glands**: addressed with platysma slings

# Surgical Techniques

## Introduction

- mark patient in the upright position
- liposuction may be used for cervicofacial, submental, periparotid, and jowl regions, allows for shorter flaps and less risk of hematoma
- chemical peels can be done concurrently
- laser resurfacing techniques can be done concurrently in areas with thick flap dissection
- fat transfer can be done concurrently on undissected areas

## Superficial Plane Technique

- original technique described in late 1960s
- addresses redundant skin only
- <u>Advantages</u>: simple
- <u>Disadvantages</u>: does not address deep elements, interrupts vascular perforators to skin, higher risk of skin sloughing

## Deep Plane Technique

- sub-SMAS dissection from midface to medial melolabial crease, elevates cheek fat pad attached to skin by zygomaticus muscles, provides vertical lift
- <u>Advantages</u>: addresses melolabial crease and midface (malar fat pad) by separating SMAS from fixed bony attachments of zygomaticus muscles, provides an excellent jaw line, preserves structural integrity of facial blood supply
- <u>Disadvantages</u>: lengthy anterior dissection, persistent malar edema

## Composite Technique

- combines a deep plane technique with an orbicularis oculi muscle flap
- <u>Advantages</u>: repositions zygomaticus major to original position, healthy and thicker flap (less chance of sloughing, especially with smokers), more avascular dissection
- <u>Disadvantages</u>: persistent malar edema, requires some blind blunt dissection at curve of maxilla, unnatural tension of overlying skin of temple area

## Subperiosteal Technique

- variations of subperiosteal undermining of orbital rim, zygomatic arch, maxilla, and zygoma body

- <u>Advantages</u>: maintains perforators to skin, excellent repositioning of lateral canthus, addresses midface without causing unnatural tension on skin (places traction on periosteum)
- <u>Disadvantages</u>: causes prolonged facial edema, increases intermalar distance, limited improvement of jowling, technically more challenging

## Multiplane Technique

- combines an extended SMAS dissection and a deep plane lift (allows dissection in subcutaneous plane to release zygomatic ligaments and skin of midface)
- <u>Advantages</u>: separate dissection of SMAS allows better redraping of skin, more skin may be excised than deep plane lifts, may address melolabial crease better
- <u>Disadvantages</u>: similar to composite techniques, more compromise of vascular supply than deep plane lifts with separate SMAS and skin dissections
- **Triplane Technique**: 3 levels of dissection (subcutaneous in temple and neck, sub-SMAS in lower cheek, subperiosteal in midface), allows maximal correction of jowl while limiting the degree of sub-SMAS dissection to lower cheek, protects the facial nerve

## Minilift Technique

- limited incisions of many variations; usually indicates the lack of use of either a temporal incision, postauricular incision, or both; no extension into scalp posteriorly
- <u>Variations</u>: S-lift, short scar, minimal access cranial suspension lift (MACS lift)
- <u>Advantages</u>: limited incisions, decreased surgical time, decreased need for anesthesia, risk minimization, faster recovery
- <u>Disadvantages</u>: limited access to neck and midface, dog-ear/excess tissue, difficult visualization

## Addressing the Melolabial Crease

- deep plane and multiplane rhytidoplasty (*see previous*)
- direct fold excision
- melolabial crease liposuction
- collagen injection

## Addressing the Neck

- redrape neck skin for minor defects
- "best necklift is a facelift"
- liposuction to sculpt and redefine cervical lines (usually approached from submental incision)
- address platysma with a submental tuck (reconstruct midline by anchoring to the mandible) or vertical excision with midline plication
- correct ptotic submandibular glands with a platysma sling

# FOREHEAD LIFT AND BROW LIFT
## Anatomy

- <u>Forehead Arteries</u>: superficial temporal artery (from external carotid artery), zygomatico-orbital artery (from superficial temporal artery), supraorbital artery (from ophthalmic artery), and supratrochlear artery (from ophthalmic artery)
- "SCALP" Layers: **S**kin, sub**C**utaneous, galea **A**poneurosis, **L**oose areolar tissue, **P**ericranium
- <u>Causes of Horizontal Rhytids</u>: procerus (glabella), frontalis (forehead)
- <u>Causes of Vertical Rhytids</u>: corrugator supercilii (glabella)
- <u>Indications for Forehead and Brow Lifts</u>: elevate ptotic and asymmetric brows, address upper eyelid hooding, reduce glabellar and forehead creases

## Surgical Techniques

- **Coronal Lift**: standard for generalized brow ptosis (affords best exposure), incision placed above hairline, dissection in supraperiosteal and subgaleal plane, risk of raising anterior hairline, contraindicated with male pattern baldness or high frontal hairlines in females, does not correct brow asymmetries
- **Pretrichial Lift**: incision at anterior hairline, indicated for high hairlines (especially in women) and long vertical forehead height, causes anesthesia posterior to the incision
- **Midforehead Lift**: incision above brow; indicated for expansive foreheads (balding hair) especially in men; candidates should have prominent forehead creases with thin, dry skin to hide the skin incision; indicated for primary brow ptosis but not for forehead rhytids; risk of unsightly scar; dissection in subcutaneous plane to preserve sensation; does not help lateral brow or upper forehead

- **Direct Brow Lift**: incision directly above brow, useful for unilateral brow ptosis, does not allow resection of muscle, effect may be temporary, scar may be unsightly
- **Endoscopic Forehead Lift**: incisions in coronal scalp, less risk of nerve injury, but still some postoperative hypesthesia; contraindications include high hairline, male pattern baldness
- **Supratarsal Lift**: access through upper blepharoplasty incision, suspends brow directly

# LIPOSURGERY
## Surgical Techniques

### Overview

- hereditary and hormonal factors, diet, and exercise contribute to localized adipose tissue, which may persist despite exercise and dieting
- adipocytes increase in number until puberty, weight gain in the adult is secondary to hypertrophy (increase in size) of adipocytes, not hyperplasia (increase in number of cells)

### Lipoinjection

- 75% of adipocytes that are acquired atraumatically and injection with large cannulas (>18G) will persist after 1 year
- <u>Common Uses</u>: cheek hollows, angle of the mandible, glabella frown line, oral commissure

### Liposuction

- cannot be used for dermal defects such as rhytids
- ideally should maintain a minimum of 2 mm subdermal fat
- <u>Advantages</u>: quick, short postoperative course, minimal risk of nerve and vascular damage, minimal scarring, reduced soft tissue trauma
- <u>Disadvantages</u>: in general not used for generalized weight loss
- <u>Common Uses</u>: improve contour of submandibular (jowls), submental (wattles), cheek, malar, and parotid regions, defat pedicled or free flaps, lipoma excision
- <u>Contraindicated</u>: collagen vascular diseases, bleeding disorders, endocrine disorders

# COMPLICATIONS OF RHYTIDECTOMY, BROW LIFT, LIPOSURGERY

- **Temporal Alopecia and Unfavorable Hair Lines**: avoid poorly placed incisions or tension; <u>Rx</u>: typically temporary, for persistence, may consider scar excision for affected region or punch grafting
- **Hematoma**: most common early complication (15%) in rhytidectomy and suction lipectomy, more common in males; <u>Rx</u>: consider exploration
- **Seroma**: common, <u>Rx</u>: aspiration with pressure dressing
- **Skin Slough and Necrosis**: higher risk for smokers, longer and thinner flaps, and with hematoma; prevented by maintaining dermal–subdermal plexus (avoid overaggressive liposuction) and a tension-free closure; <u>Rx</u>: topical debridement if required, topical and oral antibiotics, should allow healing by secondary intention (requires several months of wound care)
- **Pixie Earlobe**: elongated earlobe from excessive inferior tension at lobule; <u>Rx</u>: V–Y advancement flap versus revision rhytidoplasty
- **Chronic Pain**: may be secondary to neuromas or nerve entrapment by a buried suture; <u>Rx</u>: nerve block, excision of neuroma, removal of buried suture
- **Hyperpigmentation/Hypervascularity**: thin-skinned patients are at higher risk for telangiectasia development, pigment changes may occur from postinflammatory melanocyte activation; <u>Rx</u>: usually resolve, sunblock, corticosteroid creams, may consider chemoexfoliation techniques to blend skin
- **Nerve Injuries**: may result from transection, electrocautery injury, traction and compression injury (neuropraxia), and infection
- <u>Common Nerves Injured</u>
    1. **Greater Auricular Nerve: most common** (7%), most commonly injured below tragal notch at anterior border of SCM, protect by leaving fascia overlying SCM
    2. **Frontal Branch of Facial Nerve**: most commonly injured as it lies superficially over the zygomatic arch
    3. **Marginal Mandibular Branch of Facial Nerve**: most commonly injured at anterior margin of flap elevation over mandible
    4. **Supraorbital and Trochlear Branches**: results in paresthesia and itching, avoided with dissection in the subgaleal plane
- **Cobra Neck Deformity and Other Contour Deformities**: cobra neck occurs from excess liposuction in anterior neck region; <u>Rx</u>: digastric and platysma plication or dermal grafts, select depression may be injected with autogenous fat

- **Infection**: eg, MRSA, culture immediately, antibiotics, and drain any abscess
- **Postoperative Nausea**: common in forehead lifts; <u>Rx</u>: antiemetics

# CHIN AND MALAR AUGMENTATION
## Evaluation

- chin should be at or just behind a line perpendicular to Frankfort horizontal and the vermilion border of lower lip (or nasion)
- must consider effects from adjunctive procedures (rhinoplasty, blepharoplasty, liposuction)
- ideally the malar region should appear full and should not fall below 5 mm posterior to melolabial groove
- evaluate microgenia (diminished chin eminence requiring augmentation or sliding genioplasty) versus retrognathia (retrodisplaced mandible requiring sagittal split osteotomies)

## Surgical Techniques

### Chin Implants

- implants typically gain up to 70% projection (after settling and bone resorption)
- may insert chin graft externally through submental crease or intraorally, graft is placed subperiosteally or above periosteum
- <u>Complications</u>: infection, displacement (must be removed and replaced), improper size (wait about 3 months), mental nerve injury, extrusion

### Sliding Genioplasty

- moves anterior-most mandible forward
- indicated for more severe cases (eg, retrognathia, insufficient vertical mandibular height, hemifacial atrophy, failed implant)
- more difficult, requires intraoral incision, mandibular osteotomy, advancement of segment with plates or wires
- <u>Complications</u>: lip incompetence (if mentalis is not approximated correctly), tooth injury, mental nerve injury

### Malar Implants

- may be approached intraorally (canine fossa) or subcilliary (more accurate)
- <u>Complications</u>: similar to chin implants

# FACIAL RESURFACING
## Anatomy

**Skin Layers** (*see* pp. 437–438, Figure 9–1)

- <u>Epidermis</u>: stratum corneum (dead cells), granulosum, spinosum, basale
- <u>Dermis</u>: papillary dermis, reticular dermis
- <u>Subcutaneous Tissue</u>: deep to skin, fat and fibrous tissue

## Dermabrasion

- limit to the papillary dermis (pinpoint bleeding), must avoid the parallel white fibers of the reticular layer, which houses adnexal structures required for healing (injury to the epidermis and papillary dermis does **not** result in scarring)
- preoperative topical tretinoin 2 weeks prior to dermabrasion and postoperative occlusive dressings will shorten healing from 7–10 days to 5–7 days
- freezing skin prior to abrading allows for a rigid surface and preservation of anatomic markings
- <u>Indications</u>: acne scars, adjunctive procedure with irregularization techniques (scar revisions), actinic keratosis, seborrheic keratosis, facial wrinkles, tattoos, rhinophyma
- <u>Advantages</u>: quick, local anesthesia, may be repeated, more precise level of depths
- <u>Disadvantages</u>: higher risk of scarring, more bleeding
- <u>Risks of Bad Outcome</u>: keloid, hypertrophic scar history, vitiligo (hypopigmentation in 10–20%), active herpes
- <u>Postoperative Care</u>: occlusive dressing, consider short course of oral corticosteroids to reduce edema, acyclovir for 5 days, sunblock (especially in hyper/hypopigmented skin), resume topical tretinoin

## Laser Resurfacing

### Overview

- adjustment of the power (watts) determines the energy delivered to tissues
- power density is determined by power (watts) divided by spot size (area)
- the concept of selective thermolysis is determined by the absorbance of the skin's constituents, specifically the chromophores,

oxyhemoglobin, and melanin, which have their own absorbance spectra; water absorbs infrared laser energy, which causes the thermal effect of $CO_2$ lasers

- Indications: acne scars, scar revisions, actinic keratosis, seborrheic keratosis, facial wrinkles, rhinophyma, tattoos, cutaneous vascular lesions, keloids

## Common Laser Types

- lasers may be ablative or nonablative
- **$CO_2$ Laser**: ablative; invisible beam (visible aiming beam sometimes used in conjunction with $CO_2$ laser); primarily absorbed by **water**; excellent for cutting, coagulation, or ablating (depending on area of focus); **10600 nm** wavelength; 20–60 µm depth vaporized first pass (more with additional passes); re-epithelialization in 8 days; 3–6 months of erythema; hypopigmentation is most common complication
- **Erbium:YAG Laser**: ablative, chromophore is water (12–18× absorption of $CO_2$ laser), 2940 nm wavelength, 3–5 µm depth vaporized, re-epithelialization in 5 days, 3–4 weeks of erythema, less collagen remodeling and tightening than $CO_2$ laser
- **Nd:YAG Laser**: nonablative, near-infrared beam, invisible (requires an aiming beam), primarily absorbed by pigmented tissues, penetrates to dermis (does not ablate epidermis), more scatter than $CO_2$ laser, nonspecifically absorbed, 1064 nm wavelength, may use a fiberoptic carrier, indicated for cutaneous lesions (eg, port-wine stain, telangiectasia, hemangioma)
- **KTP Laser**: visible, primarily absorbed by oxyhemoglobin, may use a fiberoptic carrier, indicated for cutaneous lesions and as a cutting tool
- **Argon Laser**: visible, broadband blue light, primarily absorbed by oxyhemoglobin, depth of penetration between $CO_2$ and Nd:YAG lasers, similar indications as the Nd:YAG laser
- **Flashlamp-Excited Dye Laser**: visible, yellow light, vascular sensitive, less scarring and hypopigmentation than Nd:YAG and argon lasers, indicated for cutaneous vascular lesions

# Chemoexfoliation (Chemical Facial Peel)

## Overview

- Indications: postacne scars, scar revision, actinic keratosis, seborrheic keratosis, rejuvenate wrinkled and aged skin, pigment irregularities, address photoaging, texture, decrease oiliness, size of pores

- <u>Depth of Penetration Factors</u>: chemoexfoliation agent, skin thickness, sebaceous gland density, use of retinoic acid or lactic acid, use of degreasing agents or prepeel agents, occluded versus unoccluded
- <u>Contraindications</u>: active herpetic lesions, pustular acne, history of keloids, collagen diseases
- <u>Postoperative Care</u>: avoid sun for 3 months (sunscreen), skin emollients to keep moist, resume topical tretinoin

## Preoperative Planning

- <u>Assess Skin</u>: darker and oilier skins have higher risk of pigment changes; evaluate for keloids, precancerous lesions, and herpetic lesions
- consider agents that remove keratin to enhance peels (eg, Lac-Hydrin, retinoic acid)
- curette actinic keratosis and seborrheic keratosis before peel
- must remove surface oils before peeling (acetone)
- preoperative photodocumentation

## Postoperative Healing Timeline

- <u>5 days</u>: epidermis regenerates
- <u>1 week</u>: epidermis loosely attached to dermis
- <u>2 weeks</u>: new collagen deposits, youthful look
- <u>1 month</u>: pigment returns
- <u>6 months</u>: epidermis at normal thickness
- <u>10 months</u>: dermis normalizes

## Peel Types

### Retinoic Acid Peel

- corrects epidermal dysplasia, reduces actinic keratosis, increases vascularization, disperses melanin granules
- <u>Indications</u>: freshening effect, enhance other peels
- <u>Advantages</u>: can be completed at home, does not induce skin injury
- <u>Disadvantages</u>: may cause drying and irritation, limited effect

### Trichloroacetic Acid (TCA) Peel

- <u>Indications</u>: superficial and medium-depth peels (depends on concentration)
- <u>Mechanism of Action</u>: coagulation necrosis limits injury to epidermis and some papillary dermis (up to the upper reticular dermis)

- Concentration Affects Depth
  1. **10–30%**: superficial, can be enhanced by retinoic acid, extend to basal cell layer
  2. **30–40%**: medium; may pretreat with Jessner's, glycolic acid, or $CO_2$; from papillary to reticular junction
  3. **45–50%**: deep, better than phenol for darker-skinned patients (less risk of permanent hypopigmentation) or patients with renal/hepatic/cardiac disease, extends to upper reticular dermis, >45% can cause scarring
- Advantages: less risk of hypopigmentation, no significant systemic toxicity
- Disadvantages: deep peels less effective than phenol peels

### *Phenol Peel*

- Indications: deep dermal peel (penetrates to middle reticular dermis)
- Mechanism of Action: liquefaction necrosis resulting in deep dermal injury (washing and degreasing skin results in deeper penetration), 75% excreted in urine
- Advantages: addresses severe pigmented lesions and deep wrinkles, typically requires only one-time therapy
- Disadvantages: systemic effects (requires pretreatment evaluation of cardiac, renal, and hepatic function and cardiac monitoring to evaluate for phenol toxicity including **arrythmia**, *see following*), **cannot** be used in conjunction with rhytidoplasty (increases chance of skin necrosis), requires premedication sedation, longer healing process
- Contraindications: areas treated with external beam radiation (may not have adnexal structures); renal, cardiac, or hepatic disease
- **Baker's Solution**: chemical or peel solution; contains liquid phenol (88% phenol concentrate), distilled or tap water, liquid soap (aids in emulsifying the solution), croton oil (enhances the keratolytic and penetrating action)
- consider tape occlusion for deeper wounding or without taped occlusion to avoid increased risk of scarring
- avoid applying to more than 25% of face and wait 10 minutes between peels to avoid cardiac toxicity
- postoperative swelling occurs for 2 days and crusting for 1 week

## Complications

- **Phenol Toxicity**: cardiac toxicity (must monitor for arrhythmias), neural (muscle weakness, slowed respiration), hepatic and renal toxicity, headache, nausea, hypotension, coma, and death; Rx: avoid by evaluating cardiac, renal, and hepatic function prior to phenol peel; avoid single large surface areas of peel; preoperatively should hydrate patient; if occurs, remove peel and address arrhythmia, hypotension, etc

- **Hypopigmentation**: normal sequela after deep peels (typically resolves), may result from melanocytic injury from deep dermabrasion; <u>Rx</u>: sunscreen, makeup, consider tattooing if severe, psoralens (increases pigmentation)
- **Hyperpigmentation**: more common in superficial peels; <u>Rx</u>: sunscreen, consider tretinoin, corticosteroid, and hydroquinone creams
- **Melasma**: hyperpigmentation in face (common with estrogen, birth control pills, pregnancy)
- **Milia**: small epidermal cysts, common 1 month postoperatively; <u>Rx</u>: mild abrasive cleaners, unroofing, tretinoin therapy
- **Scarring**: higher risk for deep peels, perioral and chin peels, keloid formers; <u>Rx</u>: compression, massage, corticosteroid injections, silicon gel sheeting
- **Ectropion**: may occur with phenol eyelid peels
- **Prolonged Erythema**: should resolve after 1 month; <u>Rx</u>: topical corticosteroids and tretinoin for prolonged erythema
- **Herpes Simplex Outbreak**: reactivation from quiescent herpetic infection (HSV-1) in the trigeminal ganglion, occurs within 24 hours; <u>Rx</u>: perioperative high-dose acyclovir for prophylaxis, topical and oral acyclovir for active outbreak
- **Telangiectasias**: may become more prominent after peel; <u>Rx</u>: electrocoagulation/laser
- **Persistent Rhytids**: may repeat peel

# FILLERS, SKIN SUBSTITUTES, AND INJECTIONS

## Injectable Fillers

### Introduction

- <u>Indications</u>: soft-tissue augmentation of facial rhytids, scars, and facial deformities
- the ideal material does not exist because most of the effects are temporary

## Materials (*see* Table 9–1)

- **Collagen**: ~3% allergic reaction, rapidly absorbed (<6 months), CosmoDerm and CosmoPlast (Inamed Corp) are human-derived collagen dermal fillers that do not require skin testing, bovine collagen (eg, Zyderm) also utilized with good results but requires skin testing (crosslinked form less reactive [Zyplast])
- **Autologous Fibroblasts**: human fibroblasts cells are cultured for 4–6 weeks from a punch biopsy of skin, requires test dose, 3–4 injections should be performed during a 3–6 month period
- **Hyaluronic Acid Derivatives (Restylane, Juvederm, Perlane)**: consists of a glycosaminoglycan biopolymer found in the dermis (identical in all species); lasts about 6–12 months depending on location with less mobile areas lasting longer; effects of injection are cumulative (smaller volumes are adequate for maintenance treatment); absorbs water; expands; injections can be painful and can cause bruising; good for lip augmentation, nasolabial folds, and

---

**TABLE 9–1.** Overview of Injectable Fillers

**Injectable Synthetic Material**

Artecoll, ArteFill (PMMA Microspheres in Bovine Collagen)

Arteplast (Polymethylmethacrylate [PMMA] Microspheres in Gelatin)

Bioplastique (Silicone Particles in Polyvinylpyrrolidone Carrier)

Radiesse (Calcium Hydroxyapatite)

Sculptra (PLLA)

Silicone

**Injectable Biologic Material**

Evolence (Porcine Collagen)

Fibrel (Plasma/Porcine Gelatin/Aminocaproic Acid)

Hyaluronic Acid Derivatives (Restylane, Hylaform, Captique, Juvederm, Perlane, Elevess, Prevelle)

Zyderm I, Zyderm II, Zyplast (Bovine Collagen)

**Injectable Homologous Material**

CosmoDerm, CosmoPlast (Human Collagen)

Cymetra (Micronized AlloDerm)

Dermalogen (Processed Dermal Suspension)

**Injectable Autologous Material**

Fat

Isolagen (Cultured Autologous Fibroblasts)

glabellar lines; reversible with hyaluronidase in the event of vascular compromise or dissatisfaction with result
- **Micronized AlloDerm (Cymetra):** injected into the subdermis, histologic evaluation of injected AlloDerm after 1 month revealed fibroblast ingrowth and collagen deposition, longevity not known (*see following*)
- **Calcium Hydroxyapatite (Radiesse):** pure synthetic identical to mineral portion of bone, placed in deep dermis, effect is permanent after fibrous ingrowth (max volume at 4–6 weeks)
- **Poly-L-Lactic Acid (PLLA) (Sculptra):** deep dermal or supraperiosteal injection, particles stimulate collagen neo-genesis; used for lipoatrophy of cheeks in thin women, men who have lost facial fat, or HIV lipoatrophy; requires multiple treatments for significant effect; effect may last years
- **Polymethylmethacrylate (ArteFill):** permanent filler, good for filling depressed scars, ArteFill is suspended in bovine collagen
- **Silicone:** previously banned by FDA, now reapproved for ophthalmologic purposes, currently may be used off-label for soft-tissue augmentation

## Complications

- allergic reaction
- **Embolization/Compression of Vasculature:** causes epidermolysis or skin necrosis; <u>Dx</u>: significant pain hours after injection, blue skin away from injection site; <u>Rx</u>: act ≤24–48 hours to prevent/minimize skin necrosis; aspirin, nitroglycerine paste, warm compress massages; dissolving product if hyaluronic acid

# Dermal Substitutes

## Introduction

- <u>Indications</u>: skin substitutes are available currently for the treatment of burns, scar revision, and chronic wounds
- the challenge of dermal substitutes is the replacement of both dermal and epidermal components

## Materials

- **AlloDerm** (LifeCell): processed human cadaveric skin from which the epidermis has been removed and the cellular components of the dermis have been extracted prior to cryopreservation, acts as a template for dermal regeneration, rare complications

- **Strattice** (LifeCell): processed porcine dermis, stretches initially (prestretch before used)
- **Apligraf** (Organogenesis): type I bovine collagen and living neonatal allogeneic fibroblasts with overlying neonatal allogeneic keratinocytes, first skin equivalent designed, one of the first commercial tissue-engineered products
- **FortaFlex** (Organogenesis): derived from tissue-engineered acellular small intestine submucosa, used for soft-tissue augmentation, including facial augmentation
- **Integra Dermal Regeneration Template** (Integra LifeSciences): collagen/chondroitin sulfate sponge with well-defined porous structure, forms a vascular neodermis in about 3–6 weeks, most widely used synthetic skin for burns

# Botulinum Toxin

## Introduction

- produced by *Clostridium botulinum*
- <u>Types</u>: onabotulinumtoxinA (Botox), abobotulinumtoxinA (Dysport), incobotulinumtoxinA (Xeomin), rimabotulinumtoxinB (Myobloc)
- Dysport:Botox conversion 3:1, Dysport has greater spread, more rapid onset (by 1–2 days), and potentially longer duration of effect (1 week)
- <u>Mechanism</u>: potent neurotoxin, inhibits release of acetylcholine at the neuromuscular junction
- improves cosmetic appearance by decreasing hyperfunctional facial lines caused by contraction of the underlying muscles
- <u>Indications</u>: glabellar lines, horizontal forehead lines, lateral orbital lines "crow's feet," platysmal bands, hyperactive mentalis muscles, essential blephorospasm, synkinesis, facial contractures, and hemifacial spasm following facial paralysis (does not address skin lines unrelated to muscular hyperfunction, such as actinic damage or skin atrophy)
- effect lasts 3–4 months
- <u>Complications</u>: mild bruising, local pain, transient weakness of adjacent muscles, eg, brow ptosis, weak smile/suck, blepharoptosis

## Technique

- document injection site, pretreatment photography
- mark hyperfunctional facial lines (the confluence of circles should completely cover the area of excess muscle function without infringing on other adjacent muscles)

- inject with tuberculin syringe with a 30, 31, or 32G needle, apply gentle pressure at injection site to prevent ecchymosis
- avoid rubbing or massaging the injected area for 6 hours to avoid excess diffusion to adjacent muscles
- **Vertical Glabellar Lines**: inject into head and tail of corrugator supercilii
- **Horizontal Glabellar Lines**: inject into central prominence of procerus when patient medializes eyebrows
- **Horizontal Forehead Lines**: inject into frontalis, stay 2 cm above brow
- **Crow's Feet**: inject lateral orbicularis oculi (avoid lower canthal area and below zygomatic arch)
- **Perioral Wrinkles**: inject orbicularis within 5 mm of vermilion, avoid corners, produces fuller lip
- **Dimpled Chin**: inject mentalis, avoid high (orbicularis) and lateral (depressor labii) injections
- **Platysmal Bands**: avoid strap muscle midline, does not correct skin laxity or fat deposits

# SURGERY FOR ALOPECIA

## Introduction

- <u>Evaluation</u>: patient age, a definitive bald area, skin-to-hair color match, hair curl, density of the donor area, and classification (*see* Table 9–2 for Norwood Classification, most popular)
- hair colors best suited for transplantation procedures include blonde, red, gray, and salt-and-pepper combination

**TABLE 9–2.** Norwood Classification of Male-Pattern Baldness

| | |
|---|---|
| Type I | Minimal to no recession of the hairline |
| Type II | Areas of recession at the frontotemporal hairline |
| Type III | Deep symmetric recession at the temples, which are bare or only sparsely covered |
| Type IV | Hair loss is primarily from the vertex; limited recession of the frontotemporal hairline |
| Type V | Vertex hair loss region is separated from the frontotemporal region but is less distinct; the band of hair across the crown is narrow |
| Type VI | Frontotemporal and vertex regions are joined together |
| Type VII | Most severe form; a narrow band of hair remains in a horseshoe shape |

- <u>Ideal patient</u>: dark skin with dark, curly hair (least ideal patient combines light pale skin with dark, straight hair)
- 12.5% of scalp available represents about 12,000 hairs

## Hair Transplant

- <u>Follicular Unit Grafting</u>: harvest from occipital scalp (less androgen-sensitive, preserved in all but most severe cases), transplant hairs in "follicular units," a term that refers to hair in its natural groupings of 1–4 follicles **(1–2 follicles is micrograft; 3–4 follicles is minigraft)**; grafts placed in a random fashion along the anterior hairline to create a natural, unoperated appearance; grafts inserted through simple stab incisions angled according to scalp subsite to allow to lie naturally; after grafting, hair follicles uniformly lose their shafts; the follicles, if viable, begin to redevelop hair shafts after several weeks (telogen effluvium)
- <u>Follicular Unit Extraction</u>: grafts harvested one at a time with 0.8-mm punches that heal with secondary intention; avoids donor site incision; best for young males who would like to shave head in future, African Americans, reconstructive work, and limited donor hair

## Scalp Reduction

- in crown-balding, allopecic area can be excised and closed with local flaps (however, male-pattern baldness will usually proceed circumferentially outward, necessitating further procedures)
- <u>Flap Designs</u>: midline sagittal ellipse, Y-pattern, paramedian pattern, and circumferential pattern
- closure is accomplished with extensive undermining and may be aided with the use of tissue expanders
- **Juri Flap**: pedicled temporoparietal–occipital transposition flap based on the superficial temporal vessels, used bilaterally to cover frontal baldness; single flap, but requires 4 stages versus 2 stages + scalp reduction; 4 cm wide, does not cross midline

# INCISION/EXCISION PLANNING AND SCAR REVISIONS

## Incision and Excision Planning

### Introduction

- initial proper planning is essential for achieving good results in excising lesions of the head and neck
- ideal angle for fusiform closure (*see following*) is **≤30°** otherwise consider a graft, flap, or adjunctive M-plasty (*see following*)
- ideally, excision should be elliptical with the long axis of the excision along a RSTL (*see following*), natural facial crease, aesthetic unit junction, or hairline
- long straight incisions (≥2 cm) are the most noticeable
- proper undermining is essential in all excisions to minimize tension along wound edges
- the principle of halves (placing sutures in a bisecting fashion) avoids "bunching" of tissues
- slight eversion of wound edges allows for a flatter scar by accounting for scar contraction

### Skin Lines

- **Relaxed Skin Tension Lines (RSTLs)**: generally run parallel to wrinkles (exceptions include the lateral orbital region) and perpendicular with the contractions of muscles, best demonstrated in upright position with active facial muscle contraction
- **Langer's Lines**: relaxation creases found on cadavers (rigor mortis), usually perpendicular to RSTLs
- **Lines of Maximum Extensibility (LME)**: run perpendicular to RSTL and represent the direction in which closure can be performed with the least tension

## Scar Revisions

### Introduction

- <u>Ideal Scar</u>: level to skin, no anatomic distortion, matching color, narrow, parallel to RSTLs, placed at junction of facial aesthetic units or nonvisible areas
- <u>Timing of Scar Revision</u>: may revise at 6–12 months (final phases of scar contracture and maturation) or at 6–9 weeks (maximal fibroblastic activity); if obviously misplaced or misdirected may consider earlier revision

- may preserve deep scar and subcutaneous tissue to preserve strength unless the revision contributes to the deformity
- broken and irregular scars are less noticeable
- may consider dermabrasion or chemoexfoliation (*see previous*)
- corticosteroids, retinoids, silicone gel sheeting, and emollient creams may be considered while awaiting scar revision or after scar revision

## Excisional Techniques

### Shave Excision

- removal of superficial lesion from skin surface
- <u>Advantages</u>: rapid, simple
- <u>Disadvantages</u>: may leave residual scar, predisposes to a locally recurrent lesion
- <u>Common Uses</u>: small elevated scars

### Fusiform Excision (Figure 9–11)

- elliptical excision with bilateral advancement for a linear closure
- <u>Advantages</u>: simplest technique
- <u>Disadvantages</u>: must be able to be designed parallel to RSTL, ideal closure angle ≤30°
- <u>Common Uses</u>: most common excisional technique, ubiquitous

### M-plasty (Figure 9–12)

- M-plasty modification at the ends of a fusiform to close a larger lesion with an ellipse and limit extent of a normal skin excision
- <u>Advantages</u>: shortens wound length, avoids extension of scars across an anatomic border
- <u>Disadvantages</u>: slightly more complex, diverges closure lines at ends away from RSTLs
- <u>Common Uses</u>: larger lesions

### Scar Repositioning

- repositioning of scar using fusiform excisions to a more favorable location (eg, junction of two aesthetic facial units, melolabial crease, hairline, preauricular crease)
- <u>Advantages</u>: scar placed in a more favorable position
- <u>Disadvantages</u>: requires sacrifice of tissue between scar and favorable site
- <u>Common Uses</u>: scars near a facial landmark

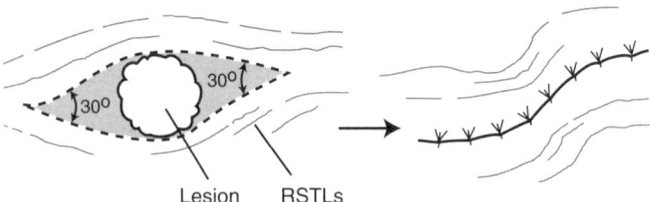

**FIGURE 9–11.** Fusiform excision for a circular lesion designed in order to allow final scar to parallel RSTLs; 30° angles are used at each end.

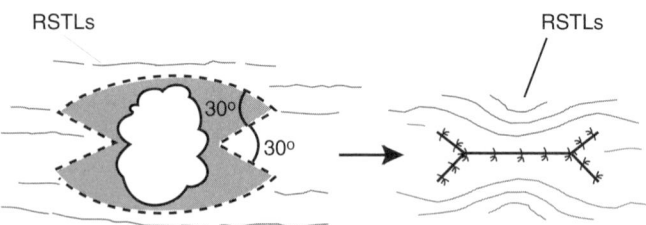

**FIGURE 9–12.** Fusiform excision with M-plasty modification on each end to allow closure of a large lesion with an ellipse; 30° angles are used to form each angle of the M-plasty.

## Serial Partial Excision

- removes part of scar with serial advancement flaps of normal adjacent skin
- concurrent tissue expanders decrease number of required excisions
- <u>Advantages</u>: may advance to hair-bearing areas or aesthetic unit junctions
- <u>Disadvantages</u>: requires multiple procedures and longer time commitment
- <u>Common Uses</u>: large-width scars, stellate lesions, skin grafts

# Irregularization Techniques

## Z-plasty (Figure 9–13)

- two flaps classically constructed with 2 same-degree angles and 3 equal limbs, peripheral limbs run parallel with the RSTL
- <u>Advantages</u>: reorients the long axis of a scar to a more favorable position (parallel to RSTLs or along an anatomic line), spreads force

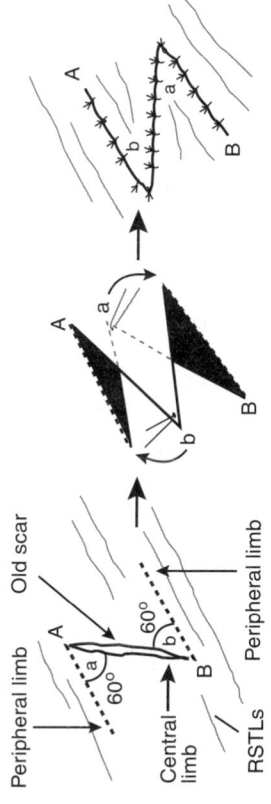

**FIGURE 9–13.** Classic Z-plasty technique utilizing 60° angles. The peripheral limbs run parallel with the RSTLs. (Adapted with permission from Lore JM. *An Atlas of Head and Neck Surgery.* 3rd ed. Philadelphia, PA: W. B. Saunders; 1988.)

of contraction in many directions to minimize distortion, most powerful leveling technique

- <u>Disadvantages</u>: lengthens scar
- <u>Common Uses</u>: contracted scars (causes distortion of landmarks), misdirected scars (crosses RSTLs or anatomic lines), webs across concavities, edges of trap door deformities, repositioning of facial landmarks (eg, pulled up eyebrow)
- angle determines gain of length: **30° angle → 25% gain in length; 45° → 50%; 60° → 75%, 90° → 120%**
- final direction of central limb predicted by connecting free ends of peripheral limbs
- Z-plasty angle <20° increases risk of tip necrosis, angle >75° increases risk of a dog-ear deformity

## W-plasty (Figure 9–14) **and Geometric Broken-Line Closure** (Figure 9–15)

- **W-plasty**: excises scar with mirrored W-pattern, each leg <6 mm with 60° angles (regularly irregular)
- **Geometric Broken-Line Closure**: random, irregular patterns (triangles, rectangles, semicircles, and squares between 5–7 mm) with mirrored opposite side, more effective in camouflaging scar than W-plasty (irregularly irregular)
- <u>Advantages</u>: avoids straight-lined scar (less noticeable)
- <u>Disadvantages</u>: more complex closure, time-consuming, requires excision of small amount of normal tissue
- <u>Common Uses</u>: long scars not parallel to RSTLs, convex lines (mandible border, forehead, cheek)

## Tissue Sealants and Platelet Gels

### Tissue Sealants

- <u>Indications</u>: close incisions, seal and secure skin flaps, promote hemostasis, and enhance wound healing
- <u>Advantages</u>: fibrin sealants improve hemostasis reducing blood loss and complications
- <u>Disadvantages</u>: autologous fibrin tissue requires lengthy preparation time (collected from cryoprecipitate), donor cryoprecipitate may cause disease transmission

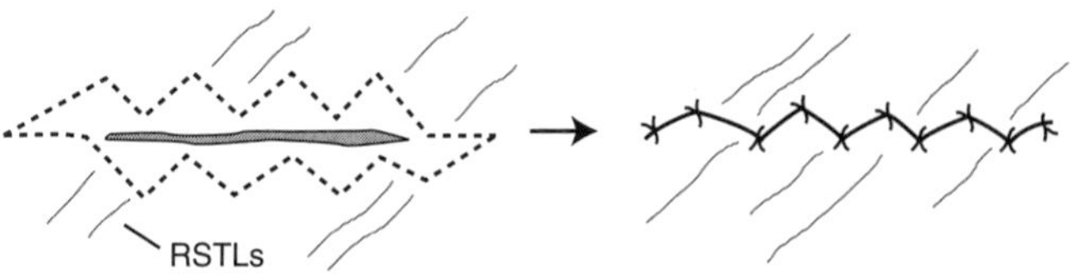

**FIGURE 9–14.** W-plasty technique utilizes a regularly, irregular mirrored W-pattern to camouflage the scar by avoiding a long single straight line.

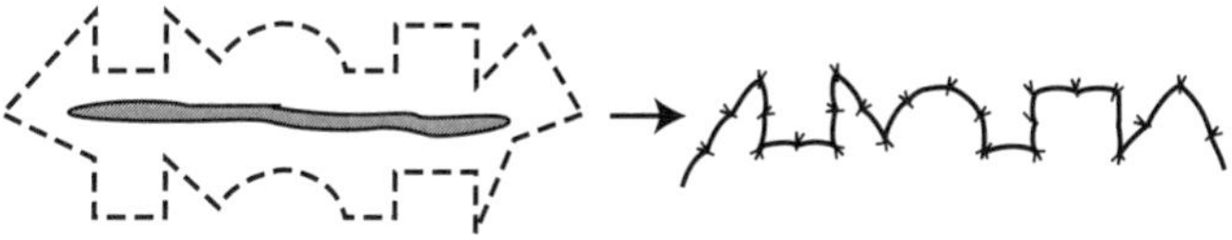

**FIGURE 9–15.** Geometric broken line closure technique utilizes mirrored random patterns to camouflage a scar.

## Platelet Gels, Platelet-Derived Growth Factor (PDGF), Platelet-Rich Plasma (PRP)

- platelet gels release PDGF and TGF-ß, which aids in wound healing (stimulates the formation of a blood clot)
- platelet gels are prepared from autologous whole blood obtained in the immediate preoperative period
- <u>Indications</u>: facelifts, necklifts, chronic skin wounds (diabetic ulcerations, venous stasis ulcers, and pressure sores)
- <u>Advantages</u>: improves wound healing, no risk of disease transmission
- <u>Disadvantages</u>: requires blood draw, expensive

# Hypertrophic Scars and Keloids

## Introduction

- scar contracture is the result of a contractile wound-healing process occurring in a scar that has already been re-epithelialized and adequately healed
- keloids and hypertrophic scars are fibrous tissue outgrowths that result from a derailment in the normal wound-healing process
- a combination of biochemical factors, skin tension, endocrinologic factors, and genetic factors are the likely culprits
- keloids and hypertrophic scars are histologically similar under light microscopy (differences are demonstrated with scanning electron microscopy)

- <u>Risks</u>: darker complexion, sebaceous skin, wounds closed under tension, genetic predisposition (5–15% incidence in Blacks and Hispanics)
- <u>Areas</u>: more common in areas such as deltoid, sternum, and over bony prominences, tendency to spare midface

## Hypertrophic Scar

- overactive inflammation and collagen synthesis resulting in an enlarged scar **confined** to the boundaries of surgical trauma, typically flattens and softens over time, often precipitated by closure under tension, infection, or wound dehiscence
- does not recur when excised, responds well to steroid treatments
- <u>SSx</u>: pruritus (from histamine release during active inflammation), pain, erythema, induration
- <u>Rx</u>: excision

## Keloid

- deposition of collagen that **extends beyond** the limits of the scar, does not regress over time
- recurs frequently following single modality treatment, marginal response to steroid injection when used as a single modality of treatment
- <u>SSx</u>: expansile soft tissue mass
- <u>Management</u>
  1. gentle massage with intralesional corticosteroid injections (triamcinolone acetonide) with repeat injections every 3 weeks
  2. if no response, may consider excision (with corticosteroid injections)
  3. pressure delivery devices, silicone gel applications
  4. radiation therapy for severe cases may be considered but must weigh risk of malignant transformations

***Acknowledgment:*** *We wish to acknowledge and thank Gabriel Calzada and Anthony E. Brissett for their contributions to this chapter.*

# CHAPTER

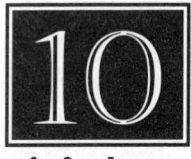

# Pediatric Otolaryngology

Valerie Cote, Jeremy D. Prager, Henry Ou, Peggy E. Kelley, Raza Pasha, and Justin S. Golub

# THE PEDIATRIC ENCOUNTER
## Pediatric History and Physical Exam

### History

- <u>Prenatal</u>: maternal infections, complications, ultrasound findings, alcohol/drugs consumption, maternal smoking
- <u>Perinatal</u>: gestational age at birth, spontaneous vaginal delivery versus Cesarean section, breastfeeding, intubation (endotracheal tube size, duration), use of antibiotics, significant jaundice, prolonged oxygen supplementation (duration)
- <u>Otologic</u>: neonatal hearing screening, otorrhea, previous infections, previous myringotomies, hearing or speech delays
- <u>Nasal</u>: rhinorrhea, epistaxis, congestion, stertor, allergy
- <u>Oral/Pharyngeal</u>: snoring, apneas, restless sleep, enuresis, hyperactivity, sleepiness, previous tonsillitis, dysphagia, excessive drooling, stertor
- <u>Laryngeal</u>: stridor (inspiratory, expiratory, biphasic), cyanosis, retraction, previous croup/pneumonia/bronchiolitis, hoarseness, voice abuse, choking, coughing, throat clearing
- <u>Neck</u>: masses
- <u>Neurologic</u>: alertness, facial symmetry, cerebral palsy, stroke, seizures
- <u>Risk Factors</u>: parental smoking, daycare/school, other siblings, ethnicity
- <u>Constitutional Symptoms</u>: weight loss or gain, fever
- <u>Other History</u>: congenital diseases, syndromes, neuromuscular diseases, surgery, family history (acute otitis media, hearing loss, hereditary diseases, bleeding or anesthesia issues)

### Physical Exam

- <u>Vital signs</u>: weight, temperature at a minimum
- <u>Appearance</u>: hydration status, well versus toxic-looking, energetic versus tired
- <u>Head/Face</u>: dysmorphic features, craniosynostosis, asymmetry
- <u>Eyes</u>: ocular mobility, proptosis, glasses
- <u>Ears</u>: external (tags, pits, sinuses, auricular deformities, patency of the external canal), middle (integrity of the tympanic membrane, presence of retraction, middle ear status)
- <u>Nose</u>: nasal mucosa, turbinate size and color, hypo/hypernasality, nasal air escape, septal deviation, discharge
- <u>Oral/Pharyngeal</u>: presence of ankyloglossia, tongue mobility, tonsil size (*see* p. 525), single versus notched uvula, presence of cleft/zona pellucida/palatal notch, postnasal drip

- <u>Laryngeal</u>: flexible laryngoscopy (adenoid size, velopharyngeal function, base of tongue position, larynx and vocal fold movement, vocal fold appearance)
- <u>Neck</u>: palpable nodes (mobility, size, level), masses (movement with swallowing or tongue protrusion), thyroid (size, tenderness, nodule), skin discoloration/pits

# GENERAL PEDIATRIC OTOLARYNGOLOGY AND PEDIATRIC SLEEP

## Adenotonsillar Anatomy

### Tonsils

- **Waldeyer's Ring**: circle of lymphoid tissue consisting of palatine/faucial tonsils (referred to simply as "tonsils"), pharyngeal tonsils (adenoids), lingual tonsils, and **tubal tonsils of Gerlach** (near fossa of Rosenmüller); lateral bands and the posterior pharyngeal wall complete the ring
- tonsils increase in size between 6 months–3 years old (after exposure to antigens), peak between 3–7 years old, and may involute after puberty
- <u>Arterial Supply</u> (branches of external carotid)
  1. lingual artery → dorsal lingual branch (anterior lower pole)
  2. facial artery → ascending palatine and tonsillar arteries (main supply, posterior and middle inferior lower pole)
  3. ascending pharyngeal artery (posterior upper pole)
  4. maxillary artery → greater palatine and descending palatine arteries (anterior upper pole)
- *NOTE:* internal carotid artery is typically 2 cm posterolateral to the deep aspect of the tonsillar fossa (medialized in some 22q11 patients)
- <u>Venous Drainage</u>: lingual and pharyngeal veins → internal jugular vein
- <u>Lymphatics</u>: no afferent lymphatics, drainage into superior deep cervical and jugular digastric lymph nodes
- <u>Innervation</u>: anterior pillar: CN X (palatoglossus); posterior pillar: CN X (palatopharyngeus); tonsillar fossa: CN IX, X (superior constrictor)
- <u>Histology/Tonsillar Zones</u>
  1. **Reticular Cell Epithelium**: foreign material presented to lymphatic cells via 10–30 crypts/tonsil, which are blind tubules of squamous epithelium → contain antigen-presenting cells

(M-cells) which transport antigens to the lymphoid germinal center → interdigitating dendritic cells and macrophages → helper T cells → memory B-cells (nasopharyngeal or systemic migration) and plasma cells (crypts); IgA most important product

2. **Extrafollicular Area**: contains T-cells
3. **Lymphoid Follicle**: composed of the **mantle zone** (mature B-cells) and the **germinal center** (active B-cells)

- tonsils are encapsulated by a specialized portion of the pharyngobasilar fascia

## Adenoids

- similar to palatine tonsils; present at birth, enlarge in childhood, usually regress during puberty
- <u>Arterial Supply</u>: ascending pharyngeal artery from the external carotid artery, minor branches from maxillary artery (ascending pharyngeal branch), facial artery (ascending palatine artery), thyrocervical trunk (ascending cervical), artery of the pterygoid canal
- <u>Venous Drainage</u>: pharyngeal veins → facial and internal jugular veins
- <u>Innervation</u>: CN IX, X
- <u>Histology</u>: ciliated pseudostratified columnar, stratified squamous, and transitional layers

# Pharyngitis (see pp. 214–218)
# Adenotonsillar Pathology

## Acute Tonsillitis

- <u>Pathophysiology</u>: often a viral infection occurs prior to a bacterial superinfection
- <u>Pathogens</u>: most commonly **Group A β-hemolytic streptococci**, **Moraxella**, and **H. influenzae**; less common organisms include *Bacteroides,* staphylococci, *E. coli,* diphtheria, syphilis, *Neisseria,* and viruses (EBV, adenovirus, influenza A and B)
- <u>SSx</u>: sore throat, fever, chills, odynophagia, trismus, cervical adenopathy, halitosis, erythematous and exudative tonsils and faucial pillars (viral infections tend to have lower grade fevers and less exudative tonsils)
- <u>Phases of Tonsillitis</u>: tonsillar erythema → exudative tonsillitis → follicular tonsillitis (yellow spots corresponding to lymphatic follicles) → cryptic tonsillitis (chronic infection)

- <u>Dx</u>: physical exam; consider throat cultures, GABHS rapid antigen test, antistreptolysin-O (ASO), or Monospot test; viral smears rarely indicated; carrier state may be detected with positive culture without a change in ASO titer
- <u>DDx</u>: peritonsillar cellulitis/phlegmon/abscess, leukemia, lymphoma
- <u>Complications</u>: acute airway compromise, peritonsillar abscess, parapharyngeal or retropharyngeal space abscess (*see* pp. 239–240, 242), sepsis; also rheumatic fever, glomerulonephritis, and scarlet fever (*see* p. 216); PANDAS (**P**ediatric **A**utoimmune **N**europsychiatric **D**isorders **A**ssociated with **S**treptococcal infections: streptococcal infections are associated with tics, obsessions and compulsions; tonsillectomy likely does not affect outcome)
- <u>Rx</u>: if suspect bacterial involvement, antimicrobials against suspected pathogens for 10 days (penicillins antimicrobial of choice, may consider β-lactamase inhibitors, clindamycin for allergic patients), bed rest, hydration, analgesics, oral hygiene, tonsillectomy

## Chronic Tonsillitis

- <u>Pathophysiology</u>: typically polymicrobial infection
- <u>SSx</u>: malaise, recurrent sore throat, fibrotic or cryptic tonsils, cervical lymphadenopathy, halitosis, tonsilloliths
- <u>Dx</u>: H&P
- <u>Rx</u>: long-term antibiotics against β-lactamase producing organisms and encapsulated organisms, tonsillectomy

## Acute Adenoiditis

- <u>Pathogens</u>: similar to tonsillitis
- <u>SSx</u>: sore throat, purulent rhinorrhea, halitosis, postnasal drip, nasal obstruction (snoring), fever, association with concurrent otitis media
- <u>Dx</u>: H&P
- <u>Rx</u>: similar to acute tonsillitis, adenoidectomy

## Chronic Adenoiditis

- <u>Pathophysiology</u>: typically a polymicrobial infection; may be related to reflux, especially in children (difficult to distinguish from sinusitis)
- <u>SSx</u>: persistent nasal discharge, malodorous breath, nasal obstruction (snoring), association with recurrent otitis media
- <u>Dx</u>: H&P
- <u>DDx</u>: chronic sinusitis
- <u>Rx</u>: similar to chronic tonsillitis, adenoidectomy

## Obstructive Tonsillar and Adenoid Hyperplasia

- Tonsillar Hyperplasia SSx: snoring, OSA, hyponasal speech, gasping at night, dysphagia
- Tonsil Grading: 0 (tonsils within tonsillar fossa), 1+ (tonsils just outside the fossa and occupying ≤25% of the width between the two anterior pillars), 2+ (26–50%) 3+ (51–75%); 4+ (>75% or touching, "kissing")
- Adenoid Hyperplasia SSx: nasal obstruction, hyponasal speech (pinching nose does not change speech, "M" words), snoring, obstructive sleep apnea, chronic mouth breathing, rhinorrhea, "adenoid facies" (open mouthed, dark circles under eyes, flattened midface, high arched palate), eustachian tube obstruction (otitis media), sinusitis
- Adenoid Grading: 0 (absent), 1+ (<25% obstruction), 2+ (25–50% obstruction), 3+ (50–75% obstruction), 4+ (>75% obstruction); abutting eustachian tube versus central mound
- Dx: visual inspection (nasopharyngoscopy); for unilateral tonsillar hyperplasia must consider neoplasms (lymphoma, leukemia, squamous cell carcinoma) or unusual infections (*M. tuberculosis*, atypical mycobacteria, actinomycosis, fungal); sleep study and lateral neck x-ray are typically not necessary
- severe obstructive presentations may have complications of OSA such as failure to thrive or cor pulmonale (*see also* p. 528); consider capillary blood gas, CXR, ECG, echocardiogram
- Rx: consider nasal trumpet for acute respiratory distress (rarely requires intubation) with a short course of corticosteroids, consider prolonged course of antibiotics (3–6 weeks) or nasal corticosteroid sprays for adenoid hyperplasia; tonsillectomy and adenoidectomy for definitive therapy

## Peritonsillar Abscess (Quinsy) and Peritonsillar Space Infection

- Pathophysiology: spread of infection outside tonsil capsule into the peritonsillar space; infection in a peritonsillar minor salivary gland (Weber gland); typically begins at superior pole
- Boundaries of Peritonsillar Space: palatine tonsil (medial border), superior constrictor muscles (lateral border), tonsillar pillars (superior, inferior, and posterior border)
- Risks: recurrent infections, dental caries
- SSx: odynophagia, trismus, uvular deviation to contralateral side, pharyngotonsillar asymmetry, unilateral soft palate swelling,

unilateral otalgia, drooling, hot-potato voice; symptoms typically exist for ≥5 days before abscess forms
- <u>Dx</u>: H&P, consider CT for atypical cases
- <u>DDx</u>: peritonsillar cellulitis or phlegmon, intratonsillar abscess
- <u>Complications</u>: airway distress, parapharyngeal or retropharyngeal abscess, Lemierre's syndrome (*see* p. 602), aspiration pneumonia
- <u>Rx</u>: urgent I&D, consider needle aspiration for minor cases, antibiotics, elective tonsillectomy after resolution of the infection (may defer until after a second occurrence); "Quinsy tonsillectomy" (tonsillectomy at time of infection) may be considered for younger children, recurrent/unresponsive cases or cases presenting with severe airway compromise

## Infectious Mononucleosis

- <u>Pathogenesis</u>: **EBV** (Epstein-Barr virus) selectively infects B-lymphocytes (90%); CMV and other viruses less commonly involved (10%); spread by oral contact
- <u>SSx</u>: high-grade fever, lymphadenopathy (posterior triangle), fibrinous exudative tonsillitis, palatal petechiae, rhinopharyngitis, general malaise, associated hepatosplenomegaly, variable rashes
- <u>Dx</u>: H&P; **heterophile antibodies** in serum (Monospot test, Paul-Bunnell test; rapid kits 85% sensitive, near 100% specific) will be 40% negative in first 2–3 weeks; presence of 80–90% mononuclear and 10% **atypical lymphocytes** on smear; levels of EBV viral capsid antigen (VCA) IgM (acute infection, first month only); levels of EBV VCA IgG (appears at 1 week, present for life); viral culture
- <u>Complications</u>: acute airway obstruction, cranial nerve involvement, meningitis, autoimmune hemolytic anemia, splenic rupture
- <u>Rx</u>: secure airway for acute obstruction with a nasal trumpet or endotracheal intubation (corticosteroids for severe obstructing tonsillitis), hydration, analgesics, oral hygiene, antimicrobials for secondary infections (ampicillin/amoxicillin may cause a severe **rash** from hypersensitivity), typically resolves after 2–6 weeks

## Surgical Management of
## Adenotonsillar Disease (*see* pp. 530–534)

# Pediatric Sleep Disorders

## Pediatric Sleep Physiology

- *see* pp. 152–156 for general sleep theory and definitions
- daytime sleepiness in children is abnormal and require investigation

### Newborn (< 2 Months)

- <u>Preterm</u>: sleep staged differently; quiet, active, and intermediate sleep; quiet is similar to NREM, active is similar to REM (about 50%), intermediate is a mix
- <u>Term</u>: sleep/wake differentiation occurs by 37 weeks gestational age
- sleep onset goes into REM until age 3 months
- normal sleep time: 16–20 hours/day with 1–4-hour sleep periods

### Infants (2 months–1 year)

- percentage of REM sleep declines
- sleep onset goes into NREM starting at age 3–6 months
- shorter sleep duration, longer sleep cycles; average 50–60 minutes
- circadian rhythms established by 2–4 months
- <u>Normal Sleep Time</u>: 15 hours by age 1, can sleep through the night, fewer daytime naps

### Toddlers (1–3 years)

- <u>1 Year</u>: 30% REM sleep, may nap 1–2 hours per day, normal sleep time 13–15 hours
- <u>2 Years</u>: 25% REM sleep similar to adults, separation anxiety and night awakenings

### School-Age–Prepubescent Children

- <u>5 Years</u>: 20% REM, naps not required, adult-like sleep cycles (90–110 minutes)
- <u>6–12 Years</u>: slow wave sleep is maximal, then abruptly drops off in puberty and declines throughout adulthood; circadian phase preferences develop (morning versus evening); parasomnias may develop

### Adolescents

- phase delay increases with Turner staging
- <u>Normal Sleep Time</u>: nine hours; at risk for behavior induced insufficient sleep syndrome

## Pediatric Sleep-Disordered Breathing (SDB)

- <u>Definition</u>: abnormal respiratory pattern during sleep that includes snoring, mouth breathing, and pauses in breathing

- <u>Spectrum</u>: snoring (10%) → upper airway resistance syndrome → obstructive hypoventilation → obstructive sleep apnea (OSA: 1–3%)
- <u>Pathophysiology</u>: upper airway obstruction from adenotonsillar hyperplasia most common cause; obesity (25–40% SDB; also more severe and more postoperative complications); craniofacial anomalies; syndromes; prematurity; daycare exposure and frequent URIs; ethnicity (more common in African Americans); neuromuscular disorders; smoking exposure
- <u>Nighttime Symptoms</u>: snoring, apnea, or paradoxical breathing, subcostal retractions/tracheal tugging, neck hyperextension/ abnormal sleep postures, restless sleep, frequent awakenings, enuresis, parasomnias (sleep terrors, sleep walking)
- <u>Daytime Symptoms</u>: hyperactivity, sleepiness, poor school performance, neurocognitive deficits, behavior problems (anxiety, aggression, depression, somatization), unrefreshing sleep/difficulty waking in the morning, mouth-breathing/dental or craniofacial changes, dysphagia
- <u>Dx</u>: indications for polysomnography (PSG) in children with SDB (AAO-HNS Clinical Practice Guidelines, 2011):
  1. laboratory-based PSG is the gold standard for the diagnosis of OSA in children; portable monitoring devices may be used if pediatric sleep centers are not accessible or based on a strong parental preference
  2. prior to tonsillectomy in presence of obesity, Down syndrome, craniofacial anomalies, neuromuscular disorders, sickle cell disease, mucopolysaccharidoses
  3. discordance between tonsillar size and SDB symptoms
- <u>OSA Complications</u>: developmental delay, failure to thrive (increased energy expenditure, feeding impairment, reflux from high negative intrathoracic pressures), cardiorespiratory complications (cor pulmonale, pectus excavatum), behavioral disorders
- <u>Rx</u>: *see following* for treatment options

## Pediatric Polysomnography Sleep Scoring

- **Apneic Events**: do not need to last 10 seconds but rather the duration of 2 baseline breaths
- **Hypopneic Events**: nasal air pressure decreases by ≥50% lasting the duration of 2 breaths and must be associated with a ≥ 3% oxygen desaturation or an arousal/awakening
- **Respiratory Effort Related Arousals (RERAs)**: nasal air pressure flattens and decreases in amplitude but **not** ≥50% and is associated with snoring, noisy breathing, increased work of breathing, or elevation of end-tidal or transcutaneous $PCO_2$

- **AHI**: apnea–hypopnea index, number of obstructive apneas and hypopneas per hour of sleep
- Obstructive Sleep Apnea Syndrome Scoring Scale
  1. **Normal**: AHI ≤1, oxygen saturation nadir >92%
  2. **Mild OSA**: AHI >1 and ≤5
  3. **Moderate OSA**: AHI >5 and ≤10
  4. **Severe OSA**: AHI >10, oxygen saturation nadir <80%
- **Hypoventilation Syndrome**: if end tidal $CO_2$ >50 mmHg for >10% of the total sleep time
- **Central Sleep Apnea:** similar to adults but the event must last ≥20 seconds or 2 missed breaths with an arousal/awakening or with a ≥3% desaturation; consider medical causes, Arnold-Chiari malformation, metabolic disorders, cardiac disease, medications (opioids), high altitude
- **Primary Sleep Apnea of Infancy**: central apnea of ≥20 seconds associated with immaturity of brainstem respiratory control centers; lead to bradycardia and hypoxemia, may require resuscitation or stimulation; more common in preemies
- **Periodic Breathing**: series of 3 episodes of central apneas lasting >3 seconds each occurring within 20 seconds; frequent in Arnold-Chiari patients
- **Congenital Central Hypoventilation Syndrome (Ondine's Curse):** PHOX2b gene mutation causing a failure of autonomic central control of breathing at night; <u>Rx</u>: tracheotomy and long-term ventilation during sleep/naps

## Other Sleep-Related Disorders

- *see also* pp. 176–184
- **Sudden Infant Death Syndrome (SIDS)**: abrupt, unanticipated death of unknown etiology; <u>Risk Factors</u>: male, preemie, prone position sleep, multiple births, maternal young age (teen), family history; prevent by supine position sleep ("back to sleep"), firm mattress, no bed sharing, removal of surrounding soft objects
- **Behavior Insomnia of Childhood**: <u>Types</u>:
  1. **Sleep-Onset**: caused by reliance on an inappropriate sleep association and inability to "self soothe" (eg, rocking, bottle, parents' bed); <u>Rx</u>: CBT, extinction ("crying it out"), gradually reduced parent intervention, daytime naps, discontinued feeding after 6 months, consider preemptive scheduled awakenings (15 minutes before anticipated awakening)
  2. **Limit-Setting**: characterized by parents' inability to establish appropriate sleep behaviors, "child stalling" or refusals; <u>Rx</u>: CBT,

consistent bedtime, parent education, may provide a **transitional object** (eg, stuffed animal, blanket)

# Surgical Management of Adenotonsillar Disease

## Tonsillectomy and Adenoidectomy Overview

- second most common ambulatory surgical procedure in children
- tonsils with chronic or recurrent tonsillar infections may have developed immunological impairment; excision has therapeutic benefit
- <u>Depth of Excision</u>: extracapsular excision most common, intracapsular partial tonsillectomy (**tonsillotomy**) typically for obstructive symptoms only
- <u>Instruments Employed</u>: electrocautery, "cold knife" (metal blade), ultrasonic (Harmonic) scalpel, laser, Coblator, microdebrider, radiofrequency reduction; all are debated regarding pain and risk of hemorrhage
- <u>Patient Care Recommendations</u> (AAO-HNS Guidelines, 2011)
  1. **Preoperative Care**: avoid anxiolytics or sedatives in SDB children, if required, then monitor closely for hypoventilation and hypoxemia
  2. **Intraoperative Care**: intraoperative IV dexamethasone reduces postoperative nausea/vomiting; SDB children are at increased risk of airway collapse and delayed emergence; avoid or reduce intraoperative opioids for SDB children; local anesthesia injections should **not** be used
  3. **Postoperative Care**: SDB children require more intensive nursing care and monitoring; in SDB children, pain needs to be controlled with less potent opioids in smaller divided doses or with smaller doses in combination with nonopioid analgesics; strong recommendations **against** perioperative antibiotics (not shown to reduce postoperative hemorrhage, pain, or return to normal function significantly)
- <u>Pain Control</u>: postoperative opiates, especially codeine, should be avoided or used with caution (FDA warning); codeine metabolism related to liver microenzyme CYP2D6 (also metabolizes tramadol, hydrocodone and oxycodone), some patients have duplication of the gene and produce morphine more quickly, resulting in respiratory depression and potentially death; replace with acetaminophen and ibuprofen; ketorolac is relatively contraindicated

- <u>Monitored Overnight Stay</u>: considered in <3 years old, syndromic, comorbidities, obesity (>99th percentile BMI), live >1 hour from hospital, unreliable parents, bleeding disorder, or severe OSA (AHI ≥10, oxygen saturation nadir <80%, or both); "REM rebound" may occur in severe OSA patients after 18 hours which may cause hypoventilation and hypoxemia
- <u>ICU admission</u>: severe OSA, children with comorbidities that cannot be managed on a ward, children with significant airway obstruction and oxygen desaturation in the recovery room that were unresponsive to repositioning and oxygen
- frequent catch-up growth and weight after tonsillectomy; improvement in behavior, attention, quality of life, neurocognitive functioning, enuresis, parasomnias and restless sleep

## Tonsillectomy Indications and Contraindications

### *Absolute Indications*

- tonsillar hyperplasia resulting in SDB or OSA associated with cor pulmonale
- suspected malignancy
- tonsillitis resulting in febrile convulsions (may require a Quinsy tonsillectomy)
- persistent or recurrent tonsillar hemorrhage
- failure to thrive (not attributable to other causes)

### *Relative Indications (AAO-HNS Guidelines)*

- <u>Recurrent Acute Tonsillitis</u>
    1. **Paradise Criteria**: 5–7 infections in 1 year, 5 infections/year × 2 years, or 3 infections/year × 3 years, or >2 weeks of missed school or work in 1 year (infections defined as sore throat with 1 or more of fever >38.3°C, cervical adenopathy, tonsillar exudate, or positive strep test)
    2. full 1-year period of observation is recommended for all patients but not necessary if complications occur (hospital admission, Lemierre syndrome, family history of rheumatic heart disease, numerous infections in a single household)
- recurrent acute tonsillitis not meeting above criteria but with multiple antibiotic allergy/intolerance, PFAPA, aphthous stomatitis, pharyngitis and adenitis, or history of peritonsillar abscess
- peritonsillar abscess (usually wait for second occurrence)
- chronic tonsillitis with persistent sore throat, halitosis, or cervical adenitis

- dysphagia (not attributable to other causes)
- drooling within the context of severe tonsillar hyperplasia
- tonsillolithiasis
- orofacial or dental disorders (results in a narrow upper airway)
- *Streptococcus* carrier unresponsive to medical management
- recurrent or chronic otitis media

### Contraindications

- leukemia, hemophilia, agranulocytosis, uncontrolled systemic disease (diabetes, TB)
- Relative Contraindications: cleft palate, acute infection

## Adenoidectomy Indications and Contraindications

### Absolute Indications

- adenoid hyperplasia resulting in SDB or OSA associated with cor pulmonale
- nasal obstruction associated with orofacial abnormalities
- failure to thrive (not attributable to other causes)

### Relative Indications

- recurrent acute adenoiditis (5–7 infections in 1 year, 5 infections/year × 2 years, or 3 infections/year × 3 years, or >2 weeks of missed school or work in 1 year)
- chronic adenoiditis with persistent sore throat, halitosis, or cervical adenitis
- swallowing difficulties (not attributable to other causes)
- drooling within the context of adenoid hyperplasia
- recurrent or chronic otitis media (second set of PE tubes) or rhinosinusitis

### Contraindications

- cleft palate; if sleep-disordered breathing or OSA can consider superior partial adenoidectomy
- **velopharyngeal insufficiency** (submucous cleft palate, hypernasal speech, nasal regurgitation)

## Tonsillectomy and Adenoidectomy Complications

### General Complications

- throat pain, otalgia, postop nausea/vomiting, delayed feeding, voice changes, hemorrhage, death

- <u>Mortality rate</u>: 1:16,000–35,000 (anesthetic complication and hemorrhage)
- <u>Traumatic Complications</u>: injury to eyes, lips, tongue, teeth, nerves, local vascular structures, larynx, pharyngeal wall, soft palate; jaw dislocation and fracture of the mandibular condyle

## Hemorrhagic Complications

- most common serious complication (0.5–5%)
- <u>Types</u>
  1. **Intraoperative**: arterial injury such as aberrant carotid artery, retained tonsillar tissue, tears in posterior pharyngeal wall
  2. **Immediate Postoperative** (<24 hours; 0.2–2.2%): similar to intraoperative, may be due to inadequate hemostasis during surgery
  3. **Delayed** (>24 hours; 0.1–3%): usually 5–10 days postop, due to eschar sloughing
- <u>Rx</u>: intraoperative pressure packing, hemostatic agents (eg, thrombin, cellulose, microfibrillar collagen), suction cautery, sutures, posterior nasopharyngeal pack (for recalcitrant intraoperative bleeding), external carotid artery ligation (life-threatening bleeding), embolization; very mild delayed postoperative bleeding may sometimes be addressed in the treatment room in a cooperative patient with topical hemostatic agents, if unsuccessful proceed to operating room

## Nonhemorrhagic Complications

- **Anesthetic Complications**: airway fire (<u>Rx</u>: avoid airway leaks, remove endotracheal tube, water irrigation), laryngospasm, difficult intubation, endotracheal tube kinking, iatrogenic premature extubation, postoperative opioid overmedication
- **Postoperative Airway Compromise**: rare, may occur from dislodged clot, dislodged adenotonsillar tissue, postoperative oropharyngeal edema, or retropharyngeal hematoma; <u>Rx</u>: manage airway (reintubation, surgical airway), corticosteroids, address retropharyngeal hematoma
- **Dehydration**: typically due to pain; <u>Rx</u>: analgesics, parenteral hydration
- **Pulmonary Edema**: caused by the sudden relief of airway obstruction from long-standing adenotonsillar hyperplasia resulting in a sudden drop of intrathoracic pressure, increased pulmonary blood volume, and increased hydrostatic pressure; may occur immediately or after a few hours; <u>Rx</u>: positive end-expiratory pressure ventilation, mild diuresis

- **Velopharyngeal Insufficiency**: results from an incompetent velopharyngeal inlet; increased risk with the presence of a submucosal cleft palate, history of nasal regurgitation, or preoperative hypernasality; <u>Rx</u>: speech therapy (typically resolves), pharyngeal flap or palatal lengthening for persistent problems; if persistent consider testing for 22q11 del

- **Nasopharyngeal Stenosis**: rare complication from scarring; <u>Rx</u>: difficult to treat (high rate of recurrence), may consider pharyngeal flaps or stents

- **Eustachian Tube Dysfunction**: from scarring and stenosis of the eustachian tube orifice; <u>Rx</u>: pressure equalization tubes, prevent by avoiding curettage or cautery near torus tubarius

- **Aspiration Pneumonia**: rare, occurs from aspiration of blood clots of adenotonsillar tissue

- **Atlantoaxial (C1–C2) Subluxation (Grisel Syndrome)**: spread of inflammation from the oropharyngeal to the cervical ligaments resulting in laxity and spinal cord compression; rare, increased risk with **Down syndrome**; <u>Rx</u>: orthopedic consult, may need antibiotics, cervical collar

- **Eagle Syndrome**: long styloid process previously covered by the tonsils or new osteitis and reactive styloid calcification, which gives symptoms of unilateral neck pain, sore throat, and dysphagia after tonsillectomy; <u>Rx</u>: NSAIDs, pain control, local steroid injection, partial styloidectomy

- **Sickle Cell Crisis**: consider a preoperative CBC and sickle cell screen in African American children; if positive, consult hematology and avoid hypoxia and hypothermia perioperatively to preven a crisis; <u>Rx</u>: if a crisis occurs, treat with oxygen, pain control, and blood transfusions; monitor for strokes, ischemic attacks, seizures

- **Nonresolution of Symptoms**: parental counseling on this possibility is important; more common in Down syndrome, obese patients (60–80% persistent SDB)

# Other Surgical Treatments for Obstructive Sleep Apnea

## Nasal Surgery

- consider septoplasty at ~15–16 years old, earlier if nasal septal deviation is very severe and is the obvious cause of OSA

**Base of Tongue and Tongue Reduction** (*see* p. 173)

**Mandibular Distraction Osteogenesis (MDO)**

- progressive elongation of native mandible and soft tissue envelope by performing bilateral sagittal osteotomies and placement of internal or external distraction devices
- Indications: **micrognathia/retrognathia**, airway obstruction and feeding difficulties, tracheostomy decannulation, severe obstructive sleep apnea, hemifacial microsomia; commonly performed for Pierre-Robin Sequence and Treacher Collins, Nager, velocardiofacial and Pfeiffer syndromes; frequently allows patient with neonatal airway obstruction related to micrognathia/retrognathia to avoid tracheostomy or prolonged intubation as it relieves the supraglottic obstruction
- Phases: **latency** (1–5 days; shorter in toddlers/young children, wait 5–7 days in adults; allows hematoma formation and platelet-derived growth factor production; if too short may lead to fibrous union and if too long may lead to callus), **active distraction** (1–2 mm/day until supraglottic obstruction relieved), **consolidation** (4–12 weeks), **hardware removal**
- Complications: infection, scarring, nerve injury (marginal mandibular, inferior alveolar, facial nerve), dental injury (tooth bud injury with tooth loss, dentigerous cysts), malocclusion (anterior open bite), poor healing (malunion, nonunion, relapse), device failure, TMJ ankylosis
- Workup: required laryngoscopic airway assessment and **jaw thrust** maneuver (a distance of ≤3 mm between the posterior pharyngeal wall and the lingual root can be used as criterion to perform distraction), lateral cephalometric x-ray +/– 3D CT of facial bones

**Midface Advancement Techniques** (*see* p. 173–174)

**Tracheotomy** (*see* pp. 551–552)

# Vascular Anomalies of the Head and Neck

## Vascular Tumors

### *Infantile Hemangioma*

- most common benign pediatric tumor; most common head and neck neoplasm in children; **endothelial** origin

- presents at birth as a white spot (**Herald Patch**) or a superficial small spot; usually discovered a few weeks after birth if deep
- more common in females (3:1 ratio); 10% population incidence
- <u>Pathophysiology</u>: unknown, possibly from disrupted placental cells or stem cells
- <u>Histopathology</u>: immunohistochemical markers: GLUT1 (glucose transporter-1 protein) and LeY (Lewis Y antigen); biologic markers: β-fibroblast growth factor, urokinase
- <u>Stages</u>
  1. **Proliferative**: ≤12 months old, endothelial cell **hyperplasia**, elevated mast cells, multilaminar basement membrane
  2. **Involuting**: 50% regress by 5 years old, 70% by 7 years; fibrosis, decreased cellularity
  3. **Involuted:** soft mass of excess skin and fibrofatty tissue, scarring, telangiectasias, atrophy
- <u>Types</u>
  1. **Superficial/Cutaneous (Strawberry or Capillary Hemangioma)**: bright strawberry-red color
  2. **Deep (Cavernous Hemangioma)**: covered by skin, appear blue
  3. **Compound**: also known as mixed
- <u>Classification</u>
  1. **Focal**: localized
  2. **Segmental**: CN V distribution (beard distribution), 60% airway involvement, low threshold for endoscopy; ocular involvement can lead to blindness; PHACES (*see following*)
  3. **Disseminated**
- **PHACES Syndrome**: **P**osterior cranial fossa anomalies (requires MRI), **H**emangioma (facial segmental), **A**rterial/carotid anomalies, **C**ardiac anomaly/**C**oarctation of the aorta (requires cardiac echo), **E**ye anomaly, **S**ternal pit; consider PHACES workup in all patients with large segmental hemangiomas; more common in females (90%)
- **Maffucci Syndrome**: multiple deep hemangiomas +/- visceral vascular lesions; dyschondroplasia; chondrosarcoma in 25% of patients
- <u>Complications</u>: in 20%; cosmetic deformity, amblyopia (eye involvement), ulceration (10%), infection, bleeding (rare, reassure parents that it will not "burst"), airway compromise (laryngeal), thrombocytopenia, and high output cardiac failure (rare)
- <u>Dx for Subglottic Hemangioma</u>: endoscopy (avoid biopsy), CT and MRI may confirm diagnosis; PA and lateral neck x-rays may show unilateral subglottic lesion or posterior subglottic lesion

**H&N SSx**

- **Cutaneous**: may present anywhere in the head and neck, (concerning in the eyelid and orbit); common in the parotid and oral cavity (lip), 1% of children with a cutaneous lesion will have a subglottic hemangioma
- **Laryngeal**: polypoid or sessile lesions, present with inspiratory or biphasic stridor within the first few months of life that is worse with crying (engorgement), dysphonia, dysphagia, seldom causes bleeding in the larynx, cyanosis; most common in the left posterolateral **subglottic** quadrant, **50% of children with a subglottic hemangioma will have a cutaneous lesion**
- **Nasal**: most commonly in Little's area (Kiesselbach's plexus) or inferior turbinate
- **Ear/Periauricular**: may deform the ear (CHL)
- **Parotid**: 50% parotid hemangiomas associated with cutaneous hemangiomas
- 20% have multiple hemangiomas

**Management**

- if >3 hemangiomas, consider abdominal ultrasound for occult lesions (eg, liver)
- management depends on complications (**VASCO**: impaired **V**ision or hearing, **A**irway compromise, impaired **S**wallowing, important **C**osmetic effect or with ulceration, high **O**utput cardiac failure)
- Hemangiomas Without Complications: observation, propranolol, oral steroids, intralesional steroids, interferon, vincristine, photocoagulation, surgical excision (cold or pulsed dye laser 585 nm)
- Hemangiomas With Complications: **propranolol** is new standard of care for hemangiomas in the proliferative stage, consider trial of oral steroids if >12 months old, consider vincristine or interferon for severe cases
- Propranolol Considerations: requires baseline vital signs, recent normal cardiovascular and pulmonary exams (contraindications: cardiogenic shock, sinus bradycardia, hypotension, greater than first-degree heart block, heart failure, bronchial asthma, drug hypersensitivity), ECG; no need for routine glucose screening, avoid prolonged fasting while on drug; usually responds within 2–12 weeks; continue until age 8–12 months; in patients with PHACES, higher stroke risk

### Congenital Hemangioma

- Classification
    1. **Rapidly Involuting (RICH)**: fully mature at birth and involutes by 6–14 months; typically GLUT-1 negative
    2. **Non Involuting (NICH)**: present at birth but does not involute; GLUT-1 negative; <u>Rx</u>: surgery; for large lesions, preoperative angiography with embolization can be helpful

### Tufted Angioma (TA) and Kaposiform Hemangioendothelioma (KHE)

- vascular tumor of arteries and veins that is **GLUT-1 negative**; considered a **spectrum** from TA to KHE
- congenital or acquired, >50% present before 1 year old; variable growth and regression patterns
- **KHE** is **aggressive** permeating muscle, soft tissue and bone
- <u>Histopathology</u>: hypercellular tufts of capillaries in the reticular dermis; may be associated with dilated lymphatic vessels; deeper spindle cells indicate KHE; positive for D2-40 (lymphatic marker)
- <u>SSx</u>: macules/patches (mottled red), plaques (red-purple, indurated), annular patterns of presentation; tenderness; hyperhidrosis, hypertrichosis
- visceral involvement almost always associated with platelet trapping (*see following*)
- <u>Dx</u>: **biopsy**; may need to be in more than 1 location
- <u>Rx</u>: observation, cryotherapy, pulse-dye laser, surgical excision, and more recently aspirin
- **Kasabach-Merritt Phenomenon**: sequestration of platelets and severe thrombocytopenia, microangiopathic hemolytic anemia, and consumptive coagulopathy in KHE or TA (not infantile hemangioma); suspect with rapidly enlarging lesion; can be life-threatening; <u>Rx</u>: drug combinations/chemotherapy or surgery, avoid blood products

## Vascular Malformations (VM)

- vascular channel malformations secondary to a defect in morphogenesis; characterized as **high flow** (arteriovenous) or **low flow** (lymphatic, capillary, venous) malformations
- differ from hemangiomas in that VM present at birth (although may manifest later secondary to hormonal changes, severe infections near vessels or trauma); grows with child (endothelium **hypertrophies**); and does not regress; sudden increase in size is concerning

- <u>Histopathology</u>: mature endothelium with normal mitosis (versus hemangioma, which has increased mitosis in the proliferative phase)
- <u>Associated Syndromes</u>: **Sturge-Weber syndrome** (SWS; unilateral port-wine stain in the $V_1$ distribution with extension to the leptomeninges), **Klippel-Trenaunay syndrome** (KTS; combination of capillary, venous, and lymphatic types of VM), **Parkes-Weber syndrome** (arteriovenous and capillary malformation in association with skeletal/soft tissue hypertrophy), blue rubber bleb (venous malformation with associated GI lesions)

### *Low Flow Vascular Malformations*

#### Lymphatic Malformation

- 90% present <3 years old (65% present at birth), may persist in adulthood
- associated with venous malformations (lymphatics and venous system develop concurrently)
- <u>Histopathology</u>: abnormal development or obstruction of primitive jugular lymphatics that undergo irregular growth with lymphoendothelial hyperplasia; increase in mast cells during proliferative phase, fewer mast cells during the involutional stage
- <u>Classification</u>: **macrocystic** (≥1 cysts, ≥2 mL), **microcystic** (<2 mL), **mixed;** (formerly called **cystic hygroma** and **lymphangioma**)
- <u>Staging (Modified de Serres)</u>: I: unilateral infrahyoid; II: unilateral suprahyoid; III: unilateral infrahyoid and suprahyoid; IV: bilateral suprahyoid; V: bilateral infrahyoid and suprahyoid; VI: bilateral infrahyoid, VII; retropharyngeal; M: mediastinal extension (I–III typically macrocystic and IV–VI typically microcystic)
- <u>SSx</u>: **soft painless compressible mass** (lymphatic dilation) **with** skin discoloration (macrocystic); soft noncompressible masses with mucosal or skin vesicles (microcystic); both types may cause dysphagia, dyspnea; may remain dormant; may become painful with acute infection
- <u>Dx</u>: physical exam, MRI
- <u>Complications</u>: respiratory distress from respiratory tract compression, infection (common, presents as a rapid enlargement of the malformation), disfigurement, spontaneous hemorrhage
- <u>Rx</u>: early conservative excision when symptomatic (spare vital structures), low rate of recurrence if completely removed (only 50% if gross tumor remains), sclerotherapy; if detected

prenatally and airway concerns, may require EXIT procedure
(*see* p. 554)

- <u>Sclerotherapy</u>: effective for lymphatic and venous
  malformations; agents include ethanol, bleomycin,
  doxycycline, polyvinyl alcohol; OK-432 not currently used in
  United States

### Capillary Malformation

- also called port-wine stain, stork bite, salmon patch (nape of the
  neck) or angel kiss (forehead)
- <u>Classification</u>: **medial** (salmon patch, usually lightens and
  disappears with time) or **lateral** (port-wine stain, always persists,
  usually follows CN V on face; involvement of lateral thigh and
  knee indicates Klippel-Trenaunay syndrome)
- <u>SSx</u>: bright red, scarlet at birth fades to pink in infants but then
  gradually enlarges and deepens to dark purple by adulthood;
  medial type is lighter at birth
- <u>Rx</u>: pulse-dye laser

### Venous Malformation

- **ectatic** venous channel network which has a tendency to grow
  slowly in childhood, then expand rapidly with hormonal changes
  or trauma; often involve the aerodigestive tract
- <u>SSx</u>: **compressible** mass, skin discoloration (none to dark blue/
  purple); airway obstruction, dysphagia; symptoms often get worse
  with recumbent position or Valsalva
- <u>Dx</u>: physical exam, MRI
- <u>Complications</u>: congestion, thrombosis and **phleboliths**, pain,
  distal emboli (large lesions)
- <u>Rx</u>: surgery, laser, sclerotherapy (small lesions); heparin can be
  used to reduce thrombosis

## *High Flow Vascular Malformations*

### Arteriovenous Malformation (AVM)

- **shunting** between the arterial and venous systems via
  anomalous capillary beds
- typically small and stable in childhood, then rapid growth in
  2nd–3rd decade of life with puberty and/or trauma
- <u>Staging (Schobinger)</u>: stage I: quiescent; stage II: expansion
  (bruit, thrill, warm throbbing); stage III: destruction (ulcers,
  bleeding, bony changes); stage IV: systemic (congestive heart
  failure, left ventricular hypertrophy)

- <u>SSx</u>: warm, pulsatile intermittently growing lesion with skin discoloration; **bruit**
- <u>Dx</u>: physical exam, pulsed Doppler, CTA, MRA and sometimes still digital angiography
- <u>Complications</u>: local tissue destruction, hemorrhage
- <u>Rx</u>: embolization; some require surgical excision

# PEDIATRIC RHINOLOGY

## Nasal Disease

### Congenital Nasal Disorders and Neonatal Nasal Obstruction

- newborns are **preferential nasal breathers** for 6–20 weeks (variable)
- nasal obstruction considered in newborns with tachypnea, **cyclical cyanosis** (worse with feeding, improve with crying), difficulty with feeding, failure to thrive, rhinorrhea, unable to pass 6 French flexible suction catheter
- <u>Dx</u>: assessment for dysmorphisms (telecanthus, broad nasal bridge, nasal pits), ocular discharge, periocular infection/edema, anterior rhinoscopy, nasal endoscopy, oral exam (palate arching or clefting), CT or MRI if tumor suspicion
- <u>DDx</u>: rhinitis of the newborn, viral rhinitis, dacryocystocele, piriform aperture stenosis, midnasal stenosis, choanal atresia, tumors (encephalocele, glioma, dermoid, teratoma, hemangioma), septal deviation (birth trauma, rare)
- <u>Rx</u>: address underlying cause, for bilateral obstruction or airway distress consider an oral cannula (McGovern nipple, oral airway) prior to intubation; tracheostomy reserved for severe cases

### Idiopathic Rhinitis of the Newborn

- consider after negative full investigation for nasal obstruction
- <u>Pathophysiology</u>: unclear; maternal estrogen, infectious (congenital syphilis ["snuffles", *see* pp. 577–578], chlamydia, other), early allergic rhinitis (high prevalence of familial atopy), ciliary dyskinesia, hypothyroidism
- <u>SSx</u>: abundant rhinorrhea (mucoid), nasal mucosal edema, stertor, tachypnea, poor feeding
- <u>Rx</u>: culture, frequent suctioning, nasal saline sprays, nasal steroid drops, avoid stenting if possible

# Allergic Rhinitis (AR)

- *see* pp. 32–40 and the following pediatric considerations
- <u>Associated SSx</u>: decreased energy and stamina, sleep disruption, limitations in organized sports and outdoor activities, poor school performance
- <u>Risk Factors</u>: urban living, obesity, no breast feeding, environmental tobacco smoke
- <u>Complications</u>: asthma exacerbation (united airway, asthma in 48% of patients with AR, but rhinitis in 80% of patients with asthma), sinusitis, otitis media, sleep disorders, craniofacial abnormalities (upturned nose or "allergic salute," elongated "adenoid" facies), decreased cognitive functioning
- immunotherapy protective against new sensitivities, helps prevent the development of asthma

# Nonallergic Rhinitis (*see* pp. 40–45)

## Choanal Atresia

- <u>Pathophysiology</u>: persistence of the bucconasal membrane or abnormal migration of neural crest cells into the nasal vault resulting in a complete bony (30%), mixed bony-membranous (70%), or membranous (rare) defect of the posterior nasal cavity; bony components are from the pterygoid plate (lateral) and vomer (medial)
- more common in females
- unilateral (65%, right-side predominance) more common than bilateral
- <u>SSx</u>: unilateral presents with rhinorrhea, anosmia, nasal obstruction; bilateral presents within first days of life with cycles of apnea and cyanosis followed by crying due to obligate nasal respiration in neonates
- <u>Dx</u>: mirror to detect condensation, attempt transnasal passage of 6 French catheter, attempt nose blowing with an occluded nostril, nasal endoscopy, CT
- <u>Associated Syndromes</u>: **CHARGE** syndrome (most common concurrent syndrome in bilateral atresia, 50%), Apert, Treacher Collins, Crouzon, trisomy 21, 22q11 deletion
- <u>Rx</u>: surgical repair via **transnasal (usually endoscopic)**, **transantral** (creation of large cavity for recurrent cases), **transseptal**, or **transpalatal** (classic operation, may interrupt orthodontic growth, less common today) approach; postop stenting less common with endoscopic repair; unilateral atresia may be repaired electively;

bilateral atresia must be addressed during first weeks of life, early measure includes establishing an oral airway (eg, with a McGovern nipple, which can also be used for feeding, or if needed a finger inserted into the oral cavity), intubation not usually required

# Nasal and Nasopharyngeal Masses

## Differential Diagnosis of Unilateral Pediatric Nasal Mass (*see* Table 10–1)

### Neurogenic Tumors

- **Fonticulus Frontalis**: embryologic space that normally fuses during the development of the frontal bones
- **Prenasal Space**: embryologic space between the nasal bone and nasal cartilage
- **Foramen Cecum**: region between ethmoid and frontal bones, connects with prenasal space
- Pathophysiology: dura projects through the foramen cecum, the fonticulus frontalis (**intranasally**), or the prenasal space into skin (**extranasally**) with failure of anterior neuropore closure
- Dx: MRI/CT to evaluate intracranial extension, do not biopsy

**TABLE 10–1.** Differential Diagnosis of a Unilateral Pediatric Nasal Mass

| | |
|---|---|
| Vascular | Juvenile nasopharyngeal angiofibroma (JNA) |
| | Hemangioma |
| | Arteriovenous malformation (AVM) |
| Infectious/inflammatory | Polyp |
| | Rhinolith |
| Neoplastic/mass | Encephalocele |
| | Glioma |
| | Neurofibroma |
| Drug-related | |
| Idiopathic | |
| Congenital | Nasolacrimal duct cyst |
| Autoimmune/allergic | |
| Traumatic | Foreign body |
| Endocrine | |

### Encephalocele

- Pathophysiology: failed closure of neuropore or failed migration of neural crest cells results in ependymal-lined meninges herniation through the base of skull; communicates with subarachnoid space (CSF filled)
- more common in lumbar-sacral region; may have associated anomalies
- Types by Contents
  1. **Meningocele**: meninges only
  2. **Meningoencephalocele**: meninges and brain elements
  3. **Meningoencephalocystocele**: meninges, brain, and a part of the ventricular system
- Types by Location
  1. **Occipital**: most common (75%)
  2. **Sincipital (Frontoethmoidal)**: defect occurs between frontal and ethmoid bones at the foramen cecum; **nasofrontal** (glabellar lesion), **nasoethmoidal** (lateral nose lesion), and **nasoorbital** (medial orbital wall lesion) subtypes
  3. **Basal**: transethmoidal, sphenoethmoidal, transsphenoidal, and sphenomaxillary subtypes
- SSx: bluish, soft, pulsatile, compressible mass that changes with straining and crying, transilluminates; intranasal encephaloceles often confused with nasal polyps
- Dx: CT and/or MRI reveals a bony defect, positive **Furstenburg test** (compression of the internal jugular vein causes increase in the size of the mass due to increased CSF pressure)
- Complications: meningitis, nasal obstruction, cosmetic deformity, hydrocephalus
- Rx: surgical excision similar to gliomas, must also close the dural defect to prevent CSF leak and brain herniation (neurosurgical consultation)

### Nasal Glioma

- Pathophysiology: sequestered glial tissue or "pinched-off encephalocele" results in unencapsulated collection of heterotopic glial cells
- 15% connect to dura by a fibrous stalk
- Location: extranasal (60%) or intranasal (30%), typically not midline
- SSx: firm, nonpulsatile mass, skin-covered, does not change in size with straining, noncompressible, does not transilluminate, may present as an intranasal polyp, broad nasal dorsum
- Dx: CT and/or MRI to evaluate for intracranial extension (15%), negative Furstenburg test

- <u>Complications</u>: meningitis, nasal obstruction, cosmetic deformity
- <u>Rx</u>: surgical excision (intranasal approach for small tumors, extranasal approach for larger tumors), may require craniotomy for intracranial involvement (neurosurgical consultation)

### Nasal Dermoid

- **most common midline nasal mass**
- <u>Pathophysiology</u>: defective obliteration of dural tissue in prenasal space or fonticulus frontalis forms a dermal cyst
- may contain both **mesodermal and ectodermal components**, including adnexal tissue (hair follicles, sweat glands, sebaceous glands)
- <u>Location</u>: most commonly at nasal dorsum but may occur anywhere from glabella to nasal tip (extranasal, intranasal, or intracranial)
- <u>SSx</u>: presents at birth; forms a fistulous tract, pit, or cyst; firm, noncompressible, does not transilluminate; tuft of hair may protrude from pit
- <u>Dx</u>: CT and/or MRI to evaluate for intracranial extension (25%), negative Furstenburg test
- <u>Complications</u>: meningitis, CSF leak, repeated local infection, cosmetic deformity
- <u>Rx</u>: meticulous excision, must excise complete tract (usually subcutaneous although may dive deep into nasal bone or intracranially)

## Rathke's Pouch Cyst

- <u>Pathophysiology</u>: persistent craniopharyngeal canal from failure of the obliteration of Rathke's pouch (a diverticulum of ectoderm that invaginates to form the anterior lobe of the hypophysis [pituitary] and pars intermedius)
- <u>Location</u>: nasopharynx
- <u>SSx</u>: typically asymptomatic, smooth mass in nasopharynx, may enlarge and impinge on the pituitary
- <u>Dx</u>: CT or MRI, biopsy
- <u>Rx</u>: endoscopic removal or marsupialization for symptomatic lesions, add antibiotics if infected

## Dacryocystocele (Nasolacrimal Duct Cyst)

- <u>Pathophysiology</u>: failure of opening of the distal nasolacrimal duct with cyst formation from accumulation of secretions
- <u>Location</u>: nasolacrimal duct (anteriorly in the inferior meatus)

- <u>SSx</u>: usually asymptomatic, epiphora, nasal obstruction, may cause respiratory distress and difficulty feeding in infants with large obstructive cysts (obligate nasal breathing)
- most (~85%) spontaneously resolve by 9 months of age
- <u>Dx</u>: nasal exam, nasal endoscopy, CT or MRI
- <u>Rx</u>: endoscopic marsupialization for symptomatic cysts (if presence of infection, respiratory obstruction, feeding difficulties) or antibiotics with excision for infected lesions (consider ophthalmology consultation)

## Thornwaldt's Cyst

- <u>Pathophysiology</u>: arises from a pharyngeal notochord remnant (pharyngeal bursa or pouch of Luschka)
- <u>Location</u>: **nasopharynx** (midline, surrounded by adenoid tissue)
- <u>SSx</u>: asymptomatic, smooth mass found in nasopharynx; rare infection, postnasal drip, referred otalgia, or otitis media with effusion
- <u>Dx</u>: CT or MRI, biopsy
- <u>Rx</u>: observation, antibiotics with marsupialization or excision for infected lesions

*NOTE: see also* inflammatory nasal masses (pp. 14–16), juvenile nasopharyngeal angiofibroma (JNA; pp. 17–18), keratotic papilloma (pp. 16–17), other benign tumors (pp. 18–19, 537), rhabdomyosarcoma (pp. 605–606), other malignancy (p. 607)

# Paranasal Sinus Disease

## Pediatric Rhinosinusitis

- typically involves maxillary and anterior ethmoid sinuses (sphenoid and frontal sinuses are less developed)
- <u>Most Common Bacterial Pathogens</u>: *Streptococcus, S. aureus, M. catarrhalis, H. influenzae* (acute); α-hemolytic *Streptococcus*, coagulase negative *Staphylococcus, P. aeruginosa, Peptostreptococcus, Bacteroides* (chronic)
- <u>Most Common Viral Pathogens</u>: rhinovirus, adenovirus, influenza, parainfluenza
- <u>SSx</u>: similar presentation to URI; however, tends to include cough, halitosis, persistent nasal obstruction, rhinorrhea, and fever; less facial pain than adults

- <u>Dx</u>: similar to adults; however, for persistent rhinosinusitis must consider adenoid hyperplasia, cystic fibrosis (presence of polyps), immunodeficiencies (IgG subclasses), asthma, and GERD; if recurrent sinusitis, pneumonia, and bronchiectasis, perform an immune workup
- <u>CT Indications</u>: severe illness/toxic, acute episode not resolving in 48–72 hours with treatment, immunocompromise, suppurative complications

## *Management*

- <u>Antibiotics</u>: similar to adults
- <u>Adjunctive Medical Agents</u>: saline irrigations, nasal corticosteroids, oral decongestants, mucolytics
- <u>Allergy Management</u>: (*see previous*)
- **Antral Lavage**: controversial efficacy, addresses only maxillary sinus, typically requires multiple lavages; useful for culture-directed medical therapy, reserve for failure of therapy (after 72 hours), severely toxic or immunocompromised patient or workup for fever of unknown origin
- **Adenoidectomy**: may harbor pathogens and block drainage, symptom improvement in ≤50%
- **Functional Endoscopic Sinus Surgery (FESS)**: <u>Indications</u>: select patients who fail extensive medical management and have significant effect on quality of life, cystic fibrosis (*see following*), sinusitis complications (orbital, intracranial), mucocele or antrochoanal polyps, fungal rhinosinusitis; <u>Anatomy</u>: the relationships of the anterior ethmoids, middle meatus, uncinate process, ethmoid infundibulum, semilunar hiatus, and bulla ethmoidalis are relatively constant landmarks throughout life, sphenoid and frontal sinuses typically do not need to be explored since they do not develop until 8–12 years old, may also consider balloon catheterization techniques (*see* p. 56)
- **Mini-Functional Endoscopic Sinus Surgery (Mini-FESS)**: fewer complications, involves removing the uncinate process, opening the maxillary os (or just identifying the opening), and taking down the ethmoid bulla or anterior ethmoids

# Cystic Fibrosis and Rhinosinusitis

- **Cystic Fibrosis (CF)**: autosomal recessive disorder caused by a mutation in the CF transmembrane conductance regulator (CFTR) gene (chromosome 7) that leads to impaired transmembrane chloride ion transport; results in abnormal exocrine gland function; manifests as a progressive pulmonary disorder with associated pancreatic (eg, type I diabetes), hepatobiliary, genitourinary, and sinus disease

- <u>Pathophysiology</u>: thick tenacious mucus keeps bacteria from being cleared and leads  to ciliary dyskinesia and prevents antibiotics from being effective
- universally develop chronic pansinusitis; 10% associated obstructive nasal polyps
- <u>Dx</u>: sweat chloride test (>60–90 mmol per liter), genetic testing
- <u>Pathogens</u>: higher risk for pseudomonal infections, *Burkholderia capacia, S. aureus* (including methicillin-resistant varieties), *E. coli,* and *Aspergillus fumigatus*

## Medical Management

- aggressive nasal hygiene with mucolytics, topical corticosteroids, and **saline irrigations** (consider irrigation with hypertonic saline and antipseudomonal antibiotics such as tobramycin)
- consider sinus aspirate for culture to detect *Pseudomonas*
- long-term antibiotics including possible parenteral administration
- aerosolized antibiotic inhaled treatment with gentamicin or tobramycin

## Surgical Management

- in general, avoid surgical management (high recurrence rate, increases nasal scarring, patients do not tolerate long-term general anesthesia due to retained pulmonary secretions, higher risk of bleeding from liposoluble vitamins deficiency)
- <u>Indications</u>: uncontrolled pain, persistent nasal obstruction, mucoceles, unresolved fevers, fungal infections, pulmonary exacerbations that correlate with sinonasal disease
- <u>Surgical Considerations</u>: may be vitamin K deficient (supplement), surgery should be kept <1 hour to avoid respiratory compromise; recurrence rates are high, thus perform polypectomy for relief of obstruction and not for cure (keep landmarks); wide maxillary antrostomies (endoscopic medial maxillectomy under investigation)
- <u>Postoperative Care</u>: hospitalize postoperatively, aggressive irrigations, postoperative sinus debridement (in operating room for younger patients)

# Primary Ciliary Dyskinesia (*see* p. 52)

# PEDIATRIC LARYNGOESOPHAGOLOGY
## Anatomy and Embryology

- *see also* pp. 94–96

## Pediatric Airway Anatomy

- neonatal epiglottis engages the soft palate forming a central tunnel for airway and the lateral sides for food to allow simultaneous respiration and deglutition (infant epiglottis is omega shaped)
- neonates are obligate nasal breathers until age 2 months because of lack of coordination of oral/respiratory functions and epiglottis location with uvula overlap
- infant's larynx is at the level of C2–3, descends during infancy and sits at C6–7 by adulthood
- location of the smallest cross-sectional area in the infant airway is the subglottis, whereas in adults it is the glottis inlet (rima)
- **1 mm** of subglottic edema in the neonate can reduce airway by **more than 50%**
- **approximate endotracheal tube size = (age + 16)/4**

## Laryngeal Embryology

### *Development of the Respiratory Primordium*

1. at the fourth week of development the respiratory primordium appears as an outgrowth (**laryngotracheal groove**) from the ventral wall of the foregut (primitive pharynx)
2. the laryngotracheal groove evaginates to form the **laryngotracheal diverticulum** dividing the foregut into a dorsal portion (esophagus) and ventral portion (larynx, trachea, and lung) separated by the **tracheoesophageal septum**
3. the respiratory primordium (ventral portion) maintains open communication with the pharynx through the laryngeal orifice
4. epithelial proliferation obliterates the laryngeal lumen, **recanalization** occurs by the 10th week (no recanalization results in stenosis)
5. 3 tissue swellings (1 median swelling behind the hypobranchial eminence which forms the epiglottis, and 2 lateral swellings that form the arytenoid cartilages) surround the laryngeal orifice

### Branchial Arch Derivatives

- **II**: lesser horn and upper portion of the hyoid bone
- **III**: greater horn and lower portion of the hyoid bone
- **IV**: supraglottic structures (thyroid cartilage), superior laryngeal nerve (SLN) structures (cricothyroid muscle and pharyngeal constrictors)
- **V/VI**: glottic/subglottic structures (cricoid, cuneiform, corniculate, and arytenoid cartilages) and recurrent laryngeal nerve (RLN) structures (all intrinsic laryngeal muscles except the cricothyroid)

## Esophageal Embryology

- epithelial proliferation obliterates the lumen, recanalization occurs by 8th–10th week (abnormal recanalization results in congenital stenosis)

# Evaluation of the Stridulous Child

## Initial Management

- *see also* pp. 102–106
- **Evaluate Airway**: clinical determination of severity/stability of problem, rate of progression, associated conditions (eg, polytrauma); establishes need for immediate management
- **Establish Airway**: if emergent condition then bag mask, intubate (oral/nasal), or perform surgical airway

## Initial Exam

- consider initial airway evaluation and treatment in OR if suspected foreign body aspiration or epiglottitis
- <u>History</u>: onset of stridor, speed of progression, witnessed choking episode, order of birth, delivery history, history of intubation, medications and allergies, associated symptoms (drooling, hoarseness, cough, feeding problems, failure to thrive)
- <u>H&N Exam</u>: respiratory rate, retractions, neck landmarks, cutaneous lesions (eg, hemangioma), consider passing suction catheter/flexible endoscope through both nares, flexible nasopharyngoscopy, and laryngoscopy
- **inspiratory stridor** suggests supraglottic or glottic pathology, **biphasic stridor** suggests glottic or subglottic, **expiratory stridor** alone suggests distal tracheal or bronchial

## Ancillary Testing

- **CXR**: evaluate for unilateral subglottic lesion (eg, hemangioma), foreign body aspiration (**inspiratory/expiratory CXR** may demonstrate the foreign body and/or diaphragmatic flattening and mediastinal shift), other causes
- **CT Neck/Chest**: vascular compression
- **MRI Neck/Chest**: extrinsic compression, best for lymphovascular malformation workup
- **Modified Barium Swallow (MBS)**: for concern about aspiration exacerbating airway symptoms
- **Flexible Endoscopic Evaluation of Swallow (FEES)**: for concern of aspiration exacerbating airway symptoms
- **Pulmonary Function Testing**: evaluate for a fixed obstruction and airway reactivity
- **Labs**: consider arterial blood gas for long-standing airway obstruction

## Pediatric Microlaryngoscopy and Bronchoscopy

- performed under general anesthetic with **spontaneous ventilation** (can consider apnea with jet ventilation in certain circumstances)
- topical anesthetic (lidocaine) is often applied to the vallecula and larynx to reduce laryngospasm
- a telescope or ventilating bronchoscope is advanced through the vocal folds and the more distal airway is examined after supraglottic findings noted; evaluate for **malacia** (intrinsic or extrinsic), **stenosis** (location, length, etiology), **fistulae** and/or laryngeal **cleft**, complete **rings**, **masses**, other lesions
- airway may be sized with endotracheal tubes placed into the subglottis; appropriate tube for the patient will leak air around it at less than **capillary perfusion pressure** (approximately 20–30 cmH$_2$O); note **Cotton-Myer grading scale** (*see* Figure 10–1)

## Pediatric Tracheotomy

- prolonged intubation (often for months) with properly sized uncuffed endotracheal tube is generally preferred over tracheotomy in premature infants and full term neonates; exception is a patient known to have a chronic ventilation need (then performed after patient >2 kg)
- hyoid overlies superior laryngeal cartilage
- <u>Technique</u>: small vertical or horizontal incision (~1 cm), limited fat removal, divide strap musculature in the midline and retract

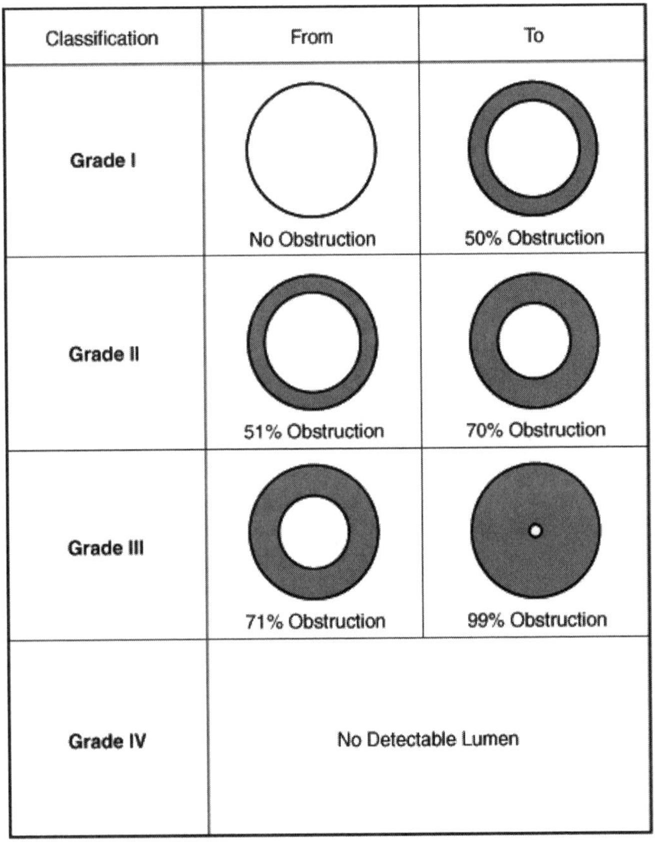

| Classification | From | To |
|---|---|---|
| **Grade I** | No Obstruction | 50% Obstruction |
| **Grade II** | 51% Obstruction | 70% Obstruction |
| **Grade III** | 71% Obstruction | 99% Obstruction |
| **Grade IV** | No Detectable Lumen | |

**FIGURE 10–1**. Cotton-Myer grading system for subglottic stenosis (Used with permission. Myer CM III, O'Connor DM, Cotton RT. Proposed grading system for subglottic stenosis based on endotracheal tube sizes. *Ann Otol Rhinol Laryngol* 1994;103:319).

laterally, stay sutures placed laterally through trachea on either side of proposed tracheotomy incision and labeled "right" and "left," consideration of "maturation sutures" in 4 quadrants approximating the skin to the pretracheal fashion, tracheotomy incision most commonly at 2nd or 3rd tracheal ring, ICU care until first trach tube change on postop day 5–7

- consider endoscopy to evaluate for subglottic stenosis or suprastomal granuloma prior to downsizing or decannulating trach tube
- pediatric trach tubes do not have inner cannulas, raises the risk of plugging and airway obstruction

# Evaluation of the Dysphagic or Aspirating Child

## Initial Evaluation

- <u>History</u>: coughing/choking with feeds, reflux behavior, chronic cough, nasopharyngeal regurgitation, recurrent pneumonia, suspicion of aspiration (neurologic condition, syndrome associated with cranial neuropathy or decreased tone/sensation, known vocal fold mobility issue); family or personal history of atopy, eczema, and reactive airway disease
- <u>Physical Exam</u>: similar to exam for the stridulous child (*see previous*); attention to cranial nerve exam, flexible laryngoscopy while awake (vocal fold mobility, handling of secretions)

## Ancillary Testing

- **Modified Barium Swallow (MBS)**: confirm aspiration and evaluate for what consistencies are safe to consume and whether swallowing maneuvers are beneficial
- **Flexible Endoscopic Evaluation of Swallow (FEES)**: provides information on upper aerodigestive tract structure and function, secretion management, and aspiration
- **CXR**: evaluate for pneumonia
- **Chest CT**: evaluate for bronchiectasis in the case of long-standing aspiration
- **Barium Esophagram**: evaluate for H-type tracheoesophageal fistula
- **Brain MRI** considered if no obvious etiology for aspiration and a normal operative aerodigestive evaluation (*see following*)

## Consultation

- **Pulmonary Medicine**: for confirmed aspiration to assist in protection of the end organ
- **Gastroenterology**: for reflux behavior, dysphagia, family/personal history of atopy, evaluation of esophageal condition such as GERD associated with aspiration and reflux esophagitis, *H. pylori* infection, and eosinophilic esophagitis
- **Feeding Team**: for dysphagia/food refusal behavior with no aspiration or atopic concerns

## Operative Aerodigestive Evaluation

- patients with confirmed aspiration and/or refractory dysphagia and no obvious cause (eg, vocal fold immobility after PDA ligation) may undergo microlaryngoscopy and bronchoscopy to evaluate for a structural abnormality of the aerodigestive tract such as a laryngeal cleft or H-type tracheoesophageal fistula

- if possible, patients may also undergo simultaneous pulmonary flexible bronchoscopy for bronchoalveolar lavage for cytology and microbiology as well as esophagogastroduodenoscopy with biopsy and pH impedance probe placement by gastroenterology

## Pediatric Management Options

- <u>Medical Management</u>: includes thickening agents and swallowing rehabilitation
- **Feeding Tube**: for severe and/or irreversible swallowing dysfunction and aspiration
- **Fundoplication**: for confirmed GERD associated aspiration pneumonia unresponsive to more conservative interventions
- <u>Salivary Management</u>: if excessive sialorrhea and/or aspiration of saliva causing respiratory illness
  1. **Botulinum Toxin**: injection into submandibular and parotid glands
  2. **Submandibular Gland Excision and Parotid Duct Ligation**: for severe cases (surgical rerouting of submandibular ducts also an option in patients who do not aspirate)
- **Vocal Fold Medialization**
- **Tracheotomy**: provides access for pulmonary hygiene
- **Laryngotracheal Separation**: chronic, severe, life-threatening aspiration; prevents vocalization; considered in neurologically devastated patient

# Congenital Disorders of the Aerodigestive Tract

## Congenital High Airway Obstruction Syndrome (CHAOS)

- identified on prenatal ultrasound and confirmed on MRI
- <u>Etiology</u>: includes obstruction by congenital mass, such as teratoma, epignathus (teratoma arising from the basisphenoid region and filling the oral cavity; often protruding through the hard palate), lymphovascular malformation
- may be delivered by **EX** utero **In**Trapartum (**EXIT**) procedure with efforts to secure the airway at delivery

# Laryngomalacia

- most common congenital laryngeal anomaly
- most common cause of **stridor** in neonates and infants
- associated with secondary airway lesions (eg, subglottic stenosis, tracheomalacia)
- <u>Pathophysiology</u>: immature, constricted laryngeal anatomy with poor structural support and/or tone
- <u>SSx</u>: **intermittent inspiratory stridor that may improve in prone position**; exacerbated with feeding, crying, or when placed on back; retractions, poor weight gain, failure to thrive; presents within weeks of birth; normal voice; usually self-limited and resolved by 18 months
- <u>Dx</u>: H&P, flexible laryngoscopy
- <u>Most Common Laryngeal Findings</u>
    1. inward collapse of A–E folds and arytenoid cartilage into laryngeal inlet during inspiration
    2. epiglottis collapse into laryngeal inlet during inspiration
    3. short aryepiglottic folds
- <u>Rx</u>: observation (typically resolves with growth), antireflux medication may improve symptoms, supraglottoplasty (release short A–E folds +/- remove excess mucosal tissue from arytenoids)

# Congenital Bilateral Vocal Fold Immobility

- <u>Etiology</u>
    1. **Neurologic: Arnold-Chiari Malformation and Meningomyelocele**
    2. **Iatrogenic:** birth trauma, increased risk with complicated deliveries or forceps delivery (traction injury, may be temporary)
    3. **Idiopathic**
- **Arnold-Chiari Malformation**: compression of fourth ventricle → decreased CSF outflow → compression of brainstem or increased intracranial pressure (ICP) → brainstem herniation → traction against vagal rootlets in foramen magnum → stretch injury to vagus nerves; always consider in neonate; types of varying severity exist (eg, syringomyelia, Dandy-Walker malformation); <u>Rx</u>: decompression to relieve tension
- **SSx: stridor,** feeding difficulties, strong voice, cyanosis, apnea
- <u>Dx</u>: flexible laryngoscopy, MRI to evaluate for Arnold-Chiari malformation, consider operative evaluation for vocal fold fixation if etiology suggests traumatic intubation, consider genetics consultation, laryngeal EMG (investigational); evaluate for aspiration

- <u>Rx</u>: may spontaneously resolve, consider observation, various surgical options from tracheotomy to direct vocal fold management (lateralization, arytenoidopexy, arytenoidectomy, posterior cordotomy, posterior cricoid cartilage grafting, laryngeal reinnervation; *see also* p. 123)

## Congenital Webs

- most commonly **anteriorly** based, thin or thick
- <u>Pathophysiology</u>: incomplete recanalization of the airway at 10th week of embryologic development
- <u>Types</u>: supraglottic (2%), **glottic** (75%), subglottic (7%)
- <u>SSx</u>: weak cry at birth, aphonia, variable degrees of respiratory obstruction (inspiratory or biphasic stridor)
- <u>Dx</u>: flexible nasopharyngoscopy, direct laryngoscopy
- <u>Rx</u>: genetics evaluation (eg, 22q11 deletion); endoscopic lysis +/- brief period of intubation or endoscopic keel placement, open lysis via laryngofissure with keel placement, may require tracheotomy

## Congenital Subglottic Stenosis

- <u>Pathophysiology</u>: incomplete recanalization; small diameter or elliptical cricoid cartilage (less than 3.5 mm diameter is considered abnormal); first tracheal ring partially telescoped under cricoid cartilage (trapped ring)
- <u>Types</u>
  1. **Membranous:** circumferential, thickened mucous glands or fibrous tissue
  2. **Cartilaginous:** abnormal cricoid, trapped ring
  3. **Mixed**
- <u>Cotton-Myer Grading Scale</u>: **I**: ≤50% obstruction; **II**: 51–70%; **III**: 71–99%; **IV**: 100% (no detectable lumen) (*see* Figure 10–1)
- <u>SSx</u>: **biphasic stridor**, may mimic croup or recurrent URI, failure to thrive
- <u>Dx</u>: microlaryngoscopy and bronchoscopy

### *Management*

- <u>Medical Management</u>: antireflux medication (consider GI referral if symptomatic)
- consider observation with airway surveillance if less symptomatic (eg, grade I, some grade II) as normal/appropriate subglottic growth occurs

- <u>Surgical Management</u>: endoscopic intervention; open surgical procedures for symptomatic grade I–II failing conservative management and grade III–IV inappropriate for endoscopic management
- **Anterior Cricoid Split +/- Augmentation**: originally described as alternative to tracheotomy for infants with subglottic stenosis who are <40 weeks gestation and no longer require ventilation, recent descriptions include use of anterior cartilage graft for augmentation
- **Posterior Cricoid Split:** endoscopic or open, indicated for posterior glottis/subglottic stenosis, may use costal graft, usually requires a period of intubation or stent placement unless performed in an older child, may also be used concurrently with an open anterior cricoid split +/- augmentation
- **Laryngotracheoplasty with Anterior and/or Posterior Lumen Augmentation**: requires cartilage grafts, may be used to reconstruct cricoid and tracheal rings
- **Cricotracheal Resection**: resection and reanastomosis technique involving resection of portion of cricoid and affected upper trachea
- **Tracheotomy**

## Congenital Tracheal Stenosis

- rare congenital cause of airway obstruction
- often due to **complete tracheal rings**
- associated with congenital cardiac abnormalities (eg, pulmonary artery sling)
- <u>Rx</u>: may be managed expectantly for less symptomatic patients; surgical correction includes tracheal resection and reanastomosis, slide tracheoplasty, augmentation procedures (pericardial patch)

## Tracheomalacia

### *Intrinsic*

- less common than laryngomalacia
- associated with premature infants and tracheoesophageal fistulas
- <u>Pathophysiology</u>: poor cartilaginous strength, low tone
- <u>SSx</u>: expiratory or biphasic stridor, barky cough, exacerbated with infection, usually self-limiting as cartilage stiffens with growth over years but may persist in children with tracheoesophageal fistula and a large pouch
- <u>Dx</u>: history, flexible tracheoscopy, bronchoscopy

- <u>Rx</u>: observation (typically resolves with growth), may require noninvasive ventilation, stenting, splinting, but often require tracheotomy for associated ventilation support

### Extrinsic

- extrinsic mass effect (eg, lymphovascular malformation)
- <u>Vascular Compression</u>
  1. **Double Aortic Arch**: most common vascular anomaly to cause stridor; right aortic arch persists, wraps around esophagus and trachea
  2. **Right Aortic Arch**
  3. **Anomalous Innominate Artery**
  4. **Anomalous Left Common Carotid**
  5. **Pulmonary Artery Sling**: left pulmonary artery originates from right pulmonary artery, slings around right mainstem bronchus, then between trachea and esophagus, associated with complete tracheal rings
  6. **Retroesophageal Right Subclavian Artery (Dysphagia Lusoria)**
- <u>SSx</u>: biphasic stridor (external compression of trachea), barking cough, dyspnea with feeding
- <u>Dx</u>: barium esophagram, CT with contrast, MRI
- <u>Rx</u>: symptomatic compression requires surgical intervention with thoracic surgery

## Laryngeal Cleft and Laryngotracheoesophageal Cleft

- absence of tissue between larynx/trachea and hypopharynx/esophagus
- <u>SSx</u>: mild clefts may present with stridor and dysphagia/aspiration/recurrent pneumonia; more severe clefts may present with respiratory distress at birth
- <u>Associations</u>: Opitz G/BBB syndrome, Pallister-Hall, tracheoesophageal fistula, esophageal atresia, laryngomalacia, congenital heart defects
- <u>Dx</u>: endoscopy
- <u>Ancillary Testing</u>: Modified barium swallow to evaluate for aspiration, CXR
- <u>Benjamin-Inglis Classification</u>: **I**: interarytenoid defect; **II**: cricoid involvement; **III** cervical trachea involvement; **IV** thoracic trachea involvement
- <u>Rx</u>: goal is securing airway and avoiding chronic aspiration; symptomatic type I–II and certain type III clefts can be repaired endoscopically, most type III and all type IV require open repair

### Tracheoesophageal Fistula (TEF)

- Pathophysiology
  1. **Congenital**: failure of recannulation of the esophagus or developmental failure of the tracheoesophageal septum
  2. **Acquired**: secondary to tracheostomy, long-term intubation, tumor, inflammation, trauma; results in communication between lumen of the esophagus and the trachea
- Types
  1. **Esophageal Atresia with Distal TEF: most common** (~85%)
  2. **Isolated Esophageal Atresia without TEF**: second most common (~10%), associated with polyhydramnios
  3. **Isolated Tracheoesophageal Fistula (H-type)**: rarely remains asymptomatic until later in life
  4. **Esophageal Atresia with Proximal TEF**
  5. **Esophageal Atresia with Proximal and Distal TEF**
- SSx: immediate gagging and cyanosis after birth, gas-filled stomach; may present later in life with cough, recurrent aspiration pneumonia, gagging; long-term symptoms include issues associated with tracheomalacia and poor esophageal motility
- Dx: barium esophagram, endoscopy
- Rx: division (and reconstruction of the trachea/esophagus as needed)

### Subglottic Hemangioma (*see* pp. 536–537)

## Acquired Laryngeal and Tracheal Lesions

### Acquired Glottic and Supraglottic Stenosis

- Causes: blunt trauma, endotracheal tube trauma, infection, caustic ingestion, foreign body
- SSx: inspiratory or biphasic stridor, dyspnea, cough
- Dx: flexible laryngoscopy, endoscopy
- Rx: endoscopic and open techniques described depending on degree of problem

### Angioedema (*see* p. 115)

### Acquired Subglottic and Tracheal Stenosis

- typically more common and more severe than congenital

- Etiology
  1. **Endotracheal Intubation**: pressure necrosis results in ulceration and cartilage exposure, healing occurs by secondary intention causing fibrosis and stenosis
  2. **Postoperative**: pressure necrosis from a high tracheotomy, cricothyroidotomy, or **failed previous airway surgery**
  3. **Granulomatous Disease**: tuberculosis (most common granulomatous disease of larynx), sarcoidosis, rhinoscleroma (*Klebsiella*), granulomatosis with polyangiitis (Wegener's)
  4. **Infectious**: leprosy (epiglottic and vocal fold ulceration), syphilis, blastomycosis, coccidiomycosis, histoplasmosis
  5. **Idiopathic**: amyloidosis, unknown
  6. **Trauma**: foreign body, caustic ingestion, blunt trauma, hematoma, thermal injury
  7. **Systemic**: connective tissue disorders, GERD (presumed cause), radiation effects
  8. **Neoplasia**: chondroma, fibroma, malignancy
- SSx: dyspnea, biphasic stridor, cough, dysphagia, cyanosis, exercise limitation
- Dx: endoscopy, CT of neck, directed labs for various etiologies
- Rx: surgical management similar to congenital subglottic stenosis

## Subglottic Cyst

- cause of stridor in a previously intubated infant
- Rx: consider unroofing endoscopically +/- cauterization of the base of the lesion
- propensity for recurrence

## Unilateral Vocal Fold Immobility

- most commonly iatrogenic from birth trauma, intubation, PDA ligation or aortic arch anomaly repair, or tracheoesophageal fistula repair
- *see also* pp. 119–123

# Infectious Laryngotracheal Airway Disorders

## Croup (Acute Laryngotracheobronchitis, LTB)
(*see* Table 10–2)

- most common infectious cause of stridor in children
- common in 1–5 year olds during fall and winter seasons
- primarily involves the subglottic region

**TABLE 10–2.** Contrasting Acute Laryngotracheobronchitis (Croup) and Epiglottitis

|  | Acute Laryngotracheobronchitis | Acute Epiglottitis |
| --- | --- | --- |
| Pathogen | Parainfluenza virus 1 | *Haemophilis influenzae b* |
| Age | <5 years old | 2–6 years old |
| Location | subglottic | supraglottic |
| Onset | gradual (days) | sudden onset (hours) |
| Cough | barky | normal |
| Posture | supine | upright |
| Drooling | no | yes |
| Fever | low-grade | high fevers |
| Radiographs | steeple sign | thumbprinting |
| Treatment | supportive | airway management and antibiotics |

- <u>Pathogen</u>: **parainfluenza 1 (most common cause)**, parainfluenza 3, influenza A, rhinovirus, respiratory syncytial virus
- <u>SSx</u>: inspiratory or biphasic stridor, **gradual** onset, long course (3–7 days), low-grade fever, relief in the recumbent position, **brassy/barky cough** (worse at night), hoarse, nontender larynx, no dysphagia, no drooling
- <u>Dx</u>: H&P, plain neck x-rays ("**steeple**" sign = narrowed subglottis on PA neck x-ray), flexible nasopharyngoscopy (not required)
- <u>Complications</u>: airway compromise
- <u>Rx</u>
  1. **Assess Airway**: intubation or tracheotomy rarely required unless there is a coexisting laryngeal abnormality (subglottic stenosis)
  2. **Medical Management**: humidified oxygen, corticosteroids, nebulized racemic epinephrine, antibiotics not required unless suspect bacterial superinfection
  3. **Endoscopy**: if no resolution with conservative management

## Bacterial Tracheitis (Exudative Tracheitis, Membranous Laryngotracheobronchitis)

- <u>Pathophysiology</u>: bacterial superinfection following viral URI prodrome
- <u>SSx</u>: thick secretions in airway, fibrinous sloughing (exudative) membrane in trachea, high fever, tender larynx and trachea

- <u>Dx</u>: clinical suspicion, lateral neck x-ray may show shaggy appearance of the trachea (membranes), flexible laryngoscopy may reveal exudative membranes in the subglottis and upper trachea, microlaryngoscopy and bronchoscopy
- <u>Rx</u>: aggressive pulmonary hygiene, parenteral antibiotics, microlaryngoscopy and bronchoscopy with membrane clearing and culture, may require intubation

## Diphtheria

- uncommon since immunization (milder form may present despite immunization)
- <u>Pathogen</u>: *Corynebacterium diphtheriae*
- <u>Risks</u>: nonimmunized children >6 years old
- <u>SSx</u>: sore throat; progressive airway obstruction; **thick, gray-green plaques; membranous, friable exudate on tonsils, pharynx, and larynx;** low-grade fever; acetone breath
- <u>Dx</u>: flexible nasopharyngoscopy, culture and smears
- <u>Complications</u>: nephritis, airway obstruction, death (secondary to neurologic toxin)
- <u>Rx</u>: microlaryngoscopy and bronchoscopy for diagnosis and airway cleaning, may need to establish airway via tracheotomy, avoid intubation (may dislodge exudative plaques precipitating an airway emergency), diphtheria antitoxin, antibiotics (penicillin, erythromycin), humidity

## Acute Supraglottitis (Epiglottitis) (*see* Table 10–2)

- <u>Pathogen</u>: classically **Haemophilis influenzae b**; older children and adults may have infection with gram-positive bacteria (*see* p. 109 for adult supraglottitis)
- <u>Risks</u>: children >1 year old to adult (most common between 2–6 years old), rare since Hib vaccine
- <u>SSx</u>: sudden onset (hours) and short course, **high fever**, odynophagia, dysphagia, **drooling**, dyspnea, "sniffing position" (neck flexed and head extended), no cough, normal voice, tender larynx
- <u>Dx</u>: H&P, plain neck x-ray ("**thumbprint sign**" swollen epiglottis on lateral neck x-ray) if needed, serum Hib capsule antigen, cultures
- <u>Complications</u>: bacteremia/sepsis, acute airway obstruction (death)

### Management

- **avoid aggravating patient and precipitating airway collapse** (if high clinical suspicion and patient symptomatic, establish airway in operating room); for mild symptoms and stable patient with diagnosis in question, consider plain x-ray, flexible laryngoscopy to rule out epiglottic/supraglottic edema

- <u>Establish Emergency Airway</u>: intubation performed in the operating room with preparation for a tracheotomy
- <u>Endoscopy</u>: examine and culture epiglottis
- <u>Postoperative Care</u>: monitored bed, parenteral antibiotics and corticosteroids for 7–10 days, consider extubation when clinical improvement and decreased epiglottic edema

## Recurrent Respiratory Papillomatosis

- <u>SSx</u>: progressive dysphonia, inspiratory or biphasic stridor, dyspnea
- rare malignant change (higher risk in adults and with less common **HPV types 16, 18**)
- <u>Pathophysiology</u>: commonly **HPV types 6, 11**
- <u>Risks</u>: younger, child of first-time mother (longer second stage of delivery in the birth canal), lower socioeconomic status; **50%** born from mothers with genital HPV infection and active condylomas, oral sex, multiple sexual partners; most likely route of transmission from mother to child during labor
- <u>Lesion</u>: wartlike, irregular, exophytic, between any **junction of ciliated and squamous epithelium** (limen vestibuli, midzone epiglottis, ventricle margin, and undersurface of true vocal fold), nasopharyngeal, tracheal, and bronchial lesions are potentially from contamination
- <u>Types</u>
  1. **Juvenile Onset**: presents <12 years old, multiple sites, recurrent, may resolve spontaneously
  2. **Adult Onset**: presents >12 years old, may involve single site, recurrence less common, identical histology
- <u>Dx</u>: flexible nasolaryngoscopy, videostroboscopy, endoscopy with biopsy
- <u>Complications</u>: pulmonary involvement (rare), may cause hemorrhage and abscess formation, respiratory compromise

### Management

- <u>Endoscopic Excision</u>: frequent microlaryngoscopy and bronchoscopy with conservative excision employing cold techniques, microdebrider, lasers
- **avoid tracheotomy**, may seed lower airway or stoma
- biopsy to evaluate for dysplasia/malignancy at least once, consider yearly biopsy for patients requiring regular surgical management

- consider CXR to evaluate pulmonary involvement
- <u>Adjunctive Therapy</u>: (*controversial*) cidofovir, interferon
- <u>Prevention</u>: HPV vaccine (*see* Appendix C)

# Esophageal Disorders Affecting the Airway

## Tracheoesophageal Fistula (*see* p. 559)

## Gastroesophageal Reflux (GER)

- *see* pp. 194–196 and the following pediatric considerations
- associated with otitis, sinusitis, laryngotracheal stenosis, pneumonia (causation difficult to prove)
- laryngopharyngeal reflux (LPR) may trigger laryngospasm leading to apnea and/or spasmodic croup presentation, exacerbate laryngomalacia, or cause hoarseness and vocal fold nodules
- <u>Dx</u>: H&P, laryngoscopy, consider adult diagnostic tools (eg, 24-hour multichannel intraluminal impedance [MII] with pH monitoring), short trial of antireflux medication

## Cricopharyngeal Dysfunction (*see* p. 199)

## Eosinophilic Esophagitis

- implicated as a cause of airway surgery failure when uncontrolled
- associated with atopy
- <u>SSx</u>: feeding intolerance, failure to thrive, vomiting and abdominal pain, food impaction, rhinitis and rhinosinusitis, voice complaints, noisy breathing, reactive airway disease, aspiration, airway edema/subglottic stenosis
- <u>Dx</u>: clinicopathologic disease characterized by esophageal symptoms and characteristic histopathology of ≥15 eosinophils per high-powered field in the absence of routine GERD or eosinophilia throughout the GI tract
- <u>Rx</u>: various allergic treatments including oral corticosteroids, elimination diets, and immune-modulators (*investigational*)

# Foreign Body and Caustic Ingestion

## Foreign Body of the Esophagus

- most common objects in pediatrics are **coins**; food impaction in the absence of known esophageal pathology should raise possibility of eosinophilic esophagitis
- most common objects in adults are fish bones, dentures, and meat

- most common location is the **cricopharyngeus** (also gastroesophageal junction, indentation from the aortic arch, and left mainstem bronchus)
- SSx: respiratory complaints in young child, dysphagia, drooling, weight loss, chest pain, fever
- Dx: chest/neck/abdominal x-ray to identify object (if radiopaque)
- Complications: esophageal perforation, mediastinitis, pneumomedi-astinum, pneumothorax, aspiration

### Management

- initial observation may be considered for an esophageal coin at the cricopharyngeus
- obtain description of object to aid removal strategy
- **Rigid Esophagoscopy**: remove objects not passing within 24 hours or those causing significant symptoms (except disk **batteries** which must be emergently removed), always check for second foreign body

## Foreign Body of the Airway

- most common aspirated object is **food** (eg, vegetable matter, nuts)
- most common locations are right > left mainstem bronchus or subsegmental bronchi
- SSx: choking episode, cough (may become chronic), wheeze, decreased breath sounds, stridor
- Dx: CXR with inspiratory/expiratory phases (evaluate for air trap-ping if object not radiopaque, object may produce ball-valve effect causing the affected side to be hyperinflated; alternatively atelectasis may cause affected side to be hypoinflated) or left/right lateral decubitus phases (affected lung may not undergo normal collapse when dependent), neck x-ray
- Complications: airway compromise, death, airway edema, pneumonitis, postobstructive penumonia, pneumothorax, chronic lung infection, bronchiectasis

### Management

- obtain description of object and obtain similar object to aid removal strategy
- preparation for bronchoscopy is essential (communicate plan with anesthesia)
- **Rigid Bronchoscopy**: light sedation, jet ventilation may be considered though do not want to push material more distally, intraoperative corticosteroids may be used to minimize edema

- <u>Postoperative Rx</u>: consider oral corticosteroids for presence of edema and prophylactic antibiotics, close follow-up, may require multiple endoscopies

## Caustic Ingestion

- alkali exposure (pH >7) causes **liquefaction** necrosis (deeper penetration, more severe damage to esophagus) and is often odorless and tasteless (initially better tolerated)
- acid exposure (pH <7) causes **coagulation** necrosis, a coagulum forms on the mucosa and leads to more superficial penetration than alkali exposure, rapid transit results in skip areas and more severe damage to the stomach
- bleach exposure (pH-7) causes irritation but no significant morbidity
- <u>Common Alkali Agents</u>: laundry detergent, lime, hair straightener, **disk/button batteries**
- <u>Common Acidic Agents</u>: battery fluid, toilet cleaners, sulfuric acid
- <u>SSx</u>: drooling, mouth pain, stridor, dysphagia; chest and abdominal pain (do not reliably predict severity)
- <u>Complications</u>: stricture (circumferential burns), pneumonia, tracheoesophageal fistula, laryngeal edema, mediastinitis, perforation, esophageal carcinoma (increases risk 1000×), death

### *Stages of Esophageal Caustic Injury*

- <u>≤24 Hours</u>: dusky submucosal edema +/− ulceration
- <u>2–5 Days</u>: submucosal inflammation (gray coagulum) with thrombosis
- <u>5–7 Days</u>: sloughing of superficial layer
- <u>1 Week</u>: fibrosis of deep layers and formation of scars and strictures
- <u>2–5 Weeks</u>: contraction

### *Management*

- assess vitals and evaluate airway status (be aware that edema may cause airway compromise quickly)
- have patient drink water or irrigate mouth with water, **do not lavage or induce emesis**
- identify agent, determine pH if possible
- <u>Direct Esophagoscopy</u>: required to evaluate esophageal and gastric injury (ideal between 24–48 hours), if performed too early (<12 hours) may miss severity of damage, if performed >48 hours esophagus may be too damaged risking perforation

- barium swallow (esophagram) is first diagnostic tool if >48 hours; also obtain for progressive dysphagia to evaluate for stricture formation and to confirm perforation
- <u>Grading</u>
  1. **First Degree esophageal burn**: superficial mucosal injury
  2. **Second Degree esophageal burn**: transmucosal injury
  3. **Third Degree esophageal burn**: transmural injury
- <u>Corticosteroids:</u> considered for prevention of circumferential stenosis, contraindicated in transmural injuries, not required in injuries limited to mucosa
- <u>Antibiotic</u>: controversial, considered in transmural injuries
- <u>Initial Management</u>: remove granules and powder with water, maintain nothing by mouth with IV hydration, do not induce emesis, do not neutralize (causes a harmful exothermic reaction)
- <u>Evaluate for Complications</u>: CXR (mediastinitis), abdominal series (gastric perforation), arterial blood gas (acid–base disturbance)

## *Management Based on Endoscopic Findings*

### First Degree Esophageal Burn

- <u>Endoscopic Presentation</u>: mild hyperemia and edema of mucosa
- <u>Immediate Management</u>: irrigation, observation
- <u>Long-Term Management</u>: consider antireflux regimen, follow-up in 2 weeks (consider esophagram if symptomatic at follow-up)

### Second Degree Esophageal Burn

- <u>Endoscopic Presentation</u>: white exudate, erythema, injury to mucosa, submucosa, and possible extension to muscle layer
- <u>Immediate Management</u>: observation overnight
- <u>Long-Term Management</u>: corticosteroids, consider antireflux regimen, consider antibiotics
- <u>Followup</u>: esophagram at followup (evaluate for esophageal stricture formation)
- if circumferential consider nasogastic tube or Silastic stent placement as a place holder

### Third Degree Burn

- **high mortality**
- <u>Endoscopic Presentation</u>: full-thickness burn, black coagulum, extension beyond the esophagus
- <u>Immediate Management</u>: airway management (may require tracheotomy), may require esophagectomy/gastrectomy with

exploratory laparotomy to remove necrotic tissue, for minimal necrosis may consider nasogastric tube placement or Silastic stent, monitored bed, second look at 24 hours

- Long-Term Management: broad-spectrum antibiotics, reflux regimen, corticosteroids are contradicted (may mask infection, increase risk of perforation, cause poor healing), may consider lathyrogenic agents
- Followup: esophagram after 1 month from injury, then every 3 months × 4 (evaluate for esophageal stricture formation)

**Stricture**

- most common long-term complication
- Immediate Management: serial dilation, esophagectomy for severe cases
- Follow-up: monitor with esophagrams for circumferential, all third-degree injuries, all symptomatic patients

# PEDIATRIC SALIVARY GLANDS

## Embryology

- derived from the **first pharyngeal pouch**
- 4th Week: parotids formed from the posterior stomodeum (ectodermal) forming cords through the mesenchyme, which later forms the capsule; parotid encapsulates late allowing entrapment of lymphoid tissue within the parotid fascia
- 6th Week: submandibular glands form as buds in the floor of mouth then grow into the submandibular triangle (endodermal)
- 9th Week: sublingual glands form as multiple buds in the floor of mouth (endodermal)
- Pathology: aberrant salivary gland tissue, accessory glands (most common in the parotid), diverticuli

## Salivary Gland Dysfunction

### Sialorrhea and Ptyalism (Drooling)

- **Sialorrhea**: excessive saliva production
- **Ptyalism**: drooling
- can be physiologic until 2 years old (inefficient or infrequent swallowing)
- Pathophysiology: neurologic (cerebral palsy, immature neurologic system with poor oromotor control, developmental delay),

hypersecretion (inflammatory, parasympathomimetic medications, GERD), psychogenic, anatomic (macroglossia, oral incompetence, orthodontic problems, nasal obstruction), postural
- <u>Dx</u>: history (need to change clothes or wipe many times a day, recurrent pneumonia), physical exam (skin infections, signs of dehydration)

## *Management*

- **Speech Therapist and Orthodontist**: evaluate swallowing function and techniques for improving oral motor function and consideration of orthodontic appliances; behavior therapy can be considered
- **Botulinum Toxin A:** local injection into major salivary glands; botulinum toxin B can be used in failures
- **Anticholinergic Medications** (**Glycopyrrolate**, **Scopolamine**): blockade of parasympathetic innervation
- **Submandibular Gland Excision**: straightforward procedure, risk of marginal branch of facial nerve injury
- **Parotid Duct Ligation**: simple, risk of sialocele, often combined with bilateral submandibular duct excision, risk of dental caries
- **Chorda Tympani Transection** (**Jacobson's Nerve Neurectomy**): transtympanic route is quick, however, with neural regeneration results in return of salivary function (needs to be repeated in 6–18 months), consider in elderly
- **Submandibular Duct/Parotid Duct Rerouting**: reroutes to posterior mouth, combined with sublingual gland excision, rare procedure
- **Radiation Therapy**: consider in severe cases in adult/elderly patients too ill to undergo surgery, risk of secondary malignancy

# Salivary Gland Nonmalignant Pathology

*NOTE:* for pediatric salivary gland neoplasms, *see* p. 608; for salivary gland enlargement, *see* pp. 77–81 and the following considerations; for salivary gland cysts and minor salivary gland lesions, *see* pp. 81–82

## Mumps

- presents at 4–6 years old, uncommon due to MMR vaccine
- <u>Pathogen</u>: mumps virus (a **paramyxovirus**)
- <u>SSx</u>: 75% bilateral, painful parotid swelling (may involve submandibular and sublingual glands); initially may present with malaise, fever, trismus, and sore throat

- <u>Dx</u>: mumps titers; hemeagglutination antigens; virus may be cultured from saliva, urine, or CSF; PCR
- <u>Complications</u>: sudden SNHL (CN VIII involvement), infertility (orchitis), encephalitis, pancreatitis, and nephritis
- <u>Rx</u>: self-limiting, supportive care (hydration, analgesics), audiologic evaluation, vaccine for prevention

## Juvenile Recurrent Parotitis

- second most common salivary gland disease of childhood (first is obstructive sialadenitis); idiopathic, recurrent, unilateral parotid inflammation
- <u>SSx</u>: nonobstructive, nonsuppurative, widened Stenson's duct, yellow plaques in saliva
- <u>Dx</u>: sialography (sialectasis, combination of dilations, strictures, and kinks)
- <u>Rx</u>: conservative (gland massage with warm compresses, hydration, sialagogues), surgical (duct probing and dilation +/− duct lavage with saline and corticosteroids, duct ligation, parotidectomy)

# PEDIATRIC OTOLOGY

## Pediatric Audiology and Hearing Screening

### Pediatric Audiology

- *see pp. 349–357 for general audiology principles*
- <u>Pediatric Considerations</u>: pediatric audiology involves specialized tests depending on the patient's age and developmental level (*see* Table 10–3)
- **Pediatric Tympanometry**: normal EAC volume 0.4–1 mL

### *Pediatric Hearing Loss Levels*

- ≤20 dB HL: normal (different from adult)
- 21–25 dB HL: borderline (different from adult)
- 26–40 dB HL: mild
- 41–55 dB HL: moderate
- 56–70 dB HL: moderately severe
- 71–90 dB HL: severe
- ≥91 dB HL: profound
- *NOTE:* for adult levels, *see* p. 350

| TABLE 10–3. Pediatric Audiometric Testing | |
| --- | --- |
| **Age Range** | **Appropriate Audiometric Test** |
| **Birth–6 months** | **ABR (BAER):** ear specific, frequency response |
| | **OAE:** ear specific, frequency specific response (DPOAE) |
| | **Behavioral Observation Audiometry (BOA):** narrow band of tones (warble tones) are introduced via speaker and the examiner observes for a response (eg, eye widening, startle, head turn) to provide a means for grossly estimating an infant's auditory thresholds, tests the better ear |
| **6 mos–3 years** | **Visual Response Audiometry (VRA):** child between speakers (sound-field testing) or wearing headphones is trained to turn head toward auditory signal with visual stimulus (toy animation, etc), used to reinforce an appropriate response |
| | **Visual Reinforcement Operant Conditioning Audiometry (VROCA):** like VRA except child conditioned to push button or other device in response to sound, rewarded with visual stimulus (toy animation, etc), typically for >2 years of age |
| | **ABR** and **OAE** may also be considered |
| **3–5 years** | **Conditioned Play Audiometry (CPA):** child performs a task in response to an auditory stimulus, ear specific and frequency specific |
| **6 years and older** | Standard Audiometry |

# Neonatal Hearing Screening

- universal screening of neonates is employed in many centers, screening based only on risk factors will miss large percentage of congenital hearing loss
- <u>High Risk Factors</u>: **TORCH** infections (**T**oxoplasmosis, **O**ther infections [Syphilis], **R**ubella, **CMV**, **H**erpes simplex) or bacterial meningitis, family history, presence of other head and neck abnormalities, birth weight <1500 g, neonatal hyperbilirubinemia, Apgar score <4 at 1 minute or <6 at 5 minutes, hypoxia, prolonged stay at the neonatal intensive care unit, ECMO, mechanical ventilation, prematurity
- <u>Example Model for Universal Screening</u>: otoacoustic emission (OAE) screening or ABR by 1 month of age; if fail, ABR by 3 months of age; amplification (if necessary) and **early intervention** by 6 months of age

- in the United States, all states now implement newborn screening programs, nearly all states have mandatory compliance (unfunded federal mandate)

# Approach to Pediatric Hearing Loss

## Overview

- **Congenital Hearing Loss**: hearing loss that is present at birth, may be hereditary (**50%**) or acquired (**50%**, eg, infection, birth trauma)
- congenital hearing loss occurs in ~1–3:1000 neonates
- **Hereditary (Genetic) Hearing Loss**: hearing loss that presents at or after birth whose cause is in the **genetic** code
- hereditary hearing loss may be **syndromic (1/3)** or **nonsyndromic (2/3)**
- **80%** of hereditary hearing loss is autosomal recessive, **18%** is autosomal dominant, 2% is X-linked or mitochondrial
- most common prenatal cause of hearing loss is **intrauterine infection**; common causes of perinatal hearing loss are **hypoxia, hyperbilirubinemia, infection**, and **medication toxicity**

## History

- <u>Character of Hearing Loss</u>: age of onset, progression of hearing loss, communication skills
- <u>Prenatal and Perinatal History</u>: term of delivery, birth weight, prenatal infections, bilirubinemia, Apgar score, maternal drug and alcohol abuse, ICU stay, ventilation, ECMO
- <u>Contributing Factors</u>: syndromic features; family history of hearing loss; history of neurologic (seizures), cardiac (Jervell and Lange-Nielsen), thyroid (Pendred), renal (Alport's), sickle cell anemia, infections (recurrent otitis media, meningitis), or other congenital disease; delayed development (growth history); surgical history (otologic, neurologic); medications (ototoxic); recent trauma
  <u>Associated Symptoms</u>: delayed speech development, imbalance or gait disturbances, vision problems, other neurologic complaints

## Physical Exam

- <u>Otoscopy/Microscopy</u>: inspect auricle, EAC, TM, pneumatoscopy
- <u>Inspection and Palpation</u>: inspect auricle, periauricular pits and appendages, and other facial malformations
- <u>Other Physical Exam</u>: vestibular testing; orofacial deformities (palate and lip deformities, mandible and maxilla abnormalities);

goiter (Pendred); ocular exam (Stickler, Usher, osteogenesis imperfecta); telecanthus, hetereochromia iridis, and white forelock (Waardenburg); branchial anomalies (branchio-oto-renal); other syndromic defects (limbs, phalanges, café-au-lait spots, etc)

## Diagnostic Tests

- in the absence of signs suggesting a specific etiology, workup should begin with higher yield tests (connexin 26, temporal bone CT, CMV PCR) prior to testing for less common etiologies
- <u>Genetic Testing</u>: **connexin 26** is first line test in nonsyndromic recessive hearing loss, other genetic tests can be performed based on clinical suspicion and radiographic findings
- **CT Temporal Bone**: to evaluate for inner ear disorders, cholesteatoma, and osteodysplasias (only 20% of congenitally deaf individuals have radiologically anomalous ears)
- **CMV Test**: congenital CMV is a common cause of nongenetic hearing loss, can test with serology or PCR
- **ECG**: screen for **Jervell and Lange-Nielsen syndrome** (uncommon, but noninvasiveness of test and possibility for intervention makes ECG worthwhile), **Refsum disease** (retinitis pigmentosa, hypertrophic peripheral neuropathy, SNHL, arrythmias)
- **Ophthalmology Consult**: due to importance of vision in a hearing impaired child and to monitor for associated ophthalmologic conditions
- **Multigene Testing**: increasing availability with multiple platforms for simultaneous testing of numerous gene mutations associated with hearing loss

## Other Diagnostic Studies

- only when indicated by H&P
- **CBC**: may suggest leukemic process, labyrinthitis, active inflammation
- **Spirochete Studies**: Lyme titers and VDRL/FTA-ABS (luetic labyrinthitis)
- **Pendred and Thyroid Function Tests**: genetic test now preferred (older study is **perchlorate test**: administer radioactive iodine, if infusion of perchlorate causes excessive release of iodine from thyroid then test is abnormal)
- **Lipid Profile**: evaluate for hyperlipidemia (associated with hearing loss)
- **Immune Function Tests**: may suggest an autoimmune disorder (Cogan's)

- **Urine Analysis, BUN, Serum Creatinine, Renal Ultrasound**: screen for Alport's and branchio-oto-renal syndromes
- **TORCH Studies**: IgM assay which investigates common intrauterine infections

## General Management Concepts

- key concept is **early detection** and **early intervention** by 6 months of age
- consider genetic evaluation and counseling
- hearing amplification devices and early intervention services to prevent speech and developmental delays
- serial audiograms to evaluate for progression
- even mild, unilateral hearing loss can affect school performance
- surgical correction may be feasible for some types of CHL (eg, stapes fixation, auricular and external ear canal abnormalities, chronic otitis media)
- counsel on preventive strategies, particularly avoidance of noise trauma
- consider treatment with ganciclovir to prevent hearing loss in symptomatic congenital CMV infection

# Hearing Device Considerations

- *see also* pp. 357–359 for conventional hearing aids

## Bone-Anchored Hearing Aid (BAHA; Auditory Osseointegrated Implant)

- *see also* p. 360
- two-stage procedure preferred in children to allow more time for osseointegration
- **BAHA Softband**: nonimplanted bone-conduction hearing aid, may be used initially prior to BAHA surgery for younger children
- <u>Eligibility</u>: ≥5 years old and ≥3 mm of calvarial cortical bone thickness, if performed at earlier age, high rate of fixture (implant) loss (40% versus 8%)
- <u>Indications</u>: congenital aural atresia, chronic ear disease/otorrhea preventing use of conventional hearing aids, congenital ossicular anomalies and other significant conductive/mixed hearing loss, unilateral profound hearing loss
- if repair of microtia is planned, place the fixture more posterior and superior than usual
- because of thin skull, exposure of dura or sigmoid sinus in up to 70% of pediatric cases

- "sleeper screw" (second screw) often placed in the event the original implant is dislodged

## Cochlear Implant

- *see also* pp. 360–362
- <u>Pediatric Indications</u>: ≥1 year old, bilateral, profound (severe to profound if >18–24 months) cochlear hearing loss with minimal benefit from hearing aids (>90 dB HL, <20% word recognition score with hearing aids if >5 years old), ability to participate in rehabilitation; may be **pre- or postlingual**; may be implanted <1 year old if deafness is due to meningitis (to avoid labyrinthine ossification); expanding criteria for children <1 year old and children with residual hearing
- **vaccinate for *S. pneumoniae*** to reduce risk of meningitis (*see* Appendix C)
- optimize middle ear function prior to implantation; no current evidence that placement of ear tubes increases risk of cochlear implant-related meningitis, however, otitis media in context of cochlear implant should be managed aggressively
- children with severe developmental delay or other disabilities can still benefit from cochlear implantation despite more limited speech and language outcomes
- bilateral implantation associated with more accurate sound localization and hearing in noise for children

# Inner Ear Dysmorphologies

## Michel Aplasia (Complete Labyrinthine Aplasia with Absent Cochlea)

- <u>Pathophysiology</u>: complete failure of the development of the inner ear at week 3 of gestation, autosomal dominant
- <u>SSx</u>: anacusis, normal middle and outer ear
- <u>Dx</u>: CT reveals a hypoplastic petrous pyramid and an absent cochlea and labyrinth
- <u>Rx</u>: consider vibrotactile devices for bilateral involvement

## Mondini Dysplasia (Incomplete Partition)

- most common cochlear malformation (likely because of ambiguous definition)
- <u>Pathophysiology</u>: developmental arrest of the bony and membranous labyrinth at week 7 of gestation; can be autosomal dominant

- <u>SSx</u>: congenital or progressive SNHL
- associated with an increased risk of perilymphatic gusher and meningitis from a dilated cochlear aqueduct
- <u>Dx</u>: CT reveals a 1.5 turn (variable) cochlea with no interscalar septum/deficient modiolus, semicircular canals may be absent or wide, enlarged vestibular aqueduct
- <u>Rx</u>: amplification, cochlear implant

## Enlarged (Large) Vestibular Aqueduct

- <u>Pathophysiology</u>: multiple hereditary mechanisms
- associated with early onset SNHL (40%) and Mondini dysplasia; also seen in *DFNB4*-associated hearing loss, Pendred syndrome, branchio-oto-renal syndrome
- <u>SSx</u>: fluctuating SNHL or mixed HL with rapid stepwise decline after mild head trauma (eg, sports), variable vestibular symptoms
- <u>Dx</u>: typically defined as >1.5 mm vestibular aqueduct diameter as measured at the midpoint between the common crus and the operculum on temporal bone CT
- <u>Rx</u>: prevent decrements in hearing by avoidance of head trauma (judicious helmet use, no contact sports), amplification, cochlear implant

## Scheibe Dysplasia (Cochleosaccular Dysplasia)

- <u>Pathophysiology</u>: partial or complete **membranous aplasia of the pars inferior** (cochlea and saccule) with a **normal pars superior** (semicircular canals and utricle); can be autosomal recessive
- syndromic association including Usher and Waardenburg, also associated with congenital rubella
- <u>SSx</u>: SNHL
- <u>Dx</u>: difficult to diagnose by CT since primarily a membranous defect, definitive diagnosis may only be determined by histologic examination
- <u>Rx</u>: amplification

# Acquired Prenatal (Congenital Infectious) Hearing Loss

## Congenital Toxoplasmosis

- <u>Pathophysiology</u>: maternal *Toxoplasmosis gondii* infection crosses the placenta, or rarely transmitted at birth
- <u>Otologic SSx</u>: delayed onset, progressive SNHL

- <u>Other SSx</u>: jaundice, low birth weight, vision problems, hydrocephalus, cerebral palsy, intracranial calcifications
- <u>Dx</u>: serology (IgM, IgG), physical exam
- <u>Rx</u>: maternal treatment with spiramycin; infant treatment with pyrimethamine and sulfadiazine

## Congenital Rubella

- rare since vaccine and prenatal testing
- <u>Pathophysiology</u>: maternal rubella causes atrophy of the organ of Corti, loss of hair cells, and thrombosis within the stria vascularis
- <u>Otologic SSx</u>: ossicular and cochlear disorders, severe to profound SNHL, may cause delayed endolymphatic hydrops
- <u>Other SSx</u>: cardiac malformation, congenital cataracts, anemia, mental retardation, deformities of the lower extremities, microcephaly, thrombocytopenia
- <u>Dx</u>: antirubella IgM; PCR; or culture of virus from urine, throat, or amniotic fluid

## Congenital Cytomegalovirus

- ~0.64% of newborns contract; 10% of those have symptoms, including SNHL
- <u>Pathophysiology</u>: spread from maternal primary CMV
- <u>Otologic SSx</u>: hearing loss (mild to profound, unilateral SNHL), may be progressive
- <u>Other SSx</u>: hemolytic anemia, microcephaly, mental retardation, hepatosplenomegaly, jaundice, cerebral calcifications, retinitis
- <u>Dx</u>: serum anti-CMV IgM, presence of intranuclear inclusions ("owl eyes") in renal tubular cells found in urinary sediment; PCR for viral DNA from neonatal bloodspot or saliva
- <u>Rx</u>: consider ganciclovir, valganciclovir

## Congenital Syphilis

- <u>Pathophysiology</u>: maternal *Treponema pallidum* infection that crosses the placenta
- often fatal
- <u>Otologic SSx</u>: deafness occurs within first 2 years of life or may present in a delayed form that manifests at 2nd or 3rd decade of life, **Hennebert's sign** (positive fistula test in delayed congenital syphilis), may present with endolymphatic hydrops
- **Hutchinson's Triad**: abnormal central incisors (Hutchinson's teeth), interstitial keratitis of the eye, SNHL
- <u>Dx</u>: VDRL (nonspecific), FTA-ABS (specific), audiogram

- <u>Rx</u>: long-term penicillin, ampicillin, tetracycline, or erythromycin; consider corticosteroids for associated hearing loss

# Autosomal Recessive Causes of Hearing Loss

## Nonsyndromic Autosomal Recessive Disorders

- more common than syndromic
- identified by genetic loci, denoted with DFN**B**- prefix (nonsyndromic autosomal dominant hearing loss with DFN**A**-prefix; X-linked with DFN**X**- prefix)
- by definition, no other physical or systemic findings (nonsyndromic)

### Connexin Mutations

- most common cause of hereditary nonsyndromic hearing loss
- **DFNB1** accounts for ~50% of congenital severe-to-profound autosomal recessive nonsyndromic hearing loss
- *GJB2* gene (encodes **connexin 26** protein, most common) and *GJB6* gene (encodes connexin 30) reside at DFNB1 locus
- **35delG** is most common connexin 26 mutation.
- <u>SSx</u>: mild to profound SNHL, usually normal vestibular function

## Syndromic Autosomal Recessive Disorders

### Usher Syndrome

- most common cause of **autosomal recessive syndromic** hearing loss
- most common cause of deaf-blindness (dual sensory impairment)
- <u>Etiology</u>: genetically heterogeneous with several responsible genes, primarily autosomal recessive (may also be autosomal dominant or X-linked recessive) results in variable expression of SNHL and progressive retinitis pigmentosa
- <u>Otologic SSx</u>: congenital SNHL, vestibular dysfunction (variable)
- <u>Other SSx</u>: **progressive retinitis pigmentosa** (delayed tunnel vision and blindness), mental retardation, cataracts, delayed walking
- <u>Types</u>: **I**: profound congenital SNHL, vestibular areflexia, adolescent-onset retinitis pigmentosa; previously thought to be most common form; **II**: moderate to severe congenital SNHL, legally blind by mid-adulthood, normal vestibular function; most common form (likely underdiagnosed) **III**: progressive SNHL, varied progression of blindness, progressive vestibular dysfunction
- <u>Dx</u>: ophthalmologic evaluation including electroretinography, genetic testing, vestibular testing showing areflexia should raise suspicion

### *Pendred Syndrome*

- second most common cause of autosomal recessive syndromic hearing loss
- <u>Etiology</u>: mutation in gene (usually *SLC26A4 [PDS]*) producing the pendrin protein resulting in defective iodine metabolism and organification; *SLC26A4* mutation can cause spectrum of disease ranging from Pendred syndrome to DFNB4 (nonsyndromic hearing loss)
- <u>Otologic SSx</u>: mild to profound SNHL (can be mixed HL due to third window effect), normal middle and outer ear, associated with Mondini deformity and enlarged vestibular aqueduct, variable vestibular dysfunction
- <u>Other SSx</u>: euthyroid **multinodular goiter** at 8–14 years old
- <u>Dx</u>: genetic testing, positive **perchlorate test** (increased iodine release from thyroid in response to perchlorate)
- <u>Rx</u>: exogenous thyroid hormone if necessary (suppress goiter growth, no effect on hearing), thyroidectomy typically not required; risk of progression with head trauma (avoid contact sports)

### *Jervell and Lange-Nielsen Syndrome*

- third most common cause of autosomal recessive syndromic hearing loss
- <u>Etiology</u>: genetically heterogeneous with several responsible genes resulting in severe SNHL and cardiac defects; most commonly associated with mutations in *KCNQ1*
- <u>Otologic SSx</u>: severe to profound bilateral SNHL
- <u>Other SSx</u>: **cardiac abnormalities**, recurrent **syncope** (may be misdiagnosed as epilepsy), sudden death
- <u>Dx</u>: ECG (prolonged QT, large T-waves)
- <u>Rx</u>: β-blockers, defibrillator

### *Goldenhar Syndrome (Oculoauriculovertebral Spectrum, Hemifacial Microsomia)* (*see* p. 591)

# Autosomal Dominant Causes of Hearing Loss

## Nonsyndromic Autosomal Dominant Disorders

- identified by genetic loci, denoted with DFNA-prefix
- often will have 1 parent with hearing loss

- examples include DFNA2A (mutation in *KCNQ4* gene) causing predominantly high frequency SNHL; DFNA6 (mutation in *WFS1* gene) causing predominantly low frequency SNHL

## Syndromic Autosomal Dominant Disorders

### Waardenburg Syndrome

- most common cause of autosomal dominant syndromic hearing loss
- <u>Etiology</u>: mutation in *PAX3* gene (in types I and III)
- <u>Otologic SSx</u>: unilateral or bilateral SNHL, may have vestibular dysfunction
- <u>Other SSx</u>: **pigmentary abnormalities** (heterochromia iridis, white forelock, patchy skin depigmentation), craniofacial abnormalities (dystopia canthorum [widely spaced medial canthi, telecanthus], synophrys [confluent eyebrows], broad nasal root)
- <u>Types</u>: **I**: dystopia canthorum, 50% have SNHL; **II**: no dystopia canthorum, 80% have SNHL; **III**: skeletal abnormalities, unilateral ptosis; **IV**: Hirschprung disease
- <u>Dx</u>: H&P, family history

### Stickler Syndrome (Progressive Arthro-Ophthalmopathy)

- <u>Etiology</u>: mutation in collagen-producing genes (*COL2A1* in Stickler type 1)
- <u>Otologic SSx</u>: progressive SNHL (may have mixed HL)
- <u>Other SSx</u>: ocular abnormalities (myopia, retinal detachment, cataracts), Marfanoid habitus (tall and thin), arthritic abnormalities (joint hypermobility, early arthritis), Pierre-Robin sequence (micrognathia, glossoptosis, cleft palate)
- <u>Dx</u>: H&P, family history

### Branchio-Oto-Renal Syndrome (Melnick-Fraser Syndrome)

- <u>Etiology</u>: mutation most commonly in *EYA1* gene (chromosome 8q) causing abnormal development of branchial arches (including ears) and kidneys
- <u>Otologic SSx</u>: pinna deformities; preauricular ear pits, fistulas, or tags; varied mixed hearing loss with ossicular and cochlear malformations; may have an associated Mondini deformity or enlarged vestibular aqueduct
- <u>Other SSx</u>: varied renal abnormalities (agenesis, mild dysplasia); branchial anomalies; lacrimal duct stenosis
- <u>Dx</u>: renal involvement may be asymptomatic and only detectable with pyelography or renal ultrasound

### Other Syndromic Autosomal Dominant Disorders

- **Treacher Collins Syndrome (Mandibulofacial Dysostosis)** (*see* p. 595)
- **Neurofibromatosis 1 and 2** (*see* pp. 404–405)
- **Apert Syndrome (Acrocephalosyndactyly)** (*see* p. 588)
- **Crouzon Syndrome (Craniofacial Dysostosis)** (*see* p. 590)

# X-Linked Causes of Hearing Loss

## Nonsyndromic X-Linked Disorders

- identified by genetic loci, denoted with DFN**X**-prefix

### X-Linked Stapes Gusher

- <u>Etiology</u>: mutation in the *POU3F4* gene
- <u>Otologic SSx</u>: congenital stapes fixation with perilymphatic gusher, enlarged IAC, mixed HL
- <u>Other SSx</u>: typically nonsyndromic but may be associated with choroideremia and mental retardation
- <u>Dx</u>: CT temporal bone
- <u>Rx</u>: consider stapes surgery cautiously

## Syndromic X-Linked Disorders

### Alport Syndrome

- <u>Etiology</u>: X-linked (or autosomal dominant) mutation in type IV collagen gene (most commonly *COL4A5*); effects in the glomerular basement membrane result in progressive renal disease; also associated with SNHL
- <u>Otologic SSx</u>: slowly progressive SNHL (bilateral degeneration of organ of Corti and stria), presents in first decade of life
- <u>Other SSx</u>: renal dysplasia/agenesis, **progressive nephritis** (hematuria, proteinuria, chronic glomerulonephritis, uremia), ocular disorders (myopia, cataracts)
- <u>Dx</u>: urinalysis, renal ultrasound, BUN, serum creatinine, immunohistochemistry
- <u>Rx</u>: dialysis and renal transplant

### Otopalatodigital Syndrome

- <u>Etiology</u>: mutation in *FLNA* gene
- <u>Otologic SSx</u>: ossicular malformation (CHL)

- <u>Other SSx</u>: craniofacial deformities (supraorbital deformity, flat midface, small nose, cleft palate, hypertelorism), digital abnormalities (broad fingers and toes), short stature, mental retardation

### Other Syndromic X-Linked Disorders

- **Norrie Syndrome**: progressive SNHL with onset in 2nd–3rd decade, congenital/rapidly progressing blindness (cataracts, leukoria, retinal detachment), mutation in *NDP* gene
- **Wildervanck Syndrome (Cervico-Oculo-Acoustic Syndrome)**: SNHL or mixed HL due to bony inner ear malformation, CN VI paralysis, fused cervical vertebrae (Klippel-Feil malformation), suspected X-linked dominant (seen in females, embryonic lethality in males)

# Other Hearing Disorders

- **Auditory Neuropathy** (*see* p. 404)
- **Central Auditory Processing Disorder** (*see* p. 404)
- **Sudden Sensorineural Hearing Loss (SSNHL)** (*see* pp. 401–402)
- **Noise-Induced Hearing Loss** (*see* pp. 402–403)
- **Ototoxin-Induced Hearing Loss:** (*see* p. 403)

# Otitis Media

## Introduction

- *see also* pp. 372–383
- <u>Definition of Acute Otitis Media</u>
  1. moderate to severe bulging of the tympanic membrane, or
  2. new onset of otorrhea of middle ear origin, or
  3. mild bulging of the tympanic membrane and new-onset (<48 hours) ear pain, which can be seen as holding/tugging/rubbing of the ear, or intense erythema of the tympanic membrane

## Medical Treatment of Otitis Media

<u>Acute Otitis Media (2013 American Academy of Pediatric Guidelines)</u>
  1. **<6 months old** with SSx of nonsevere or severe acute otitis media should be treated with antibiotics
  2. **≥6 months old** with severe SSx of acute otitis media (moderate–severe otalgia, otalgia ≥48 hours, temperature ≥39° C) should be treated with antibiotics

3. **6–23 months old** with nonsevere bilateral acute otitis media (mild otalgia <48 hours, temperature <39° C) should be treated with antibiotics

4. **6–23 months old** with nonsevere unilateral acute otitis media should be offered antibiotics or observation with close follow-up; if observation chosen, antibiotics should be given if symptoms worsen or fail to improve within 48–72 hours of onset of symptoms

5. **≥24 months old** with nonsevere unilateral or bilateral acute otitis media should receive either antibiotics or observation

6. <u>First-Line Antibiotics</u>: amoxicillin (80–90 mg/kg/day) if not allergic, not received antibiotics in <30 days, no purulent conjunctivitis (more likely non-typeable *H influenzae* which is resistent) and no history of recurrent AOM unresponsive to amoxicillin; amoxicillin-clavulanate (14:1) if not allergic and does not meet other criteria to receive amoxicillin; cefdinir (14 mg/kg/day), cefuroxime (30 mg/kg/day), cefpodoxime (10 mg/kg/day) or ceftriaxone (50 mg IM/IV per day for 1–3 days) if allergic to amoxicillin

7. <u>Second-Line Antibiotics</u>: amoxicillin-clavulanate, ceftriaxone first-line for failure of initial treatment; clindamycin (30–40 mg/kg/day) +/– third-generation cephalosporin and consider tympanocentesis for failure of second antibiotic

- <u>Chronic Otitis Media with Effusion</u>: no evidence that decongestants, antihistamines, or antibiotics reduce duration; potential small benefit from steroids
- <u>Recurrent Otitis Media</u>: prophylactic antibiotics not generally recommended

# Myringotomy with Pressure Equalization Tubes (PETs)

- *see also* p. 376
- Indications
  1. recurrent otitis media (~3 episodes/6 months, ~4 episodes/1 year) with effusion present at the time of evaluation
  2. persistent bilateral middle ear effusion > 3 months (consider 6 months for unilateral effusion)
  3. complications of acute otitis media (eg, mastoiditis, meningitis, etc)

# Adenoidectomy

- *see also* pp. 376, 530–534

- for children >1–4 years old (age criteria controversial) with chronic otitis media with effusion needing a second set of PETs, performing adenoidectomy with PETs may reduce the duration of effusion and reduce (up to 50%) the need for additional surgery
- some consider performing in children >1 year old whose recurrent ear infections start with nasal symptoms (*controversial*)
- adenoid size alone does not correlate with the need for additional surgeries, laterally abutting adenoid pads seem more significant than a central adenoid mound

## Mastoidectomy (*see* pp. 376–377)

## Ossicular Chain Reconstruction (*see* pp. 378–379)

## Complications of Otitis Media (*see* pp. 379–383)

# Other Disorders of the Ear and Temporal Bone

## Foreign Body and Cerumen Impaction

- *see also* p. 385
- always perform bilateral aural examination and confirm complete removal of foreign bodies (a second may be present)
- disk batteries are a true emergency because of the generation of electrolytic currents and potential leakage of alkaline contents; necrosis of the EAC can occur rapidly; irrigation is contraindicated because it can spread the corrosive substance further
- <u>Rx</u>: remove with cerumen loop/curette, angle hook, Frazier/Baron suction, alligator forceps, etc, then inspect for injury to the external auditory canal and tympanic membrane

## Tympanic Membrane Perforation

- *see also* pp. 387–388
- **Tympanoplasty**: success rate in children (35–94%) lower than in adults; factors include the higher rate of URIs, ongoing eustachian tube dysfunction (especially cleft palate, Down syndrome, craniofacial anomalies) and inconsistent postoperative care; success of surgery improves with age until 13 years, best to wait until adenoid pad is regressing (age 7) or regressed (age 10); otherwise consider adenoidectomy and treating nasal disease first; also should wait for both ears to be without effusion, retraction, or recurrent infections; *see also* pp. 377–378

## Congenital Stapes Fixation

- most common congenital isolated ossicular anomaly (20–35%)
- fixation between the lamina of the stapes and the annular ligament
- nonprogressive conductive hearing loss, usually bilateral
- <u>Rx</u>: stapedectomy or stapedotomy

## Other Disorders

- **Aural Atresia and Microtia** (*see* pp. 610–613)
- **Noninfectious Disease of the External Ear** (*see* pp. 385–387)
- **Infections of the External Ear** (*see* pp. 369–372)
- **Congenital and Acquired Cholesteatoma** (*see* pp. 388–389)
- **Tympanosclerosis** (*see* p. 388)
- **Infections of the Inner Ear** (*see* pp. 383–384)
- **Fibrous Dysplasia** (*see* pp. 225, 398)
- **Langerhans Cell Histiocytosis** (*see* pp. 398, 608–609)
- **Osteogenesis Imperfecta** (*see* p. 390)
- **Barotrauma** (*see* p. 400)
- **Temporal Bone Fractures** (*see* pp. 658–662)

# Vestibular Pathology

## Overview

- *see also* pp. 405–420
- <u>Vestibular Development</u>: vestibular end organs are responsive at birth, however maturation continues postnatally such that they become typically responsive at 6–12 months of age
- <u>SSx</u>: children can present with either gross motor delays as a result of congenital or early acquired loss of vestibular end organ function or they can present with episodic vertigo in a fashion similar to adults
- <u>Dx</u>: careful history, complete neurotologic, gross motor, and audiologic exam, *see* pp. 405–412 for vestibular evaluation

## Pediatric Vestibular Disorders

- **Otitis Media**: otitis media-related imbalance
- **Benign Paroxysmal Vertigo of Childhood (Benign Recurrent Vertigo of Childhood)**: not the same as benign paroxysmal positional vertigo (BPPV); occurs in early childhood; presents with episodic vertigo lasting seconds to minutes with associated imbalance, nausea, and vomiting; migraine variant; normal

audiometry and vestibular end organ testing; diagnosis of exclusion; typically self-limiting, proportion develop migraine later on in life
- **Peripheral Vestibular Dysfunction Associated with SNHL**: >50% of children with SNHL have significant vestibular dysfunction; risk highest in meningitis, ototoxicity, cochleovestibular anomalies, CMV
- **Recurrent Vestibulopathy**: recurrent, episodic vertigo lasting minutes to hours without auditory or neurologic signs/symptoms, not provoked by changes in head position
- **Ménière's Disease**: similar to adults, uncommon in children
- **Central Causes**: migraine-associated vertigo, temporal lobe seizures, posterior fossa and CPA tumors, Chiari malformation
- **Other Causes**: metabolic diseases, toxicity, perilymphatic fistula
- *see* also **Vestibular Neuronitis and Labyrinthitis** (pp. 383–384), **Labyrinthine Concussion** (p. 417), **Perilymph Fistula** (p. 417), **Cogan Syndrome** (pp. 417–418), **Other Peripheral Vestibular Disorders** (p. 418)

# Facial Nerve Disorders

## Introduction

- facial nerve has more superficial and inferior course and mastoid is absent until 2 years old
- *see also* pp. 420–423 for anatomy, pp. 424–427 for evaluation, and pp. 431–433 for nerve repair/reanimation

## Congenital and Developmental Causes of Facial Paralysis

- **CHARGE Syndrome** (*see* p. 589)
- **Mobius Syndrome**: wide spectrum of abnormalities secondary to central brainstem defects (possibly due to prenatal stroke-like event) and peripheral neuromuscular defects; <u>SSx</u>: bilateral or unilateral CN VII and VI palsies; club foot (talipes equinovarus), micrognathia, arched or cleft palate, tongue weakness, mental retardation, mixed hearing loss, external ear deformities, ophthalmoplegia
- **Albers-Schoenberg Disease**: autosomal recessive, disorder of bone metabolism resulting in osteopetrosis of the bony IAC causing compression of nerves (CN III, VII, and VIII)
- **Congenital Unilateral Lower Lip Palsy (Asymmetric Crying Facies)**: most common congenital cause of facial paralysis, presents with hypoplasia of the depressor anguli oris muscle, associated with cardiac defects (~10%)

## Birth Trauma

- most common cause of neonatal unilateral facial paralysis
- <u>Pathophysiology</u>: facial nerve is at risk for injury during delivery as it courses through the underdeveloped mastoid process
- <u>Risks</u>: forceps delivery, prolonged delivery, large infant
- <u>SSx</u>: asymmetric crying facies, hemotympanum, periauricular ecchymosis
- <u>Dx</u>: EMG (preserved neuromuscular activity suggests inherited or developmental etiology), electrophysiologic testing, ABR (evaluate for associated hearing loss)
- <u>Rx</u>: observation (usually recovers)

## Infectious, Idiopathic, and Other Causes of Facial Palsy

- **Idiopathic Facial Paralysis (Bell's Palsy)** (*see* pp. 427–428)
- **Herpes Zoster Oticus (Ramsay Hunt Syndrome)** (*see* p. 428)
- **Lyme Disease** (*see* p. 429)
- **Otitis Media** (*see* p. 429)
- **Necrotizing Otitis Externa** (*see* p. 429)
- **Melkersson-Rosenthal Syndrome** (*see* pp. 428–429)
- **Trauma (Post-birth)** (*see* p. 430)

# PEDIATRIC SYNDROMES AND CONGENITAL DISORDERS

## Overview

### Terminology

- **Association:** multiple congenital anomalies occurring at a high frequency together
- **Sequence:** a single anomaly or mechanical factor leading to multiple anomalies
- **Syndrome:** a specific trigger causing a predictable combination of anomalies

## Syndromes and Congenital Disorders

### 22q11 Syndrome

- includes **DiGeorge syndrome**, **Velo-cardio-facial syndrome**, **Schprintzen syndrome** (slight differences, part of spectrum)

- Etiology: chromosome 22q11.2 hemizygous microdeletion, leads to a disorder of **third and fourth branchial pouch development**
- H&N SSx: elongated face, almond eyes, long and wide nose with bulbous tip, low-set ears with overfolded helix or other auricle anomalies, malar flattening and hypoplastic mandible, open-mouthed, hypotonia, submucous cleft palate and velopharyngeal insufficiency (poor mobility of the palate and lateral pharyngeal walls), anterior glottis web (15%), medialized carotid arteries
- **CATCH22 Mnemonic**: **C**ardiac (**C**ongenital heart disease, **C**onotruncal defects), **A**bnormal facies, **T**hymic aplasia (immunodeficiency), **C**left lip/palate, **H**ypoparathyroidism (**H**ypocalcemia, agenesis of parathyroid glands), **22**q11

## Achondroplasia

- Etiology: mutation in *FGFR3* gene (chromosome 4p16.3); autosomal dominant, majority sporadic mutations
- affects endochondral bone and results in short limb dwarfism; normal IQ
- H&N SSx: midface hypoplasia, frontal bossing, hearing loss (conductive in 60%)

## Alport Syndrome (*see* p. 581)

## Apert Syndrome

- Etiology: mutation in *FGFR2* gene (chromosome 10q26); autosomal dominant, may be sporadic
- acrocephalosyndactyly (skull and extremity malformations)
- Otologic SSx: middle and inner ear affected; **stapes fixation** (primarily CHL), can also have cochlear and vestibular dysplasia, patent cochlear aqueduct
- Other H&N SSx: craniosynostosis, midface hypoplasia, hypertelorism, proptosis, strabismus, low nasal bridge (saddle nose), parrot-beaked nose, choanal atresia, class III malocclusion, high arched palate, trapezoid mouth (downturned corners), cleft palate, cervical fusion, syndactyly (lobster claw hands)
- Other Sx: extremity malformations (syndactyly), mild developmental delay

## Beckwidth-Wiedemann Syndrome

- Etiology: chromosome 11p15 mutation, may include *IGF2* gene; autosomal dominant, mostly sporadic

- <u>H&N SSx</u>: macroglossia, ear lobe creases
- <u>Other SSx</u>: organomegaly, omphalocele, visceromegaly, cytomegaly of the adrenal cortex
- monitor for hypoglycemia in the perioperative period

## Binder's Syndrome

- <u>Etiology</u>: unclear
- <u>H&N SSx</u>: midface hypoplasia (maxillonasal dysplasia), class III malocclusion, flattened nose, broad philtrum, cervical vertebral anomalies; obstructive sleep apnea

## Blue Rubber Bleb Nevus Syndrome (*see* p. 539)

## Branchiootorenal Syndrome (Melnick-Fraser Syndrome) (*see* pp. 580–581)

## CHARGE Syndrome

- <u>Etiology</u>: *CHD7* gene mutation (chromosome 8q, 70%)
- **C**oloboma (iris keyhole defect), **H**eart disease (endocardial cushion), **A**tresia (choanal), **R**etardation (CNS), **G**enital hypoplasia, **E**ar anomalies (microtia, ossicular malformations, inner ear anomalies)
- <u>H&N SSx</u>: square asymmetric face with broad forehead, flat midface, wide nasal bridge and thick nostrils; can have CN I, VII, IX, X deficiencies; sometimes tracheoesophageal fistula, cleft lip/palate

## Cornelia de Lange Syndrome

- <u>Etiology</u>: multiple genes involved, almost exclusively sporadic
- <u>H&N SSx</u>: microcephaly, synophrys (unibrow), long eyelashes, nasal anomalies (short upturned nose, long philtrum), thin and downturned lips, hypertrichosis, low-set ears, hearing loss, cleft palate, micrognathia, developmental delay

## Cri-du-chat Syndrome

- <u>Etiology</u>: chromosome 5p deletion
- severe developmental delay
- <u>H&N SSx</u>: microcephaly, hypertelorism, cleft lip/palate, high-pitched stridor resembling a cat's cry, diamond-shaped endolarynx, interarytenoid muscle paralysis, hypotonia

# Crouzon Syndrome (Craniofacial Dysostosis)

- <u>Etiology</u>: *FGFR2* gene mutation (chromosome 10q26); autosomal dominant
- normal IQ; skull, maxilla, eye, and external ear affected
- <u>Otologic SSx</u>: predominantly **CHL** from external auditory canal and ossicular deformities, can have SNHL component and microtia
- <u>Other H&N SSx</u>: craniosynostosis, midface hypoplasia, hypertelorism, proptosis, strabismus, low nasal bridge, parrot-beaked nose, choanal atresia, class III malocclusion, high arched palate, short upper lip, cleft palate, mandibular prognathism, cervical fusion

## Down Syndrome *(Am J Med Genet C Semin Med Genet.* 2006;142C(3):131–140)

- <u>Etiology</u>: trisomy of chromosome 21 (1 in 800 live births in the United States)
- <u>Risk Factors</u>: older maternal age (1:100 if >40 years versus 1:1500 if <30 years), although 80% born to women <35 years
- <u>H&N SSx</u>: brachycephaly and midface hypoplasia, flat occiput, small auricles with very narrow EACs, upslanting palpebral fissures and epicanthic folds, small nose and shortened nasopharynx especially in the AP dimension, large and fissured lips/tongue, dental anomalies, short neck, small larynx, cervical spine anomalies (atlanto-axial instability in 25%, subluxation of the cervical spine in 2% with significant risk of spinal cord compression with hyperflexion or hyperextension; cervical spine x-rays not sensitive/reliable to predict those at risk, protect cervical spine of every patient instead)
- <u>Complications</u>
  1. **Otitis Media**: increased risk (up to 3× chronic infection); due to eustachian tubes more collapsible, hypotonia of the tensor veli palatini, craniofacial features with narrow nasopharynx, and immunodeficiency; see all Down patients every 6 months with audiograms, or every 3 months if stenotic ear canals
  2. **Obstructive Sleep Apnea**: muscular hypotonia, increased obesity, increased susceptibility to URI; cor pulmonale more likely; <u>SSx</u>: poor sleep habits, frequent waking, unusual sleeping positions (sitting up, head hyperextended, bent forward); <u>Rx</u>: manage nasal congestion, oxygen, weight loss, oral appliances, CPAP, adenotonsillectomy (can fail to normalize in more than 50%; failure because of macroglossia, glossoptosis, recurrent adenoids, enlarged lingual tonsils, hypopharyngeal collapse), lingual tonsillectomy and midline posterior glossectomy, genioglossus advancement, maxillo-mandibular distraction

3. **Subglottic Stenosis**: intubate with endotracheal tube that is 2 sizes (1 mm) smaller
4. **Sinusitis**
5. <u>Other</u>: cardiovascular (40–50%), pulmonary (pulmonary hypertension), gastrointestinal (congenital duodenal atresia, Hirschsprung's), endocrine (hypothyroidism), hematologic (polycythemia, leukemia)

- <u>AAP Guidelines (2011)</u>
  1. **Hearing**: ABR by 3 months old, behavioral audiograms every 6 months until ear-specific testing is achieved, yearly audiograms if hearing normal once ear-specific testing is achieved
  2. **OSA**: baseline sleep study at 4 years old
- <u>AAO-HNS Guidelines (2011)</u>: sleep study prior to adenotonsillectomy for OSA

# Goldenhar Syndrome (Oculoauriculovertebral Syndrome, Hemifacial Microsomia)

- <u>Etiology</u>: multifactorial, possibly related to an early injury to the stapedial artery, affecting the 1st and 2nd branchial arch structures
- autosomal dominant or recessive
- usually unilateral and more common on the right side
- <u>Grading</u>
  1. **OMENS+**: **O**rbit, **M**andible, **E**ar, **N**erves, **S**oft tissues, + (extra-craniofacial features); a subclassification exists for each component
  2. **Pruzansky/Kaban Mandible Grading**: **I**: minimal hypoplasia; **II**: functioning but deformed TMJ with anteriorly/medially displaced condyle (**IIa**: glenoid fossa in acceptable functional position; **IIb**: TMJ anterior/medial with no articulation with temporal bone and can not be incorporated in surgical construction); **III**: absence of ramus and glenoid fossa
- <u>Otologic SSx</u>: preauricular appendages; microtia/anotia; aural atresia; ossicular malformation or absence (CHL); abnormal development of CN VII, stapedius, semicircular canals, oval window (SNHL)
- <u>Other H&N SSx</u>: variable microsomia of the hemiface affecting the mandible, orbit, muscles, and vertebrae; **ocular** (epibulbar dermoid, **coloboma** of the upper eyelid) and **vertebral** abnormalities (fusion or absence of cervical vertebrae), mild developmental delay

# Jervell and Lange-Nielsen Syndrome (*see* p. 579)

# Klippel-Feil Syndrome

- congenital fusion of cervical vertebrae

- <u>H&N SSx</u>: short, poorly mobile neck; low hairline in the posterior neck; cleft palate; hearing loss

## Klippel-Trenaunay Syndrome (*see* p. 539)

## Maffucci Syndrome (*see* p. 536)

## Mobius Syndrome (*see* p. 586)

## Mucopolysaccharidoses

- **Hunter's Syndrome:** <u>Etiology:</u> deficiency of iduronate-2-sulfatase; X-linked; <u>H&N SSx</u>: macrocephaly, broad features with low nasal bridge, short neck, bulging forehead, macroglossia, recurrent URIs and otitis media, adenotonsillar enlargement, mucosal membrane hypertrophy, dwarfism
- **Hurler's Syndrome:** <u>Etiology</u>: deficiency of α-L-iduronidase which normally breaks down heparin-, dermatan- and keratan-sulfates; death in the first decade; autosomal recessive; <u>H&N SSx</u>: facial dysmorphisms, macroglossia, progressive neurologic dysfunction, corneal clouding, hearing loss, short neck, recurrent URIs and otitis media, adenotonsillar enlargement, dwarfism; obstructive sleep apnea in >80%

## Muenke Syndrome

- <u>Etiology:</u> *FGFR3* gene mutation; autosomal dominant
- <u>H&N SSx</u>: craniosynostosis (mostly coronal), telecanthus, low-set ears, hearing loss

## Nager Syndrome

- <u>Etiology</u>: unknown underlying cause, disrupted development of first and second branchial arches
- <u>H&N SSx</u>: malar hypoplasia, micrognathia, antimongoloid palpebral fissures, absent eyelashes, lower eyelid coloboma, short soft palate, ear anomalies (microtia, hearing loss), cleft palate

## Neurofibromatosis 1 and 2 (*see* pp. 404–405)

## Noonan Syndrome

- <u>Etiology</u>: many possible signaling pathway gene mutations; autosomal dominant

- <u>H&N SSx</u>: hypertelorism, pale eyes (blue or green), flat nasal bridge, low-set ears, frequent otitis media, high-arched palate, wide philtrum, micrognathia, short neck, neck webbing, dysphagia, failure to thrive, speech and language delay; recurrent epistaxis, excessive bruising and prolonged bleeding

## Norrie Syndrome (see p. 582)

## Opitz G/BBB Syndrome

- former names include **Opitz-Frias Syndrome**, **G-syndrome**
- <u>Etiology</u>: *MID1* gene mutation (chromosome 22); X-linked
- <u>SSx</u>: midline defects, hypertelorism, cleft lip/palate, hypospadias, laryngeal cleft

## Osteogenesis Imperfecta (van der Hoeve) (see p. 390)

## Otopalatodigital Syndrome (see pp. 581–582)

## Pallister-Hall syndrome

- <u>Etiology</u>: *GLI3* gene mutation
- <u>H&N SSx</u>: laryngeal cleft or bifid epiglottis, hypothalamus abnormalities (hamartoblastoma, panhypopituitarism);
- <u>Other SSx</u>: imperforate anus, postaxial polydactyly

## Parkes-Weber Syndrome (see p. 539)

## Pendred Syndrome (see p. 579)

## Pfeiffer Syndrome

- <u>Etiology</u>: *FGFR2* gene mutation (chromosome 10q26); autosomal dominant
- acrocephalosyndactyly (skull and extremity malformations)
- <u>H&N SSx</u>: craniosynostosis, midface hypoplasia, hypertelorism, exophthalmos, strabismus, low nasal bridge, parrot-beaked nose, choanal atresia, class III malocclusion, high arched palate, cleft palate, cervical fusion
- <u>Other SSx</u>: digital broadening, severe developmental delay

## Pierre-Robin Sequence (PRS)

- triad of micrognathia, glossoptosis/airway obstruction, and cleft palate

- cleft palate (U-shaped instead of classic V-shaped) is a collateral from the glossoptosis preventing the lateral palatal processes from descending and fusing
- autosomal recessive or sporadic; nonsyndromic or syndromic
- <u>Nonsyndromic Etiology</u>: in utero positional deformation (oligohydramnios, twins, tumors)
- <u>Syndromic Etiology</u>: associated with Stickler (18%), 22q11 (7%), Treacher Collins (5%), Goldenhar (3%), Nager syndromes
- <u>H&N SSx</u>: stertor, retractions, cyanosis (worse supine); failure to thrive (poor swallow, increased caloric needs, aspiration); may have pulmonary hypertension; associated ear anomalies (external: low-set ear, microtia; middle: CN VII, ossicular anomalies; inner: hypoplasia, Mondini); hypotonia (in syndromic cases)
- <u>Dx</u>: clinical triad, prolonged/difficult feeds, high bicarbonate levels/ $CO_2$, CT facial bones; always perform direct or flexible airway assessment for airway narrowing and rule out other anomalies (eg, laryngomalacia, subglottic stenosis); may need sleep study
- catch-up growth can occur in nonsyndromic cases over 6 months– 4 years (controversial)
- <u>Rx</u>: usually conservative management (prone or decubitus positioning, constant monitoring, oxygen, feeding supplementation, nasopharyngeal airway, CPAP, intubation with laryngeal mask); surgical options include bilateral sagittal osteotomy and mandibular distraction osteogenesis, tongue–lip adhesion, floor of mouth muscular release, tracheostomy

## Saethre-Chotzen Syndrome

- acrocephalosyndactyly (skull and extremity malformations)
- <u>Etiology</u>: *TWIST1* gene mutation (chromosome 7p21)
- <u>H&N SSx</u>: craniosynostosis along the coronal suture, asymmetrical face with high forehead, ptosis, telecanthus, microtia, hearing loss

## Smith-Lemli-Opitz Syndrome

- <u>Etiology</u>: deficiency in 7-DHC reductase (final enzyme in cholesterol synthesis); autosomal recessive
- <u>H&N SSx</u>: microcephaly, cleft palate, hypotonia, feeding difficulties
- <u>Other SSx</u>: developmental delay

**Stickler Syndrome** (*see* p. 580)

**Sturge-Weber Syndrome** (*see* p. 539)

## Treacher Collins Syndrome (Mandibulofacial Dysostosis)

- Etiology: *TCOF1* gene mutation most common (chromosome 5q, treacle protein) which is involved in early craniofacial development; malformation of the 1st and 2nd branchial arches; autosomal dominant, sporadic in 60%
- typically normal intelligence (may have developmental delay from hearing loss)
- Otologic SSx: auricular deformities, atresia or stenosis of EAC, preauricular fistulas, malformed ossicles (**CHL**), bony plate replacement of the TM, widened aqueduct, aberrant facial nerve
- Other H&N SSx: zygomatic and mandibular hypoplasia, lower eyelid coloboma, antimongoloid palpebral fissures, "fishmouth," possible cleft lip/palate and choanal atresia
- Rx: bone conduction aids, auditory osseointegrated implant (BAHA), consider surgical correction of aural atresia

## Uniparental Disomy Syndromes

- both alleles of a chromosome pair are inherited from the same parent
- **Prader-Willi Syndrome:** Etiology: chromosome 15q11-q13 anomaly; either maternal uniparental disomy or paternal deletion; H&N SSx: hyperphagia and morbid obesity, which frequently leads to OSA, hypotonia, short stature, cognitive deficiencies, high pain thresholds; Rx: for OSA, maximize weight loss, oxygen, and CPAP/BiPAP before considering adenotonsillectomy
- **Angelman Syndrome:** Etiology: chromosome 15q11-q13 anomaly; either paternal uniparental disomy or maternal deletion; H&N SSx: microcephaly, coarse facial features, seizures, severe speech and developmental delay, poor swallow, insomnia, ataxia; hand-flapping, frequent laughter and fascination with water

## Usher Syndrome (*see* pp. 578–579)

## VACTERL Association

- Etiology: unclear, various genetic and environmental factors
- **V**ertebral, **A**nal, **C**ardiac (PDA or valve problems), Tracheo**E**sophageal Fistula, **R**enal/**R**adial bone, **L**imb (extra digits, shortened limbs) anomalies

## Van der Woude Syndrome

- <u>Etiology</u>: *IRF6* gene mutation (chromosome 1p)
- <u>H&N SSX</u>: cleft lip/palate, lip pits (related to the location of embryonal developmental grooves on the lower lip)

## Von Hippel-Lindau Syndrome

- <u>Etiology</u>: *VHL* gene mutation (tumor suppressor, chromosome 3p25.3); autosomal dominant
- **HIPPEL Mnemonic:** **H**emangioblastoma (CNS, retina; ataxia, blindness), renal cysts/carc**I**noma, **P**heochromocytoma, **P**ancreatic cysts, **E**pididymal papillary cystadenomata, endo**L**ymphatic sac tumor (11%)

## Waardenburg's Syndrome (*see* p. 580)

## Wildervanck Syndrome (*see* p. 582)

# PEDIATRIC HEAD AND NECK SURGERY
## Anatomy of the Neck (see pp. 230–231)
## Embryology of the Neck, Thyroid, and Parathyroids

### Branchial Apparatus

#### Components of the Branchial Apparatus

- **Branchial Arch**: composed of a cartilaginous bar, brachiometric nerve, muscular component, and aortic arch artery
- **Branchial Grooves or Clefts**: external, lined with ectoderm
- **Branchial Membrane**: formed between branchial groove and pouch
- **Branchial Pouches**: internal, linked with endoderm, contains a ventral and dorsal wing

#### Branchial Arches

##### I (Mandibular Arch)

- **Meckel's Cartilage**: malleus head and neck, incus body and short process, anterior malleal ligament, mandible (formed from intramembranous ossification)
- **CN V$_3$**: muscles of mastication, tensor tympani, tensor veli palatini, mylohyoid, and anterior digastric muscles

- **Maxillary Artery**
- <u>Hillocks of His</u>: 1. tragus; 2. helical crus; 3. helix

## II (Hyoid Arch)

- **Reichert's Cartilage**: manubrium of malleus, long process and lenticular process of the incus, stapes (except vestibular part of footplate), styloid process, stylohyoid ligament, lesser cornu and upper half of hyoid
- **CN VII**: muscles of facial expression, stapedius, stylohyoid, and posterior digastric muscles
- **Stapedial Artery** (degenerates; if too early causes microtia/atresia)
- <u>Hillocks of His</u>: 4. antihelix crus; 5. scapha; 6. lobule

## III

- <u>Cartilage</u>: greater cornu and lower half of hyoid
- **CN IX**: stylopharyngeus muscle, superior and middle constrictors
- **Common Carotid and Internal Carotid Arteries**

## IV

- <u>Cartilage</u>: thyroid and cuneiform cartilage
- **Superior Laryngeal Nerve**: cricothyroid muscles and inferior pharyngeal constrictors
- **Aorta** (left); **Proximal Subclavian Artery** (right)

## V/VI

- <u>Cartilage</u>: cricoid, arytenoid, and corniculate cartilage
- **Recurrent Laryngeal Nerve**: intrinsic laryngeal muscle (except cricothyroid muscle)
- **Ductus Arteriosus** and **Pulmonary Artery** (left); **Pulmonary Artery** (right)

## *Branchial Clefts (Grooves)*

I:      external auditory canal, outer tympanic membrane (dorsal part)
II–V:   obliterates

## *Branchial Pouches*

I:      eustachian tube, middle ear (mastoid air cells), inner tympanic membrane
II:     supratonsillar fossa, palatine tonsils, middle ear
III:    epithelial reticulum of thymus, inferior parathyroids
IV:     parafollicular cells (C-cells) of thyroid, superior parathyroids

## Thyroid Embryology

- endoderm between the **first and second branchial arch** on the floor of pharynx (**foramen cecum**) invaginates around the fourth week and descends into mesenchymal tissue along the path of the thyroid duct (anterior to the hyoid bone), forming a ventral diverticulum that differentiates at the distal end into the thyroid anlage; the proximal portion typically atrophies by the 6th week
- <u>Embryologic Pathology</u>: **athyreosis** (rare), **ectopic thyroid** (may be found anywhere along the thyroid duct from the tongue as a lingual thyroid to the sternal notch), **thyroglossal duct cyst** (*see* pp. 600–601)

## Parathyroid Embryology

- **third dorsal branchial pouch** → inferior parathyroids and thymus
- **fourth dorsal branchial pouch** → superior parathyroids and C-cells of the thyroid
- <u>Embryologic Pathology</u>: **supernumerary parathyroids, aberrant parathyroids** (most common location at the **anterior superior mediastinum**)

# Evaluation of the Pediatric Neck Mass

- *see also* pp. 230–232
- 80–90% of pediatric head and neck masses are **benign**
- <u>DDx</u>: based on the **location** of the neck mass
- <u>DDx Lateral Neck Mass</u>: congenital (branchial anomaly, laryngocele); inflammatory (lymphadenitis); vascular (hemangioma, lymphatic malformation, venous malformation); neoplastic (thyroid malignancy, thymic cyst, lipoma, neuroblastoma, lymphoma); traumatic (pseudotumor of infancy)
- <u>DDx Midline Neck Mass</u>: congenital (thyroglossal duct cyst, ectopic thyroid, dermoid cyst, teratoma, thymic cyst); inflammatory (lymphadenitis, plunging ranula); neoplastic (thyroid malignancy)
- <u>DDx Submandibular Mass</u>: inflammatory (plunging ranula, sialadenitis, lymphadenitis); vascular (lymphatic malformation); neoplastic (salivary gland neoplasm)
- **PFAPA Syndrome**: **P**eriodic **F**ever, **A**phthous stomatitis, **P**haryngitis, cervical **A**denitis; idiopathic condition in <5 years old, ≥3 monthly episodes lasting 5–7 days that include fever/chills/malaise, pharyngitis, aphthous stomatitis, tender cervical lymphadenopathy; <u>Rx</u>: corticosteroids in the acute phase and consider tonsillectomy

# Congenital Neck Masses

## Branchial Cleft Anomalies

- <u>Pathophysiology</u>: developmental alterations of the branchial apparatus result in **cysts** (no opening), **sinuses** (single opening to skin or digestive tract), **fistulas** (opening to skin and digestive tract), or cartilaginous remnants
- <u>SSx</u>: anterior neck mass (anterior to SCM, deep to platysma); may have an associated subcutaneous palpable cord; fistulas and sinuses may express mucoid discharge; secondary infections (commonly after URI) cause periodic fluctuation of size, tenderness, and purulent drainage; cartilaginous remnants appear as small horns or firm bumps
- <u>Dx</u>: physical exam, CT with contrast (may consider injecting contrast into fistula, poor sensitivity), MRI, laryngoscopy to visualize internal opening if there are associated symptoms or if it will change the surgical approach
- <u>Histopathology</u>: lined by squamous epithelium

### First Branchial Cleft Cyst

- <u>SSx</u>: usually presents as a preauricular cyst (type I) or at the mandibular angle or submandibular region (type II)
- <u>Types and Fistula Pathways</u>
  1. **Type I: ectodermal elements only**; duplicated EAC; typically begins periauricularly → passes lateral (superior) to CN VII → parallels the EAC → ends as a blind sac near the mesotympanum
  2. **Type II**: more common; **ectodermal and mesodermal elements**; duplicated membranous EAC and pinna; presents near angle of mandible → passes lateral or medial to CN VII → ends near or in the EAC
- <u>Rx</u>: full excision after resolution of infection (risk of facial nerve injury), may need superficial parotidectomy, avoid I&D

### Second Branchial Cleft Cyst

- **most common branchial cleft abnormality** (95%)
- <u>SSx</u>: cyst along anterior border of the SCM
- <u>Fistula Pathway</u>: external opening at anterior neck → along carotid sheath → **between** external and internal carotid arteries → **deep** to CN VII and **superficial** to CN XII and CN IX → internal opening at middle constrictors or in **tonsillar fossa**

- the course of the second branchial cleft cyst runs deep to second arch derivatives and superficial to third arch derivatives
- <u>Rx</u>: full excision after resolution of infection, avoid I&D

### Third Branchial Cleft Cyst

- <u>SSx</u>: cyst in lower anterior neck (less common); majority on left side; presents as abscess, neck mass (stridor, dysphagia, feeding difficulties), recurrent acute suppurative thyroiditis (late presentation, usually only presents with slight variation in thyroid function); often associated with thymic cysts
- <u>Fistula Pathway</u>: external opening at lower anterior neck → superficial to CN X and common carotid artery → superficial to CN XII → deep to CN IX → pierces thyrohyoid membrane staying above superior laryngeal nerve → internal opening at **upper (base of) piriform sinus**
- <u>Rx</u>: treat infection with antibiotics; full excision after resolution of infection, avoid I&D; excision must include partial thyroidectomy (superior pole of affected side); endoscopic obliteration of the piriform opening increasingly popular

### Fourth Branchial Cleft Cyst

- extremely rare
- <u>SSx</u>: similar to third branchial cleft cyst
- <u>Fistula Pathway</u>: external opening at lower anterior neck → loop around CN XII→ posterior to common carotid artery → thoracic component with loop below the aorta (left) or around subclavian artery (right) → posterior to thyroid gland → tracheoesophageal groove → pierces cricothyroid membrane beneath superior laryngeal nerve → **apex of piriform sinus**; recurrent laryngeal nerve remains deep to tract
- <u>Rx</u>: similar to third branchial cleft cyst, follow the tract

## Thyroglossal Duct Cyst (TGDC)

- <u>Pathophysiology</u>: failure of complete obliteration of thyroglossal duct (created from tract of embryologic thyroid descent: from floor of embryologic pharynx [**tuberculum impar**], which later forms the **foramen cecum,** down to midline neck)
- <u>SSx</u>: midline neck mass with cystic and solid components, elevates with tongue protrusion (attached to hyoid bone), typically inferior to hyoid bone and superior to thyroid gland, may have fibrous cord, dysphagia, globus sensation

- <u>Dx</u>: neck ultrasound (especially to confirm the presence of a thyroid gland; in 1% of patients, the TGDC contains the only functional thyroid tissue)
- <u>Histopathology</u>: lined with respiratory and squamous epithelium, possible thyroid follicles and colloid
- <u>Complications</u>: rare malignant potential, secondary infection
- <u>Rx</u>: **Sistrunk procedure** (excision of cyst and tract, including cuff of tongue base and mid-portion of hyoid bone, 3% recurrence; without hyoid resection 20–50% recurrence)

## Lingual Thyroid

- failure of thyroid gland to descend from the foramen cecum; presents as a posterior tongue mass, usually in females; in 75% it is the only functional thyroid tissue; potential malignant transformation
- <u>SSx</u>: dysphagia, dysphonia, stertor; frequently hypofunctioning
- <u>DDx</u>: thyroglossal duct cyst, lymphatic malformation, vallecular cyst, midline tumors (dermoid, teratoma)
- <u>Dx</u>: CT and/or neck ultrasound (identify caudal thyroid tissue), thyroid function tests, consider I-123 or technetium scan
- <u>Rx</u>: may observe if asymptomatic (watch closely for malignancy); ablative radioactive iodine considered in older adults; excision (transoral or transcervical) with possible thyroid tissue transplantation; almost all options require thyroid hormone supplementation or suppression

## Thymic Cysts

- <u>Pathophysiology</u>: remnant of **third pharyngeal pouch** between angle of mandible and midline neck
- <u>SSx</u>: unilateral (usually left) neck mass
- <u>Dx</u>: biopsy, serum calcium (associated parathyroid disorders, DiGeorge syndrome/22q11), CT/MRI
- <u>Rx</u>: excision (may require thoracic surgery)

## Dermoid Cysts and Teratomas

- <u>Pathophysiology</u>: derived from pluripotent embryonal stem cells
- <u>Types</u>
  1. **Teratoma**: composed of all 3 embryologic layers
  2. **Dermoid Cyst**: ectodermal and mesodermal elements only, most common type
  3. **Teratomoma**: differentiated to organ structure (usually fatal)
  4. **Epignathi**: differentiated to body parts (usually fatal)

- <u>SSx</u>: soft midline neck mass, may be associated with tufts of hair
- <u>Dx</u>: biopsy
- <u>Complications</u>: rare malignant potential
- <u>Rx</u>: excision

## Congenital Torticollis (Fibromatosis Colli, Sternocleidomastoid Tumor of Infancy, Pseudotumor of Infancy)

- <u>Pathophysiology</u>: intrauterine or birth trauma causing muscle injury, hematoma, and resultant fibrosis (typically of the SCM)
- <u>SSx</u>: presents 2–4 weeks after birth; head and neck held to diseased side, chin toward healthy side; firm thickened mass confined to SCM (may be tender)
- <u>Dx</u>: H&P (if biopsied looks malignant because of muscle cell death and regeneration with necrosis and mitotic figures)
- <u>Rx</u>: physical therapy, observation

# Infectious and Inflammatory Neck Masses

- *see also* pp. 233–236 for other infectious/inflammatory neck masses, pp. 238–243 for neck space infections, and pp. 131–133 for thyroid nodules and cysts

## Acute Suppurative Lymphadenitis and Neck Abscess

- <u>SSx</u>: rapidly enlarging, painful, mobile, fluctuant neck mass; malaise and fever (often in picket-fence [spiking] pattern)
- most common organisms are *S. aureus* and *S. pyogenes*; *S. anginosus* (formerly *S. milleri*)
- <u>Dx</u>: H&P, CT neck with contrast, culture, PCR
- <u>Rx</u>: antibiotics (may be resistant requiring longer course), I&D if abscess and/or nonimprovement with antibiotics (may trial 48 hours of IV antibiotics in pediatric neck abscess, whereas adults usually require prompt I&D)
- **Lemierre's Syndrome**: thrombophlebitis of the internal jugular vein following pharyngitis, peritonsillar abscess, or suppurative lymphadenitis; systemic microemboli leading to dyspnea and cough, pleuritic chest pain, pneumonia, arthralgia, endocarditis, meningitis, sepsis; usually caused by *Fusobacterium necrophorum;* <u>Dx</u>: CT with contrast or MRI; <u>Rx</u>: I&D; IV antibiotics for 3–6 weeks; anticoagulation controversial

## Atypical Mycobacterial Infection

- <u>SSx</u>: slowly enlarging, nontender, indurated neck mass with progressive skin discoloration (purplish), skin fixation, and possible fistulization; common in the anterior neck triangle and parotid region; corneal ulceration is the most common head and neck manifestation; does not cause pulmonary involvement but may colonize the respiratory tract; natural history is to suppurate and drain for 3 years then "burn out"
- <u>Subtypes</u>: *M. avium intracellulare, M. scrofulaceum, M. kansasii*
- <u>Dx</u>: culture (requires 2–4 weeks for growth), PCR, PPD (weak or negative)
- <u>Rx</u>: triple antibiotic therapy (clarithromycin, rifampin, ethambutol for 6 months); full surgical excision versus I&D with curettage

## Kawasaki Disease (Mucocutaneous Lymph Node Syndrome)

- <u>Pathophysiology</u>: uncertain etiology, results in acute vasculitis of multiple organ systems in children
- <u>Stages and Symptoms</u>
  1. **Acute**: high fevers (up to 40° C), cervical lymphadenopathy, conjunctivitis, red and dry blistering lips, desquamating rash, "strawberry tongue" (prominent papillae), oropharyngeal mucosal hyperemia, anterior uveitis, perianal erythema
  2. **Subacute:** decreased fever, more irritable and anorexic, thrombocytosis, acral desquamation, formation of coronary aneurysms
  3. **Convalescent/Chronic**: expansion of aneurysm and risk of MI
- <u>Dx</u>: H&P (must have 5 of the following: fever ≥5 days [absolute criteria], erythematous rash, conjunctival injection, oropharyngeal changes, peripheral extremity changes [erythema, edema, induration, desquamation], and cervical lymphadenopathy); echocardiogram and ECG
- <u>Complications</u>: coronary aneurysms in 20–25% (acute myocardial infarction in 0.5%), vasculitis
- <u>Rx</u>: hospital admission for high-dose IVIG while febrile, aspirin or dipyridamol for coronary aneurysms

## Plunging Ranula

- *see also* pp. 81–82
- <u>DDx</u>: lymphatic malformation, branchial cleft cyst

- <u>Dx</u>: usually component superior to mylohyoid and appears as translucent bluish swelling under tongue; CT/MRI/ultrasound (unilocular water density with smooth capsule, no septations, may have a "tail sign" between sublingual and submandibular spaces; macrocystic lymphatic malformations will have indistinct margins, septations, and infrequent communication with sublingual space); fine needle aspiration (mucus and high amylase)
- <u>Rx</u>: excision including involved sublingual gland (reduces recurrence from 50% to 2%)

## Rosai-Dorfman Disease

- rare idiopathic inflammatory disease characterized by massive, bilateral, nontender cervical lymphadenopathy in children <10 years old
- can present in the nasal cavity or paranasal sinuses
- <u>Rx</u>: endoscopic debulking for nasal disease; if dissemination, can consider targeted surgery, chemo/radiation

# Pediatric Head and Neck Malignancy

## Introduction

- 5–10% of malignant tumors in children arise from the head and neck
- squamous cell carcinoma is relatively rare in the pediatric population compared to adults
- neck is most common presenting anatomic location

## Hematologic Malignancy

- **lymphoma** is most common pediatric malignancy of the head and neck (excluding retinoblastoma and central nervous system malignancy), *see also* pp. 327–330
- both Hodgkin's and non-Hodgkin's lymphoma are more common in boys, Burkitt's lymphoma almost exclusively affects children; 60% of lymphomas in children are non-Hodgkin's

### Hodgkin's Lymphoma (HL)

- more common in adolescents; EBV may play a role in some cases
- airway compromise from mediastinal involvement (66%) or adenotonsillar enlargement; 30–40% will present with "B" symptoms (systemic symptoms such as fever, night sweat, weight loss)

- <u>Dx</u>: excisional lymph node biopsy; avoid giving steroids prior to the biopsy (affects ability to make diagnosis), must send as a fresh specimen

## Non-Hodgkin's Lymphoma (NHL)

- more common in males
- <u>Histopathology</u>: majority of children with NHL have high grade lesions (**Burkitt**/small noncleaved: diffuse B-cell malignancy, starry sky pattern; lymphoblastic: immature T-cells with convoluted nuclei; immunoblastic/large cell: equal number of B- and T-cells in children, heterogeneous group of lymphocytic and histiocytic tumors)
- <u>Burkitt Lymphoma SSx</u>: nasopharyngeal mass, unilateral otitis media, dysphagia, dyspnea, fatigue, weight loss
- <u>Burkitt Lymphoma Dx</u>: flexible laryngoscopy, CBC with differential, liver function tests, LDH level, CT neck/chest/abdomen/pelvis, barium swallow (up to 10% of patients can have an associated GI lesion), bone marrow biopsy, LP

# Soft Tissue Malignancy

## Rhabdomyosarcoma

- most common soft tissue malignancy in children, 35–40% are in head/neck
- within head/neck most common **ONES** are in the **O**rbit, **N**asopharynx, middle **E**ar/mastoid, **S**inonasal cavity
- <u>Parameningeal Sites</u>: middle ear/mastoid, sinonasal, nasopharyngeal, infratemporal fossa; may spread into meninges, less favorable prognosis
- 20% regional lymph node involvement (rare for orbital tumors), rare distant metastasis (lungs, bones, bone marrow)
- <u>Types</u>
  1. **Embryonal**: 75%, more common in infants and young children; poorly differentiated, **botryoid type**, consists of spindle-shaped, round, and "tadpole"-shaped cells; best prognosis
  2. **Alveolar**: 20%, more common in adolescence; composed of round cells with reticulin-staining trabeculae; worst prognosis
  3. **Pleomorphic**: 5%, more common in adults; well-differentiated, consists of spindle and "strap" cells
- <u>Pediatric Staging</u>: Stage 1: head and neck, no parameningeal involvement, no metastases; Stage 2: parameningeal involvement, ≤5 cm; Stage 3: parameningeal involvement, >5 cm or nodal metastasis; Stage 4: distant metastasis

- <u>SSx</u>: commonly misdiagnosed early due to vague symptoms; rapidly progressive proptosis, vision loss, unilateral otitis media, nasal obstruction, headache, cranial nerve palsies
- <u>Dx</u>: CT/MRI, FNA, open biopsy
- <u>Rx</u>: chemotherapy (either as a primary regimen, with radiation therapy, or less commonly as postoperative adjuvant therapy), surgical debulking may be required without causing morbidity and if full excision is expected (several ongoing trials through the **Intergroup Rhabdomyosarcoma Study Group [IRS]** have led to a tripling of the 2-year survival rate in the last 30 years)
- <u>Prognosis</u>: Stage 1: 80% survival if all disease removed plus chemoradiation; Stage 2: 72% survival if microscopic disease left behind plus chemoradiation; Stage 3: 50% survival if gross disease left behind plus chemoradiation; Stage 4: 20% survival if distant metastasis and chemoradiation)

### Ewing's Sarcoma

- malignant bone sarcoma; second most common malignant bone tumor in children; usually affects long bones and pelvis
- 1–9% are in head and neck; skull base and mandible most common sites
- <u>Histopathology</u>: high grade **small round blue cell tumor**, PAS+
- locally aggressive and frequent metastases
- <u>SSx</u>: slow-growing, firm enlarging mass with or without pain
- <u>Dx</u>: biopsy
- <u>Rx</u>: chemotherapy, wide local resection (if complete resection possible and no intracranial involvement), radiotherapy (if large tumor and surgery not possible or residual tumor)
- <u>Prognosis</u>: **Intergroup Ewing Sarcoma Study (IESS)** found a 3-year survival rate of 80% with 3–4 drug chemotherapy

### Others

- fibrosarcoma, chondrosarcoma (less common in pediatrics)

## Thyroid Malignancy

- *see also* pp. 133–137
- majority of thyroid nodules are solitary in children
- nodules more likely malignant than in adults (20–40%)
- FNA in children less accurate than in adults (90% versus 97%)
- follicular adenoma is most common benign diagnosis

- <u>Risk Factors for Malignancy</u>: age (pediatric age range; most common 10–20 years old), previous H&N XRT, family history of thyroid cancer or MEN
- in children, more likely to have locoregional (40–80%) and metastatic spread (7–25%, lung most common); high recurrence rate; more sensitive to $^{131}$I; overall survival rate near 100%
- <u>Histopathology</u>: papillary (85–90%), medullary (5%)
- <u>Rx</u>: lowest radioactive iodine dose possible because of lifetime risks of secondary neoplasms; surgery for malignancy must include central compartment neck dissection at a minimum if no obvious locoregional disease on ultrasound; if locoregional disease present, full neck dissection on involved side
- **Multiple Endocrine Neoplasia (MEN):** MEN 2a: total thyroidectomy at ~6 years old; MEN 2b; total thyroidectomy in infancy (>90% risk of medullary thyroid carcinomas over lifetime)

## Nervous System Malignancy

### *Neuroblastoma*

- malignant tumor of the sympathetic nervous system; arises from **neural crest cells**
- most common extracranial solid malignancy in childhood; 8–10% of all pediatric malignancies
- <u>SSx</u>: typically originates from sites below the diaphragm; presents as a painless cervical mass with possible **Horner's** syndrome, dysphagia (local pressure on aerodigestive tract), and heterochromia iridis; frequent bone metastases (60%, including skull and facial bones)
- <u>Dx</u>: urine catecholamines, MRI
- <u>Rx</u>: surgical resection if complete excision possible (incomplete excision can be therapeutic in some cases), chemotherapy; neoadjuvant chemotherapy if unresectable

## Other Malignancy

### *Nasopharyngeal Carcinoma*

- typically nonkeratinizing, undifferentiated subtype
- children have more advanced disease at presentation
- <u>Rx</u>: chemotherapy (cisplatin, 5-FU) with radiotherapy at lower dose than adults to avoid secondary malignancies

# Salivary and Other Pediatric Head and Neck Tumors

## Pediatric Salivary Gland Tumors

- **infantile hemangioma** and **pleomorphic adenoma** are the most common **benign** parotid tumors of childhood
- excluding hemangioma, salivary gland infection, and lymphatic malformations, >50% of parotid solid masses are malignant
- well-differentiated **mucoepidermoid** tumors are the most common salivary gland malignancies in children
- **acinic cell** carcinoma is second most common salivary gland cancer in children
- <u>Rx</u>: surgery; adjuvant radiation if high grade, locoregional disease or involving nerves

## Lipoblastoma

- rare benign, rapidly growing neoplasm of **embryonic fat**
- <u>Histopathology</u>: encapsulated (lipoblastoma, usually unifocal); diffuse (lipoblastomatosis); lobulated tumor of immature fat with connective tissue septae, a myxoid background, and absence of atypia
- more common in <3 years old (including infants), males
- very high rate of **recurrence** (≤25%; average within 3 years) if surgical resection not complete; lack of malignant transformation; spontaneous regression/transformation to lipoma reported
- <u>SSx</u>: often asymptomatic; stertor/stridor/obstructive sleep apnea, Horner's syndrome, hemiparesis
- <u>Dx</u>: MRI, biopsy
- <u>Rx</u>: function-preserving wide local resection

# Benign Oral Cavity Lesions (see pp. 203–217)

# Odontogenic, Jaw, and Bone Pathology (see pp. 217–229)

# Head and Neck Manifestations of Systemic Diseases (see pp. 243–252)

## Langerhans Cell Histiocytosis

- obsolete terminology includes histiocytosis X and reticuloendotheliosis
- **noninfectious granulomatous disease**

- affects 0.5–5 children per million per year
- <u>Pathophysiology</u>: granulomatous disease of unknown etiology, manifests as a proliferation of bone marrow-derived histiocytes
- <u>Histopathology</u>: sheets of polygonal histiocytes, Birbeck granules ("zipper" pattern), rod-shaped cytoplasmic organelles with a central linear density and a striated appearance ("tennis-rackets")
- otologic manifestations may mimic a wide range of disease (otitis externa/media, aural polyps, mastoiditis, temporal bone metastases)
- modern classification scheme based on organs and sites involved, classic terminology follows

## Eosinophilic Granuloma

- **localized form**, excellent prognosis
- presents in children and young adults
- <u>SSx</u>: monostotic or polyostotic osteolytic bone lesions (predilection for temporal and frontal bones, ribs, long bones), proptosis (sphenoid involvement), acute mastoiditis, **middle ear granulation tissue**, tympanic membrane perforation, facial paralysis
- <u>Rx</u>: surgical excision; radiation therapy reserved for recurrence, inoperable sites, and high-risk patients

## Hand-Schüller-Christian Disease

- **chronic disseminated form**, 30% mortality (higher risk with heart, lung, brain involvement)
- presents in children and young adults (rare in elderly)
- <u>SSx</u>: polyostotic osteolytic lesions (skull), exophthalmos, diabetes insipidus (from erosion of sphenoid into sella turcica), facial paralysis, EAC polypoid lesions
- <u>Rx</u>: radiation, chemotherapy, corticosteroids

## Letterer-Siwe Disease

- **acute disseminated form**, uniformly fatal
- presents in children <3 years old
- <u>SSx</u>: fever, proptosis, splenomegaly, hepatomegaly, exfoliative dermatitis, thrombocytopenia
- <u>Rx</u>: same as Hand-Schüller-Christian disease

## Congenital Self-Healing Reticulohistiocytosis (Hashimoto-Pritzker Syndrome)

- mucosal and cutaneous form with dark nodules on face, trunk, and scalp

**Infectious Granulomatous Diseases** (*see* pp. 245–248)

**Congenital Syphilis** (*see* pp. 577–578)

# PEDIATRIC RECONSTRUCTIVE AND FACIAL PLASTIC SURGERY

## Fundamentals of Wound Healing
(see pp. 437–442)

## Aural Atresia and Microtia

### Evaluation

- <u>H&P</u>: examine mandible, oral cavity, spine, eyes, skin quality, hairline, position of ear remnant, facial nerve function
- <u>Hearing</u>: audiogram, ABR; usually 40–60 dB CHL; 10–15% have SNHL
- if unilateral microtia/atresia and the other ear passes newborn screening, more extensive testing of the affected ear can be delayed until 6–7 months; if it fails, do ABR
- CT temporal bone (*see* atresia grading systems *following*)

### Aural Atresia

- 90% nonsyndromic, 10% syndromic; 20–30% bilateral
- <u>Associations</u>: cholesteatoma (4–7%), malformed cochlea (5%), malformed semicircular canals (10%), stapes fixation (4%), **microtia** (55–93%)
- fusion of malleus/incus is most common middle ear anomaly, footplate is usually normal
- otitis media should be treated aggressively to preserve hearing in the normal contralateral ear
- no need to perform CT before age 4 for congenital cholesteatoma as cholesteatoma usually slow growing (CT performed early must be repeated anyway before ultimate atresia repair)
- <u>Candidacy for Surgical Repair Grading Systems</u>
  1. **Jahrsdoerfer Grading**: 10-point system based on CT findings; better atresiaplasty candidate if ≥6 points; **stapes** present (2 points), oval window open (1), middle ear space (1), facial nerve normal (1), malleus-incus complex present (1), mastoid

well-pneumatized (1), incus-stapes connection (1), round
window normal (1), appearance of external ear (1)

2. **De la Cruz Classification**: **minor malformations** (better
surgical candidate): normal mastoid pneumatization, normal oval
window/footplate, reasonable facial nerve–footplate relationship,
normal inner ear; **major malformations** (poor surgical candidate;
hearing aid better option): poor pneumatization, abnormal or
absent oval window/footplate, abnormal facial nerve course,
abnormalities of inner ear

- <u>Rx</u>: early bone conduction hearing aids if bilateral; definitive
treatment controversial; traditional hearing aids or auditory
osseointegrated implants (BAHA; particularly if bilateral atresia)
versus eventual surgical repair; if repair then perform at age 7
after microtia repair; 3 surgical approaches: mastoid, anterior, and
modified anterior

- <u>Prognosis</u>: 30 dB HL or better with surgery in 50–75% cases; air–
bone gap closure with BAHA in 85%

- <u>Surgical Complications</u>: lateralization of the tympanic membrane
graft (25%), canal stenosis (8%), TMJ pain/trauma (2%), facial
nerve injury (1%), SNHL (2–5%)

## Microtia

- congenitally malformed auricle, often associated with atresia;
degree of auricular malformation usually correlates with degree of
middle ear deformity; associated inner ear abnormalities more rare
(vestibular dysplasia most common)

- <u>Causes</u>: genetic, teratogens (vitamin A/isotretinoin, thalidomide),
vascular insults

- 25% bilateral, right side more common, M:F ratio of 2.5:1,
highest rate in Japanese, Hispanic, and Native American; may have
syndromic association (eg, hemifacial microsomia)

- <u>Classification</u> (multiple systems exist)
  1. **Grade I:** auricle slightly smaller but all subunits present (**lop ear**:
  auricular cartilage angled inferiorly; **cup ear**: deep conchal bowl,
  anterior protrusion of auricular cartilage)
  2. **Grade II:** auricle smaller than grade I, more rudimentary; some
  subunits severely underdeveloped or absent; lower half of ear often
  more developed than upper half
  3. **Grade III:** small piece of cartilage in the superior remnant,
  anteriorly deflected inferior lobule (**peanut ear**)
  4. **Grade IV:** anotia (complete absence of auricle and lobule)

- <u>Rx</u>: surgical repair (typically at 5–6 years old in girls and at 10 years old in boys, timing also influenced by coexisting atresia), cosmetic prosthesis (may be bone anchored, *see following*)

## Total Auricular/Microtia Reconstruction Techniques

- **Costal Cartilage Autograft**: rib is popular cartilage source due to suitable integrity, sufficient quantity, and minimal morbidity with harvest (*see* Brent *and* Nagata *techniques following*)
- **Alloplastic Implant**: includes Medpor (porous polyethylene) implant, technically easier, does not tolerate trauma well, risk of extrusion
- **Auricular Prosthesis**: prosthesis is anchored by magnets (previously clips) to titanium posts, which are connected to osseointegrated implants placed in the mastoid bone, often very realistic
- **Tissue Engineering**: cartilage grafts constructed from cultures of autologous chondrocytes or stem cells (*experimental*)

### *Brent Cartilage Autograft Technique*

- 2–4 stages separated by 3 months (some stages may be combined)

#### 1st Stage

- contralateral 6th–7th rib cartilage framework is carved and placed in a postauricular subcutaneous pocket (thin overlying skin as much as possible), 8th rib approximates helical rim
- contours are exaggerated to anticipate flattening
- include scaphoid and triangular fossae carve-out

#### 2nd Stage

- lobule transposition: lobule is rotated (use ear vestige in microtia) and often filleted to receive the end of the cartilage framework

#### 3rd Stage

- construct is elevated to achieve projection of the helical rim
- ear position can be stabilized by placing a piece of banked cartilage posteriorly beneath the framework in a fascial pocket
- retroauricular scalp advancement flap and STSG used to close the postauricular defect

#### 4th Stage

- tragus construction, conchal excavation, symmetry adjustments

## *Nagata Cartilage Autograft Technique*

- 2 stages separated by 6 months

### 1st Stage

- 6th–9th rib cartilage framework, which incorporates a tragal component, is placed in a subcutaneous pocket and the lobule is transposed
- roughly corresponds to the first two stages in Brent's sequence

### 2nd Stage

- construct is elevated using a crescent-shaped piece of cartilage harvested from the 5th rib
- **temporoparietofascial flap** is elevated and tunneled subcutaneously to cover the posterior surface of the cartilage graft, reconstructed auricle, and the mastoid surface; STSG also used

## *Complications of Cartilage Autograft Reconstruction*

- **Hematoma**: may result in loss of cartilage, must investigate severe pain by removing dressings; prevented with suction drains; <u>Rx</u>: immediate exploration with removal of clot, hemostasis, and antibiotics
- **Chondritis**: presents with pain, may result in loss of cartilage; <u>Rx</u>: aggressive antibiotic regimen, drainage and debridement if required
- **Skin Necrosis and Cartilage Exposure**: may be secondary to excessive tension, hematoma, or infection; <u>Rx</u>: small areas may be treated with topical antibiotics, debridement should be limited to obvious necrotic tissue, cartilage exposure requires coverage (may consider FTSG)
- **Hypertrophic Scars and Keloids, Scar Contracture**: avoid by providing a tension-free closure
- **Poor Contouring or Poor Positioning**: poor cosmetic outcome
- **Pneumothorax and Atelectasis**: rare potential risk from rib harvest

# Craniosynostosis

## Overview

- premature ossification of 1 or more of the fibrous skull sutures, resulting in abnormal head shape
- <u>Normal Closure of Sutures</u>: metopic at 9 months; lambdoid, sagittal, coronal at 22–39 months; most common early closure is sagittal followed by coronal, metopic, lambdoid (*see* Figure 10–2)

- Etiology: **fibroblast growth factor receptor** (FGFR) defect involved in 1/3 of nonsyndromic and most syndromic cases
- Classifications
  1. **Nonsyndromic (Isolated) or Syndromic**: 15–40% syndromic, eg, Apert, Crouzon, Pfeiffer, Saethre-Chotzen, Muenke
  2. **Simple (1 Suture) or Complex**
  3. **Phenotype-Based: brachycephaly**: coronal sutures on both sides, wide head with flat occiput; **dolichocephaly/scaphocephaly**: sagittal suture, long narrow head; **plagiocephaly**: anterior (coronal suture on 1 side; forward displacement of the ipsilateral ear and face, unilateral bulging forehead) or posterior (lambdoid suture on 1 side; occipital asymmetry with posterior displacement of the ipsilateral ear); **trigonocephaly**: metopic suture, triangular head shape with narrow forehead; **turricephaly/oxycephaly**: coronal suture and 1 other suture; **bathrocephaly**: mendosal suture (accessory suture in occipital bone), posterior skull deformity; **pansynostosis**: 3 or more sutures, can present as microcephaly or cloverleaf skull anomaly (Kleeblattschädel)
- SSx: increased intracranial pressure that can lead to hydrocephalus, developmental delay, vomiting, bulging fontanelles, obstructive sleep apnea (midface hypoplasia), as well as visual (papilledema), sleep, and eating disturbances
- Dx: physical exam (eye/ear position, mastoid bulge), skull x-ray, CT, head circumference, fundoscopy

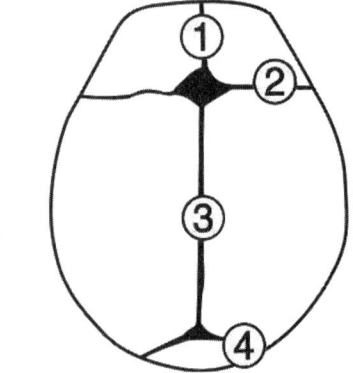

1. Metopic
2. Coronal
3. Sagittal
4. Lambdoidal

**FIGURE 10–2.** Cranial sutures.

- <u>Rx</u>: surgical repair, ideally between 6–12 months
- **Positional Plagiocephaly**: skull deformation secondary to extrinsic forces, normal sutures; <u>Rx</u>: physiotherapy, parent education, "tummy time" when awake, helmeting controversial

## Craniofacial Clefts

- classified using the Tessier classification (*see* Figure 10–3) around the central facial landmarks (numbers 0 to 14, with possible combinations), transverse/lateral clefts are most common type
- <u>Etiology</u>: failure of mesoderm fusion, lateral clefts could be explained by amniotic bands

## Parry Romberg Disease (Hemifacial Progressive Atrophy)

- acquired, idiopathic, self-limited, unilateral atrophy of the face (95% cases), variably involving the skin, subcutaneous tissues, fat, muscles, and bones
- onset slow and progressive (begins first 2 decades of life, 2–10 year course)

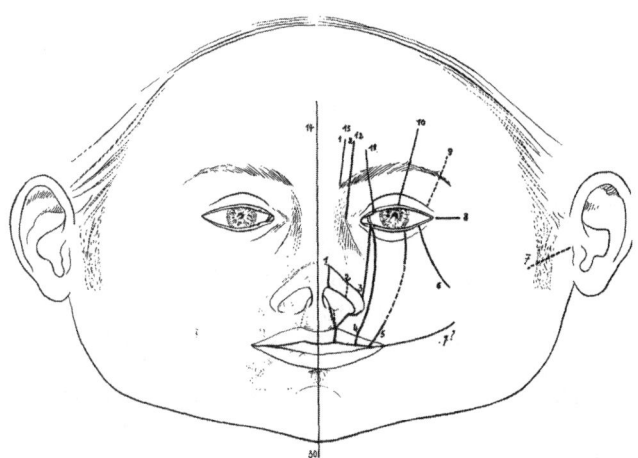

**FIGURE 10–3.** Craniofacial clefts (Used with permission. Tessier P. Anatomical classification facial, cranio-facial, and latero-facial clefts. *J Maxillofac Surg* 1976;4:69–92).

- unknown etiology; possibly an autoimmune neurovasculitis, localized scleroderma (morphea), or neuritis
- can be associated with CNS manifestations (neurologic, ophthalmologic, or intravascular disorders)
- <u>Types</u>: **I:** very mild, thinness of soft facial tissues (noticed by patient and family only); **II:** deformity noticeable to others; **III:** soft tissues/bone/cartilage thinner than type II; **IV:** most severe, associated with functional problems
- <u>Rx</u>: I–II: lipoinjection; III–IV: cartilage, bone, dermis, fat grafts; galeal flaps or free flaps

# Cleft Lip and Palate

## Anatomy

- **Primary Palate (Premaxilla):** anterior to incisive foramen, formed first, wedge-shaped, houses 4 incisors
- **Secondary Palate:** nonpremaxilla portion of hard palate and the soft palate
- <u>Soft Palate Muscles</u>
  1. **Tensor Veli Palatini:** (CN V₃) opens eustachian tube and depresses and tenses soft palate
  2. **Levator Veli Palatini:** (CN X, pharyngeal plexus) elevates palate
  3. **Musculus Uvulae:** (CN X, pharyngeal plexus) moves uvula up and forward
  4. **Palatoglossus:** (CN X, pharyngeal plexus) draws palate down, narrows pharynx
  5. **Palatopharyngeus:** (CN X, pharyngeal plexus) draws palate down, narrows pharynx

## Embryology

- **Frontonasal Prominence:** first phase (**4th–5th weeks**); medial; anterior labial component → philtrum; anterior palatal/medial component → midline alveolus; posterior component → palate anterior to incisive foramen (**primary palate**); also contributes to nasal anatomy
- **Maxillary Prominence:** second phase (**8th–9th weeks**), **secondary** palate; medial growth and fusion of the mesodermal palatal shelves from the lateral maxilla; fusion begins rostral → caudally beginning at incisive foramen; process complete by the 12th week
- **Mandibular Prominence:** mandible

# Epidemiology

- second most common congenital malformation (club foot is most common)
- cleft lip and palate occurs in 1/1000 births, cleft palate 1/2000 births
- 45% both cleft lip and palate; 30% secondary palate only; 25% lip only; cleft lips (with or without associated cleft palate) and isolated cleft palates occur in distinct genetic lines
- Risk Factors: Asian, Native American, males have more cleft lips, females have more isolated palates
- Etiology: unknown (most common), genetic, environmental (folate deficiency, maternal diabetes, amniotic band syndrome, teratogens [ethanol, thalidomide, vitamin A derivatives])
- genetic concordance for cleft lip/palate is 25–40% in monozygotic twins, 3–5% in dizygotic twins
- associated heart anomalies up to 10% (cleft palate most common, also in combined cleft lip and palate); theory is that medial edges of epithelium fail to fuse because of failure of epithelium to transform into mesenchyme, as happens with several heart defects; a theory of failure of apoptosis also exists

# Evaluation

- prenatal consultation
- immediate concerns at birth are airway and feeding

## *Define Type of Defect*

- **Lip**: unilateral, bilateral; complete, incomplete (presence of Simonart band), microform (forme fruste)
- Unilateral Cleft Lip Defect: orbicularis oris muscle is directed superiorly in complete cleft or is hypoplastic in incomplete cleft; floor of nose communicates with oral cavity; maxilla is hypoplastic on cleft side; lower lateral cartilage is inferior on cleft side; nasal ala is retrodisplaced on cleft side; nasal columella is displaced toward normal side; dome is lowered, horizontal nares on cleft side; cartilaginous nasal septum and nasal spine are deflected away from cleft; alveolar defect passes through developing dentition
- Bilateral Cleft Lip Defect: floor of nose communicates with oral cavity bilaterally; central part of alveolar arch is rotated forward and upward; prolabium skin for the lip is underdeveloped; central lip has no muscle or vermilion; nasal columella is short, nasal tip is widened, cartilaginous nasal septum and nasal spine are deflected forward

- **Palate**: unilateral, bilateral; complete (primary and secondary palates), incomplete (secondary palate, posterior to incisive foramen), submucous
- Veau Classification of Cleft Palate: **I**: isolated cleft of soft palate; **II**: cleft of soft/hard palates, extending into the incisive foramen; **III**: complete unilateral cleft of the lip, alveolus and soft/hard palate; **IV**: complete bilateral clefts of the lip, alveolus, soft/hard palates
- Submucosal Cleft: minor form of a secondary cleft palate defect causing a midline diastasis of the levator muscles with the mucosa remaining intact; deficient musculature of the palate causes a blue streak (zona pellucida), associated with a bifid uvula and loss of posterior nasal spine (palatal notch); higher risk of velopharyngeal insufficiency after adenoidectomy

## *Examine for Other Defects*

- **Craniofacial**: Pierre-Robin sequence (U-shaped cleft palate, secondary palate only), facial clefts, telecanthus, maxillary/malar hypoplasia, craniosynostosis
- **Nasal**: with unilateral cleft lip findings are inferolateral displacement of the alar base and lateral crus, dome flattening and downward rotation, horizontal positioning of the nostril on the cleft side and a short columella
- **Otologic**: microtia, atresia, ear tags/pits, CN VII dysfunction, eustachian tube dysfunction (hypoplastic levator and tensor veli palatini; eustachian tube more horizontal and hypercompliant; increased reflux leads to chronic otitis media)
- **Complete Pediatric Assessment**: evaluate for heart, genitourinary, limb, other anomalies

## *Determine if Syndromic*

- **Family History**: positive in 26%
- **Genetic Evaluation**: isolated cleft palates have 8% association with a syndrome (eg, Stickler, Treacher Collins, Pierre-Robin sequence, Apert, 22q11, Down, Smith-Lemli-Opitz, van der Woude)

## *Evaluate Feeding Assistance*

- poor suction, lengthy feeds, inadequate intake, excessive air intake, nasal regurgitation, poor airway protection
- if feeding >25–30 minutes consider feeding assistance because too much energy is being expended and will cause failure to thrive
- breast feeding may be possible with isolated cleft lip

## Management

- **Feeding/Lactation**: special nipples help with difficulty obtaining a seal (preemie nipples: Mead-Johnson, McGovern's cross-cut; unidirectional feeders: Haberman, Pigeon); frequent rests and burps, upright feeding with chin support, palatal prosthesis/obdurator or preoperative nasoalveolar molding (PNAM)
- **Otologic**: PE tubes (on average 3 sets needed by age 7; 90–100% incidence of middle ear effusion by 1 month old); yearly audiogram; palatoplasty improves eustachian tube dysfunction
- **Speech/Swallow Therapy**: follow closely for feeding/swallow, speech development, and assistance with velopharyngeal dysfunction
- **Psychology and Social Work**: parental counseling and assistance is important starting prenatally; child and family will need ongoing support throughout childhood
- **Pediatrics**: involvement of a pediatrician familiar with cleft care is important to help with global development
- **Dental**: prostheses/molding (*see* previous), latham appliance, orthodontic appliances, oral hygiene and care, dental restoration
- **Surgical Repair**: *see* following

## Surgical Repair

### *Timeline*

- <u>Birth</u>: lip repair (especially wide clefts); consider taping, lip adhesion, or nasoalveolar molding (needs adjustments every 2 weeks), Latham appliance
- <u>3–4 Months</u>: cleft lip repair, tip rhinoplasty, close nasal floor, PE tubes (if did not pass newborn hearing screening); perform slightly later if primary lip adhesion
- <u>1 Year</u>: palate repair, PE tubes
- <u>3–5 Years</u>: columellar lengthening (bilateral clefts), nasal tip revision
- <u>6–8 Years</u>: speech surgery
- <u>8–16 Years</u>: orthodontics
- <u>10 Years</u>: alveolar cancellous bone grafts (iliac crest or bone morphogenic protein (rhBMP-2)
- <u>14 Years</u>: definitive rhinoplasty and orthognathic surgery

### *Cleft Lip Repair*

- repair at 10–14 weeks (**rules of 10: >10 weeks, >10 pounds, Hb >10**)

- <u>Goals</u>: correct cupid's bow, normal orbicularis oris muscle function, symmetric repair of vermilion, create nasal floor and vestibular sill, placement of nasal alar base and columella
- bilateral defects may be staged within months
- varying degrees of primary rhinoplasty can be performed at the time of primary cleft lip repair (controversial)
- **Lip Adhesion**: produces an incomplete cleft, performed at 2–4 weeks for severe clefts; reduces tension when definitive repair is performed (postponed to 4–6 months), scar band may interfere with definitive repair

### Common Techniques

- **Millard Repair**: rotation-advancement technique for unilateral lip repair, limited tissue loss, reconstructs the philtrum and nasal sill, may be difficult to close large clefts
- **Mohler Repair**: modification of Millard repair, extension and backcut into columella
- **Noordhoff Repair**: incorporates triangles from the cleft side above the vermilion and at the lip red line to improve lip symmetry
- **Triangle Cleft-Lip Repair (Tennison-Randall)**: modification of the original stencil method by Tennison; utilizes the rotation, advancement, and interposition of triangular flaps
- **Rose-Thompson**: first described technique; straight line repair, simple design, favorable suture line, risk of vertical line contracture, difficult to close large clefts
- **Anatomical Subunit Repair (Fisher)**: repair along lines of anatomical subunits, combines Rose-Thomson and Noordhoff techniques; very reliable but technically challenging

## Cleft Palate Repair

- repair at 10–14 months (after lip repair)
- may require orthodontic treatment (NAM, latham, taping) to move premaxilla or to realign maxillary segments

### Common Techniques

- **Von Langenbeck Palatoplasty**: incision along the cleft and alveolar margins producing 2 bipedicle mucoperiosteal flaps that are advanced maintaining the anterior attachment at the alveolar margin; used in isolated complete cleft palate repair
- **Two-Flap Palatoplasty (Bardach)**: modification of the von Langenbeck with complete incisions at the alveolar margin, flap based on the greater palatine vessels; indicated for complete

unilateral and bilateral clefts of the primary and secondary palate; modifications allow closure of wide clefts and include the use of vomer mucosal flaps and neurovascular bundle skeletonization and lengthening; detachment of the velar muscle fibers from the posterior palate and reconstruction of the muscular sling is key (intravelar veloplasty)

- **Furlow Palatoplasty**: opposing Z-plasty, elongates soft palate
- **V–Y Pushback (Veau-Wardill-Kilner)**: retroposition of the mucoperiosteal flap and soft palate, provides additional palate length
- **Schweckendick's Primary Veloplasty**: early soft palate closure with hard palate closure delayed until 12–14 years old; can improve midfacial growth

### Complications

- <u>Early</u>: bleeding, airway obstruction, dehiscence (reduce with soft or pourable liquid diet for 2 weeks postop, no pacifier, use of arm restraints, feeding by sippy-cup or syringe)
- <u>Late</u>: fistulae (various types), velopharyngeal insufficiency, maxillary growth disturbance

## Velopharyngeal Dysfunction/ Insufficiency (VPI)

- lack of coordinated or complete closure of the **soft palate** to the **posterior pharyngeal wall**; also involves movement of the **lateral pharyngeal walls**
- speech abnormalities should be addressed early (leads to pervasive problems in socialization, education, and global development)
- <u>Etiology</u>: syndrome (eg, **22q11**), submucous cleft palate, iatrogenic (after adenoidectomy or cleft palate repair)
- <u>SSx</u>: nasal air emission, **hypernasal speech**, increased nasal resonance, nasal regurgitation, impaired speech intelligibility, decreased speech volume, **facial grimacing**; plosive sounds (consonants) are most difficult, also watch for glottic stops
- <u>Dx</u>: speech language pathology assessment, nasometry, nasopharyngoscopy, or multiview speech fluoroscopy (either or both, debated)
- <u>Rx</u>: **speech therapy** (usually >3–6 months to correct maladaptive speech patterns before considering surgery; crucial postoperatively); targeted **surgery** should take into consideration the velopharyngeal gap size and pattern of closure (palatal length deficiency versus central defects versus lateral pharyngeal wall immobility versus palate

scarring and immobility); <u>Surgical Techniques</u>: Furlow palatoplasty, superior-based pharyngeal flap, sphincter pharyngoplasty, posterior pharyngeal wall augmentation; prosthetic obduration

- consider repair as early as 4 years old in severe cases; earlier repair associated with better long-term speech outcomes

- <u>Complications</u>: **obstructive sleep apnea**, aspiration/pneumonia, hemorrhage (palpate for medialized carotids; MRA preoperatively for 22q11 deletion patients), infection, dehiscence, scarring, nasopharyngeal stenosis, neck stiffness, hyponasality

# Other Pediatric Reconstructive and Plastic Surgery Considerations

## Rhinoplasty

- *see also* pp. 476–485
- usually wait until age 15–16 years to avoid growth disturbances, especially for procedures disturbing the cartilaginous vault; bony pyramid osteotomies, tip work, alar base work, and transcolumellar incisions considered safe; cartilage grafting can give unpredictable results

## Otoplasty

- *see also* pp. 485–487
- auricle mature size at 13 (female) or 15 (male) years old; 95% of adult size at 6 years old
- usual timing for otoplasty is just before entering school at ~6 years old to avoid social stigma (incisionless technique can be performed at a younger age)

## Lipoinjection

- *see also* p. 499
- fat harvest and injection/grafting for facial recontouring and defect reconstruction
- low-pressure syringe-assisted fat harvesting methods preferred in children; washing the graft may be harmful; graft nutrition by **imbibition** occurs up to 1.5 mm from vascularized edge; resorption 20–50% depending on technique used
- <u>Pediatric Indications</u>: congenital facial dysmorphism, scars, acquired lipodystrophy, Treacher Collins, hemifacial microsomia, hemangioma scars, Parry Romberg disease

- <u>Complications</u>: minor: contour irregularities, hematoma; major: fat necrosis, infection, ocular or cerebral embolism (avoid by using blunt needles)

## Incision/Excision Planning and Scar Revisions and Scar Resurfacing (*see* pp. 512–518)

## Tissue Fillers (*see* pp. 506–509)

# PEDIATRIC HEAD AND NECK TRAUMA
## Overview
### Introduction

- children susceptible to head and neck trauma because of their disproportionately large heads, decreased motor coordination and low awareness of environmental hazards
- maxillofacial fractures less common (15%) in pediatric trauma (retruded face in relation to cranium, additional horizontal buttresses from **unerupted teeth**, higher cancellous-to-cortical-bone ratio leading to **greenstick**-type fractures, undeveloped sinuses, thick soft tissue)
- low-velocity trauma in young children; fractures increase in incidence after age 13 with high-velocity trauma; more common in males; nose and mandible fractures most common
- reduce/stabilize fractures that need treatment quickly (children heal faster than adults)
- long-term followup required due to effects of fracture and method of repair on growth and development of the face

### Evaluation

- *see* also pp. 628–635
- do not rely on child's vital signs or urinary output to assess for hypovolemic shock; assess for **pediatric dehydration** instead (lethargy, sunken eyes, sunken fontanelles, dry mucous membranes, prolonged capillary refill, mottled extremities, absence of tears, etc)
- **Initial Resuscitation**: 20 mL/kg bolus, use a warm isotonic crystalloid solution
- **Blood Transfusion**: routine amount is 10 mL/kg (normal blood volume is ~70 × patient's weight in kg)
- **Maintenance Fluid**: use **4:2:1 formula** (4 mL/kg/hr for the first 10 kg of weight, 2 mL/kg/hr for the second 10 kg of weight, 1 mL/kg/

hr for any additional weight; if child is obese, use the estimated lean weight)

- **Airway:** avoid surgical cricothyroidotomy in infants and young children (high rate of subglottic injury and subsequent stenosis)
- **Nonaccidental Trauma (NAT):** ie, abuse; always consider possibility; 30% involve children <6 months; risk factors include socioeconomic status, single parent, young parental age, parental substance abuse

# Traumatic Injuries

## Caustic Ingestion (*see* pp. 566–568)

## Mandibular Fractures

- *see also* pp. 635–642
- most common in **condyle**, symphysis, alveolus (younger children), or angle of mandible (older children)
- in general prefer conservative management (soft diet, observation with followup, joint exercises), usually can tolerate some malocclusion, which adjusts with growth
- may treat with maxillomandibular fixation for 3 weeks only for open bite deformity or severe trismus (TMJ ankylosis may lead to facial distortion from altered joint growth)
- children 6–12 years old may need direct skeletal/circummandibular wires or piriform aperture suspension, as primary (deciduous) teeth are difficult to wire
- pediatric subcondylar fractures are more prone to ankylosis and mandibular growth abnormalities and therefore require long-term followup
- damage to tooth buds after ORIF is a concern; remove hardware after 2–3 months at sites of facial skeleton and dental development

## Maxillary Fractures

- *see also* pp. 642–646
- less common in children (protected by unerupted teeth, trauma usually low velocity)
- treatment with maxillomandibular fixation preferred over ORIF (ORIF can lead to growth compromise of midface)

## Zygomaticomaxillary and Orbital Fractures

- *see also* pp. 646–651
- orbital floor fracture with **inferior rectus entrapment** must be reduced within 24 hours to avoid muscle fibrosis

- follow closely for nonunion, which could lead to entrapment and permanent damage

## Frontal Sinus and Naso-Orbitoethmoid Fractures

- *see also* pp. 651–656; in general management similar to adults
- monitor for appropriate healing, risk of nonunion and associated complications (eg, encephalocele) with ongoing skull growth
- risk of subsequent abnormal frontal sinus pneumatization and contour abnormalities

## Nasal Fractures

- *see also* pp. 656–658
- children usually have dislocated or greenstick fractures
- higher risk of septal hematoma and fractures (septum is more rigid than the cartilage of the anterior nose)
- most require closed reduction under general anesthesia

## Temporal Bone and Otologic Trauma (*see* pp. 658–662)

## Penetrating Head and Neck Trauma

- *see also* pp. 662–664
- majority of injuries are in zone 2
- **oropharyngeal injuries** are relatively common and are usually due to falls while holding an object in the mouth (eg, toothbrush, pencil); complications include subcutaneous **emphysema** (monitor for airway compromise), **hemorrhage** (aspiration, shock, direct carotid injury, most concerning area is retromolar trigone), **neurological insults** (carotid injury [pseudoaneurysm, dissection, thrombosis], penetrating intracranial trauma); CT angiogram useful to rule out carotid injury

## Laryngeal Trauma

- *see also* pp. 664–667
- laryngeal ossification starts with hyoid (age 2), then cricoid; thyroid cartilage remains cartilaginous during childhood
- children less at risk for laryngeal trauma because of more superior position of the larynx in the neck and cartilaginous structures are more flexible
- blunt trauma more common than penetrating trauma in children

## Soft Tissue Trauma

- *see also* pp. 667–673

### *Facial Dog Bites*

- 80% of all dog bites occur in the head and neck (nose, lips, cheeks)
- involved in nearly 1% of all ER visits in the United States; 41% of dog bites occur in children
- >75% due to provoked events, including playing/petting; usually the dog is known to the victim
- superficial lacerations, avulsions, and shearing may harbor deeper injuries due to **crush injuries**
- documentation important for medicolegal reasons; counsel family on appropriate expectations because of need for revision surgery in 75% of cases and frequency of permanent cosmetic deformity
- <u>Rx</u>: profuse wound irrigation; broad-spectrum antibiotics +/- rabies prophylaxis (depending on rabies status of dog); debridement and simple closure (no advantage to delayed closure); CN VII management and fracture reduction as needed

**Acknowledgment:** *Many thanks to Sharon L. Cushing, MD, Msc, FRCSC from The Hospital for Sick Children in Toronto, Canada, for her review of the Vestibular Pathology section.*

# CHAPTER

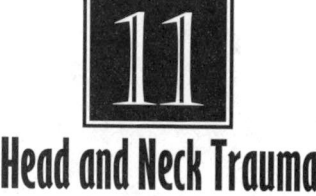

# Head and Neck Trauma

Cody A. Koch, Timothy D. Doerr, Robert H. Mathog, and Raza Pasha

# EVALUATION OF THE HEAD AND NECK TRAUMA PATIENT

## Resuscitation (ABCs)

### A: Airway and Cervical Spine

- anoxia can result in death in 4–5 minutes
- establish airway without mobilizing cervical spine (immobilize neck, maintain axial traction, avoid hyperextension)
- **do not** precipitate an airway crisis, any attempt at endotracheal intubation should also have a backup plan for an emergent surgical airway
- initially suction blood, clots, and secretions from the oropharynx (remove foreign bodies and teeth)
- overcome pharyngeal collapse with forward traction of the tongue, jaw lift, chin lift, or reduction of an unstable mandible or maxillary fracture
- **Masked Ventilation**: may provide adequate oxygenation until able to secure airway (*see* p. 103, Table 3–2)
- **Nasopharyngeal or Oral Airway:** indicated for a conscious or obtunded patient or as a temporary airway for an obstruction at the level of the tongue base and nasopharynx (oral airways are not tolerated by conscious patients, nasal airways can be placed in conscious patients)
- **Nasotracheal Intubation:** generally better tolerated in awake patients and can be accomplished without extension of the neck, intubation approach of choice for severe mandible fractures

- **Orotracheal Intubation:** higher risk of cervical spine injury, consider video laryngoscopes for better visualization or other specialized laryngoscopes
- **Intubation Over a Flexible Bronchoscope:** consider in any potentially "difficult airway," anesthetize nasal airway, oropharynx, and hypopharynx with 4% topical lidocaine, place anterior traction on tongue and advance scope through oral cavity (for oral intubation) or through naris (for nasal intubation), pass scope through vocal folds into trachea and advance endotracheal tube over scope into place, verify placement of endotracheal tube using visualization with scope; can be performed awake
- **Needle Cricothyrotomy (Cricothyroidotomy):** establishes a temporary airway until a more secure surgical airway can be established (may be maintained for 30 minutes until hypoventilation results in toxicity), a #12 or larger IV catheter is placed through the cricothyroid membrane, the needle is removed, leaving the sheath, which is connected via IV tubing to $O_2$ (1 second of $O_2$ injection, 4 seconds of exhalation)
- **Cricothyrotomy:** make a vertical skin incision, incise horizontally through the cricothyroid membrane, spread airway open with curved clamp, place endotracheal tube
- **Urgent Tracheostomy:** consider in an emergent situation in pediatric patients, laryngeal trauma, or tracheal disruption (laryngeal blunt trauma may require a surgical airway to avoid worsening the airway; however, penetrating laryngeal trauma may undergo intubation over a flexible bronchoscope due to lower risk of laryngeal skeletal injury) (*see also* pp. 106–108)

## B: Breathing

- severe head trauma commonly results in decreased respiratory drive (opioids, alcohol, and other medications may also depress respiratory drive)
- after establishing a secure airway, ease of ventilation and maintenance of oxygenation should be evaluated
- hypoventilation may be caused by tension or sucking pneumothorax, hemothorax, or severe pulmonary contusions
- tension pneumothorax occurs with a tear in the pleura or tracheobronchial tree, resulting in entrance of air without means of egress; <u>Rx</u>: needle thoracocentesis and chest tube placement
- sucking pneumothorax results from a larger defect in the chest wall allowing exchange of air through opening; <u>Rx</u>: occlude defect, provide positive pressure ventilation

## C: Circulation and Hemorrhage Control

- identify and control hemorrhage with direct pressure or packing (severe oral bleeding that does not resolve with pressure may require oral packing with rolled gauze after establishing an airway)
- essential to recognize shock (inadequate perfusion of end organs) by tachycardia, hypotension, skin pallor, lethargy, decreased urine output; assess class of hemorrhage (*see* Table 11–1)
- adult blood volume is ~7% of total body weight (5 L in a 70 kg patient)
- establish circulation with 2 large-bore intravenous lines (minimum 18 gauge), resuscitate with crystalloid solutions (normal saline or lactated Ringer's solution) initially with 2 L in adults and 20 mL/kg in children
- replacement of blood loss with crystalloid solution requires 3 times the volume of the estimated blood loss
- packed red blood cells are indicated for blood volume >30% (hemorrhage class III and IV), specified blood should be utilized (usually available <15 minutes), for emergencies type O

## D: Disability

- determine Glasgow Coma Scale (GCS, *see* Table 11–2)
- GCS ≤8 suggests severe head injury; 9–12 moderate head injury, ≥13 mild head injury

## E: Exposure and Secondary Survey

- remove clothing for complete physical exam
- complete history (**AMPLE: A**llergies, **M**edications, **P**ast illnesses, **L**ast meal, **E**vents preceding injury)
- <u>Screening Radiographs</u>: chest, C-spine (must visualize C1–7, T1), and pelvic x-rays
- <u>Initial Labs</u>: type and screen (type and cross for severe blood loss), CBC, electrolytes, coagulation studies, urine analysis, ethanol level, pregnancy test
- <u>Other Tests as Needed</u>: ABG, sickle prep, ECG, urine toxicology, cardiac enzymes, serum amylase, thoracic and lumbar spine radiographs, FAST (focused assessment with sonography for trauma), or diagnostic peritoneal lavage
- <u>Infection Prophylaxis</u>: tetanus status, antibiotics for facial fractures (amoxicillin/clavulanate, clindamycin), antibiotic ointment to wounds

**TABLE 11-1.** Hemorrhage Classes

| Class | Loss of Blood | Symptoms | Treatment |
|-------|---------------|----------|-----------|
| Class I | 10% (500 mL) | asymptomatic | maintain urine output of 30–60 mL/hour |
| Class II | 20% (1000 mL) | mildly anxious, narrowed pulse pressure | replace blood loss with crystalloid fluids (33 estimated blood loss) |
| Class III | 30–40% (1500–1700 mL) | tachycardia, diaphoresis, hypotension, confusion | rapidly bolus with crystalloid fluids, replace blood loss with packed red blood cells |
| Class IV | >40% | lethargy, coma, tachycardia, diaphoresis, hypotension | rapidly bolus with crystalloid fluids, replace blood loss with packed red blood cells, address acid/base/electrolytes |

| TABLE 11–2. Glasgow Coma Scale (GCS) | | |
| --- | --- | --- |
| | **Response** | **Score** |
| **Eye Opening** | spontaneous | 4 |
| | responds to speech | 3 |
| | responds to pain | 2 |
| | no eye opening | 1 |
| **Verbal Response** | oriented | 5 |
| | confused | 4 |
| | inappropriate | 3 |
| | incomprehensible sounds | 2 |
| | none | 1 |
| **Motor Response** | moves to command | 6 |
| | localizes to pain | 5 |
| | withdrawals from pain | 4 |
| | decorticate posturing (flexion) | 3 |
| | decerebrate posturing (extension) | 2 |
| | no movement | 1 |

# History and Physical Exam

## Head and Neck History

### Nature of Injury

- **W**hen: elapsed time since injury
- **W**here: motor vehicle, pedestrian, etc
- **W**hat was the mechanism of injury: assault (fists, bat, etc), penetrating trauma (gunshot wound, stab wound), blunt injury (motor vehicle accident), vector of force (anterior versus lateral impact), fall
- <u>Motor Vehicle Accidents</u>: speed of injury, restrained, air bag deployment
- <u>Gunshot Wound</u>: caliber of gun, distance fired, number of gunshots

### Review of Systems

- <u>Ocular</u>: change in vision (acuity), diplopia
- <u>Otologic</u>: vertigo, hearing loss, otalgia, otorrhea

- <u>Nasal</u>: nasal obstruction, epistaxis, rhinorrhea
- <u>Laryngeal</u>: hoarseness, difficulty breathing, odynophagia, stridor
- <u>Oral</u>: malocclusion, missing/chipped teeth, dysarthria, trismus
- <u>Neurologic</u>: loss of consciousness, numbness, weakness
- <u>General</u>: facial pain, shortness of breath, chest tightness

## Head and Neck Physical Exam

### *Otologic*

- <u>Inspection</u>: otoscopic exam, foreign bodies, hemotympanum, CSF otorrhea, tympanic membrane perforation, Battle's sign (mastoid ecchymosis)
- <u>Palpation</u>: auricular hematoma
- <u>Assess Function</u>: hearing (tuning forks for CHL versus SNHL), balance

### *Ocular*

- <u>Inspection</u>: enophthalmos (globe sunken in posteriorly), proptosis (globe bulges anteriorly), **hypoglobus** (hypophthalmos; globe sits too inferior), ptosis, extraocular movements, "raccoon eyes" suggest basilar skull fracture (cribriform fracture), eyelid lacerations, telecanthus (increased distance between medial canthi), hyphema (blood in anterior chamber), subconjunctival hemorrhage, chemosis (conjunctival edema)
- <u>Palpation</u>: palpate bony rim (crepitus, tenderness, step-offs, mobility), periorbital soft tissue, assess entrapment (**forced duction test**, apply topical ocular anesthetic, use forceps on conjunctiva to move globe), assess medial and lateral canthus (**lid torsion test**, tests for medial canthal ligament by palpating ligament while pulling lid laterally)
- <u>Assess Function</u>: visual acuity, diplopia, nystagmus, hypesthesia of infraorbital and supraorbital nerves, assess lacrimal system (epiphora), pupil response (equal, reactive, consensual response, Marcus Gunn pupil)

### *Nasal*

- <u>Inspection</u>: epistaxis, septal hematoma, septal dislocation, mucosal tears, external deformity, edema, ecchymosis, open fracture, CSF leak (**halo sign**, peripheral clear zone with a central pigmented spot appears when fluid placed on a gauze)
- <u>Palpation</u>: palpate for nasal fractures (crepitus, tenderness, step-offs, mobility)

### Mandible and Oral Cavity

- <u>Inspection</u>: floor of mouth hematoma, dental exam (missing teeth, condition of dentition, dental fractures), palatal fracture, intraoral and lip lacerations, interincisal opening (normal 4–5 cm), occlusion (open bite, cross-bite)
- <u>Palpation</u>: palpate for mandible fractures (tenderness, step-offs, mobility), palatal mobility
- <u>Assess Function</u>: hypesthesia of lower lip (inferior alveolar nerve) and chin (mental nerve), occlusion

### Face and Facial Skeleton

- <u>Inspection</u>: lacerations, hematomas, ecchymoses
- <u>Palpation</u>: bimanual palpation for facial fractures (crepitus, tenderness, step-offs, mobility), mobility of maxilla
- <u>Assess Function</u>: cranial nerve exam, sensory deficits, salivary gland and ductal injuries

### Larynx and Neck

- <u>Inspection</u>: lacerations, hematomas, ecchymoses, vocal fold mobility
- <u>Palpation</u>: crepitus, tenderness, subcutaneous emphysema, bruit
- <u>Assess Function</u>: hoarseness, stridor, airway obstruction

# Head and Neck Radiologic Exams

## Facial Plain Radiographs

- largely replaced by CT except for mandible
- **Panorex (Orthopantomogram)**: requires patient to be able to sit erect, poor view of symphyseal region and the lingual surface of the mandible

## Computed Tomography (CT)

- best radiographic exam for head and neck trauma
- axial and coronal facial (maxillofacial) CT with bone and soft tissue windows, <2 mm slice thickness, 3D reconstructions; CT of head for intracranial injury, CT of neck for laryngeal trauma
- <u>Inspect Areas of Concern</u>: skull base, orbit (walls, floor, retrobulbar hematoma, muscle entrapment), horizontal and vertical buttresses, zygomatic arch, bony palate, mandible (condyles), soft tissue (fluid in sinuses, subcutaneous air, hematomas, etc)

## Special Radiologic Exams

- **CTA, MRA, or Standard Angiography**: indicated for possible vascular injury
- **Magnetic Resonance Imaging (MRI)**: consider for intracranial injury and complications
- **Modified Barium Swallow and Esophagram**: evaluate for esophageal perforation

# MANDIBULAR FRACTURES

## Overview

### Introduction

- most common in young males (ages 18–30)
- <u>Causes</u>: assault, motor vehicle accidents, sports, falls, and gunshot wounds
- <u>Most Common Fracture Sites</u>: varies based on study and mechanism of injury
- <u>Risks</u>: impacted teeth, osteoporosis, edentulous, pathologic lytic lesions

### Physical Examination

- can give clues to the type of fracture
- **Anterior Open Bite:** displaced bilateral condylar or angle fractures
- **Posterior Open Bite:** anterior alveolar process or parasymphyseal fracture
- **Chin Deviation:** typically deviates to side of subcondylar fracture, associated with open bite on opposite side
- **Inability to Open Jaw:** coronoid process fracture or impingement on coronoid by zygoma fracture

## Classification

### Classification by Site

- **Symphyseal/Parasymphyseal**: between canines
- **Body**: between canine and anterior attachment of masseter, weakened by the mental foramen
- **Angle**
- **Ramus**: protected by the "sling" of pterygoid and masseter muscles

- **Coronoid Process**: protected by zygoma, rarely fractured
- **Condyle**: neck (subcondylar region; **weakest point**) and head (TMJ)
- **Alveolar Process**: teeth-bearing region

## Classification by Favorability (Figure 11–1)

- favorable versus unfavorable determined by direction of fracture line and result of muscle force on the mandibular segments
- **Favorable**: vector forces from muscles pull fragments together
- **Horizontally Unfavorable**: vector force of masseter and temporalis muscles pulls fragments apart (angle)
- **Vertically Unfavorable**: vector force of anterior muscles and pterygoid muscles pulls fragments apart (body and symphyseal fractures)

### Anterior Muscles

- weaker force
- mylohyoid, geniohyoid, genioglossus, platysma, anterior digastric muscles
- muscle action depresses and retracts (opens mandible)

### Posterior Muscles

- **stronger force**
- **Temporalis**: raises and retracts mandible
- **Masseter**: raises and retracts mandible
- **Medial Pterygoid**: attaches to medial ramus, raises mandible
- **Lateral Pterygoid**: attaches to condylar neck, **protrudes** and **depresses** mandible

## Other Classifications

- <u>Open Versus Closed</u>: **open** (compound) has exposed bone, **closed** (simple) has intact overlying skin and mucosa
- <u>Fracture Pattern</u>: comminuted (multiple fragments), oblique, transverse, spiral, greenstick (incomplete fracture through only one cortical surface)
- <u>Pathologic</u>: fractures secondary to bone disease (eg, tumors, osteoporosis)

## Dental Evaluation

- <u>Adult</u>: 32 permanent (secondary) teeth (8 incisors, 4 canines, 8 bicuspids or premolars, 12 molars), numbering begins with

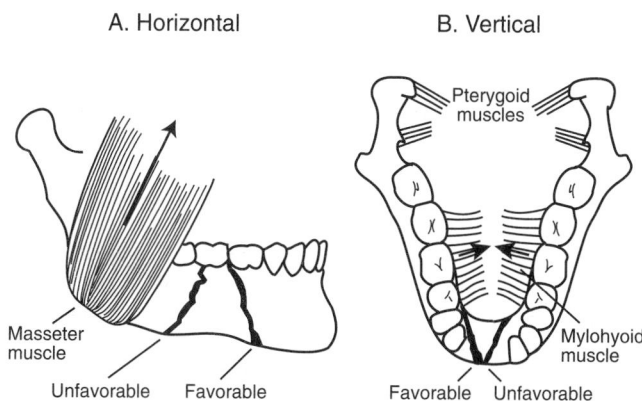

**FIGURE 11–1.** *Horizontal* favorable and unfavorable fractures of the mandible are determined by the action of the masseter muscle. **B.** *Vertical* favorable and unfavorable fractures of the mandible are determined by the actions of the pterygoid and mylohyoid muscles.

maxillary right third molar (#1) to maxillary left third molar (#16) then from mandibular left third molar (#17) to mandibular right third molar (#32)

- <u>Children</u>: 20 deciduous (primary) teeth (8 incisors, 4 canines, 8 molars), numbered A to T, all deciduous teeth are typically gone by age 12

### *Dental Classification*

- **Class I**: teeth on both sides of fracture line, dentulous
- **Class II**: fracture has teeth on 1 side (partially dentulous)
- **Class III**: completely edentulous

### *Angle's Classification*

- **Class I**: normal bite, the **mesiobuccal cusp of the maxillary first molar lies in the buccal groove of the mandibular first molar**
- **Class II**: retrognathic (**overjet**)
- **Class III**: prognathic (**underjet**)

# Management

## Management Concepts

- <u>Goals</u>: restore occlusion, establish bony union, return of function, avoid TMJ ankylosis

- repair within first week, delayed repair increases complications
- consider prophylactic antibiotics
- when placing into occlusion must match wear facets of the mandibular and maxillary teeth (do not assume class I occlusion, recreate the premorbid occlusion)
- **Compression Stress**: force on lower border of mandible, pushes segments together, compensated with a rigid compression plate placed inferiorly
- **Tension Stress**: force on upper border of mandibular angle and body that causes distraction (separation), compensated by placing a thinner, monocortical miniplate superiorly or leave arch bars in place
- <u>Postoperative Care</u>: antibiotics (penicillins, clindamycin), analgesics, oral hygiene (eg, sodium bicarbonate, chlorhexidine gluconate), soft diet

### Indications to Remove Tooth

- tooth within fracture line interferes with occlusion
- infected tooth within fracture line
- fractured tooth, nonviable tooth, or exposed pulp
- <u>Disadvantages</u>: an extracted tooth leaves a point of entry for infection and a point of weak fixation (dental occlusion prevents upward drift at angle), second and third molars also make up a significant portion of mandibular height

### Maxillo-Mandibular Fixation (MMF; Intermaxillary Fixation, IMF)

- <u>Indications</u>: initial intraoperative stabilization of occlusion prior to exposure of the fracture (provides a tension band), may use MMF alone for favorable minimally displaced fractures, selected condylar fractures
- <u>Methods</u>: arch bars (stronger), interdental eyelet wires (Ivy loops), rapid IMF screws, or circumferential wiring of dentures or teeth
- arch bars may employ metal wires (rigid) or rubber bands (flexible, allows easy removal and resetting, allows for exercise, less risk of injury to surgeons)
- requires an intact maxilla
- typically MMF may be removed after 2–8 weeks depending on age and type of injury (eg, children 2–4 weeks, adults 4–6 weeks, elderly >8 weeks, condylar fractures 1–2 weeks, body and angle fractures 4–6 weeks)
- <u>Complications</u>: airway compromise, dental injury, weight loss, loss of fixation (malunion, nonunion), TMJ dysfunction, aspiration

### *Open Reduction Internal Fixation (ORIF)*

- <u>Indications</u>: unfavorable and comminuted fractures, elderly, poor pulmonary reserve (unable to endure MMF), noncompliant patients (alcoholics), pregnant women, multiple fractures, bilateral fractures, or seizure disorders
- MMF needed to establish occlusion prior to placement in ORIF
- **Transoral Approach**: avoids injury to marginal mandibular nerve and no external scar; easy access to symphyseal, parasymphyseal, and body regions (more posterior fractures may be approached intraorally with percutaneous drilling techniques)
- **External Approach**: indicated for more posterior fractures that cannot be accessed intraorally or severely comminuted fractures
- <u>External Approach Types</u>
  1. **Submandibular (Risdon Incision):** allows exposure of posterior body, angle, ramus, and sometimes condyle; incision ~2 cm below inferior border of mandible; incise platysma avoiding marginal mandibular nerve; isolate, clamp, cut, and tie the facial artery and vein as low as possible at the mandibular notch and retract superiorly to protect nerve, dissect to the pterygomasseteric sling and incise at inferior border of mandible, elevate in sub-periosteal plane
  2. **Retromandibular:** allows exposure of angle, ramus, and condyle; incision placed 0.5 cm inferior to earlobe continues inferiorly just behind posterior border of mandible, may be extended anteriorly along inferior border of mandible; blunt dissection through SMAS and parotid in direction of facial nerve branches; may use nerve stimulator; may need to dissect marginal mandibular nerve; dissection continues to pterygomasseteric sling which is divided to expose fracture segments
  3. **Rhytidectomy:** variant of retromandibular approach, incision is same as used for facelift
  4. **Preauricular:** allows exposure of TMJ; pretragal incision from helical root to earlobe, blunt dissection from just superior to zygomatic arch down to just below TMJ, limited exposure due to facial nerve

## Management by Type

- **Coronoid, Greenstick, Unilateral Non-displaced Fractures**: observation with soft diet, analgesics, oral antibiotics, and close follow-up; physiotherapy exercises for 3 months

- **Favorable, Minimally Displaced Non-condylar Fractures**: consider closed reduction and 4–6 weeks of MMF, ORIF treatment of choice

### Displaced Fractures

- **Symphyseal and Parasymphyseal Fractures**: tend to be vertically unfavorable from the force of anterior muscle groups
- **Body Fractures**: almost always unfavorable due to the obliqueness of the fracture and pull of pterygoid and masseter muscles
- **Angle Fractures**: highest complication rate by site because of location posterior to dentition, thin-walled bone, and vector forces from the masseter muscle
- **Ramus Fractures**: isolated ramus fractures are rare (protected by the masseter muscle), displacement is typically minimal, ORIF may be considered for multiple fragments or marked displacement
- Management Options
  1. **Rigid Fixation with Tension Band**: two plates, inferiorly placed plate on inferior border of mandible with bicortical screws, superiorly placed miniplate just below tooth roots with monocortical screws acts as tension band, provides stable fixation for early removal of MMF and early oral intake (may also consider using 2 miniplates)
  2. **Rigid Fixation with MMF**: one plate placed on inferior border of mandible, arch bars left on to act as tension band, MMF does not necessarily need to be maintained (eg, fish loops or rubber bands)
  3. **Eccentric Dynamic Compression Plate (EDCP)**: single plate provides compression and tension forces, not commonly used
  4. **Interosseous Wires with MMF**: wires placed on either side of the fracture to provide fixation with MMF
  5. **Lag Screws**: bicortical screws; drill through superficial cortex, through fracture line, and into deep cortex of opposite bone, then overdrill proximal segment; brings fracture together; indicated to stabilize fixation for oblique symphyseal or body fractures
  6. **External Fixation (Ex Fix)**: indicated for "difficult" fractures (comminuted, multiple, osteomyelitis, elderly), requires 2 fixation points on either side of an unstable area

### Condylar Fractures

- **Observation**: for nondisplaced fractures (typically high condylar fractures) consider observation with close follow-up, soft diet, analgesics, oral antibiotics, and physiotherapy exercises for 3 months

- **Closed Reduction**: displaced fractures (typically subcondylar fractures) may be addressed with closed reduction followed by MMF using rubber bands for 2–3 weeks
- **ORIF**: employ when condyle displaced into middle cranial fossa, lateral extracapsular displacement of condyle, unable to obtain good occlusion (no occluding teeth), foreign body in TMJ, bilateral condylar fractures with gross displacement, need to re-establish vertical height of the mandible, other associated fractures in the mandible or maxilla
- **Bilateral Condylar Neck Fractures**: risk of airway compromise (may need intubation or tracheostomy), associated with anterior bite deformity, consider MMF for 2–3 weeks if minimal displacement; however, must encourage movement of jaw to prevent TMJ ankylosis

### Comminuted Fractures

- in general should retain as many fragments as possible
- <u>General Management Options</u>: MMF for 6 weeks, reconstruction plate, external fixation, bone grafts (for significant nonviable bone, typically from iliac crest)

### Pediatric Patients

- in general prefer conservative management
- *see* p. 624

### Edentulous Patients

- typically have atrophic mandibles from decreased loading effects from loss of dental support (also secondary to osteoporosis in the elderly)
- ORIF with plates should be procedure of choice to prevent reduction of jaw opening
- other options include applying arch bars directly to dentures (circumdenture wires), transosseous wires, or external fixation

### Surgical Complications

- **Chin and Lip Hypesthesia**: inferior alveolar or mental nerve injury (mental nerve is a continuation of the inferior alveolar nerve), **most common complication**; spontaneous regeneration occurs in the majority of cases
- **Osteomyelitis**: increased risk from poor oral hygiene, devitalized teeth, infected teeth within fracture line, improperly repaired fracture

(nonunion), loose hardware; Rx: initially should remove unstable hardware followed by long-term IV antibiotics to avoid bone loss; infected teeth should be removed; surgical debridement of nonviable bone should be replaced with fixation with later consideration of bone graft for large defects

- **Malunion/Malocclusion**: healing of bone in malalignment caused by inadequate immobilization, inaccurate reduction, infection, gross loss of bone, compromised blood supply, malnutrition, osteogenesis imperfecta, or osteopetrosis; Rx: address underlying cause (infection, malnutrition, etc), consider orthodontic realignment for subtle defects or osteotomy with repositioning and refixation
- **Nonunion**: failure of bone to produce osteogenic tissue, nonosteogenic matrix produced (**fibrous union**); Rx: initial excision of fibrous tissue and nonviable bone with refixation (may require bone grafting)
- **Plate Exposure**: similar causes as malunion; Rx: address underlying cause (infection, malnutrition, etc), oral antibiotics, local application of antibiotic ointment, and 3% hydrogen peroxide; plate should be retained as long as possible then removed with completion of healing
- **Marginal Mandibular Nerve Injury**: increased risk with external approaches; Rx: direct anastomosis if noticed intraoperatively
- **Necrosis of Condylar Head (Avascular Necrosis)**: compromised vasculature to the condylar head with damage to the condylar neck; Rx: debridement of necrotic bone with reconstruction
- **TMJ Ankylosis**: defined as inability to open jaw >5 mm between incisors, in children may cause facial deformities from growth disorders occurring at joint; Rx: if fibrotic ankylosis has occurred treat with passive jaw opening exercises, if skeletal ankylosis occurs must resect with reconstruction of the TMJ
- **Dental Injury**: may be secondary to improper placement of arch bars and MMF

# MAXILLARY FRACTURES

## Introduction

- Causes: assault, motor vehicle accidents, sports, falls, gunshot wounds
- the maxilla absorbs energy with impact, thereby protecting the orbit, intracranial contents, and nose from total destruction
- severe maxillary fractures are associated with a high incidence of intracranial and orbital injuries

- sinusitis is a potential complication and is generally avoided with prophylactic antibiotics and early removal of nasal packing; persistent sinusitis may require surgical intervention to address structural abnormalities

# Classification

## Buttress System (Figure 11–2)

### *Vertical Buttresses*

- strong, developed to withstand load from mastication
- Types
    1. **Naso-Maxillary (NM)**
    2. **Zygomatico-Maxillary (ZM)**: bears the strongest load, begins above maxillary first molars
    3. **Pterygo-Maxillary (PM)**: projects into skull base

### *Horizontal Beams*

- weaker, reinforces vertical buttresses and provides width and projection of the face
- Types
    1. **Frontal Bar**: essential support, made from superior orbital rim and glabellar area, suspends the nasomaxillary and zygomaticomaxillary struts
    2. **Inferior Orbital Rims**
    3. **Maxillary Alveolus and Palate**
    4. **Zygomatic Process**
    5. **Greater Wing of the Sphenoid**
    6. **Medial and Lateral Pterygoid Plates**
    7. **Mandible**

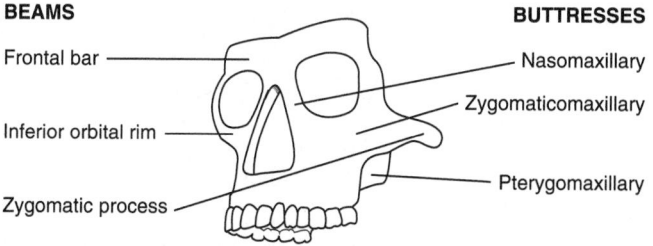

**BEAMS**                                    **BUTTRESSES**

Frontal bar ———                              ——— Nasomaxillary

                                             Zygomaticomaxillary

Inferior orbital rim ———

                                             ——— Pterygomaxillary

Zygomatic process ———

**FIGURE 11–2.** Facial skeleton buttress system of vertical buttresses and horizontal beams.

## Le Fort Classification (Figure 11–3)

- based on patterns of fractures ("lines of minimal resistance"), classified according to the highest level of injury
- in many cases Le Fort classification is incomplete for maxillary fractures
- may present in many combinations or on one side (hemi-Le Fort)
- all involve fracture of **pterygoid plates**

### Le Fort I (Low Maxillary)

- transverse maxillary fracture (upper alveolus becomes separated from upper maxilla) typically caused by a low anterior-to-posterior force
- involves anterolateral maxillary wall, medial maxillary wall, pterygoid plates, septum at floor of nose

### Le Fort II (Pyramidal)

- typically caused by a superiorly directed force against the maxilla or an anterior-to-posterior blow along the Frankfort plane
- involves the nasofrontal suture, inferior orbital foramen, orbital rim, orbital floor, frontal process of lacrimal bone, zygomaxillary suture, lamina papyracea of ethmoid, pterygoid plate, and high septum

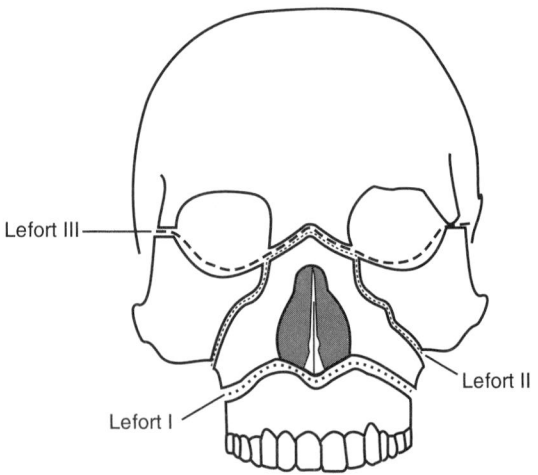

**FIGURE 11–3.** Classification of Le Fort fractures: Le Fort I or low maxillary, Le Fort II or pyramidal, Le Fort III or craniofacial disjunction.

### Le Fort III (Craniofacial Dysjunction)

- separates facial skeleton from base of skull, typically caused by high velocity impacts, motor vehicle accidents, oblique forces
- involves nasofrontal suture; medial and lateral orbital wall and floor; zygomaticofrontal suture; zygoma and zygomatic arch; pterygoid plates and nasal septum

# Management

## Principles

- <u>Goals of Reconstruction</u>: re-establish midfacial height, width, and projection; restore soft tissue contour; restore function and occlusion
- <u>Exposure</u>: gingival labial sulcus incision, degloving approach, coronal incision, periorbital incisions (transconjunctival, subciliary incisions)
- <u>Timing</u>: most favorable operative time is within first 24–48 hours prior to significant facial edema; however, direct fixation techniques allow repair up to 2 weeks after injury prior to the onset of significant scarring, fibrosis, and bony resorption
- <u>Panfacial Fractures</u>: **"work from a stable base"**; begin with MMF and management of associated mandible fractures; work lateral (zygoma and ZM buttress to establish anterior projection) to medial to restore buttress system; may consider repairing smaller components (eg, NOE) first then assemble them all together
- <u>Postoperative Care</u>: antibiotics, analgesics, soft diet

## Techniques

- **Plate Fixation (Miniplates)**: allow earlier removal of MMF, earlier return of function, and have biomechanical advantages over wire techniques; however, may be more sensitive to errors than interosseous wire fixation
- **Interosseous Wire Fixation**: may be considered for less displaced fractures (with 4–6 weeks of MMF), adequate for infraorbital rim
- **Bone Grafts**: indicated for significant bone loss

## Management by Le Fort Classification

- **Le Fort I**: generally may be reduced (digitally or with disimpaction forceps) and placed in MMF followed by fixation of NM and ZM buttresses; edentulous patients may require splints, circummandibular wires, or circumzygomatic fixation

- **Le Fort II**: stabilization of the ZM buttress with fixation essential after placing in MMF, may also consider fixation of the nasofrontal process or inferior orbital rim
- **Le Fort III**: usually requires coronal flap for adequate exposure for exploration and miniplate fixation

## Palatal Fractures

- must be reduced for proper dentoalveolar complex positioning
- fracture lines typically paramedian due to the stability of the vomer at midline
- after reduction (Rowe forceps, bone hooks) open reduction may be considered for anterior defects with miniplate fixation
- posterior defects may be repaired by closed reduction with MMF (although an open approach may be considered with transosseous wires or plates)
- edentulous patients may require reduction with placement of upper denture or splint (with or without MMF), may also consider miniplate fixation

## Surgical Complications

- **Malunion, Nonunion, Plate Exposure**: address similar to mandible fractures (*as previous*)
- **Palpable or Observable Plates**: avoided with thinner miniplates; <u>Rx</u>: remove after healing
- **Forehead or Cheek Hypesthesia**: injury to supraorbital or infraorbital nerves, spontaneous regeneration occurs in the majority of cases
- **Osteomyelitis**: address similar to mandible fractures (*as previous*)
- **Dental Injury**: may be secondary to reduction techniques or improper placement of arch bars and MMF

# ZYGOMATICOMAXILLARY AND ORBITAL FRACTURES

## Zygomaticomaxillary Complex (ZMC, Trimalar, Tripod, Tetrapod) Fractures

### Introduction

- <u>Sx</u>: subconjunctival and periorbital ecchymosis, depressed malar eminence, eyelid edema, epistaxis, cheek hypesthesia, diplopia, hypoglobus (hypophthalmos), enophthalmos, trismus

- rarely occur in children <5 years old (maxillary sinus not pneumatized)

### Four Sutures Involved in Zygomaticomaxillary Complex Fractures

- **Zygomaticofrontal Suture**: usually fractures cleanly
- **Zygomaticomaxillary Suture**: at the face of the maxilla, high risk of comminution
- **Zygomaticotemporal Suture**: zygomatic arch, typically fractures at midpoint or produces a double fracture
- **Zygomaticosphenoid Suture**: broad suture line, best suture to use for alignment and reduction but not as easily accessible as others

## Management

- stabilizing the zygomatic arch allows accurate anterior projection of the malar prominence
- stabilization of the zygomaticomaxillary complex requires a minimum of 2-point fixation (usually ZF and ZM)
- **Closed Reduction**: indicated for noncomminuted, simple fractures
- **Open Reduction**: indicated for trismus, orbital complications (eg, enophthalmos, diplopia), and facial asymmetry; fixation techniques include miniplates and less commonly interosseous wiring

### Common Approaches to the Zygoma

- <u>Incisions</u>: coronal incision (visualize the lateral orbital rim and zygomatic arch), periorbital incisions (transconjunctival, subciliary incisions; visualize the orbital rim and floor), upper blepharoplasty or lateral brow incisions (visualize frontozygomatic suture), gingivobuccal incision (visualize the maxillary face), behind temporal hairline
- **Gillies Approach**: indicated for isolated arch fractures with no comminution; incision behind the temporal hairline is carried through the temporoparietal fascia, superior auricular muscle, and superficial layer of the deep temporalis fascia; approach zygoma by placing elevator below the superficial layer of the deep temporalis fascia and above the temporalis muscle to avoid injuring the temporal branch of facial nerve
- **Intraoral Approach** (**Keen**): incision at gingivobuccal sulcus, tunnel lateral to the maxilla and under the zygomatic arch
- **Coronal, Hemicoronal, or Extended Pretragal Approaches**: indicated for multiple complex facial fractures (eg, Le Fort III,

frontal sinus); access to full length horizontal arc to repair a displaced middle arc segment

## Surgical Complications:

- Similar to orbital floor fractures (*see following*)

# Orbital Fractures

## Introduction

- <u>Seven Orbital Bones</u>: frontal, lacrimal, ethmoid (lamina papyracea weakest portion), maxilla, zygoma, sphenoid, palatine bones (Figure 11–4)
- <u>Optic Canal Contents</u>: optic nerve (CN II), ophthalmic artery
- <u>Superior Orbital Fissure Contents</u>: oculomotor (CN III), trochlear (CN IV), and abducens (CN VI) nerves; lacrimal and frontal divisions of CN V1; supraorbital vein; nasociliary division of CN V1
- <u>Inferior Orbital Fissure Contents</u>: zygomaticofacial and zygomaticotemporal divisions of CN V2, inferior ophthalmic vein
- <u>SSx</u>: enophthalmos (from increased orbital volume, >2–3 mm pathologic), hypoglobus, exophthalmos, proptosis, entrapment, diplopia (from entrapment or enophthalmos), hypesthesia of infraorbital nerve, pseudoptosis (enopthalmos causes upper eyelid to droop) (*see p. 633 for term definitions*)

### Theories of Orbital Floor Injury

- **Hydraulic Theory**: force to orbital region → ↑ intraocular pressure → fractures floor
- **Buckling Theory**: force on inferior rim → directly fractures floor

### Traumatic Nerve Injury

- <u>Pathophysiology</u>: injury to the optic canal and superior orbital fissure (SOF) results in compressive injury to involved nerves, **traumatic optic neuropathy** results from CN II injury
- <u>SSx</u>: vision loss (CN II), ophthalmoplegia (CN III, IV, VI), ptosis (CN III), pupillary dilation (CN III), anesthesia of upper eyelid and forehead (CN $V_1$)
- <u>Dx</u>: visual acuity, Marcus Gunn pupil (afferent injury), high-resolution CT
- sudden visual loss carries a poor prognosis (unsalvageable)
- <u>Rx</u>: for progressive loss consider high-dose corticosteroids and osmotic diuresis (mannitol), if no improvement may consider orbital

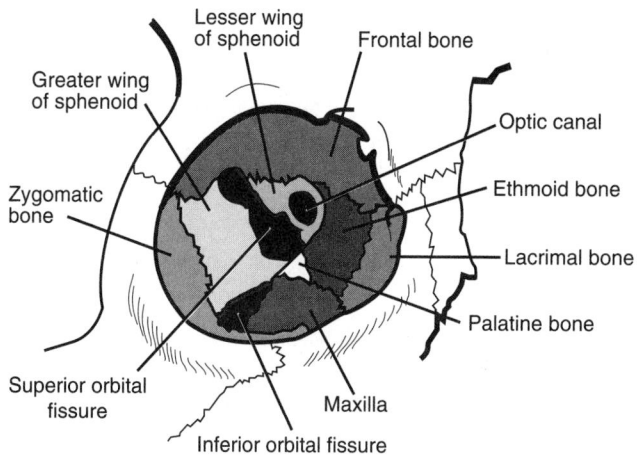

**FIGURE 11–4.** Anatomy of the bony orbit.

or optic nerve decompression; if CT reveals bony impingement may undergo urgent decompression

## Management

- <u>Indications for Surgical Intervention</u>: enophthalmos and/or hypoglobus (>2–3 mm), mechanical entrapment, diplopia, high risk of enophthalmos and/or hypoglobus (large floor defects), oculocardiac reflex (bradycardia)
- <u>Contraindications for Surgical Intervention</u>: hyphema, retinal tear, globe perforation, only seeing eye, sinusitis, frozen globe
- <u>Ophthalmologic Evaluation</u>: essential to evaluate for serious and potentially blinding problems (eg, hyphema, dislocated or subluxed lenses, retinal holes or detachment, or optic nerve contusion)
- <u>Timing</u>: ideally should be completed prior to swelling or 7–10 days after it has subsided, delayed repair may reveal bone resorption and scar contracture
- <u>Technique</u>: expose orbital rim, medial orbital wall, and floor posteriorly to the junction of the infraorbital canal and inferior orbital fissure; elevate soft tissue from the floor defect; reduce fracture; for significant defects or difficult reductions reinforce floor with grafts (eg, porous polyethylene [Medpor], Gelfilm, or bone for larger defects), always perform forced duction test at completion of procedure to ensure no entrapment, typically may repair ≤5 mm of enophthalmos without straining optic nerve, consider surgical

navigation and/or intraoperative CT to verify reduction or adequate reconstruction

- **Lateral Canthotomy**: performed urgently for **retrobulbar hematoma** (*see* pp. 60–61), decompresses the orbit and prevents ischemic injury to the optic nerve (ie, blindness)
- <u>Steps for Lateral Canthotomy/Cantholysis</u>
  1. inject lidocaine with epinephrine subconjunctivally and subcutaneously at lateral canthus, in emergency may use hemostat to clamp lateral canthus instead of injection
  2. make a 1–1.5 cm horizontal incision through the skin at the lateral canthus
  3. dissect down to the lateral orbital rim either bluntly or with needle tip cautery
  4. use a forceps to pick up the lateral aspect of the lower eyelid, then using another forceps or similar instrument feel the tight band that represents the lateral canthal tendon
  5. using a small iris scissor cut in a vertical direction to release the inferior limb of the lateral canthal tendon close to the inner aspect of the lateral orbital rim
  6. the lower eyelid should be easily distracted from the globe and should be able to be overlapped partially over the upper eyelid

## *Approaches*

1. **Subciliary Incision** (**Infraciliary**): incision placed 2–3 mm below the cilia of the lower eyelid (may extend into "crow's feet"), allows exposure to orbital floor and rim, risk of ectropion and scleral show
2. **Transconjunctival Incision**: allows exposure to orbital floor and rim, risk of entropion, no external scar, limits exposure
3. **Precaruncular Incision**: used to approach the medial orbit, incision placed immediately anterior to caruncle, dissection in a posteromedial direction to the medial orbital wall just behind posterior lacrimal crest, can be connected with transconjunctival incision to access both inferior and medial orbital walls
4. **Upper Blepharoplasty Incision**: allows exposure to posterolateral wall
5. **Lynch Incision** (**Frontoethmoidal**): allows exposure to medial wall, not commonly used
6. **Subtarsal Incision**: incision placed 5–7 mm below the cilia of the lower eyelid in a crease line, not commonly used
7. **Caldwell-Luc** (**Transantral**) **Approach**: indicated for severely comminuted and posterior fractures, completed in conjunction with an approach from above

## Surgical Complications

- **Blindness**: may be caused by injury to optic nerve, retrobulbar hematoma, and retinal artery occlusion; <u>Rx</u>: consider an urgent lateral canthotomy for a retrobulbar hematoma (*see previous*), also consider removing implant, controlling hemorrhage, and administration of corticosteroids and diuretics
- **CSF Leak**: high risk with Le Fort II and III fractures; <u>Rx</u>: *see* pp. 661–662 *for management*
- **Persistent Enophthalmos and Diplopia**: may be from inadequate repair, scarring, or motor nerve injury; <u>Rx</u>: must re-explore and establish volume/contact relationship, release scar
- **Ectropion**: risk with subciliary incision from scarring or injury to the tarsal plate; <u>Rx</u>: conservative management, upward massage, corticosteroid injections, oculoplastic surgery (lysis of scar, STSGs) if persistent
- **Entropion**: risk with transconjunctival incision; <u>Rx</u>: oculoplastic surgery
- **Epiphora**: damage to canalicular system; <u>Rx</u>: dilation and irrigation, or dacryocystorhinostomy
- **Cheek Hypesthesia**: injury to infraorbital nerve; spontaneous regeneration may occur
- **Extrusion of Grafts**: alloplastic materials have reduced incidence; <u>Rx</u>: removal of graft, if more than 3–4 weeks out may not need replacement if sufficient scar tissue has formed
- **Malunion, Nonunion, Plate Exposure**: address similar to mandible fractures (*as previous*)
- **Osteomyelitis**: address similar to mandible fractures (*as previous*)
- **Palpable or Observable Plates**: avoided with thinner or, if appropriate, resorbable miniplates; <u>Rx</u>: remove after healing

# FRONTAL SINUS AND NASO-ORBITOETHMOID FRACTURES

## Frontal Sinus Fractures

### Introduction

- <u>SSx</u>: laceration of the forehead, forehead swelling (may be confused with a subgaleal hematoma), palpable frontal defect, frontal pain, epistaxis, forehead hypesthesia
- <u>Complications of Frontal Sinus Fractures</u>: **mucocele** (from entrapped mucosa), cosmetic deformity, chronic sinusitis, CSF leak, epiphora, dystopia (if involves the roof of the orbit), intracranial infections (meningitis, brain abscess)

- Approaches: coronal (best exposure, cosmetically acceptable), endoscopic via hairline and temporal incisions, bilateral sub-brow incision ("butterfly" approach), through an existing laceration, "open sky" approach (medial canthal incisions connected with a horizontal incision)
- frontal sinus fractures are rare in children (frontal sinus does not appear until age 5–6 years old)
- frontal sinus anterior wall is thick, posterior wall and floor are thin

## Management

### Anterior Table Fractures

- Linear, Minimally Displaced: conservative measures (low risk of mucosal entrapment and cosmetic deformity), observation
- Depressed Fractures "Trap Door": explore, remove mucosa from fractured edges (may consider cutting burs), reduce fracture, may place interosseous wires, may consider endoscopic approach with reduction of fracture or reconstruction of defect with acellular human dermis or similar substance
- Comminuted or Unstable Fractures: explore, inspect posterior wall and nasofrontal recess, remove mucosa from fractured edges, reduce fracture, thin plate fixation for support, if <1 cm of total frontal bone fragments are missing consider skin covering only, if >1 cm fragments are missing use a split calvarial bone graft or mesh (eg, titanium) to reconstruct

### Posterior Table Fractures

- high risk of intracranial injury (intracranial hematoma), dural tear, CSF leak, frontal sinus outflow tract injury, and entrapped mucosa (future risk of mucocele formation)
- Isolated Nondisplaced Posterior Table Fracture: rare, conservative measures (observation), if sinus fluid does not clear within 6 weeks consider exploration
- Displaced Posterior Table Fracture: must explore frontal sinus via an **osteoplastic flap** (*see* p. 58); for more extensive fractures (comminution, dural tears, CSF leak) consider a subcranial approach (with neurosurgery consultation); repair dural tears and CSF leaks, inspect nasofrontal recess and remove all mucosa (consider drill burs); **obliterate sinus** cavity with fat, muscle (temporalis muscle galea flap), or bone; reduce fracture and repair anterior table as previous

- <u>Comminuted, Contaminated, or Through-and-Through Fractures</u>: considered a neurosurgical emergency, consider **cranialization of sinus** (remove posterior table, allows frontal lobes to fill sinus cavity, must remove all sinus mucosa via drilling or similar, eliminates sinus but risks contamination of the cranial cavity)

### Nasofrontal Recess Injuries

- most common cause of traumatic **mucocele** formation
- presents with persistent sinus fluid >10 days postinjury
- <u>Nasofrontal Recess Reconstruction</u>: indicated for limited fractures; widen the ostium and consider placement of a stent or reconstruct with adjacent nasal mucous membrane lining
- <u>Sinus Septectomy</u>: removal of the intersinus septum, indicated for injury of 1 ostium, allows drainage of damaged side to the opposite nasofrontal recess
- <u>Sinus Obliteration</u>: indicated for injury to both ducts or severe complicated fractures

## Surgical Complications

- **Mucocele, Mucopyocele**: from entrapped mucosal lining in the fracture, erodes into surrounding bone, may not appear until many years postoperatively, confirmed with CT; <u>Rx</u>; re-explore with an obliterative procedure (*see also* p. 58)
- **Sinusitis**: may be secondary to frontonasal recess injury, postsurgical contamination, or obstructing mucocele; <u>Rx</u>: consider re-exploration and obliteration (or reobliteration), repair of nasofrontal recess, or debridement with culture; aggressive antibiotic regimen (must avoid intracranial extension)
- **Forehead Contour Deformity**: may be the result of poor reduction or slipped bone flap; <u>Rx</u>: consider re-exploration, correction of the defect with recontouring, cranial grafts, or alloplastic grafts
- **Intracranial Infections**: increased risk with dural tears, wound contamination, or cranialization procedures (*see* pp. 381–383 *for management*)
- **Osteomyelitis**: address similar to mandible fractures (*as previous*)
- **CSF Leak**: (*see* pp. 661–662)
- **Forehead Hypesthesia**: higher risk with sub-brow incisions from injury to the supraorbital nerves, return of function should be expected
- **Forehead Paralysis**: from injury of the frontal branch of the facial nerve, return of function may occur

# Naso-orbitoethmoid (NOE) Fractures

## Introduction

- **NOE**: frontal process of maxilla, nasal bones, and orbital space
- <u>Common Fracture Patterns</u>
    1. nasal bones and frontal process of the maxilla are telescoped behind the frontal bone
    2. comminuted fracture with fragments into the orbital space, cranial fossa, and nasal vault
- <u>SSx</u>: flattened nasal dorsum, periorbital swelling, epistaxis, nasal obstruction, medial canthal ligament injury (telecanthus, epiphora, bowstring sign, *see following*), CSF rhinorrhea
- **Bowstring Sign**: tests the integrity of the medial canthal ligament, grasp medial eyelid near lash line and pull laterally, normally should snap back
- **Pseudohypertelorism** (**Traumatic Telecanthus**): widened intercanthal distance (>22 mm in infants and >32–35 mm in adults or the distance of the width of 1 eye), initially presents with rounding of the medial canthus from releasing the medial canthal ligament, later results in eversion of the lacrimal papilla and the appearance of flattened nasal bones
- **Fluorescein Dye Test**: assess nasolacrimal duct by placing dye within the eye and then checking for presence of dye on intranasal pledgets 1–5 minutes later

## Anatomy

### *Medial Canthal Ligament (MCL)*

- is an extension of the tarsal plates that attaches to the medial orbital wall
- receives contributions from the tendinous portion of the preseptal and pretarsal parts of the orbicularis oculi muscle, superior suspensory ligament (**Whitnall**), and inferior suspensory ligament (**Lockwood**)
- contains an anterior limb (inserts anterior to lacrimal fossa) and a posterior limb (inserts posterior to lacrimal fossa)

### *Lacrimal Collecting System*

- **Puncta**: located at the medial aspect of the upper and lower eyelids, collects tears
- **Canaliculi**: upper and lower canaliculi form the common canaliculus

- **Lacrimal Sac**: located in the lacrimal fossa, insertions of the MCL straddle the lacrimal sac and act as a pump (sac is compressed with eyelid shortening such as a blink)
- **Lacrimal Duct**: enters into the medial maxilla and exits into the inferior meatus

### Planum Sphenoidale

- radiologic term describing the area of the floor of the anterior cranial fossa that is anterior to sella turcica and posterior to fovea ethmoidalis and cribriform plate
- component of the lesser wing of the sphenoid
- laterally forms the roof of the optic foramen (high risk of optic nerve injury)

## Management

- first reconstruct medial orbital wall prior to repair of the MCL
- must consider associated injuries: ocular injury (ophthalmology consult), CSF leak, nasoseptal deformities, lacrimal duct injuries, eyelid lacerations
- may attempt closed reduction if MCL and lacrimal system are intact (rarely works)
- <u>Telescoping Nasal Bones and Frontal Process of the Maxilla</u>: requires open reduction via a coronal incision or existing laceration, reduction and maintaining reduction of NOE fractures are difficult, secure fixation with miniplates or interosseous wires

### MCL Repair

- first priority is to repair MCL, the lacrimal system may be reconstructed as a second operation
- must attempt to recreate the pull of MCL by reattaching in the direction of its initial vectors (posterior and superior)

#### Classification and Management of MCL Injuries
(*may vary by source*)

Type I:   MCL remains attached but bone fragment is detached or ligament has been severed completely; <u>Rx</u>: attempt to wire bone fragments with attached MCL to stable bone or release lateral canthal ligament then reattach the MCL to the medial wall of the orbit posterior to the lacrimal fossa (slight overcorrection is required)

**Type II**: comminuted medial orbital wall fracture; <u>Rx</u>: attach MCL with wires transnasally to the opposite side medial orbital wall (may also consider releasing the lateral canthal ligament to allow for some overcorrection)

**Type III**: bilateral medial orbital wall fractures; <u>Rx</u>: attach MCL with wires transnasally to the opposite MCL (transnasal canthoplasty), consider wiring both MCLs to the opposite frontal process

### *Lacrimal System Injury*

- the lacrimal system may be explored using surgical loupes and lacrimal dilators, stents may be placed to allow primary closure of tears (the lower canaliculus is the primary drainage system)
- **Dacryocystorhinostomy (DCR)**: indicated for injury distal to the sac
- **Conjunctivorhinostomy or Conjunctivodacryocystorhinostomy**: indicated for injuries proximal to the sac after failed recannulization

## Surgical Complications

- **Persistent Telecanthus**: avoided with accurate reattachment of MCL; <u>Rx</u>: re-exploration with repair, difficult to correct in a delayed fashion
- **Persistent Epiphora**: injury to the lacrimal system, assess with fluorescein dye test; <u>Rx</u>: repair (*as previous*)
- **Frontal Sinusitis**: may result from injury to the nasofrontal recess; <u>Rx</u>: *see* pp. 58–59
- **Scleral Show**: may occur with low placement of transnasal wires; <u>Rx</u>: reattachment of wires at higher plane or consider Z-plasty
- **Osteomyelitis**: address similar to mandible fractures (*as previous*)
- **CSF Leak**: may occur from reduction of naso-orbital injury or associated cribriform plate fracture and dural tears; <u>Rx</u>: *see* pp. 661–662

# NASAL FRACTURES

## Introduction

- most common facial bone fracture
- must differentiate bony fracture from cartilaginous injury
- anterior impacts may result in tip fractures, flattened nasal dorsum, splayed nasal bones, and septal deformities

- lateral impacts may result in a depression of the lateral nasal bone, "C-" or "S-shaped" nasal dorsum deformities, medial maxillary wall fractures, and septal deformities
- dislocated quadrangular cartilage inferiorly or "C-shaped" deformity superiorly are common septal abnormalities from trauma
- children usually have dislocated or greenstick fractures and have a higher risk of septal hematoma and fracture (septum is more rigid than the cartilage of the anterior nose)
- comminution is more common in adults
- <u>SSx</u>: palpable deformity, epistaxis, edema, nasal obstruction/ congestion
- <u>Dx</u>: clinical diagnosis (physical exam), radiographs (including CT) if additional fractures are suspected)
- <u>Complications of Nasal Fractures</u>: medial canthal ligament injury, lacrimal duct injury, cribriform plate fracture (CSF leak, anosmia), septal hematoma may cause saddle-nose deformity if untreated, persistent epistaxis

# Management

## Initial Management

- preoperative photography/x-ray may be considered for medicolegal documentation
- septal hematoma (unilateral or bilateral purple compressible bulge) requires immediate evacuation of hematoma, nasal packing, and antibiotic prophylaxis (*see* p. 22)
- open fractures require irrigation, conservative debridement, and antibiotics

## Surgical Management

- generally nasal bone depression or deviation may undergo closed reduction within first 3 hours (before swelling) or between 3–10 days (after swelling and before healing)
- <u>Closed Reduction</u>: indicated as an initial trial for most nasal fractures; should generally be avoided for cribriform plate fractures with CSF leak (to avoid nasal packing); reduction is performed with elevation and lateral motion using a Boies/Goldman elevator or Asch forceps, nasal tip should also be addressed by elevating at the anterior portion of the septum, the septum should be inspected for adequate reduction and evaluation for septal hematoma, internal and external splints should be applied (also consider nasal packing)

- <u>ORIF (Septorhinoplasty)</u>: indicated for failed closed techniques or extensive injuries that involve the maxilla or frontal bones; open septorhinoplasty techniques are utilized, fixation is achieved with interosseous wire (plates should be avoided), bone grafts may be considered for severe comminution
- <u>Pediatric Nasal Fractures</u>: generally should be treated conservatively to avoid damage to growth centers
- <u>Postoperative Care</u>: ice for 24 hours, prophylactic antibiotics, analgesics, nasal splints, nasal packing

### Surgical Complications and Associated Injuries

- **Persistent Deformity**: failed closed reduction should be addressed with an open rhinoplasty approach after healing (3–6 months)
- **Nasal Obstruction**: may occur from synechiae, scar contracture, or structural deformity obstructing the nasal vault
- **Septal Hematoma**: failure to recognize may result in septal necrosis (saddle-nose deformity); <u>Rx</u>: *see previous*
- **Septal Perforation and Deviation**: may result from open septorhinoplasty techniques
- **Cribriform Plate Fracture**: may result in anosmia or CSF leak

# TEMPORAL BONE AND OTOLOGIC TRAUMA

## Penetrating Facial Nerve Trauma (see p. 430)

## Barotrauma (see p. 400)

## Temporal Bone Fractures

### Initial Evaluation

- temporal bone fractures are associated with severe traumatic forces, initial exam includes a complete trauma workup (*see* pp. 628–635)
- <u>Focused H&P</u>: determine cause (blunt versus penetrating, lateral versus occipital impact); assess facial nerve for paralysis/paresis (partial versus complete, immediate versus delayed); hearing loss (tuning forks if stable); vertigo (nystagmus); presence of other neurologic deficits and/or cranial nerve palsies; clean EAC with suction to evaluate for CSF leak (avoid irrigation), hemotympanum, EAC lacerations; Battle's sign (ecchymosis over the mastoid process)

- <u>CT Temporal Bone</u>: imaging of choice, examine site and type of fracture (*see following*), site of potential facial nerve injuries and otic capsule involvement (indications for CT temporal bone are controversial, may not change immediate clinical management)
- <u>Audiogram</u>: assess for CHL (suggestive of ossicular discontinuity) versus SNHL (cochlear injury), perform at 6–8 weeks
- <u>Arteriography</u>: consider when injury to the carotid artery is suspected (fracture extends to foramen lacerum on CT)

## Classification Schemes

### Longitudinal Versus Transverse (*see* Table 11–3)

- **Longitudinal**: more common, lower risk of injury to facial nerve/cochlea (however because longitudinal fractures are more common overall, most facial nerve injuries are due to longitudinal fractures)
- **Transverse**: less common, higher risk of injury to facial nerve/cochlea
- most fractures are **mixed**

### Otic Capsule Sparing Versus Otic Capsule Involving

- less ambiguous classification, may correlate better to facial nerve injury
- **Otic Capsule Sparing**: less risk of facial nerve injury
- **Otic Capsule Involving**: higher risk of facial nerve injury, SNHL

## Facial Nerve Injury

- higher risk of facial nerve injury with **transverse** or **otic capsule involving** (30–50% incidence) due to the perpendicular path of the fracture with respect to the facial nerve
- most common site of injury of the facial nerve in temporal bone fractures is the **perigeniculate region** (labyrinthine and horizontal segments)
- delayed facial nerve paralysis may occur secondary to posttraumatic edema and ischemia with or without a fracture
- poor prognosis associated with immediate onset, complete paralysis, associated infection, or penetrating mechanism
- <u>Dx</u>: physical exam, for complete facial paralysis serial ENoG (electroneuronography) or EMG testing may be utilized to assess nerve integrity and function
- <u>Rx</u>: corticosteroids for any degree of facial nerve injury, surgical exploration indications are similar to idiopathic facial nerve paralysis (*see* pp. 427–428)

**TABLE 11–3.** Characteristics of Longitudinal and Transverse Temporal Bone Fractures*

| Characteristic | Longitudinal Fractures | Transverse Fractures |
|---|---|---|
| Prevalence | 75% | 25% |
| Fracture Line | parallel to long axis of petrous pyramid | perpendicular to long axis of petrous pyramid |
| Vector Force | temporoparietal blow | frontal or occipital blow |
| Relation to Otic Capsule | fracture remains anteriomedial to otic capsule | fracture may transect otic capsule and IAC |
| Hearing Loss Type | CHL (ossicular disruption, blood in the EAC) | SNHL (labyrinthine or nerve injury) |
| Signs and Symptoms | blood in EAC, Battle's sign, EAC step-off, rare vestibular signs, hemotympanum | hemotympanum, nystagmus, CSF otorrhea |
| Facial Nerve Injury | less likely | more likely |

* Pure longitudinal and transverse fractures are **not common**, most fractures are **mixed types** and follow mixed planes.

## Traumatic Hearing Loss

- SNHL more common with **transverse** or **otic capsule involving** fractures
- CHL more common with **longitudinal** fractures from ossicular injury, TM tears, or blood or CSF in the EAC
- posttraumatic profound hearing loss has poor prognosis for recovery
- surgical exploration and repair considered for persistent CHL
- <u>Ossicular Injury</u>: **incudostapedial joint separation** (most common ossicular injury with temporal bone trauma), **fractured stapes crura**, **incus dislocation**; <u>Rx</u>: ossicular chain reconstruction
- <u>TM Injury</u>: more common with longitudinal fractures; <u>Rx</u>: small TM tears typically heal spontaneously, consider paper patch procedure
- <u>SNHL</u>: may occur from a fractured labyrinth, intralabyrinthine hemorrhage, perilymph fistula, inner ear concussion, cochlear nerve injury, or acoustic trauma

## CSF Leak

- <u>SSx</u>: clear otorrhea or rhinorrhea, salty taste, "halo sign" (fluid dropped on gauze separates into a clear outer ring with blood in the center)
- <u>Dx</u>: fluid analysis (presence of $\beta_2$-**transferrin**; CSF typically has glucose >30 mg/mL, low protein, chloride ~124 mEq/L), contrast cisternography (metrizamide or iophendylate) with CT, intrathecal radioactive isotopes or fluorescein with measurements of the radioactivity of pledgets after placing at site of leak or visualization of fluorescein under ultraviolet light (more sensitive but does not localize leak)
- <u>Initial Conservative Management</u>: bed rest, head elevation, stool softeners (prevent straining), consider prophylactic antibiotics (*controversial*), >90% of posttraumatic CSF leaks stop with conservative therapy
- <u>Persistent Drainage</u>: after 2–3 days of conservative management consider lumbar drain or surgical exploration with closure

## Other Complications

- **EAC Lacerations and Stenosis**: laceration almost always associated with underlying fracture, may lead to stenosis; <u>Rx</u>: avoid stenosis by placement of an otowick, prevent otitis externa and help dissolve blood clot with antibiotic drops, complete stenosis must be repaired to avoid canal cholesteatoma

- **Cholesteatoma**: late complications from entrapped squamous epithelium from the EAC into the middle ear space, canal cholesteatoma also possible
- **Vertigo**: typically self-limiting; may be related to inner ear injury (postconcussion syndrome), injury to the vestibular labyrinth may cause a complete unilateral vestibular deficit (manage with transient vestibular suppressant course and vestibular rehabilitation), must also consider perilymphatic fistula

## Penetrating Otologic Trauma

### Penetrating TM Perforations

- posterosuperior TM quadrant high risk
- <u>Dx</u>: otoscopy, audiogram to determine CHL versus SNHL
- <u>Rx</u>: tympanoplasty with ossicular chain reconstruction, SNHL or vertigo requires urgent exploration and repair (may be due to stapes dislocation and perilymphatic fistula)

# PENETRATING HEAD AND NECK TRAUMA

## Penetrating Neck Trauma

### Introduction

- low risk of serious injury if platysma is not penetrated
- although uncommon, pharyngoesophageal injury is the most commonly missed injury to the neck

### *Symptoms*

- 5–15% of aerodigestive injuries are asymptomatic
- <u>Laryngotracheal Injury</u>: change in voice, stridor, airway obstruction, subcutaneous emphysema, pain, hemoptysis
- <u>Esophageal or Hypopharyngeal Injury</u>: dysphagia, odynophagia, hematemesis, subcutaneous emphysema
- <u>Vascular Injury</u>: shock, hematoma, diminished pulses, stroke (hemiplegia), bruit

### *Management Principles*

- <u>Pharyngoesophageal Injury</u>: primary closure if <24 hours, otherwise consider drainage (diversion) procedure, reconstruction with muscle transposition, or esophagectomy

- <u>Vertebral Artery Injury</u>: embolization preferred due to difficult exposure and control, for failed embolization consider surgical repair
- <u>Carotid Injury</u>: high mortality (10–20%); primary repair treatment of choice, otherwise consider patch grafting, bypass grafting, or ligation (ligation should not be considered if stroke suspected), intimal injuries require repair if obstructing
- <u>Laryngeal Injuries</u>: *see* pp. 664–667

## Management by Zones

***Zone I:*** sternal notch to cricoid cartilage

- high risk of injury to great vessels, trachea, and lungs
- difficult region for surgical exposure and control
- <u>Management</u>: angiography of arch, great vessels, carotids, and vertebrals (may also be used for balloon occlusion or temporary preoperative control); esophagram; direct laryngoscopy, bronchoscopy, and esophagoscopy

***Zone II:*** cricoid cartilage to angle of mandible

- high risk of injury to carotid sheath (carotid artery, internal jugular vein) and aerodigestive system
- easier region to surgically access and control
- <u>Management</u>
  1. **Mandatory Surgical Exploration**: gunshot wounds that cross midline, obvious serious injury (stridor, active hemorrhage, absent carotid pulse), active bleeding, air bubbling through wound, arteriography not available
  2. **Elective Surgical Exploration**: up to 50–70% of elective neck explorations are negative
  3. **Selective Management**: arteriography; esophagram; direct laryngoscopy, bronchoscopy, and esophagoscopy

***Zone III:*** angle of mandible to base of skull

- high risk of injury to distal carotid artery, parotid, and pharynx
- difficult region for surgical exposure and control
- <u>Management</u>: angiography, esophagram, direct laryngoscopy and esophagoscopy

# Penetrating Facial Trauma

## Management by Divisions

***Division I:*** above supraorbital rim

- high risk of intracranial complications and frontal sinus injuries
- <u>Management</u>: complete neurologic exam, facial and brain CT, neurosurgical consultation for intracranial complications, manage frontal sinus fractures (*see previous*)

***Division II:*** supraorbital rim to oral commissure

- consider parotid duct and facial nerve injuries (*see* pp. 669–670)
- disrupted globe requires ophthalmology evaluation for possible repair, otherwise consider enucleation to prevent **sympathetic ophthalmia** (autoantibodies stimulated by globe injury may result in blindness in contralateral seeing eye)
- <u>Management</u>: complete neurologic, oropharyngeal, and ophthalmologic exam; CT of brain, orbits, and paranasal sinuses; manage maxillary fractures (*see previous*)

***Division III:*** oral commissure to hyoid bone

- **Mandibular Angle Plane** (**MAP**): vertical plane from angle of mandible to base of skull, if injury crosses this plane consider carotid sheath injury
- <u>Management</u>: management similar to neck zone II (exploration versus endoscopy), panorex, angiography/embolization (if wound crosses MAP)

## Penetrating Otologic Trauma (see p. 662)

# LARYNGEAL TRAUMA
## Introduction

- blunt trauma has a higher risk of skeletal fracture than penetrating trauma
- <u>SSx</u>: dysphonia, subcutaneous emphysema, dysphagia, cough, stridor or dyspnea, hemoptysis, laryngeal pain and tenderness, neck deformity
- <u>Mechanisms of Injury</u>: motor vehicle accident, assault, "clothesline injury," strangulation, penetrating injuries (gunshot wounds, knife)
- <u>Complications</u>: airway compromise, laryngeal stenosis, vocal fold immobility (aspiration, dysphonia)
- pediatric laryngeal fractures are rare because of elasticity of cartilage and higher position of the larynx in the neck; however, children have higher risk of soft tissue injury

## Types of Laryngeal Injuries

- recurrent laryngeal nerve injury
- endolaryngeal tears, edema, and hematoma
- **Arytenoid Cartilage Subluxation (Dislocation):** presents as a fixed cord
- **Cricoarytenoid Joint Injury:** may damage recurrent laryngeal nerve
- **Cricoid Fracture:** high risk of airway compromise and injury to recurrent laryngeal nerve
- **Hyoid Bone Fracture:** risk of airway compromise
- **Cricotracheal Separation**: trachea tends to retract substernally and the larynx tends to migrate superiorly, high mortality, risk in "clothesline" injuries, may have bilateral recurrent laryngeal nerve paralysis
- pharyngoesophageal tear, cornu of thyroid cartilage may lacerate pharyngeal mucosa

# Management

## Establish Airway and Stabilize Cervical Spine (ABCs)

- must establish airway while protecting the cervical spine
- premature endotracheal intubation in blunt trauma should be avoided to prevent an airway crisis (intubation over a flexible bronchoscope may be attempted)
- a surgical airway is a safe method to establish an airway without obscuring diagnosis and potentiating an airway crisis (perform under local anesthesia)
- *see also* pp. 102–103, 628–630

## Diagnosis

- <u>Physical Exam</u>: soft tissue edema or hematoma, laryngeal tenderness and crepitus, subcutaneous emphysema
- <u>Flexible Nasolaryngoscopy</u>: first-line diagnostic test, allows visualization of the endolarynx with minimal risk to airway, evaluate vocal fold mobility (fixation, arytenoid dislocation or avulsion), endolaryngeal lacerations, airway patency, laryngeal edema and hematomas
- <u>CT of Neck</u>: diagnostic test of choice to evaluate laryngeal fractures (hyoid bone, thyroid and cricoid cartilage); however, not indicated if injury is severe enough that exploration would occur regardless of CT result
- <u>X-ray of Neck</u>: largely replaced by CT

- Esophagram: best to begin with water-soluble contrast to avoid barium sulfate-induced mediastinitis
- Direct Laryngoscopy and Esophagoscopy: consider after airway has been established to evaluate the endolarynx (allows palpation of arytenoids)

## Medical Management

- Indications for Medical Management Only: smaller soft tissue injuries (hematoma, laceration), single nondisplaced fracture (*controversial*), stable laryngeal skeleton with an intact endolarynx
- hospital observation for ≥24 hours with tracheostomy set at bedside
- nothing by mouth
- elevate head of bed, voice rest, humidified air
- prophylactic antibiotics, systemic corticosteroids, antireflux medications

## Surgical Management

- Indications for Surgical Management: large lacerations, airway obstruction, disrupted anterior commissure, exposed cartilage, progressive subcutaneous emphysema, fractured or dislocated laryngeal skeleton, dislocated arytenoids, vocal fold immobility
- Timing: ideally should be repaired within 2–3 days to avoid infection and necrosis
- Endoscopic Repair: may attempt for smaller mucosal disruptions and repositioning of arytenoids

### Open Reduction and Repair

- Approach: midline thyrotomy or infrahyoid laryngotomy
- repair mucosal injuries to provide adequate internal covering of cartilage, reapproximate tissues to reduce potential of scarring and granulation tissue formation (may require local flaps or grafts)
- reposition subluxed arytenoids (or remove for severe disruption)
- laryngeal fractures should be reduced and immobilized
- consider placing a keel or Silastic stent for unstable or comminuted fractures, disrupted anterior larynx, or massive mucosal injuries; stents increase risk of granulation tissue formation, infection, and wound necrosis
- Montgomery T-tubes may be considered for complex tracheal and subglottic injuries (eg, subglottic resections, severe cricoid fractures)
- keels may be used to prevent anterior web formation for isolated anterior commissure mucosal disruptions, keels (which possess low

tissue reactivity) are interposed between the anterior thyroid cartilage and the anterior commissure
- repair recurrent laryngeal nerve with microsurgical primary reanastomosis (prevents muscle atrophy, does not restore mobility of vocal fold since a mixture of adductor and abductor innervation results), may also consider anastomosing ansa cervicalis to distal stump of recurrent laryngeal nerve

## Complications of Surgical Management

- **Granulation Tissue**: high risk if cartilage left exposed at points of contact of the laryngeal stents; Rx: laser excision, laryngeal dilation
- **Stenosis**: avoid with proper fixation of the laryngeal skeleton; Rx: initially attempt dilation otherwise may require a revision thyrotomy with excision of scar tissue and reconstruction, severe stenosis may require tracheal resection or supraglottic laryngectomy
- **Vocal Fold Immobility**: *see* pp. 119–124

# SOFT TISSUE TRAUMA

## Introduction

### Anatomy of the Skin (*see* pp. 437–438)

### General Management of Soft Tissue Trauma

#### Local Anesthesia

- lidocaine (Xylocaine) maximum dose is **4 mg/kg** (plain) or **7 mg/kg** (with epinephrine, which enhances hemostasis and prolongs therapeutic effect); **1% lidocaine** is 1 g/100 mL = **10 mg/mL**; thus for a 70 kg patient, up to 49 mL of 1% lidocaine with epi can be subcutaneously injected
- excess local injection distorts tissue
- nerve blocks diminish volume of local anesthesia required and minimize tissue distortion

#### Cleaning and Debriding Wound

- irrigate contaminated wounds with copious saline or antibiotic solutions
- remove embedded particles, asphalt, or tattooing with a brush or forceps
- remove tar, grease, or other petroleum products with ether or acetone

- preserve all facial tissue unless unequivocally dead (facial soft tissue tends to heal well because of excellent blood supply)
- avoid use of hydrogen peroxide (causes a toxic exothermic reaction)

### *Antimicrobial Therapy*

- prophylactic antibiotics should cover skin flora (gram-positive bacteria)
- oropharyngeal exposure requires prophylactic antibiotics that cover mixed flora including anaerobes (amoxicillin/clavulanate, clindamycin)
- topical antibiotic ointments help provide moisture which aids in re-epithelialization and migration during the proliferation stage of wound healing
- **Tetanus Prophylaxis:** in general tetanus toxoid may be given for any wound if there has been no immunization in ≥10 years or as a booster for high-risk injuries; tetanus immunoglobulin may be given concurrently (at different site and with a different syringe) for tetanus-prone wounds

## Specific Soft Tissue Injuries

### Hematoma and Ecchymosis

- small asymptomatic hematoma may be observed (typically resorbs)
- larger hematoma must be evacuated to avoid pressure necrosis and infection
- early hematoma is gelatinous and cannot be aspirated (must undergo incision to evacuate), after 1 week hematoma becomes liquefied and may be aspirated

### Laceration

- facial wounds tend to resist infections and may be closed primarily up to 2–3 days ("golden hours" <8 hours) due to excellent blood supply
- always utilize atraumatic techniques (skin hooks, toothed forceps)
- reapproximate normal landmarks first (around the nose and eyes)
- initial closure of subcutaneous layer removes dead space, decreases tension, and helps with alignment
- undermining reduces tension at dermal–subcutaneous junction
- as long as minimal tissue loss, primary closure of seemingly large defects is possible because of skin laxity
- may need to freshen edges for better approximation and healing

- evert all edges (bevel wound edges outward) to allow for a flatter, less noticeable scar

## Lip Injury

- may close primarily ≤1/2 of the upper or lower lip
- mark **vermilion** (border between red lip and adjacent normal colored skin) prior to injecting local anesthetic, which will distort boundaries
- begin with a nonabsorbable "key stitch" at vermilion border to ensure it lines up
- close wound in 3 layers: mucosa (resorbable suture), orbicularis oris muscle (resorbable suture), skin (fast resorbable or nylon suture)
- for larger defects consider local flaps (*see* pp. 444–449)

## Trap-Door Deformity

- <u>Definition</u>: "U-shaped laceration," slanted, often with a beveled edge
- wound congestion occurs due to poor vascular/lymphatic drainage
- leads to pincushion deformity
- <u>Rx</u>: create a perpendicular edge to the flap, undermine surrounding tissue to allow closure in layers; if defect is small excise flap and close primarily; for larger defects a subsequent revision may be required

## Parotid Duct Injury

- must be considered with vertical lacerations posterior to the anterior border of the masseter muscle on a line from tragus to upper lip (may have an associated buccal branch of the facial nerve injury)
- <u>Dx</u>: cannulate Stensen's duct and look for cannula in wound or inject small amount of saline
- <u>Rx</u>: place a stent intraorally through Stensen's duct out the distal cut end, thread through proximal end (locate by palpating the parotid gland to express saliva), repair primarily with microscopic anastomosis around stent, remove stent after 10–14 days; may require repeated dilations; may also consider ligating duct and injection with botulinum toxin, which leads to a temporary parotitis and subsequent "burn-out" of gland
- <u>Complications</u>
  1. **Sialocele**: can occur with blunt or penetrating trauma; <u>Rx:</u> aspiration and pressure dressing with or without anticholinergic agents, consider botulinum toxin injections for persistent sialocele, also consider intraoral drain placement

2. **Salivary Fistula**: external communication of the gland with the skin; <u>Rx</u>: conservative management as previously described, surgical excision of fistulous tract with botulinum toxin injection and compression dressing, superficial or total parotidectomy

## Eyelid and Lacrimal Injury

- consider ophthalmology consult for underlying ocular injury prior to any repair
- full-thickness lacerations of the eye margin require 3-layer closure initially at the "gray line" (anterior aspect of the tarsal plate), the posterior lid margin, and the tarsal plates (avoid sutures in the orbicularis oris muscle to prevent ectropion)
- may close primarily ≤¼ of the lid without causing entropion; >¼ of lid may require full-thickness skin graft (full-thickness skin graft may be obtained from the upper eyelid)
- a lateral canthotomy may add an additional 10 mm of length
- completely avulsed eyelids should be reattached
- lacrimal duct injuries must be considered with injuries medial to puncta or through medial canthus, injury requires cannulation of duct and microscopic primary repair over a stent

## Auricular Trauma

- **Hematoma:** usually result of blunt trauma (wrestling, boxing); should be evacuated aggressively (I&D) and compression dressing applied to prevent reaccumulation, perichondritis, and "cauliflower ear;" oral antibiotics while compression dressing in place (1 week)
- **Laceration:** initial irrigation with conservative debridement; may reapproximate cartilage by placing stitches in the perichondrium; cartilage exposure requires coverage by primary closure, wedge excision, local flaps, or burial in a postauricular pocket (for later reconstruction)
- **Helical Rim Defect**: may be closed primarily if <2 cm, if >2 cm use a chondrocutaneous advancement flap
- **Avulsion**: partial avulsions usually survive with at least a 1–2 mm skin pedicle, complete auricular avulsion requires attempted replantation (microvascular techniques), may require a meatoplasty to avoid external auditory canal stenosis

## Human and Animal Bites

- human bites are considered one of the most contaminating injuries

- human bites to the face should be aggressively irrigated and debrided prior to closure, consider drain placement in large wounds or if severely contaminated
- early animal bites may be closed primarily after vigorous irrigation and debridement
- broad-spectrum antibiotics, tetanus booster (*as previous*), also consider rabies immunoglobulin

# Burns of the Head and Neck

## Introduction

- **"Rules of 9s":** used to determine total body surface area (TBSA): arm 9%, leg 18%, anterior and posterior trunk 18% each, head 9%, palms 1%
- Burn Types
  1. **Superficial (First Degree):** mild, erythema, involves **epidermis**
  2. **Partial-Thickness (Second Degree):** penetrate **into dermis** and adnexa, blisters, painful
  3. **Full-Thickness (Third Degree):** irreversible injury **through dermis**, damages nerve endings (painless), necrotic
  4. **Fourth Degree:** into **muscle, bone**

## Initial Management

- ABCs: consider early intubation if inhalation injury is suspected, avoid tracheotomies through burn regions
- History: burn agent (fire, chemical, electrical, scald), time of burn, open versus closed space (closed spaces have increased risks for inhalation injuries)
- Initial Wound Management: wash chemical burns, brush off powder, neutralization of chemical burns is not indicated (the reaction itself may become exothermic), apply surface cream (*see* Table 11–4)
- Ancillary Tests: electrolytes, ABG (with carboxyhemoglobin), CXR, ECG, urinalysis (myoglobin), renal panel, pregnancy test
- Medications: reflux regimen, consider prophylactic antibiotics, tetanus prophylaxis; corticosteroids are not indicated
- provide volume according to **Parkland formula** (volume/day = TBSA (%) × kg × 4 mL, ½ volume given first 8 hours, remaining volume given over next 16 hours), consider Foley catheter to record urine output
- assess for carbon monoxide poisoning (headaches, cherry-red skin color, mental status changes, carboxyhemoglobin >10% in a nonsmoker or >20% in a smoker)

| TABLE 11–4. Surface Creams for Burn Injuries | |
|---|---|
| **Agent** | **Comments** |
| **Silver Nitrate** | broad spectrum, may cause electrolyte imbalance, painless, poor penetration of eschar |
| **Silver Sulfadiazine (Silvadene)** | painless, no electrolyte problems, may cause neutropenia, broad spectrum (including fungal) |
| **Mafenide Acetate (Sulfamylon)** | penetrates eschar, broad spectrum (covers *Pseudomonas*), painful, may cause hyperchloremic acidosis |
| **Bacitracin Ointment** | indicated for most superficial injuries and facial wounds |

- all significant burns of the face require hospital admission for management, consider transfer to specialized burn unit

## Inhalation Injury

- significant cause of death in burned patients
- Causes: closed space exposure to chemicals, carbon monoxide, toxins in smoke (ammonia, sulfur dioxide, etc), and steam; (direct thermal injury is rare due to glottic reflex closure to heat)
- SSx: facial burns (amount of facial surface burn does not correlate with severity of inhalation injury), singed nasal hairs, soot in mouth or nose, hoarseness, wheezing, carbonaceous sputum
- Dx: direct laryngoscopy and bronchoscopy
- Complications: upper airway obstruction, pulmonary edema, chemical tracheobronchitis, carbon monoxide poisoning
- Rx: monitoring, supplemental oxygen (may require intubation), aggressive pulmonary toilet, serial ABGs, bronchodilators, **corticosteroids are contraindicated** (increases mortality)

## Facial Burns

- superficial and partial-thickness injuries require only local wound care (initial wash with soap and antibiotic ointment)
- deeper partial-thickness injuries and full-thickness injuries should be managed conservatively initially with local care, consider waiting ≤10 days before excising necrotic tissue
- skin grafting should be planned according to the aesthetic units of the face and placed over a well-perfused granulation base
- consider tissue expanders (*see* pp. 461–463)
- pressure dressings (pressure masks), massage, and corticosteroid injections reduce hypertrophic scarring
- physical therapy prevents contracture

- **Auricular Burns**: delicate, thin tissue requires gentle cleansing and avoidance of pressure to the ears (doughnut ring); <u>Rx</u>: conservative initial debridement; cover exposed cartilage with flap closure (postauricular flap) to avoid suppurative chondritis; if extensive remove auricular cartilage and place in an abdominal pocket for later reconstruction
- **Oral Burns**: oral commissure often involved with electrical injuries (pediatrics); <u>Rx</u>: initially should manage with conservative local care, may delay debridement for ≤10 days to allow areas to demarcate into regions of necrosis, to avoid microstomia from contracture consider placing an oral stent
- **Eyelid and Ocular Burns**: risks include ectropion, lid contraction, keratitis, and cataracts (electrical burns); <u>Rx</u>: ophthalmology consult; keep eye moist with artificial tears and lubricants; eyelid full-thickness burns require initial evaluation for adequate lid support (tarsal plate) prior to reconstruction; consider full-thickness skin grafts to upper and lower eyelids; require lid release for contractions or tarsorrhaphy

***Acknowledgement:*** *We thank Lawrence S. Golub, DDS for his contributions to this chapter.*

# Appendix A

## CANCER STAGING INDEX

# CRANIAL NERVES
## CN I — Olfactory

### Olfaction

- neurosensory cells (in olfactory epithelium) → lateral olfactory stria → lateral olfactory area of temporal lobe
- neurosensory cells (in olfactory epithelium) → medial olfactory stria (lesser contribution) → frontal lobe (limbic system)
- *see also* pp. 10–11

## CN II — Optic

### Vision

- ganglion cells of the retina → optic nerve → lateral geniculate body (thalamus), pretectal area (midbrain), primary visual cortex (occipital lobe)

## CN III, IV, VI — Oculomotor, Trochlear, Abducens

### Somatic Motor

- CN III: levator palpebrae superioris, superior rectus, medial rectus, inferior rectus, and inferior oblique rectus muscles (**oculomotor nucleus**)
- CN IV: superior oblique muscle (**trochlear nucleus**)
- CN VI: lateral rectus muscle (**abducens nucleus**)

### Parasympathetic

- **Edinger-Westphal nucleus** → *preganglionic parasympathetic fibers* (CN III) → **ciliary ganglion** → *postganglionic parasympathetic fibers* → ciliary muscles and sphincter pupillae muscles
- *NOTE:* sympathetic fibers to the globe and sensation from CN $V_1$ also pass through the ciliary ganglion

## CN V — Trigeminal

### Branchial Motor

- CN $V_3$ (foramen ovale) → muscles of mastication, tensor tympani, tensor veli palatini, mylohyoid, and anterior digastric muscles (**masticator trigeminal nucleus**)

## Sensory

- CN V$_1$: lacrimal (also carries parasympathetic fibers from facial nerve), frontal, nasociliary, and meningeal branches
- CN V$_2$: zygomatic, infraorbital, pterygopalatine, and meningeal branches
- CN V$_3$: buccal, auriculotemporal, lingual, inferior alveolar, and meningeal branches
- **trigeminal ganglion** (**Meckel's cave** in middle cranial fossa) → **trigeminal nucleus**

# CN VII — Facial Nerve

(*see* pp. 420–433)

# CN VIII — Vestibulocochlear Nerve

## Balance

- vestibular nerve → ipsilateral and contralateral pontomedullary (4) vestibular nuclei

## Hearing

- cochlear nerve → cochlear nucleus → superior olivary nuclei → lateral lemniscus → inferior colliculus → thalamus (medial geniculate body) → auditory cortex at sylvian fissure of temporal lobe (Brodmann's area 41)
- *see also* p. 347

# CN IX — Glossopharyngeal

## Taste

- taste from posterior 1/3 → nucleus solitarius

## Branchial Motor

- stylopharyngeus muscle (**ambiguus nucleus**)

## Parasympathetic

- **inferior salivatory nucleus** (medulla) → **glossopharyngeal nerve** (**Jacobson's nerve**) → **lesser (superficial) petrosal nerve** → **otic ganglion** → *postganglionic parasympathetic fibers* → **parotid gland**

## Sensory

- visceral sensation from carotid body (chemoreceptors for oxygen tension) → **nucleus of the tractus solitarius**
- sensation from posterior ⅓ of tongue, external auditory canal, and tympanic membrane

# CN X — Vagus

## Branchial Motor (Ambiguus Nucleus)

- **Recurrent Laryngeal Nerve:** all intrinsic laryngeal muscles except cricothyroid muscle (also sensory to laryngeal mucosa inferior to glottis)
- **Superior Laryngeal Nerve (External Branch):** cricothyroid and pharyngeal constrictors
- muscles of the pharynx (except stylopharyngeus), levator veli palatini, uvulae, palatopharyngeus, palatoglossus, salpingopharyngeus, and pharyngeal constrictors muscles

## Parasympathetic

- **dorsal motor nucleus** → *preganglionic parasympathetic fibers* → smooth muscle innervation to thoracic and abdominal viscera, secretory glands of the pharynx and larynx

## Sensory

- **Superior Laryngeal Nerve (Internal Branch):** sensory to laryngeal mucosa above glottis
- **Auricular Branch (Arnold's Nerve):** sensory from postauricular skin, external auditory canal, tympanic membrane, and pharynx
- visceral sensory from pharynx, larynx, and viscera → **nucleus of the tractus solitarius**

# CN XI — Accessory

## Branchial Motor

- sternocleidomastoid and trapezius muscles (**accessory nucleus**)

# CN XII — Hypoglossal

## Somatic Motor

- intrinsic muscles of the tongue (except palatoglossus muscle), styloglossus, hyoglossus, and genioglossus muscles (**hypoglossal nucleus**)

# Appendix C

## VACCINATIONS
### Introduction

- <u>Viral Vaccine Types</u>
  1. **Live Attenuated**: MMR, varicella, live attenuated influenza
  2. **Killed/Inactivated**: inactivated influenza, inactivated poliovirus
  3. **Viral Subunits**: HBV (composed of surface antigen)
- <u>Bacterial Vaccine Types</u>
  1. **Live Attenuated**: BCG (Bacille Calmette-Guérin, for TB, not used in U.S.)
  2. **Killed**: original pertussis vaccine, cholera
  3. **Purified Toxin**: diphtheria, tetanus, component of acellular pertussis
  4. **Bacterial Polysaccharide**: pneumococcal polysaccharide, meningococcal; ineffective <18 months of age because lack T-cell independent response
  5. **Conjugate**: pneumococcal conjugate, *H. influenzae* type b; links bacterial polysaccharide to a T-cell dependent antigen to allow immunogenicity in children <18 months
  6. **Other Bacterial Subunits**: component of acellular pertussis

### CDC Vaccination Schedule

- based on 2013 CDC guidelines (*MMWR.* 2013;62.)
- **DTaP (Diphtheria, Tetanus, Acellular Pertussis)**: series of 5 between 6 weeks–6 years, booster at 11–12 years
- *Haemophilus influenzae* **type b**: series of 3 or 4 between 6 weeks–15 months
- **Hepatitis A**: series of 2 between 12 months–2 years
- **Hepatitis B**: series of 3 between birth–18 months
- **Human Papillomavirus (Gardasil, 4-valent; Cervarix, 2-valent)**: series of 3 for females (Gardasil or Cervarix) or males (Gardasil only) between 9–12 years; Gardasil covers HPV 6, 11, 16, 18, Cervarix covers HPV 16, 18 (HPV 6, 11 cause recurrent respiratory papillomatosis and genital warts; HPV 16 causes oropharyngeal squamous cell carcinoma and cervical cancer, HPV 18 also causes cervical cancer)

- **Inactivated Poliovirus**: series of 4 between 6 weeks–6 years (oral polio vaccine discontinued in 2000 in the U.S.)
- **Inactivated Influenza**: yearly beginning at 6 months
- **Live Attenuated Influenza**: may be used instead of inactivated influenza vaccine yearly beginning at 2 years
- **Meningococcal**: single vaccine between 11–12 years with booster at 16 years (may administer at younger age if high risk)
- **MMR (Measles, Mumps, Rubella)**: series of 2 between 12 months– 6 years
- **Pneumococcal Conjugate (Prevnar 13, 13-valent)**: series of 4 between 6 weeks–15 months
- **Pneumococcal Polysaccharide (Pneunomovax, 23-valent)**: indicated for high-risk groups including **cochlear implant** recipients, administer at 2 years or older
- **Rotavirus**: series of 3 between 6 weeks–8 months
- **Varicella**: series of 2 between 12 months–6 years

# Appendix D

# Anesthesia

### Raza Pasha and Justin S. Golub

## LOCAL ANESTHESIA
### Introduction

- Uses: topical (surface), infiltration, nerve blocks, extradural and subarachnoid blocks
- Mechanism of Action: binds to the intracellular portion of neuronal sodium channels **blocking sodium influx preventing depolarization**, pain transmitting nerve fibers are thinly myelinated or unmyelinated, which allows the agent to diffuse easier into them than more heavily myelinated fibers (touch, proprioception)
- Risks: nerve injury (paresthesia), anaphylaxis, cardiotoxicity (hypotension, bradycardia, arrhythmias, cardiac arrest), CNS excitation (seizures, respiratory arrest)

### Aminoester Agents

- higher risk of allergic reaction, if allergic use an aminoamide agent
- **Cocaine**: serotonin-norepinephrine-dopamine reuptake inhibitor, abuse potential and strong sympathoadrenergic effect
- **Procaine/Novocaine**: less utilized because of allergic potential
- **Benzocaine**: common over-the-counter topical pain reliever
- **Tetracaine**: very potent, common use as a topical agent

### Aminoamide Agents

- **Lidocaine (Xylocaine)**: also an antiarrhythmic drug, short half-life (1.5–2 hrs), maximal safe dose is 4 mg/kg (70 kg adult = ~30 mL of

a 1% solution) and 7 mg/kg with epinephrine (70 kg adult = ~50 mL of a 1% solution); *see also* p. 667 *for calculations*
- **Bupivacaine**: risk of cardiotoxicity, long half-life (3.5 hrs)
- **Ropivacaine**: less cardiotoxicity, long half-life (1.6–6 hrs)
- **Mepivacaine**: rapid onset

# MALIGNANT HYPERTHERMIA
## Introduction

- rare life-threatening complication triggered by volatile inhalation agents and succinylcholine
- autosomal dominant with decreased penetrance and variable expression
- <u>SSx</u>: skeletal muscle rigidity (**masseter muscle, most common initial presentation**), increased end-title $CO_2$, tachycardia, very high temperature (late presentation), hyperkalemia, metabolic acidosis, cardiac arrhythmias
- <u>Dx:</u> muscle biopsy for those with family history
- <u>Prevention</u>: for those with known malignant hyperthermia must avoid all volatile anesthetic agents and succinylcholine, consider other agents (eg, nitrous oxide or propofol) after flushing the ventilator with 100% oxygen at maximal gas flows for 20–30 minutes as well as regional anesthetic techniques

## Acute Management

1. Call for extra help
2. Stop volatile anesthetics and succinylcholine
3. Hyperventilate with 100% oxygen
4. Give **2.5 mg/kg** of **dantrolene** sodium for injection (repeat if needed)
5. Treat acidosis with bicarbonate (if not reversed by dantrolene)
6. Address persistent arrhythmias with antiarrhythmics **except** calcium channel blockers (if not reversed by dantrolene and bicarbonate)
7. Monitor core temperature
8. Treat hyperkalemia with glucose, insulin, and calcium
9. Cool if required by nasogastric, rectal lavage, and surface cooling (avoid overcooling)
10. Continue dantrolene for at least 24 hours afterward (~1 mg/kg q 6 hours)

11. Monitor for recurrence (**25% recurrence rate**) in an ICU for 36 hours
12. Avoid parenteral potassium
13. Hydrate and give diuretics to increase urine output to avoid **myoglobinuria**
14. Monitor coagulation profile to avoid disseminated intravascular coagulation (DIC)

# Index

For index of common abbreviations, *see* p. xxv
For cancer staging index, *see* p. 675

# Author Biographies

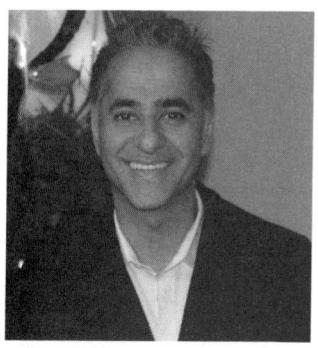

**Raza Pasha, MD**, continues to nurture his evolving private practice and ever growing family in Houston, Texas. He chooses to mime an academic career by lecturing cross-country, frequently engaging the media, and rotating students and residents alike. Dr. Pasha enjoys engaging in and contributing to research of "hot button" topics such as balloon dilation and advanced surgical sleep apnea techniques. He remains dedicated to his physician-vested projects with Altus Health Management Systems, which he cofounded. If you find yourself in the backwoods trails of Memorial Park, you may serendipitously spot Dr. Pasha on his mountain bike or more commonly ringside with his wife at a pay-per-view UFC main event.

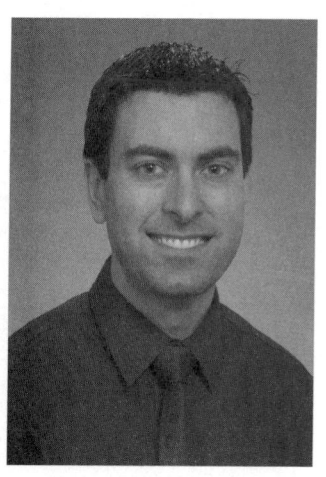

**Justin S. Golub, MD**, is an otology/neurotology/lateral skull base surgery fellow at the University of Cincinnati. He completed residency in otolaryngology-head and neck surgery at the University of Washington in Seattle and obtained his medical degree from Emory University School of Medicine. During his training, he completed research fellowships at the University of Washington and the Georgia Institute of Technology. He is the author of more than twenty peer-reviewed publications in otolaryngology and is a coeditor of *Otolaryngology Surgical Instrument Guide*. Dr. Golub's professional interests include regenerative medicine, otologic bioprostheses, and medical education. When not engaged in his perpetual training or toiling on books with Dr. Pasha, he enjoys skiing, reading, and even relaxing occasionally.

# MORE TITLES FOR OTOLARYNGOLOGY-HEAD AND NECK SURGERY RESIDENTS

## Otolaryngology Prep and Practice

*Edited by Jennifer J. Shin, MD, SM, and Michael J. Cunningham, MD*

A 1,200+ page study guide with in-depth practice cases, tiered focus questions, and multiple choice questions. The text is heavily illustrated and full color throughout.

## Comprehensive Otolaryngology Review: A Case-Based Approach

*Aaron M. Fletcher, MD*

A study guide that provides a concise review of high-yield otolaryngology topics; it is intended for preparation for the in-service training exam and the boards. The book is arranged in an interactive, topical fashion and presents questions in a case-based format with clinical vignettes, images and illustrations, radiographs, audiograms, and much more.

## Essential Paths to Life After Residency

*Edited by K. J. Lee, MD, FACS, and Yvonne Chan, MD, FRCSC, MSc*

This book covers everything from the various career routes one can take following residency, to the insurance decisions for private practices. It is the ideal reference for students currently in their residency and interested in starting a practice or entering academia. The breadth of knowledge presented by the editors and contributors, all of whom have successful, long-standing medical careers, is invaluable.

## Otolaryngology Surgical Instrument Guide

*Edited by Justin S. Golub, MD, and Nicole C. Schmitt, MD*

The definitive guide to more than 200 of the most frequently used surgical instruments in otolaryngology-head and neck surgery. Each chapter features professional photographs of instruments followed by detailed descriptions and tips for use.

**For more information, go to:**
**http://www.pluralpublishing.com**